Neurological Disorders due to Systemic Disease

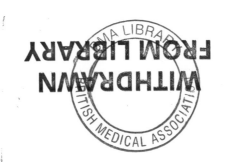

To my sons David, Michael, Adam, and Elliot, who teach me so much.

Neurological Disorders due to Systemic Disease

Edited by

Steven L. Lewis, MD
Department of Neurological Sciences
Rush University Medical Center
Chicago, Illinois, USA

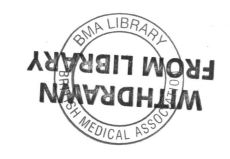
⊛WILEY-BLACKWELL

A John Wiley & Sons, Ltd., Publication

Library of Congress Cataloging-in-Publication Data

Neurological disorders due to systemic disease / edited by Steven L. Lewis.

   p. ; cm.
  Includes bibliographical references and index.
  ISBN 978-1-4443-3557-6 (hardback : alk. paper)
  I. Lewis, Steven L.
  [DNLM: 1. Nervous System Diseases–etiology. 2. Diagnosis, Differential. 3. Neurologic Manifestations. WL 141]
  616.8′0471–dc23

2012014818

A catalogue record for this book is available from the British Library.

Wiley also publishes its books in a variety of electronic formats. Some content that appears in print may not be available in electronic books.

Cover images © iStockphoto.com: Left: 'Human body with internal organs' © Max Delson Martins Santos. Right: 'Neuron Energy' ©ktsimage.
Cover Design: Sarah Dickinson

Set in 9/11.5pt, Sabon by Thomson Digital, Noida, India.
Printed and bound in Malaysia by Vivar Printing Sdn Bhd

01   2013

Contents

List of contributors

Brandon R. Barton, MD, MS
Assistant Professor
Department of Neurological Sciences
Movement Disorder Section
Rush University Medical Center
Chicago, IL, USA

Eduardo E. Benarroch, MD, FAAN
Professor
Department of Neurology
Mayo Clinic
Rochester, MN, USA

José Biller, M.D. FACP, FAAN, FAHA
Professor and Chairman
Department of Neurology
Loyola University Chicago
Stritch School of Medicine
Maywood, IL, USA

Hannah R. Briemberg, MD, FRCPC
Clinical Assistant Professor
Department of Medicine
Division of Neurology
University of British Columbia
Vancouver BC, Canada

Ted M. Burns, MD
Professor
Department of Neurology
University of Virginia
Charlottesville, VA, USA

Terry D. Fife, MD, FAAN
Director, Balance Disorders & Otoneurology
Barrow Neurological Institute
Professor of Neurology
University of Arizona College of Medicine
Phoenix, AZ, USA

Christopher G. Goetz, MD, FAAN
Professor
Department of Neurological Sciences
Head, Movement Disorder Section
Rush University Medical Center
Chicago, IL, USA

Brent P. Goodman, MD
Assistant Professor
Department of Neurology
Mayo Clinic Arizona
Phoenix, AZ, USA

Matthew T. Hoerth, MD
Assistant Professor
Department of Neurology
Mayo Clinic Arizona
Phoenix, AZ, USA

Jaffar Khan, MD, FAAN
Associate Professor and Vice Chair for Education
Department of Neurology
Emory University School of Medicine
Atlanta, GA, USA

Kevin A. Kahn, MD
Director, Clinical Care Center
Carolina Headache Institute
Clinical Associate Professor
Department of Psychiatry
Adjunct Associate Professor
Department of Anesthesiology
UNC School of Medicine
Adjunct Clinical Associate Professor
UNC School of Dentistry
Chapel Hill, NC, USA

Brendan J. Kelley, MD
Assistant Professor
Department of Neurology
University of Cincinnati
Cincinnati, OH, USA

Steven Lewis, MD, FAAN
Professor and Associate Chairman
Head, Section of General Neurology
Rush University Medical Center
Chicago, IL, USA

Michelle L. Mauermann, MD
Senior Associate Consultant
Assistant Professor of Neurology
Mayo Clinic
Rochester, MN, USA

Jennifer R. Molano, MD
Assistant Professor
Department of Neurology
University of Cincinnati
Cincinnati, OH, USA

Sarkis Morales-Vidal, MD
Assistant Professor
Director of Telemedicine
Department of Neurology
Loyola University Chicago
Stritch School of Medicine
Maywood, IL, USA

Sital V. Patel, MD
Fellow
Rush University Medical Center
Chicago, IL, USA

Janet C. Rucker, MD
Associate Professor
Departments of Neurology and Ophthalmology
Mount Sinai Medical Center
New York, NY, USA

Erik K. St Louis, MD
Consultant, Center for Sleep Medicine
Division of Pulmonary and Critical Care Medicine
Departments of Medicine and Neurology
Mayo Clinic and Foundation
Associate Professor of Neurology
Mayo Clinic
Rochester, MN, USA

Joseph I. Sirven, MD, FAAN
Professor and Chairman
Department of Neurology
Mayo Clinic Arizona
Phoenix, AZ, USA

Matthew J. Thurtell, MBBS, FRACP
Assistant Professor
Department of Ophthalmology and Visual Sciences
University of Iowa
Departments of Ophthalmology and Neurology
Iowa City Veterans Affairs Medical Center
Iowa City, IA, USA

Allison Weathers, MD
Assistant Professor
Department of Neurological Sciences
Rush University Medical Center
Chicago, IL, USA

Preface

The aim of this book is to provide an overview of the clinical presentation, pathophysiology, diagnosis, and management of the various neurological syndromes that occur in the clinical context of an underlying systemic disease or its treatment.

Although written primarily with the neurologist (generalist neurologist, subspecialist neurologist, or neurologic trainee) in mind, the material in this book should also be accessible and of interest to internal medicine and other primary care physicians, internal medicine subspecialists, and medical students. It is my hope that both neurologist and non-neurologist readers of this text will find that the unique neurologic-syndrome-based approach in the following pages will provide clinically useful insight into the wide variety of neurological disorders that occur due to systemic disease, and provide practical clinical clues to the neurological, and the underlying systemic, diagnosis and management of these patients.

I would like to thank the neurology residents and my general neurology attending colleagues at Rush University Medical Center for creating a stimulating clinical and academic milieu in our daily "work" in the inpatient and outpatient diagnosis and management of the many patients with neurologic disorders from systemic disease. Special gratitude goes to our patients with these disorders for entrusting their care to us.

I would also like to thank my publishers at Wiley-Blackwell, in particular Martin Sugden, PhD, for getting this book off the ground, and to Julie Elliott and Rebecca Huxley, for their expertise in seeing the project through to completion. Finally, a very special thank you to my wife, Julie, for all of her support.

Steven L. Lewis, M.D.
Chicago, Illinois
September, 2012

Introduction

Steven L. Lewis
Rush University Medical Center, Chicago, IL, USA

Neurological problems commonly occur in the context of an underlying systemic disease, and these neurologic presentations are a frequent source of inpatient and outpatient neurological consultation. In many patients, the neurological disorder is a manifestation of a previously diagnosed systemic illness or its treatment, but in still many others the neurological disorder is the presenting manifestation of a medical condition that has not yet been diagnosed. The aim of this book is to provide the physician with an overview of the clinical presentation, pathophysiology, diagnosis, and treatment of the various neurological syndromes that occur in the setting of systemic illnesses.

In this book, "systemic disease" and "medical disease" are used interchangeably, and refer to the kind of disease or syndrome in which the primary dysfunction involves an organ or system other than the nervous system, with the nervous system disorder occurring as a secondary—though in many cases, a potentially major—consequence. This book, therefore, focuses mostly on the neurological illnesses that occur in the setting of those primary illnesses that are typically considered to be under the purview of general internal medicine or its subspecialties. In addition, this book discusses the neurological complications that occur due to medications and other therapies typically used to treat these systemic illnesses. Conversely, this book does not focus on diseases—such as many genetic disorders—with multisystem manifestations that include both neurological and systemic complications, but where the neurological disease is not considered a complication of the systemic disease.

Unlike most books on this subject, the chapters of this book are organized and defined by neurological clinical scenarios, rather than by medical diseases. Specifically, each chapter focuses on a particular category of neurological presentation (e.g. movement disorders) and discusses the various systemic illnesses, or their treatment, that can cause dysfunction within that category of neurologic disorders. This organizational scheme, I propose, especially parallels the very common clinical scenario where the medical illness underlying the neurological syndrome is unknown; in these scenarios, the clinician needs to have some knowledge and understanding of the various systemic illnesses that can lead to these neurologic presentations.

The following major neurologic presentations define the chapters of this book: headache, encephalopathy, dementia, stroke, seizures, neuroophthalmologic disorders, neurootologic disorders, movement disorders, spinal cord disorders, peripheral nerve disorders, neuromuscular junction disorders, disorders of skeletal muscle, autonomic nervous system disorders, and sleep disorders. Each chapter, in turn, is subdivided into major categories of systemic illness that can lead to neurologic dysfunction: endocrine disorders; electrolyte and other metabolic disorders; systemic autoimmune disorders; organ dysfunction and failure; systemic cancer and paraneoplastic disorders; systemic infectious diseases; complications due to transplantation, complications of critical medical illness; drugs, alcohol, and toxins; and vitamin and mineral deficiencies. In individual chapters, some of these subheadings are excluded when they are not particularly relevant to that chapter's neurologic topic.

The book begins with the chapter on headache (Chapter 2) by Kevin Kahn, MD, from the Carolina Headache Institute, who discusses secondary headache syndromes that can be associated with systemic disease, as well as the interface between systemic illness and primary headache syndromes. Chapter 3, written by Allison Weathers, MD, from Rush University Medical Center provides an overview of the diffuse encephalopathy (delirium) syndromes that (by definition, arguably) occur within the setting of systemic dysfunction. In contrast, in Chapter 4, Jennifer Molano, MD, and Brendan Kelley, MD, from the University of Cincinnati tackle the interaction of systemic dysfunction and neurologic syndromes that more resemble dementia than typical toxic-metabolic encephalopathies; these authors also provide additional insights into the interface between the primary degenerative dementias and systemic illnesses.

In Chapter 5, Sarkis Morales-Vidal, MD, and José Biller, MD, from Loyola University Medical Center review the many systemic disorders that can be associated with, and potentially cause, cerebrovascular disease and stroke that the clinician should keep in mind in addition to the usual and well-known medical stroke risk factors. In Chapter 6, Matthew Hoerth, MD, and Joseph I. Sirven, MD, from the Mayo Clinic, Scottsdale, discuss the many medical problems that can lead to seizures; typically, recognition of these systemic causes of seizures can avoid unnecessary, or prolonged, antiepileptic drug therapy in these patients.

In Chapter 7, Matthew Thurtell, MBBS, from the University of Iowa and Janet Rucker, MD, from the Mount Sinai School of Medicine review and illustrate the many neuroophthalmological signs and symptoms that occur due to, and give clue to, the presence of an underlying potentially serious and sometimes vision-threatening systemic illness. In Chapter 8, Terry Fife, MD, from the Barrow Neurological Institute in Arizona discusses the many—and probably underrecognized by many neurologists—auditory or vestibular neurootologic syndromes that can occur due to medical illness.

In Chapter 9, Brandon Barton, MD, and Christopher Goetz, MD, from Rush University Medical Center review the many movement disorders (including parkinsonism, dystonia, tremor, chorea, myoclonus, ataxia, and tics) that can occur due to systemic disease or its treatment. In Chapter 10, Sital Patel, MD, and I, also from Rush, discuss myelopathies (whether from extrinsic compression of the spinal cord or intrinsic noncompressive spinal cord dysfunction) that can

occur as a complication of an underlying medical disorder.

In Chapter 11, Michelle Mauermann, MD, from the Mayo Clinic Rochester and Ted Burns, MD, from the University of Virginia review the many neuropathic syndromes, and their characteristic clinical patterns, that can occur due to systemic disorders. Extending the discussion further, in Chapter 12, Jaffar Khan, MD, from the Emory University School of Medicine discusses presynaptic and postsynaptic neuromuscular junction disorders and their association with underlying systemic illness. In Chapter 13, Hannah Briemberg, MD, FRCPC, from the University of British Columbia reviews the many myopathic disorders that can occur as a consequence of medical illness and certain medications.

In Chapter 14, Brent Goodman, MD, and Eduardo Benarroch, MD, from the Mayo Clinic, Rochester, review autonomic nervous system manifestations that can occur—with or without other signs of neurologic dysfunction—in the setting of systemic disease; the authors also review how to assess for these autonomic disorders. Finally, in Chapter 15, Erik St. Louis from the Mayo Clinic, Rochester, discusses the association of disorders of sleep, including the parasomnias, and underlying systemic illness.

Each chapter concludes with a list of the authors' suggestion of "Five things to remember about" that particular neurologic topic and its relation to systemic disease; these can be construed as suggested minimum "take home" points that provide some additional overall clinical perspective for the reader.

Although written primarily with the neurologist (generalist neurologist, subspecialist neurologist, or neurologic trainee) in mind, the material in this book should also be of interest and accessible to internal medicine physicians, other primary care providers, internal medicine subspecialists, and even interested medical students. It is my hope that the reader of this text will find that the unique neurologic syndrome-based approach in the following pages will provide clinically useful insight into the wide variety of neurological disorders that occur in the context of systemic disease, and provide practical clinical clues to both the neurological diagnosis and the underlying medical diagnosis and management of these patients.

2

Headache due to systemic disease

Kevin A. Kahn
Carolina Headache Institute, NC, USA

The chief complaint of headache must always be considered to have an origin in medical illness before primary headache entities may be considered. The accepted criteria for migraine and other primary headache disorders by the International Headache Society (IHS) have at their core the mandate that secondary headaches must be excluded [1]. This chapter will review the potential secondary headaches that can occur as a consequence of medical illness.

An understanding of the mechanisms through which head pain is generated is critical to appreciating how systemic illness can generate headache. Sensation within the head depends upon afferent nerves from the anterior aspect of the head and the posterior aspect of the head that converge upon the trigeminal nucleus caudalis in the pons. This nucleus then sends further input to the thalamus and higher cortical structures to process new sensory information. During primary headache disorders such as migraine, this system is activated by either peripheral or central triggers to send electrical impulses efferently to peripheral structures. The depolarization of nerves ending in the periphery results in a release of inflammatory substances causing swelling, inflammation, and pain within peripheral structures. Such structures include meningeal arteries, sinuses, skin, and musculature within the head and neck. In addition to activation of peripheral structures, there is an increase of excitatory input or lack of inhibitory control centrally that results in increased sensitivity of all senses as well as activation of brainstem emesis/nausea centers. Thus, pain generated within the head is mediated through trigeminally innervated structures. The associated features of pain are generated by trigeminally related central activation and disinhibition. The pain from other primary headache disorders such as cluster headache, tension-type headache, and the trigeminal autonomic cephalgias all generate pain via these same trigeminal pathways. The manifestation of pain is often pulsatile or throbbing but can present as burning, stinging, aching, sharp, dull, pressure, squeezing, and so on. Associated features are typically sensitivity to light (photophobia) and noise (phonophobia), nausea, and vomiting, but can also present as sensitivity to smell (osmophobia) or touch, sinus congestion, lacrimation, rhinorrhea, scleral erythema, ptosis, neck pain/tension/stiffness, and worsening with position or activity.

Since the final common pathway of head pain is trigeminally mediated, many secondary headaches seem to have features in common with the primary headaches. For instance, meningitis, an infection of trigeminally innervated membranes around the brain, can present with light/sound sensitivity, nausea, throbbing pain, and stiff neck. It is the presence of other systemic features such as fever, in addition to guidance from the patient history, that help separate the primary from secondary headaches. Thus, it is important to remember that headaches that are new to an individual or are associated with abnormal signs on exam or are a dramatic change from preexisting headaches are red flags that mandate consideration of secondary headaches. The secondary headaches can often mimic migraine since anything that can irritate central or peripheral trigeminally innervated structures will affect the same pain mechanisms as the primary headaches.

Neurological Disorders due to Systemic Disease, First Edition. Edited by Steven L. Lewis.
© 2013 Blackwell Publishing Ltd. Published 2013 by Blackwell Publishing Ltd.

Endocrine disorders

Sex hormones

Perhaps, the most common relationship between endocrine function and headache is evident in the phenomenon of hormonally mediated headache. The IHS divides hormonally mediated headaches into those from endogenous and those from exogenous hormones (see section on Drugs) [1].

Endogenous estrogen-related headache
The IHS defines this headache as being related to estrogen cycling yielding patterns of pure menstrual migraine versus menstrually related migraine. Pure menstrual migraine occurs exclusively between 2 days before onset of menses (menstrual bleeding) and 3 days after onset of menses. This pattern should be present in at least two of the three menstrual cycles. Menstrually related migraine includes the time frame of pure menstrual migraine and other times of the entire cycle [1]. The phenomenon of hormonally exacerbated headache can be one of the factors implicated in migraine chronification, defined as an increase in headache frequency from less than 15 days per month to more than 15 days per month. In such patients, with >15 days/month of headache and a history of menstrually related migraine, prevention of estrogen withdrawal during the week of menstrual bleeding has been reported to be associated with resolution of chronic migraine [2].

Hypothalamic and pituitary dysfunction

The IHS describes specific characteristics of headaches associated with altered hypothalamic and pituitary dysfunction. Headaches must be bilateral, frontotemporal, and/or retro-orbital in location. Headache should be associated with at least one of the following abnormalities: hypersecretion of prolactin, growth hormone, or adrenocorticotropic hormone with microadenoma <10 mm in diameter, or disordered temperature regulation, emotional state, thirst and appetite, and altered mental status with hypothalamic tumor. Headache must occur during the time of endocrine dysfunction and should resolve within 3 months of effective therapy for the disorder [1].

In one study of chronic migraine patients, analysis of hypothalamic function was found to be abnormal.

Chronic migraine is a condition where patients have headaches more than 15 days per month, with at least half of these headaches meeting migraine criteria. In comparison to controls, subjects with chronic migraine were found to have elevated nocturnal prolactin peaks, as well as increased cortisol concentrations and a delayed nocturnal melatonin peak. Patients with concomitant insomnia had lower melatonin levels. There was no difference between controls and subjects with chronic migraine with respect to growth hormone levels. The authors concluded that chronic migraine represents a disorder of hypothalamic chronobiologic dysregulation [3].

Hypoglycemia

Hypoglycemia is not typically associated with the complaint of headache, but head pain is more likely to occur with hypoglycemia in those patients with a history of headache. The longer the fast, the more likely headache will be present. However, hypoglycemia induced by exogenous insulin, or by intentional fasting, in patients with migraine does not induce headache. Fasting in association with caffeine withdrawal does not appear to induce headache [4]. When present, hypoglycemic headache is characterized by the International Headache Society as occurring during fasting, with resolution within 72 h of eating, and has at least one of the following features: frontal location, diffuse pain, nonpulsatile quality, and mild-moderate in intensity [1].

Hypothyroidism

Headache caused by hypothyroidism is characterized by IHS criteria as being bilateral or nonpulsatile or continuous with the presence of verified diagnostic evidence of hypothyroidism. Symptoms must have begun within 2 months of other hypothyroid symptoms being present, and must resolve 2 months after effective treatment of the hypothyroidism. The complaint of headache has been estimated to be about 30% [5] of patients with hypothyroidism. Vomiting is atypical with this headache syndrome. It is typical for patients to be female with an increased likelihood for a history of migraine in childhood [1].

Tepper et al. conducted a case–control study evaluating for thyroid dysfunction in patients presenting with new daily persistent headache ($n = 65$) compared to a cohort of migraine patients ($n = 100$) as well as individuals with chronic posttraumatic headache ($n = 69$). Hypothyroidism was more prevalent in the new daily persistent headache group compared to the migraine group (odds ratio = 16, 95% CI = 3.6–72) and chronic posttraumatic headache group (odds ratio = 10.3, 95% CI = 2.3–46.7). The authors concluded that hypothyroidism should be considered in patients who present with new daily persistent headache [6].

Hyperthyroidism

Stone et al. [7] noted that hyperthyroidism does not have its own category in IHS-defined headaches, with only sporadic descriptions of hyperthyroidism-associated headache in the medical literature; however, headache is commonly listed as a symptom of hyperthyroidism in most texts. In their small case series of three patients who presented with chronic daily headache in association with Grave's disease, the authors noted that the headache had an "unremitting quality and was not associated with sensory sensitivity." Patients with thryotoxicosis-related headaches had resolution of headache with treatment of hyperthyroidism. Stone et al. recommend that hyperthyroidism should be considered in cases of chronic daily headache of unknown origin [7].

A population-based study in Norway found that headaches were of low prevalence in subjects with high TSH values, and headaches were of much higher prevalence in subjects with low TSH values. The etiology of their findings was unclear, but the authors speculate that low beta-adrenergic activity could be a link between high TSH and low headache prevalence [8].

Adrenal dysfunction: pheochromocytoma

Pheochromocytoma is a catecholamine-producing tumor that typically is confined to adrenal tissue but can arise from extraadrenal sites in 15–20% of cases [9]. In order of prevalence, presenting symptoms/signs are as follows: headache (60–90%), palpitations (50–70%), diaphoresis (55–75%), sustained hypertension (50–60%), orthostatic hypotension (10–50%), pallor (40–45%), hyperglycemia (40%), fatigue (25–40%), weight loss (20–40%), anxiety/panic (20–40%), paroxysmal hypertension 30%, and flushing (10–20%) [9]. Additional potential presenting features of less well-defined prevalence include tremor, chest pain, nausea, vomiting, warmth or heat intolerance, polyuria, polydipsia, dizziness, hematuria, nocturia, bladder tenesmus, cardiomyopathy, constipation, Raynaud's phenomenon, and diarrhea [10].

Although pheochromocytoma is considered to be a "benign" tumor, it can cause systemic symptoms that can be life threatening. Therefore, diagnostic testing for this condition is critical [11]. The diagnosis of pheochromocytoma depends mainly upon discovery of catecholamine and metanephrine elevation via 24 h urine collection and serum plasma levels [10]. False positive testing is possible in the presence of certain medications such as tricyclic antidepressants, monoamine oxidase inhibitors, high-dose diuretics, phenoxybenzamine, levodopa, and theophylline, as well as with caffeine or nicotine use. False-negative testing may occur in the presence of reserpine and beta-blockade [9].

Once levels are discovered to be abnormal, tumors may be identified via CT or magnetic resonance imaging (MRI) imaging of the adrenal glands and abdomen, and if available, 123I-metaiodobenzylguanidine scintigraphy and/or 18F-dihydroxyphenylalanine–positron emission tomography (PET). Genetic testing is important as 25% of tumors are hereditary. Resection of tumors is done using an adrenal-sparing procedure and additional preoperative alpha-blockade [9].

The symptom of headache associated with pheochromocytoma as per International Headache Society criteria must occur with demonstrative biochemical investigations, imaging or tissue confirmation, and must resolve within 1 h of resolution of hypertension. Headache from pheochromocytoma is typically short, with 50% of patients' headaches lasting less than 15 min and 70% of patients' headaches lasting less than 1 h. It is associated with at least one of the following signs: diaphoresis, palpitations, anxiety, or pallor. The headache can range from pulsatile to constant pain with frontal or occipital location. In those patients with hypertension, it can occur to such a degree that it leads to a phenomenon of hypertensive encephalopathy (see section on headache attributed to arterial hypertension) [1]. In some patients, headache may present as "thunderclap" type, with time to peak of headache pain within 1 min of onset. Although typically such headaches occur in association with hypertension, the elevation of blood pressure may be intermittent or absent in some cases [11–13]. One explanation of the intermittent nature of symptoms is due in some cases to the need for mechanical manipulation of the tumor for provocation of symptoms. One such example is described in the case of a patient with thunderclap headache on micturation who was discovered to have a bladder wall extraadrenal tumor [14]. Other cases are described with such headaches after eating, with the tumor later discovered within the GI tract [9].

Pituitary apoplexy (hemorrhagic pituitary infarction)

This headache typically presents as a sudden onset "thunderclap headache" in association with pituitary hemorrhage or infarction. Headache from pituitary apoplexy is described by IHS criteria as being an acute, severe, retro-orbital, frontal, or diffuse headache with the presence of one of the following features: nausea and vomiting, fever, diminished level of consciousness, hypopituitarism, hypotension, ophthalmoplegia, or impaired visual acuity. Pituitary hemorrhagic infarction must be present on neuroimaging. The headache must occur simultaneously with the infarction and resolve within 1 month [1]. In a review of 400 patients with pituitary apoplexy (from multiple published case series), the following prevalence of presenting symptoms was reported: headache 63–100% (mean 93%), cranial nerve 3-4-6 palsies 40–100% (mean 68%), decreased visual acuity 40–100% (mean 75%), altered mental status and meningismus 0–42% (mean 22%), nonspecific symptoms such as nausea/vomiting 20–77% (mean 37%) [15]. Although infarction and hemorrhage is most commonly associated with the presence of an adenoma, it can occur within nonneoplastic tissue [16]. Although a specific precipitant is not usually discovered, in some cases potential precipitating events have been reported, including hypertension, sudden changes in intracranial pressure such as coughing or head trauma, history of radiotherapy, cardiopulmonary bypass surgery [17], thrombolytics [18], anticoagulants [19], estrogens, and bromocriptine [16]. Although the causes and presentations of pituitary apoplexy may be variable, it should be considered as a potential diagnosis in any patient with severe headache and neuro-ophthalmologic deficits [20]. When pituitary apoplexy is discovered it must be urgently treated with corticosteroid therapy (for both replacement and control of edema) and possible urgent surgical decompression to preserve vision and cranial nerve function, and to prevent mortality.

Electrolyte and other metabolic disorders

The IHS defines this headache group as those headaches in which there is altered homeostasis. Such headaches must occur chronologically close to the metabolic abnormality, with evidence that supports the relationship between the disturbance and the headache worsening, and evidence that when the disturbance is resolved there is corresponding headache relief [1].

Magnesium deficiency

Mauskop et al. [21] studied the relationship between the serum magnesium levels, the ionized magnesium levels, and the presence of various headache types, in addition to the effect of open label (unblinded) magnesium replacement for acute headache. Of their 40 subjects, 29 were women with headache types as follows: 16 migraine without aura, 9 cluster headache, 4 with chronic tension-type headache, and 11 with chronic migraine. All subjects were treated with 1 g of IV magnesium sulfate, with elimination of pain in 80% of subjects; 56% of these respondents had sustained freedom from pain at 24 h. There was a positive correlation between efficacy and sustained pain free rates and low serum ionized magnesium levels. The authors suggest a possible relationship between low serum and brain tissue ionized magnesium levels and predisposition to migraine [21]. In another study, Mauskop et al. showed that low serum ionized magnesium levels seemed to be correlated more strongly in patients with menstrual migraine, implicating magnesium deficiency as a possible contributing factor to menstrual migraine [22]. This finding was used as the basis for studying magnesium by Facchinetti et al. as a preventive agent in patients with menstrual migraine. They were able to demonstrate in a double-blind placebo controlled trial that not only was magnesium effective in menstrual migraine prophylaxis but also benefit was correlated directly with the degree to which intracellular magnesium levels were improved over the course of the study [23].

Bigal and colleagues performed a double-blind placebo controlled trial in patients with migraine with and without aura using IV magnesium for acute migraine. Their data supports effectiveness of IV magnesium sulfate as adjuvant therapy for acute treatment of pain and associated symptoms in migraine with or without aura [24]. In addition to the use as a menstrual migraine preventive, magnesium has been used as a preventive agent for nonmenstrual migraine in multiple double-blind placebo controlled studies with significant benefit above placebo [25–27].

Hypocalcemia and hypercalcemia

In an effort to examine the effect of calcium and parathyroid hormone on headache, several patients with these deficiencies were evaluated for headache characteristics. Compared to control subjects, calcium and parathyroid hormone levels were significantly decreased with additional decrease of phosphorous and beta-endorphin immunoreactivity. Headache was occipito-frontal in location and with migrainous features. The authors hypothesized a possible connection between headache, tetany, periodic syndromes, and hyperventilation syndromes [28]. Hypocalcemia has also been described after laryngeal/pharyngeal carcinoma resection with predominant feature of headache, altered mental status, paresthesias, and abdominal pain [29].

Patients may experience hypercalcemia in the presence of various tumor types including multiple myeloma, lung cancer, breast cancer, renal cancer, parathyroid cancer, adult T-cell leukemia, GI cancer, lymphoma, osteosarcoma, Ewing family sarcoma, soft tissue sarcoma, and melanoma. Hypercalcemia should be suspected in the presence of headache, tremor, confusion, and dehydration [30]. Headache and hypercalcemia was also reported to be the presenting symptom and laboratory finding in a patient with intracranial hypertension secondary to vitamin A toxicity [31].

Mitchondrial disease

In addition to causing significant systemic metabolic dysfunction, mitochondrial disease is associated with increased prevalence of headache. Migraine attacks are common in the syndrome of mitochondrial encephalopathy, lactic acidosis, and stroke-like episodes (MELAS) [32,33]. This syndrome is characterized as being due to a mitochondrial 3243 point mutation [34]. MELAS was thought to be a possible genetic model for migraine but the 3243 point mutation is not readily identified in patients with migraine. It has been suggested, nevertheless, that some migraine variants may be caused by other mitochondrial disease mutations [1].

Sleep apnea headache

Although the exact mechanism by which apnea relates to headache is not clear, it has been reported to be possibly due to hypoxia, hypercapnia, cerebral blood flow dysregulation, transient increases in intracranial pressure, and sleep fragmentation [35,36]. Sleep apnea headache is denoted by the IHS to occur with a Respiratory Disturbance Index > 5 by sleep study, and must be present on awakening and should resolve within 72 h of appropriate treatment to eliminate apnea. The headache must also have at least one of the following aspects: frequency more than 15 days per month, resolution within 30 min of awakening, bilateral pressing quality, and not accompanied by nausea, photophobia, or phonophobia [1,37].

Although headache on awakening is an accepted feature of sleep apnea, there does not seem to be an epidemiologic relationship between prevalence of migraine and sleep apnea [38–40]. It was noted however [38] that the complaint of snoring was elevated among headache patients. A prospective study of habitual snorers undergoing polysomnography concluded that snoring was associated with a global decrease in quality of life, increased prevalence of morning headache (23.5%), and obstructive sleep apnea (69%) [41]. A prospective study by Goksan et al. using polysomnography among 101 control subjects with AHI (apnea–hypopnea index) < 5 and 462 subjects with AHI > 5 found morning headache prevalence to be 8.9% in the control group and 33.6% in the high AHI group. The use of continuous positive airway pressure (CPAP) resulted in resolution of morning headache in 90% of subjects. Given the high morbidity associated with sleep apnea, and the increased prevalence of morning headache with increased apnea severity, the authors recommend that morning headache sufferers be considered for apnea evaluation and treatment if needed [42].

Hypercapnic headache

Headache as a consequence of hypercapnia alone can occur while diving, when a diver has insufficient ventilation intentionally (trying to breath shallowly to conserve air) or unintentionally (tight wetsuit) in combination with strenuous exercise and the decompression phase of the dive. Hypercapnia (arterial $PCO_2 > 50$ mmHg) is thought to cause headache via the known effects of elevated CO_2 with respect to relaxation of cerebrovascular smooth muscle leading to vasodilatation and increased intracranial pressure [43,44].

Systemic autoimmune disorders

Antiphospholipid antibody syndrome

Antiphospholipid antibody syndrome (APS) is defined by the presence of elevated titers of antiphospholipid antibodies (predominantly lupus anticoagulant) and anticardiolipin antibodies, possible mild-moderate thrombocytopenia, with clinical features of arteriovenous thromboses and recurrent fetal loss. Although first recognized in patients with systemic lupus erythematosus (SLE), not all patients with APS have SLE. In a cohort study of 1000 patients (820 female, 180 male) with APS, clinical features of the disorder were described, with migraine as defined by IHS criteria being present in 20.2% of patients. Female and male groups had similar profiles, with the exception that females had a greater prevalence of SLE-related APS with more frequent episodes of arthritis, livedo reticularis, and migraine. Males had more frequent episodes of myocardial infarction, epilepsy, and arterial thrombosis in the lower extremities [45].

Since APS and migraine both may present with transient neurological deficits, it has been suggested that patients with migraine be tested for antiphospholipid antibodies. Studies looking for an association between the lupus anticoagulant and the migraine have been inconclusive, with some studies positive and others negative. A prospective study in children showed no correlation between the presence of anticardiolipin antibodies and migraine. In addition, no correlation between migraine with neurological deficits and anticardiolipin antibodies has been shown. Of note, when patients with SLE are studied, there is a correlation between the presence of antiphospholipid antibodies and migraine. Headache in APS is difficult to treat and may be present for years before APS is diagnosed [46].

Systemic lupus erythematosus and headache

Recurrent headache is an extremely common phenomenon among patients with SLE. Headache is even more common in patients presenting with neuropsychological manifestations of SLE. Neuropsychological symptoms have been shown to correlate with brain injury as measured by MRI lesion burden and MR spectroscopy. It has been suggested that such findings may implicate headache as a marker for SLE activity and brain injury. In one study, using IHS criteria in a population of 40 SLE patients, recurrent headache occurred in 72.5% of SLE patients, with 45% of SLE patients meeting migraine criteria. Patients were studied from a standpoint of disease activity as measured by antibody levels, SLE symptoms other than headache, and brain disease (using MRI lesions and MR spectroscopy). Neither was there any correlation between the degree of headache and SLE activity nor was there a correlation between MRI disease, SLE activity, and headache frequency. The authors concluded that although headache is prevalent in SLE, it is not a reliable marker for SLE disease activity or brain injury, and that headache cannot be used as a surrogate marker for SLE disease activity and should not prompt the use of aggressive courses of steroids or other immunosuppressive SLE therapies. In addition, persistence of headache, with or without neurological dysfunction, should prompt consideration of other sources of headache such as infection, systemic disease, or other neurological disease [47].

Celiac disease (gluten hypersensitivity)

Celiac disease is a malabsorption condition associated with sensitivity to the gluten grains of wheat, rye, and barley. It affects approximately 1% of the population with the potential for both intraintestinal (irritable bowel) and extraintestinal (eczema, ataxia) symptoms. In addition to the effects of malabsorption, it has been postulated that there is another subset of patients with celiac disease where glutens not only affect the gut but can also affect other tissues [48]. There has been conflicting evidence regarding headache and celiac disease. In one combined retrospective and prospective study, the authors concluded that not only is headache more prevalent in celiac disease than the general population (and possibly improved with a gluten-free diet in these patients) but also patients with headache are more likely to have celiac disease [49]. In another study, there was no evidence of increased celiac prevalence in migraineurs versus control subjects (2% in both groups) with recommendation that testing for celiac disease in migraineurs may not be necessary [50].

Giant cell arteritis

Giant cell arteritis (GCA) is most commonly seen in patients more than 60 years old, and presents with new-onset headache due to inflammation predominantly involving pericranial arteries, with branches of the external carotid artery being most commonly affected. Criteria established by the IHS require that there is either biopsy evidence for temporal artery giant cell arteritis or serological evidence of elevated sedimentation rate or C-reactive protein in association with a swollen, tender, scalp vessel. The presence of jaw claudication, although classically described in GCA, is not required due to variability in presentations between patients. The headache should develop during the time of onset of arteritis and should resolve within 3 months of treating arteritis with high-dose corticosteroid treatment [1]. In practice, however, the headache from GCA usually responds very quickly to high-dose corticosteroids.

It is emphasized that this condition is an entirely preventable cause of blindness from anterior ischemic optic neuropathy. Amaurosis fugax (a "window-shade"-like description of visual obscuration) with headache requires emergent evaluation for giant cell arteritis (as well as carotid artery stenosis). Temporal artery biopsy may be falsely negative due to "skip lesions" that are common in the condition, requiring multiple sections be taken for examination [51,52]. Duplex doppler scanning may show a "halo" appearance of thickened arterial walls on axial images that could help identify the most appropriate region for biopsy [53]. If the patient loses sight in one eye, the other eye will likely lose site within 1 week if not treated with high-dose steroids [54,55]. Intracerebral vascular disease is also possible with this condition if untreated [56].

Primary and secondary cerebral angiitis

In primary and secondary cerebral angiitis, headache is typically the most common symptom, present in 50–80% of cases. Primary angiitis differs from secondary in that the former is not associated with systemic arteritis. Both conditions present with altered mental status, stroke, or seizures. Although both are treated with high-dose steroids, with expected resolution of headache within 1 month of such continuous treatment, primary angiitis may be less responsive and can often be lethal. Diagnosis is made via meningeal or cerebral biopsy. CSF pleocytosis is common, and its absence makes CNS angiitis unlikely [1,57].

Inflammatory disease and headache

The IHS gives specific criteria for headaches associated with inflammatory disease. Although not the predominant symptom, headache is often reported in systemic lupus erythematosus, Behçet's syndrome, antiphospholipid antibody syndrome, and Vogt-Koyanagi–Harada syndrome. Headache associated with these syndromes should be associated with diagnostic evidence for the syndrome in question, occur in close temporal relation to the disorder, and should resolve within 3 months of treatment of the disorder [1,58–61].

Tolosa–hunt syndrome

Tolosa–Hunt syndrome is a granulomatous condition that can affect the cavernous sinus, the supraorbital fissure, or the orbit. It presents as episodic orbital pain associated with dysfunction of one or more of the following cranial nerves: third, fourth, and sixth, with possible but rare involvement of trigeminal, optic, facial, or acoustic nerves. Although the cause is thought to be idiopathic inflammation, the differential diagnosis includes neoplastic disease, vasculitis, basal meningitis, sarcoidosis, diabetes, and ophthalmoplegic migraine (caused by a lesion in the trigeminothalamic pathway, thalamus, or thalamocortical projections). The IHS criteria for Tolosa–Hunt describes a presentation of unilateral orbital pain that lasts for weeks if untreated. The presence of the cranial nerve palsies (third, fourth, and sixth) is found on exam, and MRI or biopsy is consistent with granulomatous tissue. The onset of pain presents within 2 weeks of the presence of cranial nerve findings, and both resolve within 72 h of adequate treatment with corticosteroids. Other causes of painful ophthalmoplegia should be ruled out. Colnaghi et al. reviewed the published cases of Tolosa–Hunt syndrome from 1999 to 2007 to verify the validity of the IHS criteria. They found that MRI was positive in 92.1% of cases, with resolution of MRI findings after treatment; they suggested that the IHS criteria could

9

be improved with MRI playing a pivotal role in Tolosa–Hunt syndrome diagnosis and post-treatment follow up [1,62].

Organ dysfunction and failure (see also organ transplantation)

Kidney disease: dialysis headache

Although dialysis disequilibrium syndrome is rare, when present it commonly occurs with headache. The headache occurs during dialysis and during at least half of dialysis sessions, with resolution within 72 h of each dialysis session or after kidney transplantation. It can be prevented by changing dialysis parameters, but if not addressed can progress to obtundation and coma with or without seizures. Dialysis headache is typically considered to be due to the effect of osmotic gradients on neurologic function [1]. However, it has been suggested that there is an association of dialysis with increased levels of bradykinin and nitric oxide that may explain an increase in inflammation and vasodilation leading to the experience of headache [63].

A study by Göksan et al. prospectively reviewed patients with dialysis-induced headache and noted the following observations: the key variable for induction of dialysis headache was the difference between pre- and posttreatment urea levels and blood pressure. The larger the difference between predialysis BUN and postdialysis BUN, the more likely the presence of headache. Dialysis parameters of sodium, potassium, and creatinine were not found to be important with respect to headache. Preexisting migraine or type of dialysis solution was not found to have an impact on the likelihood of developing dialysis headache [64].

Ischemic heart disease and headache (cardiac cephalalgia)

This syndrome is defined by the IHS as headache with exertion with associated nausea, with concomitant acute myocardial ischemia, with resolution of headache with resolution of cardiac ischemia either via medical management or via a revascularization procedure. The presence of nausea and headache makes this disorder very similar to primary migraine headache. Although primary migraine can occur with exertion, cardiac cephalalgia exclusively occurs with exertion and can be diagnosed with demonstration of ischemia on treadmill testing or nuclear cardiac stress testing with simultaneous report of headache [1,65–67].

Cardiovascular risk factors and migraine

Large trials have been performed to help elucidate the risk profile for migraineurs with respect to cardiac disease. The Genetic Epidemiology of Migraine Study noted that migraineurs tend to have an increased incidence of smoking and were less likely to drink alcohol than nonmigraineurs and also were more likely to have a parental history of early myocardial infarction [68]. Subjects with migraine with aura had elevated lipid profiles, early onset heart disease or stroke, and hypertension compared to nonmigraineurs. Patients with migraine were more likely to be using oral contraceptives. The Framingham study showed a higher rate of risk factors for myocardial infarction in migraineurs compared to nonmigraineurs, although it was unclear as to what was the underlying cause for a relationship between migraine and coronary disease risk factors [69]. Kurth, et al. used the Women Health Study, a large prospective trial to evaluate which factors were most significant for migraineurs with respect to coronary disease and migraine. Major cardiovascular disease was defined as the first instance of nonfatal ischemic stroke or nonfatal myocardial infarction or death attributable to ischemic cardiovascular disease. Additional factors were studied including first ischemic stroke, myocardial infarction, coronary revascularization, and angina. Migraine without aura was not found to be associated with an increased risk of cardiovascular disease; however, migraine with aura was found to have increased hazard ratios for major cardiovascular disease of 2.15 (95% CI: 1.58–2.92; $P < 0.001$), ischemic stroke of 1.91 (95% CI: 1.17–3.10; $P = 0.01$), myocardial infarction of 2.08 (95% CI: 1.30–3.31; $P = 0.002$), coronary revascularization of 1.74 (95% CI: 1.23–2.46; $P = 0.002$), angina of 1.71 (95% CI: 1.16–2.53, $P = 0.007$), and ischemic cardiovascular death of 2.33 (95% CI: 1.21–4.51; $P = 0.01$) [70]. A similar analysis was performed using the Physician's Health Study evaluating 20084 men. Endpoints studied included first major cardiovascular event (nonfatal ischemic stroke or nonfatal myocardial infarction or death attributable to ischemic cardiovascular disease), coronary revascularization, and angina. In this trial, however, information regarding the presence of aura with migraine was not collected, and the results were analyzed solely on the basis of the variable of migraine regardless of aura history. Men with migraine, compared to nonmigraineurs, were not found to have an increased risk of angina, coronary revascularization, or ischemic cardiovascular death. There was increased hazard ratio risk, however, for major cardiovascular disease (1.24, 95% CI: 1.06–1.46; $P = 0.008$) and myocardial infarction (1.42, 95% CI: 1.15–1.77; $P < 0.001$). Suggested reasons for the association of migraine with increased cardiovascular risks include possible increased prothrombotic factors, increased inflammation related to the migraine event, shared genetics, or medications used to treat migraine. The authors conclude that regardless of the explanation it would be reasonable to carefully assess patients with migraine for coronary disease risk factors and to treat those factors that are modifiable [71].

Cardiac shunt

The issue of right-to-left cardiac shunt has been somewhat controversial with respect to its implications for headache. In patients without migraine aura, there does not seem to be an increased risk for PFO. In patients with PFO, however, the percentage of patients with migraine is 20–50% compared to the expected prevalence of migraine in the general population of 13%. Migraine with aura is described in 13–50% of patients with PFO, which is higher than the general population prevalence of migraine with aura of 4% [72–74]. Potential explanations for these findings are threefold: (1) that paradoxical emboli from right-to-left shunt reach the cortical surface and induce cortical spreading depression leading to migraine; (2) right-to-left shunt allows biogenic amines such as serotonin that are normally cleared by the lungs to bypass the lungs and reach the brain, serving as excitatory triggers for migraine initiation [75]; and (3) the association between migraine and PFO is coincidentally explained by genetic coinheritance with evidence in some family studies that there may be a genetic linkage between genes that predispose to atrial shunts and those for migraine with aura [76]. Based on the evidence in the retrospective observational studies, a number of noncontrolled retrospective studies have been done that suggest that PFO closure in patients with migraine is clinically

beneficial. Based on these studies, prospective clinical trials have been performed [69]. The Migraine Intervention with STARflex Technology (MIST-I) trial was performed in Europe and failed to meet the primary endpoint of complete migraine resolution within 91–180 days after closure and also failed secondary endpoints. North American trials are ongoing with less stringent endpoints. Pending these results, it is unclear at this time whether PFO closure will be beneficial for migraine prevention [69,77].

Liver disease

Liver disease has long been thought to be a predisposing factor for headache. In an extensive review of putative mechanisms of hepatic-related headache, Rodríguez et al. noted that there are several plausible arguments for this relationship. These include the causes of hepatic encephalopathy (inadequate clearance of substances that can act as neurotoxins such as ammonia, mercaptans, short-chain fatty acids, and amino acids), poor metabolism of intestinal toxins, endogenous benzodiazepine dysfunction, increased proinflammatory substances, medications used to treat hepatitis, and cerebral edema. However, when these hypotheses are more rigorously tested, there does not appear to be a relationship between new headache incidence with hepatic illness [78].

Lung disease

The IHS characterizes headache attributable to hypoxia or hypercarbia using hypoxia-based criteria. It is noted that the effects of hypoxia versus hypercapnia are difficult to separate. Headache occurs within 24 h after onset of acute hypoxia defined as $PaO_2 < 70$ mmHg, or in patients with chronic hypoxia persistently at or below 70 mmHg [1].

Chronic obstructive pulmonary disease
Chronic obstructive pulmonary disease (COPD) causes hypoxemia and hypercarbia due to poor ventilation and poor perfusion in lung tissue. Under similar conditions, such as sleep apnea and Pickwickian syndrome, headache is well described. A study by Ozge et al. was designed to better define the features in COPD-related headache. Of the 119 COPD patients they studied, 31.9% reported chronic headache, including the

following diagnoses using ICHDII criteria: chronic tension-type headache; frequent episodic tension-type headache; infrequent episodic tension-type headache; headache associated with arterial hypertension; migraine without aura; migraine with aura; benign cough headache; hypnic headache; symptomatic cough headache; and subdural hematoma. Of the COPD patients in this study, 54 (45.4%) reported sleep disorders, and 21 of them (38.9%) also reported headache. The authors suggest that COPD, a common disease, is responsible for a variety headache presentations given its various associated metabolic disturbances, including hypercarbia, hypoxia, and sleep disturbances [79].

Intrapulmonary right-to-left shunt
Pulmonary arteriovenous malformation (AVM) is found in one-third of patients with hereditary hemorrhagic telangiectasia (HHT) [80]. Given the potential association of intracardiac right-to-left shunt with migraine, studies have also assessed migraine prevalence and the results of treatment of pulmonary AVMs, in HHT. Thenganatt et al. found that the presence of pulmonary AVMs in patients with HHT (compared to those patients with HHT without AVMs) was significantly associated with migraine, after adjusting for age and sex [81]. In a retrospective study, Post et al. reported a reduction in migraine prevalence from 45.2% to 34.5% following therapeutic embolization of pulmonary AVMs in HHT. In those subjects with continued migraine, the frequency and severity of their headaches did not change postprocedure [82]. It is suggested that given the results of these retrospective trials, prospective trials may be useful to help discern the relationship between extracardiac shunt and migraine [69].

Systemic cancer and paraneoplastic disorders

Headaches attributed to neoplastic disease are typically associated with secondary effects of neoplasm leading to increased intracranial pressure or the direct compressive effects of neoplastic disease on pain-sensitive intracranial structures (tentorum/meninges). The IHS has established criteria for both of these clinical situations. Of note, the headache should begin in close temporal relation to the neoplasm or effects of neoplasm (hydrocephalus), with a mass lesion identified with CT or MRI. With respect to hydrocephalus-related headache with neoplasm, the pain is diffuse and nonpulsatile with at least one of the following signs: nausea or vomiting, worsening with activity, and/or Valsalva-inducing behaviors, or the headache occurs in discrete attacks. These attacks can be of sudden "thunderclap" onset with possible syncope such as sometimes seen with a cyst within the third ventricle. In headaches attributable to the direct effects of neoplasm, the headache should have at least one of the following characteristics: progressive increase of pain, localized/focal pain, worse pain in the morning, and aggravation by coughing or bending over [1].

Lung cancer and headache

Metastatic or primary lung cancer can be a source of headache. A syndrome that has been described among several case reports includes unilateral facial pain that can range from sudden-onset severe stabbing and shooting pain to a progressive continuous facial pain. Location is variable, from the hemicranium to the jaw, to the ear, with possible associated features of various cranial neuropathies. The source of the pain is considered to be compression or infiltration of the ipsilateral vagus nerve. In the cases described, not all patients had demonstrable lesions on initial chest X-ray, and it is recommended that when symptoms refer to the vagus nerve, additional evaluation including chest CT/MRI may be useful if chest X-ray is negative. It is worth noting that in most of the case studies reviewed in the literature, head pain resolves with treatment of the malignancy with chemotherapy and/or radiation therapy. The pain may be completely responsive to indomethacin or other headache treatments. However, despite the response to treatment, any new-onset headache in a previously headache-free individual should be considered a red flag for possible secondary headache. Other red flags include new-onset headache in an individual older than 50 years and an abnormal neurological examination [83–87].

Pineal cysts and headache

Pineal cysts are typically benign tumors that are usually not symptomatic unless large. They are present in 2.6% of adults. Evans et al. described that pineal cyst patients had twice the headache prevalence of controls with 26% of patients having migraine and 14% of patients having migraine with aura. Given that there is no correlation between the presence of headache and the size of the pineal cyst, the authors suggested that melatonin production may be responsible for the origin of headache in patients with pineal cysts. They suggested that patients with sleep disruption such as insomnia, delayed sleep phase syndrome, and desynchronosis be given melatonin replacement. The suggested dose is 3 mg per night increasing it up to 15 mg per night. The authors suggest further studies to investigate melatonin levels in patients with pineal cysts and to investigate the use of melatonin supplementation for treatment [88].

Systemic infectious diseases

Infection that extends intracranially to the meninges causes the classic triad of headache, neck stiffness, and photophobia. Bacteria can cause headache via direct meningeal infiltration as well as from the inflammatory effects of the products of bacteria and inflammatory mediators (bradykinin, prostaglandins, cytokines, etc). The IHS classifies headache attributable to bacterial meningitis as occurring with positive CSF findings of bacterial infection as well as during the course of the infection. Typically, the headache resolves within 3 months of resolution of the infection. The headache is typically described as diffuse severe pain with associated nausea, photophobia, and/or phonophobia [1].

If persisting more than 3 months, the headache is denoted as chronic postbacterial meningitis headache. Approximately, 32% of bacterial meningitis survivors continue to have headache. As per IHS criteria, the headache is described as having one or more of the following signs: diffuse continuous pain, dizziness, difficulty with concentration, and memory loss [1].

Encephalitic headache

When infection is infiltrative of the brain parenchyma rather than the meninges, the characteristics of the headache are the same as meningitis: diffuse, severe pain with associated nausea, photophobia, or phonophobia. Diagnosis depends on neuroimaging and CSF findings; note that PCR testing is often important for specific identification of the infective agent.

Headache from brain abscess or subdural empyema

Pain from brain abscess originates from direct compression of pain-sensitive structures (arteries, meninges) as well as possible elevation of intracranial pressure. The headache is typically described as bilateral in location with constant pain that gradually worsens from moderate to severe intensity [1].

Headache associated with subdural infection is caused by direct compression of the meninges or via increased intracranial pressure. The IHS specifies that at least one of the following signs must be present: unilateral or side-predominant pain, skull tenderness, fever, and/or stiff neck [1].

Headache attributed to systemic infection

When headache is associated with systemic infection (not originating in the brain or meninges), headache is typically not the primary complaint but rather associated with fever and malaise. The most common infection associated with headache is influenza. In some cases, headache is directly dependent on the effect of fever but may occur independent of fever. Infective organisms can irritate pericranial or intracranial pain-sensitive structures by direct infiltration, the release of endotoxins, and the immune response of inflammatory mediators. Some organisms may trigger brainstem nuclei with end result of neurogenic inflammation and headache. In HIV infection, headache is typically dull and bilateral but if the infection is associated with meningitis or encephalitis, then the headache behaves as is typical for these syndromes [1,89].

Herpes zoster

The IHS defines headache attributed to herpes zoster as head or facial pain that precedes a herpetic eruption by up to 7 days, with resolution of pain within 3 months of the skin eruption. About 10–15% of patients with herpes zoster have trigeminal ganglion involvement, with 80% of such presentations occurring in the ophthalmic division. When ophthalmic herpes zoster is present, cranial nerve palsies (including the third, fourth, and seventh nerves) are possible. The pain of herpes zoster can be constant or intermittent, and consist of any of a variety of features, including aching, burning, lancinating, allodynia (where typically nonpainful stimuli are painful), and additional itching within the region of vesicular rash.

Some patients do not present with rash (zoster sine herpete) but may still have these pain symptoms. In addition to antiviral treatment, treatment includes use of topical lidocaine, topical capsaicin, tricyclic antidepressants, and anticonvulsants; opiates may also be useful in management of this pain [1,90–91].

Complications due to transplantation

Neurological complications occur in 20–60% of organ transplant patients [92]; heart and bone marrow transplant patients tend to have the highest neurologic complication rates, while they have lower rates in kidney transplantation. Although most studies report headache as a sequela of organ transplantation, very few define the complication rate specifically attributable to headache. A review of such studies report complication of headache occurring in approximately 11% of heart transplantation patients [93], 15% of heart/lung transplantation patients [94], and 18% of liver transplantation patients [95]. A single study of 467 patients following renal transplantation reports a complication rate of headache at 3% within 3 postoperative days [96]. A retrospective study of 83 patients status post renal transplantation revealed postoperative headache prevalence of 44.5% [97]. Of note, the percentage of patients with reported IHS-defined migraine (approximately 20%) did not change pre- and postoperatively but those with headaches of other types increased from 12% to 26.5%. The authors explain that some of the higher preoperative headache prevalence may be explained by dialysis headache and metabolic dysfunction and the postoperative headache increase in nonmigraineurs may be due to cyclosporine or less easily defined causes. It was unclear whether or not beta-blockers used for treatment were effective [97]. Headaches associated with organ transplantation have generally been attributable to traditional complications of surgery versus the toxic effects of medications used for immunosuppression. Typical complications that can cause headache include fever, infection, and intracerebral hemorrhage (ICH) [98].

Given the vasoactive properties of cyclosporine and tacrolimus, these agents are thought to play a role in posttransplant headaches. However, the exact mechanism of headache induction with these agents is unknown [99]. Decreasing the dose of these medications, if possible, can sometimes ameliorate headache [98]. Of note, in a Cochrane review, patients treated with tacrolimus were found to be significantly more likely than those receiving cyclosporine to experience tremor and headache after liver transplantation [100]. Medications that slow cyclosporine metabolism such as calcium channel blockers can sometimes allow for lower immunosuppressive effective doses. Traditional preventive strategies for pain and headache can sometimes help in prevention of such headaches [98]. Given that conventional therapies can sometimes be problematic owing to drug interactions and organ toxicity, one study in six patients (five liver and one heart transplant patient) was performed using 200 mg riboflavin per day, which has been shown to be a safe and effective treatment for migraine prophylaxis. It was shown to be effective but given the small number of subjects and open-label design, it was suggested that a larger, randomized trial may be reasonable given the relative safety and tolerability of this strategy [99].

Headache can also frequently occur in the posterior reversible encephalopathy syndrome, which can occur in the setting of immunosuppressive agents used in transplantation; this syndrome is discussed below in the section on arterial hypertension and in greater detail in Chapters 3, 6, and 7.

Complications of critical medical illness
Stroke

Stroke-related headache occurs in 17–34% [101] of ischemic stroke presentations and is typically accompanied by neurological deficits and altered mental status, which separates such headache from typical migraine. Although migraine with aura can present with such deficits, without a history of multiple similar stereotyped attacks, such a presentation must be considered to be stroke unless proven otherwise. The headache location is not predictive of stroke etiology. Ischemic headache is typically related to large vessel disease as opposed to lacunar infarctions. The IHS defines ischemic stroke headache as having clinical signs and/or neuroimaging evidence of stroke where headache occurs during the time of stroke [1]. In addition to the presence of headache as an associated feature with stroke, migraine headache itself is an independent risk factor for stroke. A

2005 meta-analysis of 14 existing studies found that there is an overall increased risk of stroke in both migraine with and without aura (relative risk 2.16 with 95% CI: 1.89–2.48) [102]. The relative risk for patients without aura is 1.83 (95% CI: 1.06–3.15) and with aura is 2.27 (95% CI: 1.61–3.19). Risk is tripled among migraineurs who smoke and is increased fourfold in those using oral contraceptives. Prospective studies since the meta-analysis have found similar conclusions. The Women's Health Study (subjects age > 45) found an increased relative risk among migraineurs compared to nonmigraineurs of 1.7 (95% CI: 1.11–2.66) [70]. Migraineurs aged 45–55 have an even greater risk (odds ratio of 2.25, 95% CI: 1.30–3.91) of stroke compared to age-matched nonmigraineurs. All risk was attributable to migraine with aura as migraineurs without aura did not show increased risk. In the Atherosclerosis Risk in Communities Study (which evaluated both men and women), migraineurs were shown to have a non-significant increased risk of stroke [103]. The Stroke Prevention in Young Women Study found an increased risk for ischemic stroke for women aged 15–49 with migraine with aura of 1.5 (95% CI: 1.1–2.0) [104]. Those with aura with oral contraceptives and who smoked had odds ratio of 7.0 (95% CI: 1.3–22.8) compared to nonsmoking/nonoral-contraceptive-using migraineurs with aura. Migraineurs without aura did not have increased risk of stroke [69,104].

White matter disease in migraine

It is not unusual in the investigation into headache in patients with suspected critical medical or neurological illness to obtain an MRI of the brain. Since the utilization of this technique began, white matter lesions present within the scans of headache sufferers have been described as nonspecific or seen in "migraine." Such lesions raise the question as to the relationship between such lesions and risk of stroke or potential vascular complication [105].

A Dutch cross-sectional study of men and women aged 30–60 ($n = 435$, 295 migraineurs, 161 with aura, 140 age–gender-matched controls) evaluated MRI presence of white matter lesions and stroke. None of the subjects reported stroke symptoms. White matter lesions were found in 8.1% of migraineurs and 5% of controls, which was not statistically significant but there was a significant difference in the presence of

posterior circulation stroke seen on MRI. Migraineurs had increased odds ratios compared to controls of 7.1 (95% CI: 0.9–55; $P = 0.02$) with higher risk in those migraineurs with aura and for those migraineurs with frequent headache episodes. In those migraineurs with aura with greater than or equal to 1 attack per month, posterior circulation stroke risk was increased to 15.8 (95% CI: 1.8–140). The lesions in migraineurs tended to be in the posterior circulation (80%) and posterior watershed areas and were often multiple in numbers. The suggested etiology for these lesions include possible hypoperfusion, endothelial dysfunction, increased vascular disease risk factors among migraineurs, increased prevalence of PFO, the use of migraine medications, and a possible genetic association between migraine and stroke [105].

Transient ischemic attack headache

Headaches associated with transient ischemic attacks (TIAs) share the same chronology criteria with transient ischemic attacks. That is, headaches develop at the same time as neurologic deficits and the neurologic deficits and headaches both must be resolved within 24 h. Positive phenomena (e.g., flashing lights) are more common in migraine whereas negative phenomena are more common with TIA. TIA deficits are typically focal in a particular vascular territory, whereas migraineurs deficit tend to be progressive over several vascular territories [1,106].

Cerebral hemorrhage

Headache from hemorrhagic stroke is classified as developing simultaneously with the hemorrhage, which is much more likely to cause severe headache than ischemic stroke. If present with cerebellar hemorrhage, it can represent a neurosurgical emergency due to the increased risk of cerebellar herniation syndrome. Headache may precede neurologic deficits and can present in "thunderclap" or sudden onset fashion. Subarachnoid blood is a common cause of sudden onset secondary headache. When subarachnoid hemorrhage (SAH) is present, it typically begins suddenly, with 12% of patients dying before reaching an emergency room [107] and estimates of independence between 36% and 55% at assessments 1–12 months after onset of hemorrhage. It can have a varied presentation but typically is unilateral and associated with nausea, vomiting, and altered mental status with the potential for arrhythmia. Eighty-five percent of spontaneous SAH is caused by rupture of saccular aneurysms [108]. CT or MRI FLAIR sequences are the most sensitive diagnostic studies, but if they are not conclusive then lumbar puncture may reveal CSF xanthochromia and increased red cell count confirming the diagnosis. Given the morbidity/mortality of this condition, sudden onset severe headache should be treated as a potential neurological and/or neurosurgical emergency. Survivors of SAH with headache should experience resolution of headache within 1 month of the event.

Headache occurs in 18–36% of patients with unruptured arteriovenous malformations or saccular aneurysm [109]. Similar to SAH, headache from unruptured aneurysm may present in "thunderclap" pattern and can sometimes occur with painful third nerve palsy. This scenario (painful third nerve palsy and dilated pupil with headache) represents a potential warning sign of impending aneurysmal rupture. Neuroimaging should confirm the presence of the aneurysm, and provided it does not rupture, headache typically resolves within 72 h. Hemorrhage can be ruled out via neuroimaging and/or lumbar puncture [110].

Carotid/vertebral pain

In the event of trauma to the carotid artery or dissection of the carotid artery, headache may be triggered via autonomic and trigeminal innervation of neck structures. Headache is present in 55–100% of patients with cervical artery dissection and is the presenting symptom in 33–86% of such cases. The IHS classifies such headache as being associated with radiographic evidence of cervical vessel dissection with onset of headache in the same time frame as dissection with resolution of head pain within 1 month of the event. Radiological studies may include Doppler ultrasound, MRI, MRA, and/or helical CT. If noninvasive studies are inconclusive, then conventional angiography would be indicated. Head pain can be of variable presentation but is typically ipsilateral to the side of dissection, and with carotid artery dissection an associated Horner's syndrome or painful tinnitus is common. Cerebral ischemia and retinal ischemia are possible. Pain can mimic SAH headache with "thunderclap" sudden onset [1,111–112].

Cerebral autosomal dominant arteriopathy with subcortical infarcts and leukoencephalopathy

Cerebral autosomal dominant arteriopathy with subcortical infarcts and leukoencephalopathy (CADASIL) is a disorder caused by a mutation to the Notch 3 gene on chromosome 19. It causes migraine with aura (in a third of patients), cerebral small vessel disease with small deep infarcts, subcortical dementia, and altered mood. When aura is present it is often prolonged. The mean age of onset is 30 years old with white matter disease that could precede clinical stroke presentation by 15 years. The disease is identified clinically by the presence of migraine, prominent white matter changes on MRI T2-weighted images, and confirmation with genetic testing [1,113].

Intracranial hypertension (idiopathic intracranial hypertension and secondary intracranial hypertension)

The IHS classifies idiopathic intracranial hypertension (IIH), formerly known as pseudotumor cerebri, as having at least one of the following features including daily occurrence, nonpulsatile pain (constant and diffuse), and worsened by coughing/straining. The examination may be normal or could have papilledema, enlarged blind spots, other visual field defects, or sixth nerve palsy. Spinal fluid studies reveal recumbent opening pressure of >200 mm H_2O in nonobese patients and >250 mm H_2O in obese patients, with normal CSF chemistry and cellularity. There should be no cerebral venous sinus thrombosis or other secondary cause [1,69]. Such headache can be a neurologic emergency as the presence of visual dysfunction may indicate potential impending blindness. Treatment involving acute removal of excess CSF to obtain a standard closing pressure (100–180 mm H_2O) and the introduction of CSF pressure lowering agents are important. Patients refractory to such measures may require optic nerve sheath fenestration versus neurosurgical intervention with CSF shunting [114].

When intracranial hypertension is of a secondary cause, the headache must develop within weeks or months of the causative issue (and should resolve within 3 months of removal of the metabolic/toxic/hormonal cause) [1]. Secondary causes of intracranial hypertension include intracranial mass lesions and disorders of cerebral venous drainage. In addition, medical illnesses and medications have been associated with intracranial hypertension. Medical illnesses that have been associated with intracranial hypertension include Addison's disease, hypoparathyroidism, chronic obstructive pulmonary disease, right heart failure with pulmonary hypertension, sleep apnea, renal failure, severe iron deficiency, and anemia. Medications that have been associated with intracranial hypertension include tetracyclines; vitamin A and related compounds; anabolic steroids; corticosteroid withdrawal; growth hormone deficiency supplementation; chlordecone; nalidixic acid; lithium; and implantable progesterone [115].

Headache attributed to cerebral venous thrombosis

Although arterial disease can be a common source of headache, venous complications may induce headache as well. Cerebral venous thrombosis (CVT) often presents as a diffuse headache with progression of headache intensity and possible signs of intracranial hypertension. Headache is present in 80–90% of patients with CVT and rarely may be the only sign. However, 90% of patients with CVT also present with neurologic deficits, altered mental status, cavernous sinus syndrome, or seizures [1,116–118].

Headache attributed to arterial hypertension

Although there is little evidence for chronic mild-moderate hypertension as a causative factor for headache, conditions of paroxysmal hypertension can cause significant headache. The IHS classifies hypertensive headache with and without hypertensive encephalopathy. Both headache types occur during the hypertensive crisis. Hypertension is associated with cerebral hyperperfusion leading to headache. Headache resolves within 1 h of normalization of blood pressure and should not be caused by exogenous vasopressive agents. Sometimes, it can occur when there is a failure of baroreceptor function (e.g., neck irradiation, carotid endarterectomy, and enterochromaffin cell tumors). When encephalopathy is not present, headache is in association with a paroxysmal rise of systolic blood pressure 160 mm Hg and/or diastolic rise to >120 mm Hg. Headaches must be associated with at least of the following aspects: bilateral, pulsatile, and/or precipitation by exertion.

When hypertension exceeds the ability of cerebrovascular autoregulatory mechanisms (vasoconstriction), the blood–brain barrier becomes permeable leading to cerebral edema and encephalopathy and is termed the posterior reversible encephalopathy syndrome (PRES). This edema can be visualized on MRI and is classically, though not invariably, seen in parieto-occipital white matter regions (see Chapters 3, 6, and 7). The hypertension could be caused by endogenous dysfunction such as pheochromocytoma or exogenous vasopressive toxins such as medications [1,119–121].

Preeclampsia and eclampsia headache

The entities of preeclampsia and eclampsia require the presence of a placenta and are thought to be associated with a significant maternal immune response. Proteinuria and hypertension are typical but abnormalities in liver function can occur in addition to coagulopathy. Both conditions share the same diagnostic criteria as defined by the IHS as hypertension >140/90 mm Hg on two different blood pressure assessments at least 4 h apart, urinary protein excretion >0.3 g per 24 h, and occurring during pregnancy or up to 7 days postpartum. Eclampsia has the additional feature of seizure. Both conditions are examples of the PRES syndrome and share the same headache criteria: bilateral location, pulsatile in nature, and worsened by physical activity. The headache arises with onset of hypertension and resolves within 7 days of resolution of hypertension [1].

Drugs, toxins (including alcohol), and vitamin and mineral deficiencies

Drugs

Medications used as directed or illicitly can cause headache either via direct effect or via withdrawal effects. The mechanisms by which drugs cause headache are variable, ranging from vasodilator properties to idiosyncratic aseptic meningitic headache, to alterations in inhibitory and excitatory central pain modulatory systems. Many agents that can raise blood pressure can cause headache. The most common agents include sympathomimetic agents, monoamine

Table 2.1 Some medications that can cause headache [1]

Acetazolamide	Immunoglobulins
Ajmaline	Interferons
Amantadine	Isoniazid
Antihistamines	Meprobamate
Antiinflammatory drugs	Methaqualone
Barbiturates	Metronidazole
Beta-interferon	Morphine and derivatives
Bromocriptine	Nalidixic acid
Caffeine	Nifedipine
Calcium antagonists	Nitrates
Carbimazol	Nitrofurantoin
Chloroquine	Nonsteroidal medications
Cimetidine	Paroxetine
Clofibrate	Pentoxifylline
Codeine	Perhexiline
Didanosine	Octreotide
Dihydralazine	Omeprazole
Dihydroergotamine	Ondansetron
Dipyridamole	Primidone
Disopyramide	Prostacyclines
Disulfiram	Ranitidine
Ergotamine	Rifampicin
Estrogens	Sildenafil
Etofibrate	Theophylline and derivatives
Gestagens	Thiamazole
Glycosides	Trimethoprim sulfamethoxazole
Griseofulvin	Triptans
Guanethidine	Vitamin A

oxidase inhibitors (when taken with tyramines), and amphetamines [1].

The IHS classifies medication-induced headaches as those headaches caused by medications not used for headache therapy with onset of pain within minutes or hours of use and resolution of headache within 72 h of cessation of use [1]. Headache presentations may be variable but most are associated with diffuse location and moderate to severe, continuous dull pain. Table 2.1 lists a number of examples of medications and their classes known to cause headache.

Chemotherapy
Chemotherapy used in the treatment of neoplastic disorders can often be a source of headache. Offending agents include the alkylating agent temozolomide that is commonly used in the treatment of melanoma and primary brain tumors. Immune modulators and monoclonal antibodies used in hematological tumors are other typical agents implicated in chemotherapy-induced headache. Therapies used to suppress estrogen (such as those for breast cancer) can induce headache via the effects of estrogen withdrawal (see menstrually related migraine). Vitamin A analogues and transretinoic acid agents used in leukemia can cause elevated intracranial pressure.

Intrathecal therapies such as methotrexate and cytorabine, used in the treatment of leptomeningeal metastasis, as well as intravenous immune globulin (IVIg), can cause aseptic meningitis with features of fever, headache, nuchal rigidity, and back pain. Spinal fluid analysis in these patients will reveal lymphocytosis. Drugs that target vascular endothelial growth factor (VEGF) such as bevacizumab, sorafenib, sunitinib (used in breast, colorectal, nonsmall-cell lung cancer, glioblastoma, and renal cancer) can cause symptomatic intracerebral hemorrhage at a frequency of 1–4%. Bevacizumab can increase the risk of headache by 37% irrespective of the risk of intracerebral hemorrhage in addition to risk of stroke, systemic bleeding, and hypertension [122].

Medication overuse headache
This syndrome has been previously referred to as "rebound headache," "drug-induced headache," and "medication misuse headache," although even the current title may be a misnomer. The term applies to headache that is induced by the use of an agent for headache at a frequency of two–three times per week on a regular basis. However, as most patients will attest, there is often nothing within prescribing guidelines to prohibit such use. Nevertheless, the use of acute headache medication more than 10 times per month is associated with the potential for worsened headache frequency and severity, especially in patients with tension and migraine headache. It is noted that this syndrome does not necessarily apply to those patients with a pattern of medication use on several consecutive days followed by relatively long periods of nonmedication use. This phenomenon seems to occur regardless of mechanism of action of the drug in question and is not necessarily associated with withdrawal effects of medication. Medications specifically implicated in the ICHD II include ergotamines, triptans, analgesics, opiates, and combination medications (e.g., analgesics with opioids, butalbital,

and/or caffeine). Criteria established for these substances follow the following paradigm: medication is used equal to or more than 10 days per month for more than 3 months with the presence of headache more than 15 days per month. When the substance is removed, the headache typically resolves within 2 months. Headache typically includes at least one of the following signs: bilateral location, pressing/tightening quality, and mild to severe intensity depending on the substance in question (triptans are described to have more severe headaches with more migrainous symptoms). Diagnosis of this syndrome is crucial, as preventive therapies are rarely effective while medication overuse syndrome is present [1].

Headaches from chronic medication use

Unlike medication overuse headache syndrome, this syndrome refers to medication used not just specifically for headache. Such headache is defined by the IHS as occurring more than 15 days per month with chronic medication use for any reason. Headache resolves with medication discontinuation but, depending on the medication in question, could take several months. The etiology of this headache depends on the mechanism of the drug used but could include vasoconstriction leading indirectly to malignant hypertension, intracranial hypertension, or direct vasodilator effects. Medications known to induce intracranial hypertension include amiodarone, anabolic steroids, lithium, nalidixic acid, thyroid hormone, tetracycline, vitamin A [123], and minocycline [1].

Headaches from medication withdrawal

As opposed to medication overuse headache, this headache entity refers to the situation where medication use is on a daily basis and the headache is a direct consequence of withdrawal phenomenon. The most common agents involved in this headache type are caffeine, opioids, and estrogens. Other agents that have been suggested to cause withdrawal headache, although the evidence is insufficient, are corticosteroids, tricyclic antidepressants, selective serotonin reuptake inhibitors, and serotonin-norepinephrine reuptake inhibitors. Complete removal of these substances typically eliminates headache after various lengths of time. However, it should be noted that frequent headache would not be completely eliminated in the event of additional possible headache contributory circumstances (such as sleep deprivation, poor nutrition, toxic exposures, hormonal disturbance, etc.) [1,124].

Caffeine withdrawal headache This headache is significant in that it can be initiated after a relatively short period of time. It is defined by the IHS as requiring at least 2 weeks of caffeine use of >200 mg/day, which is then delayed or interrupted. Headache is bilateral and/or pulsatile and occurs within 24 h of the last exposure to caffeine and is relieved within 1 h of 100 mg caffeine use. Resolution of headache occurs within 7 days of caffeine cessation [1,125].

Opioid withdrawal headache Similar to caffeine withdrawal headache, this entity is also bilateral and/or pulsatile but occurs after daily use for more than 3 months is interrupted. Headache develops within 24 h of last medication use and resolves within 7 days of medication cessation [1,124].

Estrogen withdrawal headache This headache is described as being of migraine or migrainous quality in association with estrogen discontinuation after at least 3 weeks of estrogen use. Headache begins within 5 days of discontinuation and resolves within 3 days of onset [1,126].

Illicit substances

Cocaine

Cocaine-induced headache is described by IHS criteria as having at least one of the following signs: bilateral location, frontotemporal location, pulsatility, and aggravation by physical activity. Headache begins within 1 h of use of cocaine and resolves within 72 h of a single use. Headache from cocaine is not typically associated with other symptoms unless there is a vascular complication of cocaine use [1].

Cannabis

Headache associated with marijuana use is described as being associated with dry mouth, possible paresthesias, feelings of warmth, and conjunctival injection. IHS criteria mandate at least one of the following features: bilateral location, stabbing or pulsatile quality, or pressure sensation in the head. Headache should begin within 12 h of marijuana use and resolve within 72 h of a single use [1,127].

Table 2.2 Some toxins that can cause headache [1]

Arsenic	Iodine
Alcohols (long chain)	Kerosene
Aniline	Lead
Balsam	Lithium
Borate	Mercury
Bromate	Methyl alcohol
Camphor	Methyl bromide
Carbon disulfide	Methyl chloride
Carbon tetrachloride	Methyl iodine
Chlorate	Naphthalene
Clordecone	Organophosphorus compounds:
Copper	Parathion
EDTA	Organophosphorus compounds:
Heptachlor	Pyrethrum
Hydrogen sulfide	Tolazoline hydrochloride

Toxins

The IHS has defined headache from substance use or exposure as developing within 12 h of such exposure or use and resolving within 72 h of a single exposure. Headache quality is nonspecific but is generally described as diffuse in location and of dull, moderate to severe intensity and continuous headache pattern [1]. The most common inorganic and organic substances that cause headache are listed in Table 2.2 [1].

Nitric oxide donors

Drugs and some foods that serve as nitric oxide (NO) donors are often a source of headache. Headache in this situation is typically a frontotemporal bilateral pulsating pain that can arise within 10 min of the absorption of the offending agent. However, headache presentation may be variable with the quality of headache resembling that of the patient's baseline history. Those without a headache history may not experience headache at all, while migraineurs experience migraine without aura, tension-type sufferers experience tension-type headache, and cluster patients experience cluster headache. The IHS defines such headache as satisfying at least one of the features including bilateral location, frontotemporal location, pulsatile quality, and aggravated by physical activity. Headache should develop within 10 min of ingestion of the nitric oxide donor and resolves within 1 h after termination of nitric oxide release. However, some patients may have delayed onset of headache. The delayed form of nitric oxide headache is more commonly seen among patients with primary headache disorders. Migraine and tension-type headache patients experience headache onset typically within 5-6 hours of exposure, and cluster headache patients experience headache within 1-2 hours of exposure to a nitric oxide donor. Foods containing nitrates such as hot dogs may be a potential trigger. Medications such as amyl nitrate, erythrityl tetranitrate, glyceryl trinitrate (GTN), isosorbide mono- or dinitrate, sodium nitroprusside, mannitol hexanitrate, and pentaerythrityl tetranitrate may all serve as potential nitric oxide donors [1,128].

Carbon monoxide (CO)

Carbon monoxide toxicity can induce headache typically within 12 h of exposure, with resolution of headache within 72 h of elimination of carbon monoxide. Clinical signs are dependent on the level of carboxyhemoglobin concentrations. When levels range from 10% to 20%, headache is mild without GI distress. Carboxyhemoglobin levels of 20–30% induce moderate headache with irritability. Levels of 30–40% yield severe headache with nausea, vomiting, and decreased visual acuity. Levels above 40% are associated with depressed mental status and poor ability to describe symptoms. Although typically headache resolves after exposure, there is evidence to suggest that prolonged exposure may cause "chronic postintoxication" headache [1,129].

Alcohol

Alcohol typically induces headache by a delayed effect, but there are those patients who have headache via direct alcohol sensitivity. It is unclear whether, in addition to alcohol itself, other ingredients within alcoholic beverages may elicit headache.

When the effect is immediate, it is defined by IHS criteria as occurring within 3 h of ingestion and resolving within 72 h of cessation of ingestion. The pain must have at least one of the following signs: bilateral location, frontotemporal location, pulsatile quality, and aggravation by physical activity. The amount of alcohol required seems to be idiosyncratic and irrespective of the history of migraine. The more common delayed effect of alcohol has the same headache description but occurs when blood alcohol levels drop or reduce to zero. In migraineurs only modest amounts of alcohol are required, but in nonmigraineurs intoxicating amounts of alcohol are required to induce headache. Headache typically resolves within 72 h [1,130–132].

Food additives

Common foods or food additives have been attributed to being headache triggers. Although phenyl ethylamine, tyramine, and aspartame are often included in lists of headache-inducing substances, there is insufficient evidence to confirm these substances as causing headache. However, there is evidence for the syndrome of headache with exposure to monosodium glutamate (MSG), also known as Chinese restaurant syndrome. Such headache typically occurs within 1 h of ingestion of MSG but otherwise follows the pattern for food sensitivity headaches above. Headache tends to be pulsatile in migraineurs but dull or burning in nonmigraineurs. It is often associated with other symptoms including chest and facial tightness and flushing; burning sensations in the chest, neck, and shoulders; and dizziness and GI distress [1,133–136].

Vitamins

Homocysteine and vitamin B12
Elevation of homocysteine levels has been shown to be associated with an increased risk for cardiovascular disease and stroke via disordered nitric oxide metabolism and endothelial wall damage [137]. Given the relatively unexplained presence of white matter lesions in migraine [105], it has been hypothesized that there may be an association with disordered homocysteine–nitric oxide metabolism in migraine leading to the presence of such lesions. On this basis, studies have been performed showing a linkage between migraine with aura and the MTHFRC677T genotype responsible for elevated homocysteine levels [138,139]. In a clinical trial by Lea et al. utilizing folic acid, vitamin B6, and vitamin B12 in migraineurs, migraine disability was reduced from 60% to 30% within 6 months with no change in the control group. [140]. The greatest treatment effect was seen in patients with the

MTHFRC677T genotype with greatest reduction in both migraine disability and serum homocysteine levels. The authors noted that the effect was even greater in carriers of the C allele (CT/CC) form of the gene versus the "TT" form. The authors interpreted the decreased benefit in the TT genotype as due to worsened homocysteine metabolism compared to the C allele, implicating the need for possible increased vitamin supplementation in those who are homozygous (TT) for the gene. They suggest a larger clinical trial to determine if folate/B6/B12 therapy is effective in improving quality of life in all migraineurs versus whether such therapy would be indicated only if the MTHFRC77T gene is present [141].

In addition to the above research, vitamin B12 specifically has been identified as an independent scavenger molecule for nitric oxide [142]. Improvement of nitric oxide clearance should improve endothelial wall integrity that is the basis for using vitamin B12 as a possible preventive agent in migraine. It was tested in open label fashion by Vad der Kuy in 19 patients. Headache frequency was reduced by at least 50% in 53% of subjects. The authors recommend that a double-blind placebo controlled trial is warranted [141].

Vitamin D
Vitamin D deficiency has been associated with an increased risk of chronic pain and therefore a potential association has been made with headache disorders [143,144]. As vitamin D synthesis is dependent on sunlight, Prakash et al. hypothesized that there may be a correlation between latitude and headache. A review of 1-year prevalence rates of migraine and tension headache with respect to geographic latitude revealed increased headache rates with increasing latitude. In addition, headache rates also increase within the fall-/winter seasons compared to summer. The authors suggested that the presence of vitamin D receptors within the hypothalamus could explain the association between vitamin D and headache. The hypothalamus is thought to play a key role in paroxysmal neurogenic disorders such as migraine and tension headache. Vitamin D may help modulate hypothalamic activation and deficiency could possibly lower headache thresholds [145]. Despite these observations, it has also been suggested that further investigation is needed before such a link between vitamin D deficiency and headache can be confirmed [144,145].

Vitamin B2 (Riboflavin)

Riboflavin is a precursor for both flavin mononucleotide and adenine dinucleotide that function in the electron transport chain, and facilitates mitochondrial metabolism. It was observed that patients with mitochondrial disease (MELAS syndrome) have an increased prevalence of migraine than would be expected otherwise. To determine if mitochondrial metabolism may be linked to migraine pathogenesis, high dose (400 mg) daily riboflavin was given in a randomized double-blind placebo controlled fashion to 28 migraineurs and 26 placebo subjects over 4 months. Of the riboflavin-treated subjects, 56% had a >50% improvement in headache frequency ($p = 0.005$) and 59% of subjects had >50% improvement in the number of headache days ($p = 0.012$). The benefit of riboflavin begins after 1 month but is maximal only after 3 months of treatment with greatest effect on frequency and only marginal effect on attack severity and associated features of migraine [146].

Coenzyme Q10

Coenzyme Q10 has been studied for migraine headache prophylaxis similar to riboflavin given its importance as a cofactor in mitochondrial energy metabolism. In a 150 mg/day open label trial ($n = 32$), 61.3% of patients had a greater than 50% reduction in number of days with migraine headache [147]. In a 300 mg dose, double-blind, randomized, two-parallel group trial, 21 control subjects and 22 migraineurs were evaluated, with a >50% response rate of 14.4% in the placebo group and 47.6% in the coenzyme Q10 group ($P < 0.0001$) [148].

Carnitine

Carnitine is a key part of mitochondrial energy metabolism and thought to be possibly protective to the brain as well as key for fatty acid transport for all cells throughout the body. Disordered mitochondrial metabolism may present with nonketotic hypoglycemic coma, myopathy with recurrent muscle pain, myoglobinuria, and encephalopathy. Carnitine deficiency may include chronic fatigue and myalgias. In the same line of reasoning that was used to establish the relationship between mitochondrial function and migraine with riboflavin and coenzyme Q10, it has been hypothesized that carnitine may also play a similar role. To this end, carnitine was given in open label fashion to two patients (one at age 14 and the other at age 15) who presented with refractory headaches and past history of fatigue and muscle cramps. One had borderline low carnitine levels while the other was normal. Both had significantly improved headache frequency with carnitine supplementation of 330 mg three times per day in one patient and 330 mg per day in the other. The authors of this study suggested that carnitine metabolism could be a factor in migraine generation, especially when clinical presentations have some features of mitochondrial disease. Larger studies are needed to determine if carnitine metabolism is a true factor in migraine pathogenesis [149].

Vitamin E

Vitamin E inhibits the release of arachidonic acid and the conversion of arachidonic acid to prostaglandin. During menses there is a threefold increase in prostaglandin levels within the endometrium [150]. Given the antiinflammatory effect of vitamin E, it has been hypothesized that it may have an effect on menstrually related migraine. A placebo controlled double-blind trial was performed using placebo and 400 i.u. vitamin E 2 days before onset of menses and 3 days after onset of menses. Of the subjects, 67 completed 2 menstrual cycles with statistically significant differences in the pain severity ($p < 0.001$), functional disability scales ($p < 0.001$), and associated features (photophobia, phonophobia, and nausea $p < 0.05$) between the vitamin E and the control groups. The authors concluded that perimenstrual administration of vitamin E could be an effective means of controlling the symptoms of menstrual migraine, with recommendation that larger trials should be performed [151].

Five things to remember about headaches due to systemic disease

1. Secondary headaches must be excluded before primary headaches can be diagnosed, and should be suspected in patients with new-onset atypical headache or abnormal neurological exam.
2. Pheochromocytoma should be considered in patients with a combination of some or all of the following symptoms: headache, palpitations, diaphoresis, sustained hypertension, orthostatic hypotension, pallor, hyperglycemia, fatigue, weight loss, anxiety/panic, paroxysmal hypertension, and flushing.
3. Pituitary apoplexy should be considered in patients with a combination of some or all of the following symptoms: thunderclap or sudden onset headache, cranial nerve 3-4-6 palsies, decreased visual acuity, altered mental status, meningismus, and nausea/vomiting.
4. Lung cancer should be suspected and chest X-ray obtained in patients with new-onset unilateral facial pain with additional possible pain in the ipsilateral hemicranium, jaw, and ear with possible cranial neuropathies.
5. Thunderclap headache or rapid-onset severe headache with peak pain reached within 1–60 s may represent bleeding of multiple potential causes, and patients with such presentation should have CT scan and possible lumbar puncture to evaluate such etiology as a potential neurosurgical emergency.

References

1 Headache Classification Committee of the International Headache Society. The international classification of headache disorders. *Cephalalgia* 2004;24:1–160.

2 Calhoun A, Ford S. Elimination of menstrual-related migraine beneficially impacts chronification and medication overuse. *Headache* 2008;48(8):1186–1193.

3 Peres MF, Sanchez del Rio M, Seabra ML, Tufik S, Abucham J, Cipolla-Neto J, Silberstein SD, Zukerman E. Hypothalamic involvement in chronic migraine. *J. Neurol. Neurosurg. Psychiatr.* 2001;71(6):747–751.

4 Mosek AC, Korczyn AD. Yom Kippur headache. *Neurology* 1995;45:1953–1955.

5 Moreau T, et al. Headache in hypothyroidism: prevalence and outcome under thyroid hormone therapy. *Cephalalgia* 1998;18(10):687–689.

6 Tepper DE, Tepper SJ, Sheftell FD, Bigal ME. Headache attributed to hypothyroidism. *Curr. Pain Headache Rep.* 2007;11(4):304–309.

7 Stone J, Foulkes A, Adamson K, Stevenson L, Al-Shahi Salman R. Thyrotoxicosis presenting with headache. *Cephalalgia* 2007;27(6):561–562.

8 Hagen K, Bjøro T, Zwart JA, Vatten L, Stovner LJ, Bovim G. Low headache prevalence amongst women with high TSH values. *Eur. J. Neurol.* 2001;8(6):693–699.

9 Lenders JW, Eisenhofer G, Mannelli M, Pacak K. Phaeochromocytoma. *Lancet* 2005;366:665–675.

10 Reisch N, Peczkowska M, Januszewicz A, Neumann HP. Pheochromocytoma: presentation, diagnosis and treatment. *J. Hypertens.* 2006;24:2331–2339.

11 Agarwal A, Gupta S, Mishra AK, Singh N, Mishra SK. Normotensive pheochromocytoma: institutional experience. *World J. Surg.* 2005;29:1185–1188.

12 Heo YE, Kwon HM, Nam HW. Thunderclap headache as an initial manifestation of phaeochromocytoma. *Cephalalgia* 2008;29:388–390.

13 Watanabe M, Takahashi A, Shimano H, Hara H, Sugita S, Nakamagoe K, Tamaoka A. Thunderclap headache without hypertension in a patient with pheochromocytoma. *J. Headache Pain* 2010;11:441–444.

14 Im SH, Kim NH. Thunderclap headache after micturition in bladder pheochromocytoma. *Headache* 2008;48:965–967.

15 Nawar RN, Abdel Mannan D, Selman WR, Arafah BM. Pituitary tumor apoplexy: a review. *J Intensive Care Med.* 2008;23(2):75–90.

16 Semple PL, Webb MK, de Villiers JC, et al. Pituitary apoplexy. *Neurosurgery* 2005;56:65–73.

17 Pliam MB, Cohen M, Cheng L, Spaenle M, Bronstein MH, Atkin JW. Pituitary adenoma complicating cardiac surgery: summary and review of 11 cases. *J. Card. Surg.* 1995;10(2):125–132.

18 Fuchs S, Beeri R, Hasin Y, Weiss AT, Gotsman MS, Zahger D. Pituitary apoplexy as a first manifestation of pituitary adenomas following intensive thrombolytic and anti-thrombotic therapy. *Am. J. Cardiol.* 1998;81:110–111.

19 Oo MM, Krishna AY, Bonavita GJ, Rutecki GW. Heparin therapy for myocardial infarction: an unusual trigger for pituitary apoplexy. *Am. J. Med. Sci.* 1997;314(5):351–353.

20 Biousse V, Newman NJ, Oyesiku NM. Precipitating factors in pituitary apoplexy. *Neurol. Neurosurg. Psychiatr.* 2001;71:542–545.

21 Mauskop A, Altura BT, Cracco RQ, Altura BM. Intravenous magnesium sulfate rapidly alleviates headaches of various types. *Headache* 1996;36(3):154–160.

22 Mauskop A, et al. Serum ionized magnesium levels and serum ionized calcium/ionized magnesium ratios in women with menstrual migraine. *Headache* 2002; 42(4):242–248.

23 Facchinetti F, et al. Magnesium prophylaxis of menstrual migraine: effects on intracellular magnesium. *Headache* 1991;31(5):298–301.

24 Bigal M, et al. Intravenous magnesium sulphate in the acute treatment of migraine without aura and migraine with aura. A randomized, double-blind, placebo-controlled study. *Cephalalgia* 2002;22:345–353.

25 Peikert A, et al. Prophylaxis of migraine with oral magnesium: results from a prospective, multi-center, placebo-controlled and double-blind randomized study. *Cephalalgia* 1996;16(4):257–263.

26 Pfaffenrath V, et al. Magnesium in the prophylaxis of migraine: a double-blind placebo-controlled study. *Cephalalgia* 1996;16(6):436–440.

27 Wang F, et al. Oral magnesium oxide prophylaxis of frequent migrainous headache in children: a randomized, double-blind, placebo-controlled trial. *Headache* 2003;43(6):601–610.

28 Janiri L, Gallo G, Nicoletti W. Calcium deficiency and supraorbital headache: a clinical study of adult subjects. *Cephalalgia* 1986;6(4):211–218.

29 Isaacson SR, Snow JB. Etiologic factors in hypocalcemia secondary to operations for carcinoma of the pharynx and larynx. *Laryngoscope* 1978;88(8 Pt 1): 1290–1297.

30 Basso U, Maruzzo M, Roma A, Camozzi V, Luisetto G, Lumachi F. Malignant hypercalcemia. *Curr. Med. Chem.* 2011;18(23):3462–3467.

31 Sharieff GQ, Hanten K. Pseudotumor cerebri and hypercalcemia resulting from vitamin A toxicity. *Ann. Emerg. Med.* 1996;27:518–521.

32 Klopstock A, May P, Siebel E, Papagiannuli E, Diener NC, Heichmann H. Mitochondrial DNA in migraine with aura. *Neurology* 1996;46:1735–1738.

33 Ojaimi J, Katsabanis S, Bower S, Quigley A, Byrne E. Mitochondrial DNA in stroke and migraine with aura. *Cerebrovasc. Dis.* 1998;8:102–106.

34 Koo B, Becker L, Chuang S, Merante F, Robinson BH, MacGregor D, Tein I, Ho VB, McGreal DA, Wherrett JR, Logan WJ. Mitochondrial encephalomyopathy, lactic acidosis, stroke-like episodes (MELAS): clinical, radiological, pathological and genetic observations. *Ann. Neurol.* 1993;34:25–32.

35 Olson LG, King MT, Hensley MJ, Saunders NA. A community study of snoring and sleep-disordered breathing: Symptoms. *Am. J. Respir. Crit. Care Med.* 1995;152:707–710.

36 Dodick DW, Eross EJ, Parish JM, Silber M. Clinical, anatomical, and physiologic relationship between sleep and headache. *Headache* 2003;43:282–292.

37 Bigal ME, Gladstone J. The metabolic headaches. *Curr. Pain Headache Rep.* 2008;12(4):292–295.

38 Kristiansen HA, Kværner KJ, Akre H, Overland B, Russell MB. Migraine and sleep apnea in the general population. *J. Headache Pain* 2011;12(1):55–61.

39 Jensen R, Olsborg C, Salvesen R, Torbergsen T, Bekkelund SI. Is obstructive sleep apnea syndrome associated with headache? *Acta Neurol. Scand.* 2004;109:180–184.

40 Neau JP, Paquereau J, Bailbe M, Meurice JC, Ingrand P, Gil R. Relationship between sleep apnoea syndrome, snoring and headaches. *Cephalalgia* 2002;22:333–339.

41 Rains JC. Morning headache in habitual snorers. *Cephalalgia* 2011;31(9):981–983.

42 Goksan B, Gunduz A, Karadeniz D, Ağan K, Tascilar FN, Tan F, Purisa S, Kaynak H. Morning headache in sleep apnoea: clinical and polysomnographic evaluation and response to nasal continuous positive airway pressure. *Cephalalgia* 2009;29(6):635–641.

43 Sliwka U, Kransney JA, Simon SG, et al. Effects of sustained low-level elevations of carbon dioxide on cerebral blood flow and autoregulation of the intracerebral arteries in humans. *Aviat. Space Environ. Med.* 1998;69:299–306.

44 Cheshire WP, Ott MCJr., Headache in divers. *Headache* 2001;41:235–247.

45 Cervera R, Piette JC, Font J, Khamashta MA, Shoenfeld Y, Camps MT, Jacobsen S, Lakos G, Tincani A, Kontopoulou-Griva I, Galeazzi M, Meroni PL, Derksen RH, de Groot PG, Gromnica-Ihle E, Baleva M, Mosca M, Bombardieri S, Houssiau F, Gris JC, Quéré I, Hachulla E, Vasconcelos C, Roch B, Fernández-Nebro A, Boffa MC, Hughes GR, Ingelmo M, Euro-Phospholipid Project Group. Antiphospholipid syndrome: clinical and immunologic manifestations and patterns of disease expression in a cohort of 1,000 patients. *Arthritis Rheum.* 2002;46(4):1019–1027.

46 Rodrigues CE, Carvalho JF, Shoenfeld Y. Neurological manifestations of antiphospholipid syndrome. *Eur. J. Clin. Invest.* 2010;40(4):350–359.

47 Rozell CL, Sibbitt WLJr., Brooks WM. Structural and neurochemical markers of brain injury in the migraine diathesis of systemic lupus erythematosus. *Cephalalgia* 1998;18(4):209–215.

48 Ford RP. The gluten syndrome: a neurological disease. *Med. Hypotheses* 2009;73(3):438–440.

49 Lionetti E, Francavilla R, Maiuri L, Ruggieri M, Spina M, Pavone P, Francavilla T, Magistà AM, Pavone L. Headache in pediatric patients with celiac disease and its prevalence as a diagnostic clue. *J. Pediatr. Gastroenterol. Nutr.* 2009;49(2):202–207.

50 Inaloo S, Dehghani SM, Farzadi F, Haghighat M, Imanieh MH. A comparative study of celiac disease in children with migraine headache and a normal control group. *Turk. J. Gastroenterol.* 2011;22(1):32–35.

51 Gonzalez-Gay MA, Martinez-Dubois C, Agudo M, Pompei O, Blanco R, Llorca J. Giant cell arteritis: epidemiology, diagnosis, and management. *Curr. Rheumatol. Rep.* 2010;12(6):436–442.

52 Kale N, Eggenberger E. Diagnosis and management of giant cell arteritis: a review. *Curr. Opin. Ophthalmol.* 2010;21(6):417–422.

53 Kraft HE, Moller DE, Volker L, Schmidt WA. Color doppler ultrasound of the temporal arteries: a new method for diagnosing temporal arteritis. *Klin. Monatsbl. Augenheilkd* 1996;208:93–95.

54 Burde RM, Savino PJ, Trobe JD. *Clinical Decisions in Neuro-Ophthalmology*, 2nd ed. St Louis, Mo: Mosby Year Book, 1992, pp. 51–56.

55 Beri M, Klugman MR, Kohler JA, Hayreh SS. Anterior ischemic optic neuropathy, VII: incidence of bilaterality and various influencing factors. *Ophthalmology* 1987;94:1020–1028.

56 Lee AG, Brazis PW. Temporal arteritis: a clinical approach. *Am. Geriatr. Soc.* 1999;47(11):1364–1370.

57 Hajj-Ali RA, Singhal AB, Benseler S, Molloy E, Calabrese LH. Primary angiitis of the CNS. *Lancet Neurol.* 2011;10(6):561–572.

58 Farah, Al-Shubaili A, Montaser A, Hussein JM, Malaviya AN, Mukhtar M, Al-Shayeb A, Khuraibet AJ, Khan R, Trontelj JV. Behcet's syndrome: a report of 41 patients with emphasis on neurological manifestations. *J. Neurol. Neurosurg. Psychiatr.* 1998;64:382–384.

59 Glanz BI, Venkatesan A, Schur PH, Lew RA, Khoshbin S. Prevalence of migraine in patients with systemic lupus erythematosus. *Headache* 2001;41:285–289.

60 Gullapalli D, Phillips LH2nd. Neurologic manifestations of sarcoidosis. *Neurol. Clin.* 2002;20:59–83.

61 Hollinger P, Sturzenegger M. Mathis J, Schroth G, Hess CW. Acute disseminated encephalomyelitis in adults: a reappraisal of clinical CSF, EEG and MRI findings. *J. Neurol.* 2002;249:320–329.

62 Colnaghi S, Versino M, Marchioni E, Pichiecchio A, Bastianello S, Cosi V, Nappi G. ICHD-II diagnostic criteria for Tolosa–Hunt syndrome in idiopathic inflammatory syndromes of the orbit and/or the cavernous sinus. *Cephalalgia* 2008;28(6):577–584.

63 de Lima Antoniazzi AL, Corrado AP. Dialysis headache. *Curr. Pain Headache Rep.* 2007;11:297–303.

64 Göksan B, Karaali-Savrun F, Ertan S, Savrun M. Haemodialysis-related headache. *Cephalalgia* 2004; 24(4):284–287.

65 Blacky RA, Rittlemeyer JT, Wallace MR. Headache angina. *Am. J. Cardiol.* 1987;60:730.

66 Lipton RB, Lowenkopf T, Bajwa ZH, Leckie RS, Ribeiro S, Newman LC, Greenberg MA. Cardiac cephalgia: a treatable form of exertional headache. *Neurology* 1997;49:813–816.

67 Vernay D, Deffond D, Fraysse P, Dordain G. Walk headache: an unusual manifestation of ischemic heart disease. *Headache* 1989;29:350–351.

68 Scher AI, Terwindt GM, Picavet HSJ, et al. Cardiovascular risk factors and migraine: the GEM population-based study. *Neurology* 2005;64:614–620.

69 Schwedt TJ. The migraine association with cardiac anomalies, cardiovascular disease, and stroke. *Neurol. Clin.* 2009;27(2):513–523.

70 Kurth T, Gaziano JM, Cook NR, et al. Migraine and risk of cardiovascular disease in women. *JAMA* 2006;296:283–291.

71 Kurth T, Gaziano M, Cook NR, et al. Migraine and risk of cardiovascular disease in men. *Arch. Intern. Med.* 2007;167:795–801.

72 Stewart WF, Lipton RB, Celentano DO, et al. Prevalence of migraine headache in the United States: relation to age, income, race, and other socioeconomic factors. *JAMA* 1992;267:64–69.

73 Lipton RB, Stewart WF, Diamond S, et al. Prevalence and burden of migraine in the United States: data from the American Migraine Study II. *Headache* 2001;41:646–657.

74 Wilmshurst P, Nightingale S, Pearson M, et al. Relation of atrial shunts to migraine in patients with ischemic stroke and peripheral emboli. *Am. J. Cardiol.* 2006;98:831–833.

75 Gillis CN, Pitt BR. The fate of circulating amines within the pulmonary circulation. *Annu. Rev. Physiol.* 1982;44:269–281.

76 Wilmshurst PT, Pearson MJ, Nightingale S, et al. Inheritance of persistent foramen ovale and atrial septal defects and the relation to familial migraine with aura. *Heart* 2004;90:1315–1320.

77 Dowson A, Mullen MJ, Peatfield R, et al. Migraine intervention with STARFlex technology (MIST) trial: a prospective, multicenter, double-blind, sham-controlled trial to evaluate the effectiveness of patent foramen ovale closure with STARFlex septal repair implant to resolve refractory migraine headache. *Circulation* 2008;117:1397–404.

78 Rodríguez RR, Saccone J, Véliz MA. Headache and liver disease: is their relationship more apparent than real? *Dig. Dis. Sci.* 2004;49(6):1016–1018.

79 Ozge A, Ozge C, Kaleagasi H, Yalin OO, Unal O, Ozgür ES. Headache in patients with chronic obstructive pulmonary disease: effects of chronic hypoxaemia. *J. Headache Pain* 2006;7(1):37–43.

80 Gossage JR, Kanj G. State of the art: pulmonary arteriovenous malformations. *Am. J. Respir. Crit. Care Med.* 1998;158:643–661.

81 Thenganatt J, Schneiderman J, Hyland RH, et al. Migraines linked to intrapulmonary right-to-left shunt. *Headache* 2006;46:439–443.

82 Post MC, Thijs V, Schonewille WJ, et al. Embolization of pulmonary arteriovenous malformations and decrease in prevalence of migraine. *Neurology* 2006;66:202–205.

83 Abraham PJ, Capobianco DJ, Cheshire WP. Facial pain as the presenting symptom of lung carcinoma with normal chest radiograph. *Headache* 2003;43(5):499–504.

84 Grosberg BM, Lantos G, Solomon S, Bigal ME, Lipton RB. Multiple cranial neuropathies, headache, and facial pain in a septuagenarian. *Headache* 2004;44(10):1038–1039.

85 Robbins MS, Grosberg BM. Hemicrania continua-like headache from metastatic lung cancer. *Headache* 2010;50(6):1055–1056.

86 Capobianco DJ. Facial pain as a symptom of nonmetastatic lung cancer. *Headache* 1995;35(10):581–585.

87 Evans RW. Hemicrania Continua-like headache due to nonmetastatic lung cancer: a vagal cephalalgia. *Headache* 2007;47(9):1349–1351.

88 Evans RW, Peres MF. Headaches and pineal cysts. *Headache* 2010;50(4):666–668.

89 De Marinis M, Welch KM. Headache associated with noncephalic infections: classification and mechanisms. *Cephalalgia* 1992;12:197–201.

90 Pavan-Langston D. Herpes zoster antivirals and pain management. *Ophthalmology* 2008;115(2 Suppl.): S13–S20.

91 Liesegang TJ. Herpes zoster ophthalmicus natural history, risk factors, clinical presentation, and morbidity. *Ophthalmology* 2008;115(2 Suppl.):S3–S12.

92 Patchell RA. Neurological complications of organ transplantation. *Ann. Neurol.* 1994;36:688–703.

93 Cemillan CA, Alonso-Pulpon L, Burgos-Lazaro R, Millan-Hernandez I, del Ser T, Liano-Martinez H. Neurological complications in a series of 205 orthotopic heart transplant patients. *Rev. Neurol.* 2004;38:906–912.

94 Goldstein L, Haug M, Perl J, Perl M, Maurer J, Arroliga A, Mehta A, Kirby T, Higgins B, Stillwell B. Central nervous system complications after lung transplantation. *J. Heart Lung Transpl.* 1998;17:185–191.

95 Frank B, Perdrizet GA, White HM, Marsh JW, Leman W, Woodie ES. Neurotoxicity of FK 506 in liver transplant recipient. *Transplant. Proc.* 1993;25:1887–1888.

96 Adams HP, Dawson G, Coffman TJ, Corry RJ. Stroke in renal transplant recipients. *Arch. Neurol.* 1986;43:113–115.

97 Maggioni F, Mantovan MC, Rigotti P, Cadrobbi R, Mainardi F, Mampreso E, Ermani M, Cortelazzo S, Zanchin G. Headache in kidney transplantation. *J. Headache Pain* 2009;10(6):455–460.

98 Carson KL, Hunt CM. Medical problems occurring after orthotopic liver transplantation. *Dig. Dis. Sci.* 1997;42(8):1666–1674.

99 Stracciari A, D'Alessandro R, Baldin E, Guarino M. Post-transplant headache: benefit from riboflavin. *Eur. Neurol.* 2006;56(4):201–320.

100 Webster A, Woodroffe RC, Taylor RS, Chapman JR, Craig JC. Tacrolimus versus cyclosporin as primary immunosuppression for kidney transplant recipients. *Cochrane Database Syst Rev.* 2005; (4):CD003961.

101 Ferro JM, Melo TP, Oliveira V, Salgado AV, Crespo M, Canhao P, Pinto AN. A multivariate study of headache associated with ischemic stroke. *Headache* 1995;35:315–319.

102 Etminan M, Takkouche B, Isorna FC, et al. Risk of ischaemic stroke in people with migraine: systematic review and meta-analysis of observational studies. *Br. Med. J.* 2005;330:63–65.

103 Stang PE, Carson AP, Rose KM, et al. Headache, cerebrovascular symptoms, and stroke: the Atherosclerosis Risk in Communities Study. *Neurology* 2005;64:1573–1577.

104 MacClellan LR, Giles W, Cole J, et al. Probable migraine with visual aura and risk of ischemic stroke: The Stroke Prevention in Young Women Study. *Stroke* 2007;38:2438–2445.

105 Kruit MC, van Buchem MA, Hofman PA, Bakkers JT, Terwindt GM, Ferrari MD, Launer LJ. Migraine as a risk factor for subclinical brain lesions. *JAMA* 2004;291(4):427–434.

106 Martsen BH, Sorensen PS, Marquardsen J. Transient ischemic attacks in young patients: a thromboembolic or migrainous manifestation? A ten-year follow-up of 46 patients. *J. Neurol. Neurosurg. Psychiatr.* 1990;53:1029–1033.

107 Huang J, van Gelder JM. The probability of sudden death from rupture of intracranial aneurysms: a meta-analysis. *Neurosurgery* 2002;51:1101–1105.

108 Van Gijn J, Rinkel GJ. Subarachnoid haemorrhage: diagnosis, causes and management. *Brain* 2001;124(Pt 2):249–278.

109 Kong DS, Hong SC, Jung YJ, Kim JS. Improvement of chronic headache after treatment of unruptured intracranial aneurysms. *Headache* 2007;47(5):693–697.

110 Schwedt TJ, Matharu MS, Dodick DW. Thunderclap headache. *Lancet Neurol.* 2006;5(7):621–631.

111 Tardy J, Pariente J, Nasr N, Peiffer S, Dumas H, Cognard C, Larrue V, Chollet F, Albucher JF. Carotidynia: a new case for an old controversy. *Eur. J. Neurol.* 2007;14 (6):704–705.

112 Evers S, Marziniak M. Headache attributed to carotid or vertebral artery pain. *Handb. Clin. Neurol.* 2010;97:541–545.

113 Gladstone JP, Dodick DW. Migraine and cerebral white matter lesions: when to suspect cerebral autosomal dominant arteriopathy with subcortical infarcts and leukoencephalopathy (CADASIL). *Neurologist* 2005;11(1):19–29.

114 Ney JJ, Volpe NJ, Liu GT, Balcer LJ, Moster ML, Galetta SL. Functional visual loss in idiopathic intracranial hypertension. *Ophthalmology* 2009;116 (9):1801–1803.

115 Friedman DI, Jacobson DM. Diagnostic criteria for idiopathic intracranial hypertension. *Neurology* 2002;59(10):1492–1495.

116 Wasay M, Kojan S, Dai AI, Bobustuc G, Sheikh Z. Headache in cerebral venous thrombosis: incidence, pattern and location in 200 consecutive patients. *J. Headache Pain* 2010;11(2):137–139.

117 De Bruijn SFTM, Stam J, Kappelle LJ for CVST Study Group. Thunderclap headache as first symptom of cerebral venous sinus thrombosis. *Lancet* 1996;348:1623–1625.

118 Bousser MG, Ross Russell R. *Cerebral Venous Thrombosis: Major Problems in Neurology*, vol 1, London: Saunders, 1997.

119 Vaughan CJ, Delanty N. Hypertensive emergencies. *Lancet* 2000;356:411–417.

120 Weiss NS. Relation of high blood pressure to headache, epistaxis, and selected other symptoms: The United States Health Examination Survey of Adults. *N. Engl. J. Med.* 1972;287:631–633.

121 Zampaglione B, Pascale C, Marchisio M, Cavallo-Perin P. Hypertensive urgencies and emergencies: prevalence and clinical presentation. *Hypertension* 1996;27:144–147.

122 Goldlust SA, Graber JJ, Bossert DF, Avila EK. Headache in patients with cancer. *Curr. Pain Headache Rep.* 2010;14(6):455–464.

123 Spector RH, Carlisle J. Pseudotumor cerebri caused by a synthetic vitamin A preparation. *Neurology* 1984;34:1509–1511.

124 Tepper SJ, Tepper DE. Breaking the cycle of medication overuse headache. *Cleve Clin. J. Med.* 2010;77(4):236–242.

125 Shapiro RE. Caffeine and headaches. *Curr. Pain Headache Rep.* 2008;12(4):311–315.

126 Loder EW, Buse DC, Golub JR. Headache as a side effect of combination estrogen–progestin oral contraceptives: a systematic review. *Am. J. Obstet. Gynecol.* 2005;193 (3 Pt 1):636–649.

127 Greco R, Gasperi V, Maccarrone M, Tassorelli C. The endocannabinoid system and migraine. *Exp. Neurol.* 2010;224(1):85–91.

128 Gupta S, Nahas SJ, Peterlin BL. Chemical mediators of migraine: preclinical and clinical observations. *Headache* 2011;51(6):1029–1045.

129 Swadron SP. Pitfalls in the management of headache in the emergency department. *Emerg. Med. Clin. North Am.* 2010;28(1):127–147, viii–ix.

130 Wallgreen H, Barry A. Drug actions in relation to alcohol effects. *Action of alcohol.* New York: Elsevier, 1970, pp. 621–714.

131 Ogata S, Hosoi T, Saji H. Studies on acute alcohol intoxication. *Japanese Journal of Studies of Alcohol* 1966;1:67–79.

132 Panconesi A, Bartolozzi ML, Guidi L. Alcohol and migraine: what should we tell patients? *Curr. Pain Headache Rep.* 2011;15(3):177–184.

133 Scher W, Scher BM. A possible role for nitric oxide in glutamate (MSG)-induced Chinese restaurant syndrome, glutamate induced asthma, 'hot-dog headache', pugilistic Alzheimer's disease, and other disorders. *Med. Hypotheses* 1992;38:185–188.

134 Savi L, Rainero I, Valfrè W, Gentile S, Lo Giudice R, Pinessi L. Food and headache attacks. A comparison of patients with migraine and tension-type headache. *Panminerva Med.* 2002;44(1):27–31.

135 Kelman L. The triggers or precipitants of the acute migraine attack. *Cephalalgia* 2007;27(5):394–402.

136 Gore ME, Salmon PR. Chinese restaurant syndrome: fact or fiction. *Lancet* 1980;318:251–252.

137 Wald DS, Law M, Morris JK. Homocysteine and cardiovascular disease: evidence on causality from a meta-analysis. *BMJ* 2002;325:1202.

138 Scher AI, Terwindt GM, Verschuren WM, Kruit MC, Blom HJ, Kowa H, et al. Migraine and MTHFR C677 T genotype in a population-based sample. *Ann. Neurol.* 2006;59:372–375.

139 Rubino E, Ferrero M, Rainero I, Binello E, Vaula G, Pinessi L. Association of the C677T polymorphism in the MTHFR gene with migraine: a meta-analysis. *Cephalalgia* 2007;27:1199–1320.

140 Lea R, Colson N, Quinlan S, Macmillan J, Griffiths L. The effects of vitamin supplementation and MTHFR (C677T) genotype on homocysteine-lowering and migraine disability. *Pharmacogenet. Genomics* 2009;19(6):422–428.

141 Rajanayagam MAS, Li CG, Rand MJ. Differential effects of hydroxocobalamin on NO-mediated relaxations in rat aorta and anococcygeus muscle. *Br. J. Pharmacol.* 1993;108:3–5.

142 Farah, Al-Shubaili A, Montaser A, Hussein JM, Malaviya AN, Mukhtar M, Al-Shayeb A, Khuraibet AJ, Khan

R, Trontelj JV. Behcet's syndrome: a report of 41 patients with emphasis on neurological manifestations. *J. Neurol. Neurosurg. Psychiatr.* 1998;64:382–384.

143 Montagna P. Back to vitamins? *Cephalalgia* 2002; 22(7):489–490.

144 Yang Y, Zhang HL, Wu J. Is headache related with vitamin D insufficiency? *J. Headache Pain* 2010;11 (4):369; author reply 371.

145 Prakash S, Mehta NC, Dabhi AS, Lakhani O, Khilari M, Shah ND. The prevalence of headache may be related with the latitude: a possible role of vitamin D insufficiency? *J. Headache Pain* 2010;11(4):301–307.

146 Schoenen J, Jacquy J, Lenaerts M. Effectiveness of high-dose riboflavin in migraine prophylaxis. A randomized controlled trial. *Neurology* 1998;50(2):466–470.

147 Rozen TD, Oshinsky ML, Gebeline CA, Bradley KC, Young WB, Shechter AL, Silberstein SD. Open label trial of coenzyme Q10 as a migraine preventive. *Cephalalgia* 2002;22(2):137–141.

148 Sandor PS, Di Clemente L, Coppola G, Saenger U, Fumal A, Magis D, Seidel L, Agosti RM, Schoenen J. Efficacy of coenzyme Q10 in migraine prophylaxis: a randomized controlled trial. *Neurology.* 2005;64 (4):713–715.

149 Kabbouche MA, Powers SW, Vockell AL, LeCates SL, Hershey AD. Carnitine palmityltransferase II (CPT2) deficiency and migraine headache: two case reports. *Headache* 2003;43(5):490–495.

150 Granella F, Sances G, Messa G, et al. Treatment of menstrual migraine. *Cephalagia* 1997;17:35–38.

151 Ziaei S, Kazemnejad A, Sedighi A. The effect of vitamin E on the treatment of menstrual migraine. *Med. Sci. Monit.* 2009;15(1):CR16–CR19.

3

Encephalopathy (delirium) due to systemic disease

Allison Weathers

Rush University Medical Center, Chicago, IL, USA

The brain is highly susceptible to being adversely affected by illness elsewhere in the body and by many of the medications used in the treatment of these illnesses. If severe enough, disease processes of all other organ systems have potential central nervous system manifestations. Therefore, encephalopathy is one of the most commonly encountered neurologic manifestations of systemic illness. Consciousness is comprised of two facets, arousal, or the degree of wakefulness, and cognitive functions such as language and memory [1]. Together these result in an awareness of self and the environment. In the encephalopathic state, one or both of these aspects are usually acutely impaired with a broad range of potential neurologic outcomes, from mild lethargy to coma. As evident from the title of this chapter, delirium is used synonymously for encephalopathy, mainly by nonneurologists. Altered mental status is a less sophisticated term that is also frequently used to describe the same clinical state.

There is much similarity in the clinical picture regardless of the underlying cause of the encephalopathy. Further confusing the issue is the fact that in a systemically ill patient, there is usually more than one possible underlying cause of the encephalopathy. For example, patients with renal failure often have derangements in their electrolytes. This results in the frequent use of the catchall term "toxic-metabolic encephalopathy" by neurologists, regardless of the specific underlying etiology. However, there are numerous etiologies that result in specific and often defining clinical features; recognition of these characteristics may lead to an exact diagnosis being made, with the possibility for specific treatment interventions. This chapter will cover many of the multiple possible systemic disease processes that can result in encephalopathy, highlighting those potentially reversible systemic etiologies that result in well-defined and unique clinical signs and symptoms.

Encephalopathy due to endocrine disorders

Diabetes

Severe hypoglycemia and hyperglycemia, especially in patients with diabetes mellitus, accounts for most cases of endocrine disorder-related encephalopathy. This is due both to the very high prevalence of diabetes mellitus, especially as compared to some of the more rare endocrine disorders, and to the strong association of glucose derangements with an encephalopathic state. Neurologic manifestations regularly occur with an acute drop in serum blood glucose below 50 mg/dL [2]. A patient with longstanding, repeated episodes of hypoglycemia that occur more gradually may tolerate lower serum glucose levels without becoming symptomatic [3]. The initial manifestations of hypoglycemia are usually the systemic symptoms of tremulousness, palpitations, hunger, and diaphoresis, with anxiety as the initial neuropsychiatric manifestation [3,4]. As the patient's serum glucose level drops, the neurologic symptoms become more profound, including confusion, memory loss, lethargy, weakness, and seizures, eventually progressing to stupor and coma [3,4]. A somewhat unique feature of hypoglycemic encephalopathy is the common frequency with which focal and asymmetric neurologic deficits occur, a rare occurrence with other metabolic derangements [4].

Neurological Disorders due to Systemic Disease, First Edition. Edited by Steven L. Lewis.
© 2013 Blackwell Publishing Ltd. Published 2013 by Blackwell Publishing Ltd.

Also unique is that certain regions of the brain are much more susceptible to damage from hypoglycemia, including the cerebral cortex, basal ganglia, hippocampus, splenium of the corpus callosum, and internal capsule, with the brainstem and cerebellum usually not affected [2,5,6]. This selective sparing of the brainstem and cerebellum has been attributed to greater glucose transporter efficiency and activity in these regions [5,6]. Energy and ion pump failure, intracellular influx of calcium, other ion imbalances, intracellular alkalosis, cessation of protein synthesis, and neurotoxic amino acid release all contribute to the development of the encephalopathy [2,5,6]. Magnetic resonance imaging (MRI) is useful to exclude a structural etiology of the patient's neurologic signs and symptoms, especially when focal asymmetric findings are present. MRI may show restricted diffusion on diffusion-weighted imaging (DWI) in the regions susceptible to hypoglycemic insult, with corresponding low signal on the apparent diffusion coefficient maps [7]. Corresponding areas of hyperintensity may also be seen on the T2-weighted and fluid attenuated inversion recovery (FLAIR) sequences [2,5,6]. The radiological syndrome of reversible focal lesions of the splenium of the corpus callosum has been reported with hypoglycemic encephalopathy [8]. The classic description of this imaging finding is a well circumscribed, ovoid or "coin-shaped" lesion that is hyperintense on T2-weighted and FLAIR images, iso- to hypointense on T1-weighted images, and nonenhancing [8]. There may be corresponding high signal on the DWI and low signal on the apparent diffusion coefficient (ADC) images. This finding is not restricted to hypoglycemic encephalopathy, as will be discussed later in this chapter.

Electroencephalogram (EEG) will show increased theta activity with development of delta waves if the hypoglycemia worsens [4]. If the blood glucose level continues to drop and the patient becomes comatose, the EEG may become flat [4]. Hypoglycemic encephalopathy is treated by reversing the underlying hypoglycemia, usually with rapid intravenous infusion of hypertonic glucose, with prognosis based on the severity and duration of the hypoglycemia [2,3]. Prompt recognition of hypoglycemia is therefore crucial. Diabetes is a frequent, and often previously undiagnosed, comorbidity in hospitalized patients, and although rare, hypoglycemia may occur in non-diabetic patients. Therefore, a blood glucose level should be checked in all encephalopathic patients.

Serum glucose testing will also assess for the reverse condition, that of too much blood glucose. Diabetic ketoacidosis (DKA) and hyperglycemic hyperosmolar state (HHS) are always in the differential diagnosis of an encephalopathic patient. Despite adequate insulin dosing, a number of systemic illnesses including infection, dehydration, pancreatitis, silent myocardial infarction, and stroke may bring on DKA and HHS. In addition, DKA and HHS may be brought on by commonly administered medications, such as thiazide diuretics, corticosteroids, and antipsychotics [9]. Inadequate dosing due to noncompliance or dosing errors is a frequent cause. Patients may also present with DKA and HHS as the initial presentation of their diabetes.

DKA evolves rapidly, while HHS typically develops subacutely over days to weeks with coma occurring more rarely [9]. Frequently associated systemic signs and symptoms, including polyuria, polydipsia, tachycardia, hypotension, dry mucous membranes, and recent weight loss, may provide clues to the diagnosis. Patients with DKA may additionally have nausea, vomiting, and abdominal pain. In addition to elevated blood glucose, patients with an encephalopathy related to these diagnoses will likely have a serum osmolarity of over 330 mOsm/kg and glycosuria. As expressed in the name, patients with diabetic ketoacidosis will have a ketonuria and a metabolic acidosis. Treatment of both DKA and HHS consists of fluid administration, careful administration of insulin, and replacement, if indicated, of potassium, bicarbonate, and phosphate. Cerebral edema is a rare though often lethal complication [9].

Thyroid disease

Although referred to as an encephalopathy, steroid-responsive encephalopathy associated with auto-immune thyroiditis, also referred to as Hashimoto's encephalopathy, is actually more of a subacute dementia and therefore is discussed in Chapter 4. Once this diagnosis is excluded, true encephalopathies due to thyroid disorders are quite rare. Overt hyperthyroidism may have neuropsychiatric manifestations, including confusion, psychosis, seizures, and manic and depressive mood changes [10]. Elderly patients may have more subtle neurologic symptoms including anxiety and cognitive impairment [11]. Acute alterations in mental status and level of consciousness may occur as part of the presentation of thyrotoxic crisis. Thyrotoxic encephalopathy has been associated with a number of radiographic findings, including high signal on the DWI and reduction in the ADC in the cerebellum, white matter, and the corpus callosum [12]. These changes, with corresponding areas of hyperintensity seen on the T2-weighted and FLAIR images may be restricted only to the splenium of the corpus callosum and therefore thyrotoxicosis is another potential etiology of this distinct clinicoradiologic syndrome [12]. Park et al. reported successful treatment of this clinical and radiographic syndrome by treatment of the underlying thyrotoxicosis with glucocorticoids, propylthiouracil, and propranolol [12]. Thyroid disorders may also result in a number of other metabolic derangements, such as acute hyperammonemia, which may themselves precipitate an acute encephalopathy [13].

Parathyroid disease

Neuropsychiatric manifestations are a known complication of primary hyperparathyroidism [14]. Primary hyperparathyroidism may result in encephalopathy both from the resultant hypercalcemia (discussed in further detail in the next section) and possibly due to neurotoxic effects of parathyroid hormone itself [14]. Patients usually improve clinically with parathyroidectomy; however, encephalopathy is paradoxically becoming an increasingly recognized potential complication of this procedure [15–17]. Methylene blue selectively stains the parathyroid glands and is therefore utilized during parathyroid surgery as it improves intraoperative visualization of the glands [15–17]. It also has a number of other medical uses, ironically one being in the treatment of ifosfamide-induced encephalopathy, a topic that will be discussed in greater detail later in this chapter. Methylene blue is a monoamine oxidase A inhibitor and when administered to patients taking a selective serotonin reuptake inhibitor, a serotonin–norepinephrine reuptake inhibitor, or a tricyclic antidepressant, may result in a severe serotonin syndrome [16,17].

This syndrome is manifested by confusion, agitation, and decreased level of consciousness with the potential of coma, as well as a number of focal neurologic signs including nystagmus and opsoclonus, dilated and non-reactive pupils, myoclonus, tremor, seizures, cortical blindness, hyperreflexia, and Babinski signs [16,17]. As in classic serotonin syndrome, autonomic and neuromuscular manifestations are often present as well [16,17]. Prognosis is generally excellent with complete

recovery usually occurring in a few days with aggressive supportive care [15–17]. While increasing awareness among surgeons of this potential complication of methylene blue will decrease the incidence, prompt recognition by neurologists when it does occur will hopefully prevent costly and unnecessary testing of these patients.

Adrenal disease

Addisonian crisis may present as an acute encephalopathy with confusion, alteration in the level of consciousness, and associated psychotic features. Addison's disease is associated with more mild cognitive and psychiatric features such as fatigue, decrease in motivation, and mood changes [18]. Although the neurologic manifestations of Addison's disease have been attributed to the primary glucocorticoid-deficient state, severe electrolyte abnormalities, including hyponatremia and hypoglycemia, are very common and may compound the neurologic deficits [18,19]. Cerebral edema may result [19]. The presence of characteristic signs and symptoms of adrenal insufficiency such as hypotension, recent weight loss, gastrointestinal symptoms, hyperpigmentation, and multiple electrolyte derangements may support this diagnosis; however, these may be subtle or attributed to other diagnoses such as infection or toxin exposure [18]. Further complicating the evaluation of these patients is that Addisonian crises are often precipitated by stressors such as illness, dehydration, and thyroid replacement [18].

EEG is usually abnormal with diffuse slowing being the most frequent finding; however, this diagnosis is confirmed by the measurement of a low plasma cortisol, elevated ACTH, and abnormal corticotropin stimulation test [18,19]. Low aldosterone and high renin are supportive laboratory findings. Prognosis is excellent with prompt treatment with intravenous normal saline and dexamethasone, followed by hydrocortisone replacement therapy; if this diagnosis is suspected, treatment should be initiated empirically [18,19].

Encephalopathy is not a common manifestation of Cushing syndrome, a disorder of excess cortisol exposure. However, the severe hypertension that may occur with Cushing syndrome has been reported to precipitate posterior reversible encephalopathy syndrome (PRES) [20]. This syndrome will be discussed in further detail in the autoimmune disorders section of this chapter.

Electrolyte and other metabolic disorders

Patients with underlying systemic illnesses, especially when ill enough to be hospitalized, are prone to electrolyte and other metabolic disorders. Further complicating matters is that patients often have more than one underlying systemic illness, usually of differing chronicity and severity, such as longstanding diabetes mellitus with superimposed acute renal failure. These may have an additive effect on any electrolyte and metabolic derangements that occur. All encephalopathic patients should be screened for electrolyte and metabolic disorders due to the high frequency with which they occur, their ease of detection and correction, and high mortality rates if left undetected and untreated. Evaluation involves simple blood work in the form of a basic metabolic profile as well as serum calcium and magnesium levels.

Out of these commonly occurring disorders, hyponatremia is particularly common in hospitalized patients, and generally results in a typical encephalopathic state with few distinguishing features. The degree and the time course of the development of the hyponatremia determine the extent of the neurologic manifestations [3]. Patients with acute hyponatremia may initially present with mild confusion and lethargy, which will progress to coma if the hyponatremia remains untreated and continues to worsen. Focal weakness, ataxia, nystagmus, tremor, rigidity, and hyperreflexia may occur [21]. Chronic hyponatremia, even at levels below 130 mEq/L, may be asymptomatic or result in only mild fatigue and headache if it develops gradually enough. Seizures occur mainly with a rapid decrease in the serum sodium level to below 115 mEq/L and their presence is associated with increased mortality rates [21].

The identification of the underlying etiology, and in turn the correct subtype of the hyponatremia, often has a critical impact on treatment decisions. Hyponatremia occurs in distinct forms depending on the underlying etiology [21]. Some causes, such as acute renal failure and cirrhosis, result in a hypo-osmolar state with associated edema, while hypothyroidism and glucocorticoid deficiency may cause a hypo-osmolar hyponatremia with normovolemia [21]. Gastrointestinal fluid losses from vomiting and diarrhea may cause a hypovolemic state. Hyperglycemia may result in a hyper-osmolar hyponatremia. Patients with a normovolemic or hypervolemic state should be water restricted, while isotonic saline is usually indicated in those with a hypovolemic hypo-osmolar hyponatremia [21]. Acute, severe hyponatremia, especially once seizures occur, requires emergent treatment with the judicious use of 3% saline (4–6 mL/kg) to slowly raise the serum sodium [3,21]. Other medications, such as furosemide, may be utilized concurrently with saline solutions to enhance the excretion of free water [3].

Hypernatremia is a less commonly encountered etiology of encephalopathy than hyponatremia, occurring mainly due to dehydration in susceptible populations such as the elderly [21]. Structural hypothalamic lesions that decrease thirst, and diabetes insipidus combined with water restriction, are much less frequent causes of hypernatremia [21]. The neurologic manifestations are again most commonly that of a classic encephalopathy, with a continuum ranging from mild lethargy to coma depending on the severity and acuity of the sodium abnormality. Generally, symptoms develop at a sodium level above 160 mEq/L, with acute shrinking of brain parenchyma thought to be, at least in part, responsible [21]. There is increased risk for development of intraparenchymal and subdural hemorrhages. Seizures are not uncommon and may occur during rehydration, and abnormal movements such as tremor, myoclonus, and asterixis have been reported [21].

Hypernatremia is another potential etiology of the radiographic entity of reversible lesions of the splenium of the corpus callosum [22]. As previously discussed, this reversible imaging finding has been well described in a number of clinical scenarios, including some endocrinopathies, antiepileptic drug toxicity and withdrawal, and viral encephalitis [8,22]. MRI is usually obtained only to rule out a structural etiology of the patient's condition and this imaging finding is not in any way diagnostic of hypernatremic encephalopathy.

Hypercalcemia occurs in the settings of malignant neoplasms and hyperparathyroidism. Multiple myeloma, breast, lung, kidney, and head and neck cancers are most commonly implicated, as these are most commonly associated with osteolytic skeletal metastasis [3,21]. Many of these neoplasms are also associated with increased calcitriol and parathyroid hormone-related protein (PTH-rP) secretion [3,23]. The encephalopathic state associated with hypercalcemia tends to occur at serum calcium levels above 14 mg/dL and may range from mild lethargy to coma, and is determined heavily by the severity and acuity of onset of the calcium disturbance [3]. Seizures are rare. Long-term prophylactic bisphosphonate therapy in at-risk patients has reduced the incidence of this cancer complication. Intravenous bisphosphonate administration is a mainstay of treatment when malignant hypercalcemia occurs [3].

Less commonly occurring electrolyte disturbances that may result in encephalopathy include hypocalcemia and hypomagnesemia (the latter usually at levels below 0.8 mEq/L) [21]. Patients with hypocalcemia and hypomagnesemia will have confusion with associated signs of neurologic hyperexcitability such as seizures, tremors, myoclonus, hyperreflexia, and agitation, while patients with hypermagnesemia will have signs of nervous system depression including hyporeflexia and lethargy [21]. Potassium derangements do not usually result in encephalopathy. As patients with encephalopathy due to electrolyte abnormalities usually respond rapidly and often completely to prompt treatment, a metabolic profile should be obtained in all encephalopathic patients. In patients with multiple electrolyte derangements, the presence of classically associated peripheral nervous system manifestations may be quite beneficial in helping make the diagnosis.

Central pontine myelinolysis (CPM), now more accurately called osmotic demyelination syndrome, is a disorder associated primarily with the correction of an electrolyte disturbance, as opposed to being due to the actual disturbance itself. It is classically associated with the rapid correction of hyponatremia, and in this scenario it occurs as a result of the increase in extracellular sodium concentration occurring faster than the intracellular uptake of electrolytes and organic osmolytes [21,24,25]. Intracellular water rapidly shifts extracellularly, resulting in cell injury and neuronal demyelination. Also contributing is breakdown of the blood–brain barrier (BBB), intracellular edema, and microglia activation with cytokine release [25]. This disorder occurs with varying degrees of severity, as evidenced by the much higher incidence of this finding reported in autopsy studies as compared to that found clinically [25].

Though rapid correction of hyponatremia is the most common clinical scenario causing CPM, this syndrome has also been described in patients with hypernatremia, diabetic ketoacidosis, AIDS, hyperemesis gravidarum, systemic lupus erythematosus, Sjögren syndrome, acute intermittent porphyria, anaphylactic shock, heat stroke, and cytomegalovirus hepatitis [24–26]. Patients with CPM in the setting of hyponatremia often have a predisposing condition such as chronic alcoholism, recent liver transplantation, burns, and other electrolyte abnormalities, especially hypokalemia [25,26].

Patients with CPM due to the correction of their hyponatremia will often have an initial improvement in their encephalopathy prior to the acute decline of their neurologic status [24,25]. Pseudobulbar palsy has been well described as has dysarthria, dysphagia, nystagmus, ophthalmoplegia, ataxia, and a flaccid then spastic quadriparesis [24–26]. Patients may progress to a complete locked-in syndrome and may become stuporous or comatose [21,25]. Other more subtle neurologic manifestations suggestive of frontal lobe dysfunction, including restlessness, emotional lability, apathy, akinetic mutism, agitation, insomnia, paranoia, delusions, and disinhibited and aggressive behavior may occur [25]. The term "osmotic demyelination syndrome" is becoming more routinely used, as extrapontine involvement (most frequently the cerebellum and thalamus) is common, and pontine sparing may occur [25]. Magnetic resonance imaging may show hyperintensities in the pons, but also the midbrain, cerebellum, thalamus, external capsule, basal ganglia, cortex, and subcortical white matter on T2-weighted and FLAIR images [24,25].

Treatment is mainly supportive and includes correction of all other underlying electrolyte and metabolic disorders and management of all secondary complications such as aspiration pneumonia [24]. Plasmapheresis, intravenous immunoglobulin, and steroid administration have been anecdotally reported to be of possible benefit [26]. Unlike the usual transient encephalopathy attributed to electrolyte abnormalities, patients with CPM who survive after aggressive supportive therapy may be left with considerable neurologic deficits [24]. Patients usually require intensive rehabilitation [24,25].

Encephalopathy due to systemic autoimmune disorders

Systemic lupus erythematosus (SLE) is one of the most common autoimmune diseases in the United States. The potential neuropsychiatric manifestations of this condition are broad, including, but certainly not limited to, nonspecific headaches, seizures, strokes, transverse myelitis, aseptic meningitis, major depression, and psychosis. A majority of patients with SLE will have some neuropsychiatric involvement of their disease [27]. Acute confusional states (ACS) are another potential manifestation of neuropsychiatric involvement of SLE [28]. An acute confusional state is defined by the American College of Rheumatology as equivalent to the term delirium and is therefore equivalent to a neurologist's use of the term encephalopathy [29]. ACS may clinically range from only mild disturbances of consciousness to coma, and as with most encephalopathic states, patients may become severely agitated [29].

Any of the myriad potential neuropsychiatric manifestations of SLE, including ACS, may be the presenting symptom of the patient's disease, preceding systemic symptoms [29]. Furthermore, multiple neuropsychiatric symptoms may occur simultaneously and during periods of active disease or during periods of apparent remission. Antiphospholipid positivity has been strongly associated with certain neuropsychiatric manifestations, including ACS, stroke, psychosis, mood disorders, and transverse myelitis [27,28]. MRI abnormalities, most commonly areas of high signal in the white matter on FLAIR and T2-weighted images, may be seen in patients with neuropsychiatric involvement of their SLE [27,28]. Examination of cerebrospinal fluid (CSF) may reveal elevated protein and other signs of inflammation and is useful more for ruling out an infectious etiology of the patient's presentation. Treatment of ACS and other neuropsychiatric manifestations consists of immune suppressive treatments and symptomatic management, with anticoagulation being added when indicated [28].

In addition to being direct and presumably autoimmune-mediated complications of SLE, neuropsychiatric symptoms, especially encephalopathy, may occur through a variety of other mechanisms. Encephalopathy may occur due to lupus-mediated organ dysfunction and as an adverse effect of both symptomatic and immunosuppressive medications [27]. PRES is a well-recognized complication of SLE [30–32]. PRES is a syndrome with distinct clinical and radiologic features that over the past 15 years has been increasingly recognized to occur in a variety of clinical situations, such as with severe hypertension, eclampsia, infections, other autoimmune diseases, and exposure to certain immunosuppressants and chemotherapeutic agents [31]. Its name is now known to be something of a misnomer, as the clinical deficits and radiographic findings are not always reversible and the lesions are not always located posteriorly.

The usual clinical manifestations of PRES are seizures, headache, vision loss (including cortical blindness), and an encephalopathic state; however, patients may have no focal neurologic signs or symptoms [31,33]. MRI usually reveals abnormal high signal on the T2-weighted and FLAIR images in an appearance consistent with vasogenic edema, with often patchy, bilateral, symmetrical, frequently posterior involvement [33]. While initially thought to only involve the subcortical white matter, lesions may be seen in the cortex, basal ganglia, brainstem, and thalamus. Corresponding restricted diffusion may be seen on the diffusion-weighted images, and gadolinium enhancement may be present.

Patients with SLE often have multiple, simultaneous, potential causative factors for the development of PRES, including renal dysfunction, marked hypertension, exposure to immunosuppressants such as cyclosporine, and superimposed infections [30,31]. The proposed pathophysiologic mechanism in these clinical scenarios is failure of either cerebral autoregulation or autoregulatory-induced vasoconstriction [31,32]. Disruption of the blood–brain barrier, increased vascular permeability and leakage of blood plasma results [31,32].

Although it may be difficult, it is critical to distinguish this syndrome from an acute confusional state due to direct involvement of the central nervous system by the patient's lupus, as treatment will vary markedly between the two conditions. While treatment of a direct neuropsychiatric manifestation of SLE usually involves increased immunosuppression, PRES is usually treated by aggressive blood pressure management, withdrawal of any possible causative agents, dialysis if indicated, and supportive measures such as ventilator support if needed [30,31]. Anticonvulsants may be required if seizures persist despite the above measures and corticosteroids may be indicated if there is evidence of active, severe systemic SLE activity [31]. As the name implies, with appropriate management there is often rapid and complete improvement in the clinical and radiographic findings; however, poor outcomes may occur. Patients may also have a relapse with recurrence of the precipitating clinical situation.

Other autoimmune diseases are not as strongly associated either with the development of acute confusional states due to direct disease involvement or with PRES. Cognitive deficits have been described in Sjögren's syndrome and in Behçet's disease, including memory loss, frontal lobe dysfunction, and personality changes, but these deficits are not acute in onset, occurring more insidiously [27,28]. Systemic vasculitides and primary angiitis of the CNS may present with acute cognitive impairment and altered level of consciousness [27].

Encephalopathy due to organ dysfunction and failure

Liver disease

Overt hepatic encephalopathy will occur in almost half of all patients with cirrhosis, and even more patients may develop the subclinical form (detectable only by formal neuropsychological testing) known as minimal hepatic encephalopathy [34]. Given the high prevalence of both the precipitating systemic medical illness and the neurologic complication, hepatic encephalopathy is an entity that almost all practicing neurologists will encounter. Furthermore, the presence of this complication in patients with chronic liver disease has significant implications for prognosis, making its diagnosis even more critical.

The term hepatic encephalopathy encompasses a potentially very broad range of clinical presentations due to any number of underlying hepatic insults. Due to the confusion that resulted from this ambiguity a formal classification system was created based on the underlying etiology of the hepatic encephalopathy [35]. Type A is due to patients with acute liver failure, type B is seen in patients with portal-systemic shunting in the absence of intrinsic hepatic disease, and type C is associated with cirrhosis with portal hypertension or portosystemic shunts. Type C is further divided into the subcategories of episodic, persistent, or minimal, and then even further characterized based on the severity and presence or absence of triggering events [35].

Four grades or stages of hepatic encephalopathy have been defined based on the level of consciousness, intellectual function, extent of personality and behavioral changes, and associated neuromuscular findings [35,36]. Symptoms occur on a continuum between these stages. Patients with mild encephalopathy (grade 1) may present only with insomnia or mild fatigue. They may have mild psychiatric manifestations such as euphoria or anxiety, decreased attentiveness and concentration, and some difficulty with complex computations. Grade 2 is associated with the presence

of lethargy and mild disorientation, amnesia, confusion, and clear personality changes with inappropriate behavior. Neurological exam may reveal more pronounced dyscalculia, dysarthria, diminished reflexes, and ataxia. In severe or grade 3 encephalopathy, patients are somnolent or semistuporous with marked cognitive impairment, paranoid ideations, and hallucinations. Hyperreflexia, nystagmus, Babinski signs, clonus, and rigidity may be present on exam. Once patients are comatose they are considered to be in grade 4; opisthotonus and posturing may be seen. Asterixis is a prominent feature of grade 2 and is not seen in grade 1 or 4 [36]. In addition to the above examination findings, focal signs such as hemi- and monoplegia and paresis may occur [36]. Seizures are not a usual manifestation of hepatic encephalopathy due to chronic liver disease. The general examination in patients with hepatic encephalopathy will often reveal other evidence of advanced liver disease, including ascites, jaundice, and spider angiomas [36].

The diagnosis of hepatic encephalopathy is made through the history and physical examination findings. Ancillary testing is useful mainly to exclude differential diagnoses for the patient's encephalopathic state, such as subclinical status epilepticus. EEG findings will vary depending on the stage of the encephalopathy and may show diffuse slowing (theta waves), triphasic waves, or random, nonrhythmic, asynchronous delta waves [37]. Neuroimaging with computed tomography (CT) or MRI is helpful to exclude other etiologies such as infection or hemorrhage, not to confirm the diagnosis. MRI may show bilateral T1 high signal in the globus pallidus. This radiographic finding is thought to be due to manganese deposition and is common in patients with chronic liver disease; it is not specifically diagnostic of the clinical presence of hepatic encephalopathy.

Ammonia levels are routinely obtained in patients with suspected hepatic encephalopathy. Although it was previously believed that blood ammonia levels did not correlate well with the degree of severity of the hepatic encephalopathy, this was likely attributable to laboratory processing issues of this labile compound [36]. When processed correctly, there is a strong correlation between the blood ammonia level and the severity of the hepatic encephalopathy [36].

In addition to the direct toxic effects of ammonia in the brain, including abnormalities of neurotransmission, impaired metabolism, and abnormal gene expression, excess intracerebral glutamine production occurs due to decreased hepatic urea synthesis and results in astrocyte swelling [38,39]. Both ammonia-induced, and independent, inflammatory reactions occur with subsequent release of proinflammatory cytokines [38–40]. Oxidative stress and resultant free radical production are also contributing processes [38]. Finally, γ-aminobutyric acid (GABA), manganese, fatty acids, and other potential culprits may be involved in the pathophysiology of hepatic encephalopathy [40].

Hepatic encephalopathy is most often precipitated in patients with chronic liver disease by superimposed clinical circumstances such as dehydration, gastrointestinal bleeding, infections, intake of excessive dietary protein, electrolyte abnormalities, surgery, transjugular intrahepatic portal-systemic shunt (TIPS) placement, and further hepatic insult [36]. The first step of treatment is the recognition and correction of any and all precipitating factors [36]. This may be sufficient, but when further intervention with pharmacologic therapies is required, the nonabsorbable disaccharide lactulose and the minimally absorbed oral antibiotic rifaximin, administered either individually or in combination, are most commonly used [36,37]. Neomycin and metronidazole are also used [36]. All of these agents act by inhibiting absorption or production of ammonia. Controversy exists surrounding the efficacy of lactulose, and its adverse gastrointestinal effects (increased gas, abdominal distention, cramping, and pain, in addition to the purposeful diarrhea) are often not tolerated by patients; however, it continues to be extensively used. The starting dose of lactulose is 30 mL two to four times daily. Though initially given orally, patients with advanced stages of hepatic encephalopathy may require dosing through enemas given the risk for pulmonary aspiration [36]. This route may also be used in patients with spontaneous bacterial peritonitis and severe ascites [36]. Due to the extent of the gastrointestinal side effects, compliance with chronic lactulose treatment tends to be poor.

Rifaximin is better tolerated with less associated toxicities than other antibiotics such as neomycin. The use of neomycin is limited due to concerns over the potential ototoxicity and nephrotoxicity. Metronidazole may have potential gastrointestinal and neurologic adverse effects with long-term usage. In multiple studies rifaximin has also been shown to be better tolerated and more effective than lactulose [40]. Despite the evidence of its effectiveness as a first-line therapy, it is often administered in conjunction with lactulose. In a double-blind, placebo controlled trial, rifaximin has also been shown to be an effective prophylaxis, decreasing the risk of breakthrough episodes of hepatic encephalopathy in patients with chronic liver disease who had suffered from previous recurrent episodes of hepatic encephalopathy [41]. In this trial, the incidence of adverse events was similar in the rifaximin and the placebo group.

Other treatment strategies that have been investigated and may be of benefit are the use of benzodiazepine antagonists such as naloxone, volume expansion, and direct ammonia removal by hemofiltration [38,42]. Though protein restriction had been thought to be beneficial, restricted diets have not been shown to be of significant benefit and might be harmful in cirrhotic patients in a catabolic state [36,38]. Liver transplantation is an option to achieve successful long-term treatment in cirrhotic patients with recurrent episodic or persistent hepatic encephalopathy [36].

Encephalopathy in patients with fulminant acute liver failure is considered a neurologic emergency due to the potential for acute cerebral edema with resultant intracranial hypertension. Though this may occur with less frequency than previously believed [38], the development of an encephalopathic state in a patient with fulminant acute liver failure should still be treated as an emergent situation. Prompt neurosurgical consultation is indicated for the placement of an intracranial pressure transducer to confirm this diagnosis, which may be missed by head CT [36]. If acute intracranial pressure is confirmed, aggressive management of this complication should be undertaken.

Kidney disease

Patients with renal failure are prone to becoming encephalopathic for a myriad of reasons, with uremic encephalopathy being one of the main ones. Patients may develop electrolyte disturbances, vitamin deficiencies, hypertensive encephalopathy, dehydration, drug toxicities, and complications from the treatments themselves, including dialysis and transplantation [14,43]. Patients on hemodialysis are also susceptible to developing subdural hematomas due to a number of reasons including rapid ultrafiltration, the use of hypertonic dialysate, and concurrent anticoagulation [14,43]. These patients often present with headache and confusion.

Uremic encephalopathy is not limited to patients with acute renal failure; however, the course is worse in patients with acute renal failure both in intensity and in speed of progression [43–45] and symptoms may occur at a less severe degree of azotemia than in patients with more chronic renal failure [14]. Symptoms may develop quite rapidly but are often mild at onset. Patients may initially develop apathy, fatigue, irritability, and difficulty with concentration and attention [44–46]. Mild motor impairment in the form of clumsiness may be present [45]. Without intervention, the patient's psychiatric and cognitive symptoms will continue to progress. In the later stages, patients will have marked confusion with disorientation, delusions, and hallucinations, evolving to stupor and eventually coma [44,45]. The presence of frontal lobe dysfunction is additionally supported by the findings of gegenhalten and frontal lobe release signs on examination [45]. A hallmark of this illness is the rapid fluctuation of the clinical course; symptoms may fluctuate over hours to days [14].

In addition to the psychiatric and cognitive manifestations, motor signs are a prominent aspect of the clinical presentation of uremic encephalopathy, especially in the later stages [43–45]. A variety of abnormal movements have been described, including fasciculations, myoclonus, a course postural and kinetic tremor, and chorea [44]. Asterixis may also be seen. The motor manifestations may be quite severe and are known as "uremic twitching" or the "uremic twitch-convulsive syndrome" [43,44]. Hypertonicity, hyperreflexia, clonus, Babinski signs, and paresis may be found on neurologic examination [45]. These findings may occur unilaterally, mimicking a focal intracerebral lesion, and may even alternate sides [45]. Further confusing an already complicated clinical picture may be the presence of meningeal signs.

Seizures are another late manifestation of uremic encephalopathy. Though usually generalized tonic-clonic, multiple seizure types have been well described in this patient population including simple motor seizures with progression to epilepsia partialis continua, and complex partial seizures [44,46]. Status epilepticus may occur.

Patients with chronic uremic encephalopathy due to chronic renal failure may have more subtle symptoms including mild attention deficits, psychomotor slowing with slowed reaction time, and persistent sleep disturbances [46]. Other potential manifestations of chronic uremic encephalopathy include mild language impairment, dysarthria, headaches, decreased appetite, irritability and other mood changes, and fatigue with mild exertion [14].

Normal laboratory measures of renal function including blood urea nitrogen, creatinine, and glomerular filtration rate are not consistent with a diagnosis of uremic encephalopathy; however, the severity of the laboratory abnormalities does not correlate well with the degree of the encephalopathy [43–45]. As with hepatic encephalopathy, ancillary testing is more useful to rule out alternative diagnoses than to confirm the diagnosis of uremic encephalopathy. EEG will most often show generalized slowing, especially frontally, with delta and theta waves, seen within 48 h of the onset of renal failure [43,45]. The study may be normal if obtained very early on [46]. Triphasic waves, with an anterior predominance, may be seen. Bilateral spike-wave complexes and photoparoxysmal responses occur less commonly [46]. There is a good correlation between the EEG and the clinical course, with the EEG becoming slower and lower voltage as the clinical picture worsens [45,46]. Cerebrospinal fluid studies, especially protein level, may be mildly abnormal [45]; however, they are in no way diagnostic and are helpful only to rule out an infectious etiology of the patient's symptoms. Imaging with CT or MRI is usually obtained, but again solely to rule out an underlying structural etiology of the patient's symptoms and not to confirm the diagnosis, which has no typical neuroimaging findings.

The pathophysiology of this disorder is not fully understood. Decreased excretion and altered protein metabolism results in the accumulation of a number of potential uremic toxins [44]. Among these are urea, uric acid, and the guanidino compounds: guanidinosuccinic acid, methylguanidine, guanidine, and creatinine [44]. The guanidino compounds are hypothesized to activate the excitatory N-methyl-D-aspartate (NMDA) receptors while simultaneously acting as antagonists of the GABA receptors, in addition to other proposed pathophysiologic mechanisms of action [43,47]. Transketolase, a thiamine-dependent enzyme involved in the maintenance of myelin, may be inhibited by guanidinosuccinic acid, with resultant demyelination [43].

The lack of clear correlation of the severity of the uremic encephalopathy with the degree of azotemia is evidence that the presence of these uremic toxins is not the full answer. Renal dysfunction also results in alterations of brain metabolism with reduction in the brain metabolic rate and oxygen consumption [45]. Parathyroid hormone (PTH) may also play a significant role in the development of uremic encephalopathy [14,43,44]. The presumed mechanism is an increase in intracerebral calcium levels through PTH enhancement of calcium transport and possibly direct neurotoxic effects of the PTH itself [14,43,45]. Further supporting this theory is the finding that uremic patients improve with parathyroidectomy and by medical suppression of PTH [14].

A rare variant of the classic uremic encephalopathy is the syndrome of acute bilateral basal ganglia lesions. Initially reported only in Asian populations, this syndrome is strongly associated with the development of uremia in patients with longstanding diabetes mellitus [48–50]. This syndrome is usually monophasic with improvement of both the clinical and neuroradiographic manifestations [49]. Patients develop acute parkinsonism, characterized by severe rigidity, bradykinesia, postural instability, and a parkinsonian gait disorder, with the usual absence of a resting or postural tremor [49]. This frequently occurs in conjunction with the acute onset of cognitive impairment, including lethargy and confusion [48]. Dysarthria, dysphagia, and involuntary movements such as orofacial dyskinesias may also occur [49]. Neuroimaging reveals hypodensities in the bilateral basal ganglia on CT, with corresponding areas of signal hyperintensity on the FLAIR and T2-weighted images on MRI. Areas of signal hypointensity will be seen on the T1-weighted images as well. From a purely neurological standpoint, prognosis is good with improvement with hemodialysis and supportive care [49,50]. Unfortunately, these patients are often critically ill with an overall very poor prognosis, usually secondary to infectious complications [49,50]. It has been theorized that this unusual neurologic manifestation of uremia occurs due to chronic injury to the basal ganglia by microangiopathic changes and metabolic derangements secondary to diabetes mellitus [49]. This damage in turn may make the basal ganglia even more susceptible to the effects of uremic neurotoxins.

Uremic encephalopathy is treated either by dialysis (peritoneal or hemodialysis) or by successful kidney transplantation [43–45]. Symptoms are improved with dialysis; however, mild, though not inconsequential, cognitive deficits and alterations in sleep may persist [45].

Rarely, patients will worsen or even develop new neurological symptoms after the initiation of hemodialysis. This has classically been attributed to two different diagnoses: dialysis dementia and dialysis disequilibrium syndrome. Dialysis dementia, a progressive and often rapidly fatal illness seen in patients on chronic hemodialysis, is now considered to be mainly a historical disease. Described chiefly in the 1970s and 1980s, this disorder was characterized in the early stages by dysphasia, dysarthria, and ataxia, with subacute progression to severe psychiatric manifestations, myoclonus, seizures, and mutism [43,46]. It was attributed to aluminum toxicity secondary to both aluminum contamination of the dialysate and purposeful use of aluminum as a phosphate binder, both of which are now, in almost all cases, rigorously avoided [46].

Dialysis disequilibrium syndrome can range from mild neurologic and systemic manifestations such as mild headache, myalgias, nausea, and fatigue, to more severe manifestations including severe headaches, vision changes, nausea and vomiting, fasciculations, confusion, tremors, seizures, and rarely focal neurologic deficits [14,46]. This self-limited syndrome is attributed to the development of an increased osmotic gradient and paradoxical acidemia with subsequent development of brain edema [14]. This occurs in patients with severe azotemia who are newly dialyzed or who receive highly effective ultrarapid hemodialysis [46]. Prevention with shorter, more frequent dialysis sessions at low blood flow rates in patients at risk is considered the best management strategy [14]. Other differential diagnoses, including stroke and subdural hematomas, should be evaluated for and excluded.

Pancreatic disease

While certainly less common than hepatic and uremic encephalopathy, pancreatic encephalopathy is a well-described (although likely underrecognized) complication of pancreatic disease. Patients with pancreatic encephalopathy will present with the nonspecific encephalopathic findings of confusion with disorientation, fluctuating alterations of consciousness, agitation, paranoid ideation, and hallucinations [51–57]. The distinguishing feature of pancreatic encephalopathy is the gastrointestinal symptoms that indicate the presence of acute pancreatitis, namely, the presence of acute, severe pain of the upper abdomen [58]. Severe anorexia, nausea, vomiting, and fever may also be seen. Less frequent neurologic manifestations include depressed mood, seizures, tremor, dysarthria, aphasia, hemiparesis, clonus, signs of meningeal irritation, frontal release signs, ataxia, nystagmus, akinetic mutism, and coma [55–61]. Pancreatic encephalopathy is an acute to subacute complication of acute pancreatitis, with onset usually within the first 2 weeks of the presentation of the pancreatitis, often between the second and fifth day [53,54,58]. A hyperacute presentation has also been reported, with onset of symptoms within the first 24 h, and therefore, with neurologic manifestations present from the time of admission [51,57,61].

There appears to be no association between the occurrence of pancreatic encephalopathy and the underlying etiology of the acute pancreatitis, occurring in cases due to alcoholism, biliary disease, and other causes such as invasive procedures [52,54]. It remains unclear whether the degree of severity of the acute pancreatitis is a factor in the development of pancreatic encephalopathy. Some studies have found no relationship between the severity of the acute pancreatitis and the incidence of encephalopathy, while others have found a higher incidence in more severe cases [52,54]. The development of pancreatic encephalopathy does not seem to impact the course of the underlying pancreatitis [52].

Elevated serum amylase is the characteristic laboratory finding of acute pancreatitis, and the presence of increased serum amylase in an encephalopathic patient with severe abdominal pain and other gastrointestinal symptoms may aid in the diagnosis of pancreatic encephalopathy. However, there is no clear correlation between the amylase levels and the presence or severity of the encephalopathy [57]. EEG is usually abnormal, though in a nonspecific pattern, with diffuse slowing with bilateral theta and intermittent delta waves having been described [54,56,59]. Though routine CSF studies are often normal, mild increases in protein may occur and CSF lipase values may be higher in patients with pancreatic encephalopathy than those with pancreatitis without encephalopathy [52,53,56,62]. MRI may be normal or may show small scattered areas of signal abnormality on T2-weighted images mainly in the white matter [59], and bilateral, diffuse hyperintense lesions in the pons, middle cerebellar peduncles, and cerebral deep white matter on FLAIR and diffusion sequences [54,56,62]. Essentially, the diagnosis remains a clinical one, based on the history, the associated gastrointestinal picture, and the exclusion of other possible etiologies. The development of pancreatic encephalopathy has been postulated to be attributed to the activation of phospholipase A (PLA) by trypsin and bile acid, which in turn converts lecithin and cephalin into their hemolytic forms [54]. This in turn destroys the blood–brain barrier and results in demyelination, encephalomalacia, hemorrhage, mitochondrial injury, impaired acetylcholine release, and edema due to increased vascular permeability [53,54]. Cytokines and fat necrosis, with pulmonary fat embolism and direct cerebral fat embolism, are also thought to play a role [54,55,62,63].

As with the occurrence of encephalopathy due to any other organ failure, the differential diagnosis of pancreatic encephalopathy is quite broad and this diagnosis should be considered one of exclusion. Electrolyte, calcium, and other metabolic abnormalities, vitamin deficiencies, pH alterations, secondary liver injury, and concurrent infections may all occur in patients with acute pancreatitis [53,60]. Osmotic demyelination due to hyperosmolality, and pancreatitis-induced disseminated intravascular coagulation (DIC) syndrome, are more rare but still possible [55]. In patients with pancreatitis secondary to alcoholism, pancreatic encephalopathy may mimic delirium tremens (DT) [60].

There is no specific treatment for pancreatic encephalopathy other than symptomatic and supportive therapy including early and aggressive management of the underlying pancreatitis [59,61]. Surgical intervention, if indicated for the management of the acute pancreatitis, may improve the encephalopathy [54]. The mortality of patients with pancreatic encephalopathy is high (50%), though when improvement occurs it is often complete and usually corresponds fairly closely to the improvement of the pancreatitis [52,53,59,60].

Cardiac arrest

Neurologists are frequently consulted for the question of neurologic prognosis following cardiac arrest. This is a grave responsibility, as the primary service and other consultants often defer to the neurologist's opinion and alter their care based on it, with the resultant potential for the phenomenon of the self-fulfilling prophecy. The encephalopathy that occurs due to cardiac arrest is often severe [64,65]. This is due to the rapidity with which cerebral oxygen stores are exhausted (20 s), with energy stores of glucose and adenosine triphosphate lasting only a short while longer (5 min) [64,65]. Although a discussion of predictive factors of neurological outcome following cardiac arrest is beyond the scope of this chapter, it is important to note that therapeutic hypothermia is now considered routine care in patients who have survived out-of-hospital ventricular fibrillation cardiac arrest and this intervention may impact commonly utilized predictors, such as the physical examination and biochemical markers [64,66].

Pulmonary disease

As opposed to the often devastating clinical scenario that follows cardiac arrest, the encephalopathy associated with pure pulmonary failure is often much more gradual in its speed of onset, and subtle in its presenting symptoms. Patients with hypoventilation and resultant hypercapnea often present with a global, dull headache with initial complaints of drowsiness that progresses to lethargy and mild confusion, followed by stupor and eventually coma [1]. This pattern is not influenced by the etiology of the respiratory failure [1]. Other characteristic features of pulmonary encephalopathy include prominent asterixis and myoclonus in the absence of other motor findings, rare seizures, often small and briskly reactive pupils with preserved ocular movements, and papilledema due to increased intracranial pressure in patients with chronic, severe hypercapnea and hypoxia [1]. Patients may acutely decompensate due to a superimposed systemic illness or to treatment with benzodiazepines or other sedatives. An abnormal arterial blood gas confirming the patient's hypercapnea, followed by prompt recovery with artificial ventilation, is usually diagnostic. Improvement is typically rapid and complete [1].

Fat embolism

Pulmonary damage is also presumed to result in an encephalopathic state in the fat embolism syndrome (FES). This syndrome is a potential complication of a variety of systemic illnesses, including diabetes mellitus, burn injuries, cardiopulmonary bypass, decompression sickness, acute pancreatitis, and joint reconstruction [67]. It may also occur as a complication of liposuction procedures and of parenteral infusion of lipids, although it is most commonly associated with long-

bone fracture secondary to traumatic injury [67]. The neurologic manifestations of FES are thought to be due to chemical damage to pulmonary tissue from free fatty acids with resultant severe hypoxia and subsequent encephalopathy, as well as to direct damage from fatty emboli to the brain [67,68].

The onset of symptoms usually occurs approximately 3 days following the inciting event, with pulmonary manifestations often preceding the neurologic ones, though this is certainly not an absolute [68,69]. Patients may present with only mild dyspnea or tachycardia or in acute respiratory failure [69,70]. The neurologic symptoms, likewise, may vary from only mild disorientation to coma, with agitation, confusion, headache, and lethargy being common [68,71]. Seizures and focal neurologic signs, including hemiplegia, unilateral cranial nerve palsies, and aphasia may occur [68,72]. Other systemic manifestations include a petechial rash, fever, hematologic abnormalities, and retinal involvement [71]. High-resolution CT of the lungs and transesophageal echocardiography may be useful to detect the pulmonary abnormalities [71]. MRI of the brain may show multifocal punctate areas of hyperintensity on the T2-weighted and FLAIR images in the deep gray and subcortical white matter, and corresponding areas of restricted diffusion may be seen on the diffusion weighted images [69,72]. Neuroimaging also serves to rule out other potential differential diagnoses, especially in patients with traumatic injuries [72].

Although multiple agents, including steroids, low molecular weight dextran, nitric oxide, prostacyclins, and human albumin (although it may worsen respiratory symptoms) have been used in the treatment of FES, treatment consists mainly of supportive measures, such as respiratory support. Patients often have a rapid and full recovery, though poor outcomes may occur [68].

Encephalopathy due to systemic cancer

Cancer patients represent a particularly high-risk population for the development of encephalopathy. Encephalopathy may occur as a direct effect of the cancer, by metastatic spread to the brain or meninges, or indirectly subsequent to organ failure due to metastasis or as an adverse effect of treatment (such as in L-asparaginase-induced hepatic failure) [73]. Cancer patients are at an elevated risk for infection due to treatment-induced immunosuppression, surgical complications, and the need for often long-term vascular access. They are additionally at elevated risk for nutritional and vitamin deficiencies due to their often poor nutritional states and to chemotherapy-induced hyperemesis and appetite suppression. Electrolyte disorders may also occur in these patients due to direct effects of the cancer, treatment, or indirectly due to poor oral intake of food and hydration.

In addition to the potential adverse effects of their chemotherapeutic agents, these patients often require extensive symptomatic management with narcotics, sedatives, and anticonvulsants, all high-risk drug classes for the development of encephalopathy. Finally, this patient population is also at risk for the development of PRES (a condition discussed in detail in the section on autoimmune disorders) from a number of chemotherapeutic and antiangiogenic agents such as methotrexate, cisplatin, 5-fluorouracil, cyclosporine, and bevacizumab [74,75].

Encephalopathy due to systemic infectious diseases

Despite patients' often multiple reasons to be encephalopathic, the most frequently encountered etiology for encephalopathy in the intensive care unit setting is sepsis [76]. Septic encephalopathy may occur in up to 70% of patients with sepsis [76,77]. The timing of onset of the encephalopathic state may help distinguish between septic encephalopathy and that due to other causes. Septic encephalopathy is an early complication of sepsis, occurring within two weeks of admission and may even be the presenting sign [77,78]. The exact pathophysiology of septic encephalopathy remains unclear, with likely multiple processes contributing. Aberrant neurotransmitter function may occur secondary to alterations in amino acid production and toxic amino acid release [79]. Blood–brain barrier function may be impaired in septic patients [78]. Even if it is not, inflammatory mediators may be able to cross the BBB with resultant neurotoxic effects and additive damage from free radicals and from the brain's cytotoxic response to this inflammation [78]. Finally, direct infection of the brain may go undetected, yet may still play a role in the clinical picture [79].

While negative blood cultures are not inconsistent with this diagnosis, there should be some support by history or examination for an extracranial infection (although in some cases it is difficult to identify the septic source) [78]. In patients with evidence for severe systemic infection, an intracranial infectious process should be strongly considered as part of the differential diagnosis [77,78]. Given the broad potential differential possibilities in a critically ill encephalopathic patient, septic encephalopathy may be considered a diagnosis of exclusion [79].

Clinical features are not as helpful in distinguishing between the various possible encephalopathies in septic patients, as there are no clinical signs or symptoms distinct to or characteristic of septic encephalopathy. Patients will develop an acute impairment in their level of consciousness and confusion, with examination possibly revealing gegenhalten, tremor, myoclonus, and asterixis [79]. Focal or generalized seizures may occur; however, focal neurologic signs such as hemiparesis are rare [79]. Neuroimaging and lumbar puncture are helpful mainly in evaluating for the presence of other diagnostic considerations other than septic encephalopathy. EEG may serve as measure of the severity of the patient's encephalopathy, especially in a critically ill, ventilated patient in whom the clinical exam may be greatly limited [77,79].

Treatment of septic encephalopathy involves supportive measures, such as ventilator support when indicated, aggressive prevention and management of electrolyte derangements and organ dysfunction, and treatment of the underlying infection [77]. Mortality is higher in septic patients with encephalopathy than in those without, and higher in those with more severe encephalopathy, and typically is due to concomitant multiorgan failure [77–79].

While the specific underlying infectious organism does not seem to be a factor in the development or severity of septic encephalopathy, some infectious processes are associated with distinct encephalopathic syndromes. The recently described fulminant encephalopathy in HIV-infected drug users is a good example of this [80]. This syndrome was reported in poorly controlled HIV patients who abused cocaine (and heroin in half the cases) [80]. Patients presented with a severe encephalopathy of acute onset, with the majority also having seizures. In all patients, MRI revealed diffuse nonenhancing hyperintense lesions in the basal ganglia on the T2-weighted or FLAIR sequences and CSF studies revealed albuminocytologic dissociation (elevated protein without significant leukocytosis). Patients did not have clinical findings

41

localizable to the basal ganglia. Prognosis was very poor with high rates of mortality, though early treatment with combined antiretroviral therapy may be beneficial [80].

Encephalopathy due to transplantation

As has been true for most of the patient populations discussed in this chapter, transplant patients often have multiple possible reasons to be encephalopathic. Prior to transplantation, they are often at great risk simply due to their underlying organ failure. Posttransplantation, in addition to common surgical complications such as infections and electrolyte disturbances, the use of many of the immunosuppressant and antirejection medications (such as cyclosporine and tacrolimus) is strongly associated with the development of an encephalopathy, specifically PRES.

As described above, PRES has been particularly well described with the use of cyclosporine. Although seizures and cortical blindness may occur, patients may not have any focal neurologic findings [74,81]. Their presentation may consist only of headache followed by a severe encephalopathic state, characterized by disorientation, confusion, irritability, paranoid ideations, and abulia [81]. Fever may occur in the absence of infection. Cyclosporine levels are elevated in only approximately half of cases, and a complete cessation of the drug, rather than just a lowering of the dose, may sometimes be required before significant improvement is seen [81]. With decrease or discontinuation of the drug, prognosis is usually good. Hypocholesterolemia (in liver transplant patients), hypomagnesemia, and hypertension are risk factors for the development of cyclosporine-associated neurotoxicity [81].

While all transplant patients, despite the specific organ being transplanted, share some of the same potential causes for encephalopathy, there are a few specific clinical issues related to the organ being transplanted. Hyperammonemic encephalopathy is a more unusual, though well-described complication of both bone marrow and lung transplantation [13]. Heart transplant recipients, in addition to developing the more standard metabolic encephalopathies, are also at risk for anoxic encephalopathy, especially if more urgent transplantation, ventricular assist devices, or intraaortic balloon pumps are required [82].

Encephalopathy due to critical medical illness

This section is somewhat of an artificial distinction as all of the other potential causes of encephalopathy discussed in this chapter may be found in critically ill patients. As discussed previously, septic encephalopathy is the most commonly encountered reason for encephalopathy in critically ill patients; however, electrolyte and glucose derangements, organ failure, hypoxia, and medications are frequent etiologies as well.

The diagnosis of encephalopathy in critically ill patients has significant implications, as delirium in medical intensive care unit (ICU) patients is associated with longer hospital admissions and lower 6-month survival rates, and has been recently found to be an independent predictor of long-term cognitive impairment [83,84]. Early recognition of this complication is critical. Therefore, it is now recommended that all ICU patients be routinely monitored for the development of encephalopathy (delirium) and a number of assessment instruments now exist to aid in this task [84]. Prevention strategies including sedation protocols, daily breaks from sedation and analgesics, early mobilization, aggressive management of dehydration, removal of lines and catheters whenever possible, and frequent reorientation, are likely helpful, but this has not been proven in an ICU setting [84]. The antipsychotic agent haloperidol is frequently utilized by critical care physicians and by psychiatrists in the management of delirium in the ICU setting and may be beneficial; however, the efficacy of this treatment has not yet been proven by an adequately sized, placebo controlled, randomized study [85].

One aspect of the neurologist's role in the management of these patients is to ensure that all critically ill patients who become encephalopathic receive the appropriate evaluation. This should include laboratory studies such as complete blood count and complete metabolic screen with magnesium levels, toxin/drug screen, blood gas, and cultures of blood and urine, with consideration of CSF analysis if lumbar puncture is not contraindicated for any reason [79]. Neuroimaging with either CT or MRI should be strongly considered, particularly if there are any focal neurologic symptoms or findings on neurologic examination. EEG may be useful, especially to evaluate for the presence of subclinical status epilepticus, a differential diagnosis in critically ill patients. Regardless of the specific cause, supportive measures such as hydration, nutrition, and ventilatory support when indicated should be initiated and the underlying etiology identified as promptly as possible so that appropriate corrective actions may be taken.

Encephalopathy due to drugs, nutritional deficiencies, and vitamin deficiencies

Wernicke's encephalopathy

Although still strongly associated with chronic alcoholism, Wernicke's encephalopathy may result from any systemic condition that results in a thiamine-deficient state. Conditions manifested by protracted vomiting or prolonged diarrhea, such as hyperemesis gravidarum, inflammatory bowel disease, pyloric stenosis, and acute pancreatitis, put patients at risk for this complication if replacement therapy is not initiated [53,86,87]. Wernicke's encephalopathy may result from psychiatric illnesses that result in malnutrition, including anorexia nervosa and bulimia, and from bariatric surgeries, which have a potential risk both for protracted vomiting and for malnutrition [86–88].

Less obvious systemic illnesses that may predispose patients to the development of Wernicke's encephalopathy include end-stage renal disease (with patients on hemodialysis being most at risk), thyrotoxicosis, AIDS, chronic congestive heart failure treated with furosemide, and prolonged febrile illnesses [87–91]. In addition to furosemide, Wernicke's encephalopathy has also been attributed to the use of high-dose IV nitroglycerin and oral hypoglycemic agents, especially in susceptible patient populations [87,92]. Cancer patients, especially those with hematologic and gastric malignancies, are an exceedingly high-risk patient population. Thiamine deficiency may occur due to increased consumption of thiamine by rapidly progressive cancers, malnutrition due to inadequate intake and poor absorption, insufficient replacement in parenteral nutrition, and possibly as an adverse effect of some chemotherapies [87].

Even when Wernicke's encephalopathy is considered, the diagnosis may still be missed if physicians rely on the presence of the classic triad of ophthalmoplegia, ataxia, and mental status changes to confirm it. Only approximately 20% of patients will present with the full triad, with mental status changes the most common presenting sign [93–95]. The clinical picture may be very subtle with the mental status changes manifesting as only mild

memory impairment or emotional changes, and nystagmus being the only ocular sign [93]. Rarely, patients may present at the other extreme: in coma with absent oculocephalic and vestibular ocular reflexes [96]. Autonomic dysfunction in the form of hypotension, hypothermia, and tachycardia is a commonly associated presenting feature [87,94].

The diagnosis of Wernicke's encephalopathy is a clinical one and once made, it constitutes a neurological emergency. Treatment with thiamine replacement should not be held for any laboratory or neuroimaging ancillary studies. Direct serum thiamine levels and indirect assays of thiamine status may be measured by varying laboratory techniques; however, these tests are often not available emergently and may not be diagnostic [86,90]. Magnetic resonance imaging may show high signal intensities in the medial thalami, mammillary bodies, periaqueductal regions, and the tectum of the midbrain, seen more clearly on the FLAIR sequences than on the T2-weighted sequences [97]. Early in the course, enhancement may also be seen in the mammillary bodies along with corresponding changes on diffusion-weighted imaging [86]. Recommendations for the optimal regimen of thiamine replacement are based on anecdotal evidence and not on randomized controlled trials. As many of the patients with Wernicke's encephalopathy have diminished GI absorption of thiamine, oral replacement is not considered adequate [92]. Intravenous doses of at least 500 mg of thiamine administered up to twice daily for 3–5 days may be required for adequate treatment [90]. Patients with Wernicke's encephalopathy are often at risk for magnesium deficiency, and as magnesium is a necessary cofactor for thiamine utilization, magnesium replacement may be indicated [90]. Though adverse reactions to thiamine, including anaphylaxis, are exceedingly rare, they have been reported and therefore parenteral thiamine should be administered only in settings where intravenous or intramuscular epinephrine and cardiopulmonary resuscitation is readily available [91].

Without sufficient thiamine replacement, the mortality of this disease is approximately 20%, with approximately 80% of patients going on to develop Korsakoff syndrome, a chronic amnestic state refractory to treatment and manifested by severe anterograde amnesia, some retrograde amnesia, and confabulation [86,93]. Therefore, this diagnosis must be considered and treatment started without delay in all high-risk encephalopathic patients.

Pellagra encephalopathy

Pellagra encephalopathy shares many similarities with Wernicke's encephalopathy: it is also caused by a vitamin deficiency, in this case niacin (vitamin B3), has its own "classic" triad (dementia, diarrhea, and dermatitis), and is also strongly associated with alcoholism, with a number of other potential predisposing systemic diseases. Although there are many overlaps among the systemic illnesses that put patients at risk for Wernicke's disease and for pellagra, including psychiatric eating disorders, chronic GI illnesses, and bariatric surgery, pellagra uniquely may result from illnesses in which tryptophan is not converted to nicotinamide [98,99]. These include the genetic disorder Hartnup disease and carcinoid tumors [99]. Several drugs and supplements may interfere with the metabolism of tryptophan or niacin and cause pellagra, such as leucine, isoniazid, azathioprine, and some anticonvulsant drugs (phenytoin, carbamazepine, and phenobarbital) [100]. All at-risk patients must be deficient in protein or in a second essential vitamin for the disease to occur [100].

Patients with pellagra encephalopathy present uncommonly with the full triad [101]. In the absence of the classic dermatitis and gastrointestinal symptoms, pellagra encephalopathy may be difficult to distinguish from any other more common encephalopathy. Patients may initially have very vague and subtle neurologic and psychiatric symptoms, including headache, mild memory loss, vertigo, fatigue, insomnia, anorexia, anxiety, depression, apathy, and mood lability [102–104]. The psychiatric symptoms may become quite severe, mimicking schizophrenia, and eventually patients will develop marked confusion and fluctuations in their level of consciousness [102,104]. Other neurologic signs may develop, including spastic paraparesis and paraplegia, extrapyramidal signs, hyperreflexia, myoclonus, incontinence, gait abnormalities, and seizures [99,102,103]. When the rash does occur, it is classically a symmetrical, sharply demarcated, photosensitive, erythematous rash accompanied by desquamation, scaling, and hyperpigmentation [100,105]. Stomatitis and glossitis often accompany the other GI manifestations including diarrhea, abdominal pain, and nausea [102].

As with Wernicke's encephalopathy, pellagra is considered a clinical diagnosis with confirmatory laboratory tests considered not necessary, and possibly even harmful if they delay treatment [98,105].

Replacement therapy is therefore both diagnostic and therapeutic. Niacinamide is preferred over niacin due to its improved tolerance by patients (less GI and vasoactive adverse effects and less potential for liver toxicity) [101]. Patients should be on a diet that is high in protein, but relatively low in calories and low in dairy products, and replacement therapy of other B vitamins and magnesium should be strongly considered [101]. With prompt recognition and initiation of treatment, patients generally have an excellent prognosis [101,102].

Medication-induced encephalopathy

One of the critical first steps in the evaluation of any systemically ill encephalopathic patient is a careful review of their medication list. Medications are a major potential etiology of encephalopathy in hospitalized and systemically ill patients, both due to the detrimental effect that these patient's illnesses often have on drug metabolism and clearance and due to the sheer number of drugs that have the potential for adverse CNS effects [106]. Benzodiazepines, narcotics, and anticholinergic drugs are frequently, but certainly not always, the culpable agents [107–109]. Certain patient populations, such as patients in intensive care units, patients with malignancies, and postoperative patients are at even higher risk as they more frequently require sedation and analgesia [107]. The aforementioned categories of drugs are so pervasive and so strongly associated with mental status changes that other potential causative agents may be missed. All of a patient's medications, including those recently discontinued, should be carefully assessed for their possible contribution to the patient's encephalopathic state.

Even when recognized as the offending agent, drug classes such as antibiotics and chemotherapeutic agents are considerably more difficult to discontinue, and the risks of continued therapy need to be closely weighed against the potential benefits. When possible, substitutions should be made for alternative therapies with improved CNS adverse effect profiles. Although many of the antibiotic classes, including aminoglycosides, cephalosporins, quinolones, and penicillins, have been causally associated with the development of an encephalopathy [106], two antibiotics in particular are associated with well-described and distinct clinical presentations.

Cefepime encephalopathy

Cefepime, a fourth-generation cephalosporin with broad-spectrum efficacy, is associated with the development of an acute and rapidly progressive encephalopathic state that is frequently accompanied by myoclonus and tremors [110–112]. This neurotoxicity was initially thought to develop only in patients with renal dysfunction, but may occur even in patients with normal renal function [113,114]. Symptoms usually arise between 24 h and 7 days after administration of the drug [111]. EEG in cefepime encephalopathy may reveal findings consistent with a severe encephalopathy, such as diffuse, symmetric slowing and triphasic waves, or may reveal regular spike (or sharp) and slow wave patterns more consistent with a diagnosis of nonconvulsive status epilepticus [111,112,114]. There is often no significant difference in the clinical picture that corresponds to these respective EEG findings, and it has been hypothesized that these different manifestations simply represent varying degrees of neurotoxicity from a common pathophysiological mechanism [113]. Neuroimaging should be normal and is helpful only in evaluating for other possible diagnoses. Recognition of this syndrome is crucial as treatment first and foremost consists of discontinuing the drug. Hemodialysis may be utilized in patients with underlying renal failure [110]. The role, if any, of anticonvulsant drugs, even in patients with evidence for nonconvulsive status epilepticus remains unclear. The prognosis is usually excellent with rapid recovery, though poor outcomes have been reported [111,112,115].

Metronidazole encephalopathy

It is worth also specifically discussing metronidazole-induced encephalopathy (MIE) here. Although rare, this syndrome is notable due to its distinct imaging characteristics. This is one of the very few metabolic encephalopathy syndromes in which the imaging findings are useful more than simply to rule out another cause of the patient's symptoms. As opposed to cefepime-induced encephalopathy, the onset of symptoms in MIE may take weeks to develop, and cerebellar symptoms, including dysarthria and ataxia, are prominent clinical features [116]. The characteristic findings on brain MRI are bilateral and symmetric areas of high signal on the T2- and FLAIR images in the cerebellar dentate nuclei and less frequently in the

brainstem, basal ganglia, and corpus callosum [116]. Signal abnormalities of the inferior olivary nuclei and subcortical white matter have also been reported [116,117]. Patients have both clinical and radiological improvement with discontinuation of metronidazole [116,117]. Recognition of this rare, yet well-described syndrome, is critical; however, it is equally important to keep in mind the other potential diagnostic possibilities in the patient population that is treated with metronidazole, especially if discontinuation of the drug does not result in rapid clinical improvement. Wernicke's encephalopathy, enteroviral encephalitis, methyl bromide intoxication, and osmotic demyelination syndrome may present as an acute encephalopathy with very similar imaging findings [116].

Chemotherapeutic agents

A number of chemotherapeutic agents, including high-dose methotrexate and cytarabine, are strongly associated with the development of a chemotherapy-related encephalopathy [75]. In the case of methotrexate, prior cranial radiation is thought to be a predisposing risk factor [73]. Ifosfamide, an alkylating chemotherapeutic agent used in the treatment of a variety of cancers, such as soft tissue sarcomas, germ-cell tumors, cervical carcinoma, and lymphoma, is associated with the development of a potentially severe encephalopathy [118–120]. Presentation may range from only mild lethargy or agitation to coma, with odd behaviors, hallucinations, and personality changes being common [119–121]. Focal neurologic signs such as ataxia, hemiparesis, aphasia, and cranial nerve palsies have been described, as has a catatonic state manifested by mutism and abulia [118,120,122]. Symptom onset is usually 24–48 h following drug infusion, but can be as long as 1 week [120,121]. A hypoalbuminemic state seems to put patients at risk for developing this complication [119]. Ironically, the established treatment for ifosfamide-induced encephalopathy is methylene blue, a drug discussed earlier in this chapter as a potential cause of encephalopathy when used in parathyroidectomies. Methylene blue has been reported in a number of small uncontrolled case series to shorten recovery time and may be helpful as a prophylactic agent against further episodes of ifosfamide encephalopathy [120,121]. As prognosis is usually good, with spontaneous recovery often occurring within 48 –72 h following drug cessation, and methylene blue is not without its potential adverse effects (headache, nausea, and vomiting), treatment is usually reserved for more severe cases [118,120]. However, recovery may be delayed and patients may be left with residual neurologic deficits [118]. Rarely, this is an irreversible and even fatal condition [118].

Conclusion

Encephalopathy (delirium) is a pervasive complication of systemic disease and is actually the most common complication of hospitalization of older patients [123]. Encephalopathic systemically ill patients will often have a multitude of potential etiologies of their encephalopathy and often the most obvious cause is not the sole answer (or even necessarily a key component of the answer). It is the role of the neurologist to ensure that a thorough evaluation of the patient is performed, with the goal, whenever possible, to make a more specific diagnosis than simply that of toxic-metabolic encephalopathy. Clinical improvement and ultimately a good prognosis are possible for many of the encephalopathies discussed in this chapter, but depend on prompt recognition and the prompt initiation of the appropriate interventions. With a high index of suspicion and meticulous neurologic assessment, devastating neurologic outcomes may be prevented.

 Five things to remember about encephalopathy due to systemic disease

1. Encephalopathic systemically ill patients will often have a multitude of potential etiologies of their encephalopathy.
2. Often the most obvious cause is not the sole etiology of the patient's encephalopathy, or even necessarily a key contributor to their encephalopathic state.
3. Clinical improvement and ultimately a good prognosis are possible for many of the encephalopathies discussed in this chapter.
4. However, a good outcome is frequently dependent on prompt recognition and the prompt initiation of the appropriate interventions. For example, thiamine should be started without delay in all high-risk encephalopathic patients as empiric treatment of Wernicke's encephalopathy.
5. The evaluation of an encephalopathic patient should include a careful review of their medication list, basic laboratory studies including blood and urine cultures, and consideration of neuroimaging and CSF analysis.

References

1 Plum F, Posner JB. *The Diagnosis of Stupor and Coma*, 3rd ed. New York: Oxford, 1982.
2 Kang EG, et al. Diffusion MR imaging of hypoglycemic encephalopathy. *Am. J. Neuroradiol.* 2010;31:559–564.
3 Spinazze S, Schrijvers D. Metabolic emergencies. *Crit. Rev. Oncol. Hematol.* 2006;58:76–89.
4 Auer RN. Hypoglycemic brain damage. *Metab. Brain. Dis.* 2004;19(3/4):169–175.
5 Lee SH, et al. Lateralization of hypoglycemia encephalopathy: evidence of a mechanism of selective vulnerability. *J. Clin. Neurol.* 2010;6:104–108.
6 Aoki T, et al. Reversible hyperintensity lesion on diffusion-weighted MRI in hypoglycemic coma. *Neurology* 2004;63:392–393.
7 Mori F, et al. Hypoglycemic encephalopathy with extensive lesions in the cerebral white matter. *Neuropathology* 2006;26:147–152.
8 Gallucci M, Limbucci N, Caranci F. Reversible focal splenial lesions. *Neuroradiology* 2007;49(7):541–544.
9 Kitabchi AE, Nyenwe EA. Hyperglycemic crises in diabetes mellitus: diabetic ketoacidosis and hyperglycemic hyperosmolar state. *Endocrinol. Metab. Clin. North Am.* 2006;35:725–751.
10 Yuceyar N, et al. Thyrotoxic autoimmune encephalopathy in a female patient: only partial response to typical immunosuppressant treatment and remission after thyroidectomy. *Clin. Neurol. Neurosurg.* 2007;109:458–462.
11 Frisbie JH. Thyrotoxic cardiomyopathy and encephalopathy in a paraplegic man. *Spinal Cord.* 2009;47: 262–263.

12 Park MH, Ryu JK and Seo JA. Reversible splenial abnormality in thyrotoxic encephalopathy. *Eur. J. Neurol.* 2007;14:e23–e24.

13 U-King-Im JM, et al. Acute hyperammonemic encephalopathy in adults: imaging findings. *Am. J. Neuroradiol.* 2011;32(2):413–418.

14 Mahoney CA, Arieff AI. Uremic encephalopathies: clinical, biochemical, and experimental features. *Am. J. Kidney Dis.* 1982;2(3):324–336.

15 Mathew S, Linhartova L, Raghuraman G. Hyperpyrexia and prolonged postoperative disorientation following methylene blue infusion during parathyroidectomy. *Anaesthesia* 2006;61:580–583.

16 Pollack G, et al. Parathyroid surgery and methylene blue: a review with guidelines for safe intraoperative use. *Laryngoscope* 2009;119:1941–1946.

17 Rowley M, et al. Methylene blue-associated serotonin syndrome: a 'green' encephalopathy after parathyroidectomy. *Neurocrit. Care* 2009;11:88–93.

18 Anglin RE, Rosebush PI, Mazurek MF. The neuropsychiatric profile of Addison's disease: revisiting a forgotten phenomenon. *J. Neuropsychiatry Clin. Neurosci.* 2006;18:450–459.

19 Myers KA, Kline GA. Addison disease presenting with acute neurologic deterioration: a rare presentation yields new lessons from old observations in primary adrenal failure. *Endocr. Pract.* 2010;16(3):433–436.

20 Lodish M, Patronas NJ, Stratakis C. Reversible posterior encephalopathy syndrome associated with micronodular adrenocortical disease and Cushing syndrome. *Eur. J. Pediatr.* 2010;169:125–126.

21 Riggs JE. Neurologic manifestations of electrolyte disturbances. *Neurol. Clin.* 2002;20(1):227–239.

22 Garcia-Monaco JC, Martinez A, Brochado AP, et al. Isolated and reversible lesions of the corpus callosum: a distinct entity. *J. Neuroimaging* 2010;20(1):1–2.

23 Tudela P, et al. Hypercalcemic encephalopathy in a patient with hepatocellular carcinoma. *Dig. Dis. Sci.* 2007;52:3296–3297.

24 van der Helm-van Mil AH, van Vugt JPP, Lammers GJ, Harinck HI. Hypernatremia from a hunger strike as a cause of osmotic myelinosis. *Neurology* 2005;64(1):574–575.

25 Kleinschmidt-DeMasters BK, Rojiani AM, Filley CM. Central and extrapontine myelinolysis: then . . . and now. *J. Neuropathol. Exp. Neurol.* 2006;65(1):1–11.

26 Kumar S, et al. Central pontine myelinolysis, an update. *Neurol. Res.* 2006;28:360–366.

27 Berlit P. Neurospychiatric disease in collagen vascular diseases and vasculitis. *J. Neurol.* 2007;254(2):87–89.

28 Cho BS, et al. Comparison of the clinical manifestations, brain MRI, and prognosis between neurobehcet's disease and neuropsychiatric lupus. *Korean J. Int. Med.* 2007;22:77–86.

29 Liang MH, Corzillius M, Bae SC, et al. The American College of Rheumatology nomenclature and case definitions for neuropsychiatric lupus syndromes. *Arthritis Rheum.* 1999;42(4):599–608.

30 Leroux G, et al. Posterior reversible encephalopathy syndrome during systemic lupus erythematosus: four new cases and review of the literature. *Lupus* 2008;17:139–147.

31 Baizabal-Carvallo JF, Barragan-Campos HM, Padilla-Aranda HJ, et al. Posterior reversible encephalopathy syndrome as a complication of acute lupus activity. *Clin. Neurol. Neurosurg.* 2009;111:359–363.

32 Bag AK, et al. Central variant of posterior reversible encephalopathy syndrome in systemic lupus erythematosus: new associations. *Lupus* 2010;19:225–226.

33 Lee VH, et al. Clinical spectrum of reversible posterior leukoencephalopathy syndrome. *Arch. Neurol.* 2008;65(2):205–210.

34 Poordad FF. The burden of hepatic encephalopathy. *Aliment. Pharmacol. Ther.* 2006;25(1):3–9.

35 Ferenci P, Lockwood A, Mullen K, et al. Hepatic encephalopathy: definition, nomenclature, diagnosis, and quantification: final report of the working party at the 11th World Congresses of Gastroenterology, Vienna, 1998. *Hepatology* 2002;35:716–721.

36 Munoz, Santiago J. Hepatic encephalopathy. *Med. Clin. N. Am.* 2008;92:795–812.

37 Lockwood AH. Hepatic encephalopathy. In MJ Aminoff, editor, *Neurology and General Medicine*, 4th ed. Philadelphia, PA: Churchill Livingston, 2008, pp. 265–279.

38 Seyan AS, Hughes RD, Shawcross DL. Changing face of hepatic encephalopathy: role of inflammation and oxidative stress. *World J. Gastroenterol.* 2010;16(27):3347–3357.

39 Shawcross DL. Olde Damink SWM, Butterworth RF, et al. Ammonia and hepatic encephalopathy: the more things change, the more they remain the same. *Metab. Brain Dis.* 2005;20(3):169–179.

40 Kowdley K, McCaughan G, Trautwein C. Gut instinct: rifaximin for the prevention of hepatic encephalopathy. *Hepatology* 2010;52(2):792–794.

41 Bass NM, et al. Rifaximin treatment in hepatic encephalopathy. *New Eng. J. Med.* 2010;362(12):1071–1081.

42 Jiang Q, Jiang G, Welty TE, Zheng M. Naloxone in the management of hepatic encephalopathy. *J. Clin. Pharm. Ther.* 2010;35:333–341.

43 Brouns R, De Deyn P.P. Neurological complications in renal failure: a review. *Clin. Neurol. Neurosurg.* 2004;107:1–16.

44 De Deyn PP, et al. Clinical and pathophysiological aspects of neurological complications in renal failure. *Acta Neurol. Belg.* 1992;92:191–206.

45 Burn DJ, Bates D. Neurology and the kidney. *J. Neurol. Neurosurg. Psychiatr.* 1998;65:810–821.

46 Lacerda G, Krummel T, Hirsch E. Neurologic presentations of renal disease. *Neurol. Clin.* 2010;28:45–59.

47 De Deyn PP, et al. Guanidino compounds as uremic (neuro)toxins. *Semin. Dial.* 2009;22(4):340–345.

48 Jurynczyk M, et al. Hypoglycemia as a trigger for the syndrome of acute bilateral basal ganglia lesions in uremia. *J. Neurol. Sci.* 2010;297:74–75.

49 Wang H-C, Cheng S-J. The syndrome of acute bilateral basal ganglia lesions in diabetic uremic patients. *J. Neurol.* 2003;250:948–955.

50 Sheu Y-L, et al. The syndrome of bilateral basal ganglia lesions in diabetic uremic patients presenting with a relapsing and remitting course: a case report. *Acta Neurol. Taiwan* 2007;16(4):226–230.

51 Rothermich,NO, von Haam,E. Pancreatic encephalopathy. *J. Clin. Endocrinol.* 1941;1:872–881.

52 Estrada RV, et al. Pancreatic encephalopathy. *Acta. Neurol. Scand.* 1979;59:135–139.

53 Sun GH, et al. Pancreatic encephalopathy and Wernicke encephalopathy in association with acute pancreatitis: a clinical study. *World J. Gastroenterol.* 2006;12 (26):4224–4227.

54 Ding X, et al. Pancreatic encephalopathy in 24 patients with severe acute pancreatitis. *Hepatobiliary Pancreat. Dis. Int.* 2004;3(4):608–611.

55 Johnson DA, Tong NT. Pancreatic encephalopathy. *South. Med. J.* 1977;70(2):165–167.

56 Ruggieri RM, Lupi I, Piccoli F. Pancreatic encephalopathy: a 7-year follow-up case report and review of the literature. *Neurol. Sci.* 2002;23:203–205.

57 Bourgeois JA, Fakhri D. Pancreatic encephalopathy with prolonged delirium. *Psychosomatics* 2007;48 (4):352–354.

58 Sharf B, Bental E. Pancreatic encephalopathy. *J. Neurol. Neurosurg. Psychiatr.* 1971;34:357–361.

59 Boon P, et al. Pancreatic encephalopathy: a case report and review of the literature. *Clin. Neurol. Neurosurg.* 1991;93(2):137–141.

60 Menza MA, Murray GB. Pancreatic encephalopathy. *Biol. Psychiatry* 1989;25:781–784.

61 Bartha P, Shifrin E, Levy Y. Pancreatic encephalopathy: a rare complication of a common disease. *Eur. J. Intern. Med.* 2006;17:382.

62 Ohkubo T, Shiojiri T, Matsunaga T. Severe diffuse white mattter lesions in a patient with pancreatic encephalopathy. *J. Neurol.* 2004;251:476–478.

63 Guardia SN, et al. Fat embolism in acute pancreatitis. *Arch. Pathol. Lab. Med.* 1989;113(5):503–506.

64 Madl C, Holzer M. Brain function after resuscitation from cardiac arrest. *Curr. Opin. Crit. Care* 2004;10: 213–217.

65 Puttgen HA, Geocadin R. Predicting neurological outcome following cardiac arrest. *J. Neurol. Sci.* 2007;261: 108–117.

66 Fugate JE, et al. Predictors of neurologic outcome in hypothermia after cardiac arrest. *Ann. Neurol.* 2010;68:907–914.

67 Fabian TC. Unraveling the fat embolism syndrome. *New Engl. J. Med.* 1993;329:961–963.

68 Jacobson DM, Terrence CF, Reinmuth OM. The neurologic manifestations of fat embolism. *Neurology* 1986;36(6):847–851.

69 Hufner K, et al. Fat embolism syndrome as a neurologic emergency. *Arch Neurol.* 2008;65(8):1124–1125.

70 Van Besouw JP, Hinds CJ. Fat embolism syndrome. *Br. J. Hosp. Med.* 1989;42(4):304–311.

71 Wang HD, et al. Fat embolism syndromes following liposuction. *Aesth. Plast. Surg.* 2008;32(5):731–736.

72 Parizel PM, et al. Early diagnosis of cerebral fat embolism syndrome by diffusion weighted MRI (starfield pattern). *Stroke* 2001;32:2942–2944.

73 Sul JK, DeAngelis LM. Neurologic complications of cancer chemotherapy. *Semin. Oncol.* 2006;33:324–332.

74 Erbetta A, et al. Clinical and radiological features of brain neurotoxicity caused by antitumor and immuno-supressant treatments. *Neurol. Sci.* 2008;29:131–137.

75 Chamberlain MC. Neurotoxicity of cancer treatment. *Curr. Oncol. Rep.* 2010;12:60–67.

76 Streck EL, et al. The septic brain. *Neurochem. Res.* 2008;33(11):2171–2177.

77 Bolton CF, Young GB, Zochodne DW. The neurological complications of sepsis. *Ann. Neurol.* 1993;33:94–100.

78 Papadopoulos MC, et al. Pathophysiology of septic encephalopathy: a review. *Crit. Care Med.* 2000;28 (8):3019–3024.

79 Young GB. Neurologic complications of systemic critical illness. *Neurol. Clin.* 1995;13(3):645–658.

80 Newsome SD, et al. Fulminant encephalopathy with basal ganglia hyperintensities in HIV-infected drug users. *Neurology* 2011;76:787–794.

81 Chang SH, et al. Cyclosporine-associated encephalopathy: a case report and literature review. *Transplant. Proc.* 2001;33:3700–3701.

82 Munoz P, et al. Infectious and non-infectious neurologic complications in heart transplant recipients. *Medicine* 2010;89(3):166–175.

83 Girard TD, et al. Delirium as a predictor of long-term cognitive impairment in survivors of critical illness. *Crit. Care Med.* 2010;38(7):1513–1520.

84 Girard TD, Pandharipande PP, Ely EW. Delirium in the intensive care unit. *Crit. Care* 2008;12(3):1–9.

85 Girard TD, et al. Feasibility, efficacy, and safety of antipsychotics for intensive care unit delirium: the MIND randomized, placebo-controlled trial. *Crit. Care Med.* 2010;38(2):428–437.

86 Pearce JMS. Wernicke–Korsakoff encephalopathy. *Eur Neurol.* 2008;59:101–104.

87 Sechi G, Serra A. Wernicke's encephalopathy: new clinical settings and recent advances in diagnosis and management. *Lancet Neurol.* 2007;6:442–455.

88 Juhasz-Pocsine K, et al. Neurological complications of gastric bypass surgery for morbid obesity. *Neurology* 2007;68:1843–1850.

89 Todd KG, Hazell AS, Buttterworth RF. Alcohol–thiamine interactions: an update on the pathogenesis of Wernicke encephalopathy. *Addict. Biol.* 1999;4:261–272.

90 Thomson AD, et al. The Royal College of Physicians report on alcohol: guidelines for managing Wernicke's encephalopathy in the accident and emergency department. *Alcohol Alcohol.* 2002;37(6):513–521.

91 Wrenn KD, Slovis CM. Is intravenous thiamine safe? *Am. J. Emerg. Med.* 1992;10(2):165.

92 Cook CC, Hallwood PM, Thomson AD. B vitamin deficiency and neuropyschiatric syndromes in alcohol misuse. *Alcohol Alcohol.* 1998;33(4):317–333.

93 Victor M, Adams RD, Collins GH. *The Wernicke–Korsakoff Syndrome and Related Neurologic Disorders due to Alcoholism and Malnutrition*, 2nd ed. Philadelphia, PA: FA Davis Company, 1989.

94 Cravioto H, Korein J, Silberman J. Wernicke's encephalopathy. A clinical and pathological study of 28 autopsied cases. *Arch. Neurol.* 1961;4:510–519.

95 Harper CG, Giles M, Finlay-Jones R. Clinical signs in the Wernicke–Korsakoff complex: a retrospective analysis of 131 cases diagnosed at necropsy. *J. Neurol. Neurosurg. Psychiatr.* 1986;49:341–345.

96 Wallis WE, Willoughby E, Baker P. Coma in the Wernicke–Korsakoff syndrome. *Lancet* 1978;2(8086):400–401.

97 Bae SJ, et al. Wernicke's encephalopathy: atypical manifestation at MR imaging. *Am. J. Neuroradiol.* 2001;22:1480–1482.

98 Jagielska G, Tomaszewicz-Libudzic CE, Brzozowska A. Pellgra: a rare complication of anorexia nervosa. *Eur. J. Adolesc. Psychiatry* 2007;16:417–420.

99 Delgado-Sanchez L, Godkar D, Niranjan S. Pellagra: rekindling of an old flame. *Am. J. Ther.* 2008;15:173–175.

100 Lyon VB, Fairley JA. Anticonvulsant-induced pellagra. *J. Am. Acad. Dermatol.* 2002;46:597–599.

101 Spivak JL, Jackson DL. Pellgra: an analysis of 18 patients and a review of the literature. *Johns Hopkins Med. J.* 1977;140:295–309.

102 Spies TD, et al. The mental symptoms of pellgra: their relief with nicotinic acid. *Am. J. Med. Sci.* 1938;196(4):461–475.

103 Serdaru M, Hausser-Hauw C, Laplane D, et al. The clinical spectrum of alcoholic pellgra encephalopathy: a retrospective analysis of 22 cases studied pathologically. *Brain* 1988;111:829–842.

104 Ishii N, Nishihara Y. Pellagra encephalopathy among tuberculous patients: its relation to isoniazid therapy. *J. Neurol. Neurosurg. Psychiatr.* 1985;48:628–634.

105 Isaac S. The "gauntlet" of pellagra. *Int. J. Dermatol.* 1998;37:599.

106 Brust JCM. *Neurotoxic Side Effects of Prescription Drugs.* Boston: Butterworth–Heinemann, 1996.

107 Pandharipande P, Shintani A, Peterson J, et al. Lorazepam is an independent risk factor for transitioning to delirium in intensive care unit patients. *Anesthesiology* 2006;104:21–26.

108 Alagiakrishnan K, Wiens CA. An approach to drug induced delirium in the elderly. *Postgrad. Med. J.* 2004;80:388–393.

109 Marcantonio ER, et al. The relationship of postoperative delirium with psychoactive medications. *J. Am. Med. Assoc.* 1994;272(19):1518–1522.

110 Lam S, Gomolin IH. Cefepime neurotoxicity: case report, pharmacokinetic considerations, and literature review. *Pharmacotherapy* 2006;26(8):1169–1174.

111 Dixit S, et al. Status epilepticus associated with cefepime. *Neurology* 2000;54:2153–2155.

112 Fishbain JT, Monahan TP, Canonico MM. Cerebral manifestations of cefepime toxicity in a dialysis patient. *Neurology* 2000;55(1):1756–1757.

113 Capparelli FJ, et al. Cefepime- and cefixime-induced encephalopathy in a patient with normal renal function. *Neurology* 2006;65(11):1840.

114 Magnati R, et al. Nonconvulsive status epilepticus due to cefepime in a patient with normal renal function. *Epilepsy Behav.* 2006;8:312–314.

115 Chatellier D, et al. Cefepime-induced neurotoxicity: an underestimated complication of antibiotherapy in patients with acute renal failure. *Intens. Care Med.* 2002;28:214–217.

116 Kim E, et al. MR imaging of metronidazole-induced encephalopathy: lesion distribution and diffusion-weighted imaging findings. *Am. J. Neuroradiol.* 2007;28:1652–1658.

117 Seok JI, et al. Metronidazole-induced encephalopathy and inferior olivary hypertrophy. *Arch. Neurol.* 2003;60:1796–1800.

118 Park IS, et al. Ifosfamide-induced encephalopathy with or without using methylene blue. *Int. J. Gynecol. Cancer* 2005;15:807–810.

119 David KA, Picus J. Evaluating risk factors for the development of ifosfamide encephalopathy. *Am. J. Clin. Oncol.* 2005;28(3):277–280.
120 Patel PN. Methylene blue for management of ifosfamide-induced encephalopathy. *Ann. Pharmacother.* 2006;40:299–303.
121 Pelgrims J, et al. Methylene blue in the treatment and prevention of ifosfamide-induced encephalopathy: a report of 12 cases and a review of the literature. *Br. J. Cancer* 2000;82(2):291–294.
122 Simonian NA, Gilliam FG, Chiappa KH. Ifosfamide casues a diazepam-sensitive encephalopathy. *Neurology* 1993;43:2700–2702.
123 Young J, Inouye SK. Delirium in older people. *Br. Med. J.* 2007;334:842–846.

4 Dementia and systemic disorders

Jennifer R. Molano & Brendan J. Kelley
University of Cincinnati, Cincinnati, OH, USA

Introduction

The cognitive continuum can be seen as a spectrum between normal cognition, mild cognitive impairment (MCI), and dementia. While patients typically present with memory difficulties, other cognitive domains may be affected, including attention/executive functioning, language, and visual spatial skills. Patients with dementia tend to have impairment in at least two cognitive domains severe enough to cause functional impairments in daily activities. Patients with MCI have cognitive impairment of one or more cognitive domains, but with preserved functional abilities [1]. There are a plethora of medical conditions that may contribute to cognitive impairment and dementia. Neurodegenerative processes such as Alzheimer's disease (AD), dementia with Lewy bodies, and frontotemporal dementia cause significant cognitive decline. Importantly, systemic disorders may also result in having a detrimental effect on cognitive function, both in patients having underlying neurologic conditions and in those who would otherwise be cognitively intact.

This chapter provides an overview of the relationship between systemic disorders and cognitive dysfunction. While systemic disorders can be associated with cognitive impairment and dementia, they can also lead to encephalopathy or delirium. In this chapter, "encephalopathy" is defined as cognitive impairment that is associated with potential reversibility and possible functional decline, "delirium" refers to cognitive dysfunction associated with significant alterations in level of awareness, and "dementia" is defined as irreversible cognitive impairment that results in

functional decline. Please note that metabolic encephalopathies are discussed in detail in Chapter 3. This chapter focuses primarily on systemic illnesses that can cause a dementia or a dementia-like illness, rather than delirium. This chapter also reviews the interaction of systemic diseases and degenerative dementias.

Approach for the patient with a cognitive complaint

An accurate clinical history is paramount. Characterization of the chief cognitive complaint should address all major domains, including memory, attention/concentration, executive functioning, visuospatial skills, and language. Common memory symptoms include frequent conversational repetitions or forgetfulness for recent events. Those with attention and/or executive impairment may report problems in making decisions, planning activities, and multitasking. Visuospatial difficulties may be elicited by inquiring about increased navigational difficulties while driving, or an inability to track the lines on a page while reading. Word-finding difficulty, paraphasias, and/or anomia may indicate language dysfunction.

History taking should also focus on functional status, including the ability to drive, manage finances, and maintain basic activities of daily life. Possible neuropsychiatric, motor, and sleep issues should be addressed, as the presence of these symptoms may suggest an etiology contributing to the cognitive symptoms. Associated systemic symptoms, such as rashes, joint pain, or weight loss may also provide clues for a medical diagnosis. A thorough past medical history may help to determine if cerebrovascular disease,

Neurological Disorders due to Systemic Disease, First Edition. Edited by Steven L. Lewis.
© 2013 Blackwell Publishing Ltd. Published 2013 by Blackwell Publishing Ltd.

seizures, head trauma, systemic cancer, or infections may contribute to the cognitive impairment.

The time course of symptoms is also important. A gradual, insidious progression of symptoms may suggest a degenerative cause, while subacute onset may indicate a vascular, inflammatory, or infectious etiology. Abrupt onset of neurologic symptoms should strongly suggest the possibility of infection, stroke, or seizure.

After a history has been obtained, a general physical examination may provide additional clues to a systemic etiology. A screening mental-status examination, such as the Montreal Cognitive Assessment, Folstein Mini-Mental State Examination, or Kokmen Short Test of Mental Status [2–4], should be administered. Formal neuropsychological assessment may be useful to better characterize the breadth and severity of cognitive impairment in patients with MCI or dementia, and should include tests that sufficiently challenge a patient in each cognitive domain.

Medical laboratory tests used in the evaluation of dementia may identify medical issues that could affect cognitive function [5]. Basic laboratory tests that look for reversible causes of cognitive impairment include a complete blood count, complete metabolic panel, thyroid function tests, and vitamin B12 levels. The American Academy of Neurology guidelines for the evaluation of cognitive complaints includes a recommendation for cerebral neuroimaging [5]. Magnetic resonance imaging or computerized tomography of the brain is recommended to investigate for structural abnormalities that may contribute to symptoms. Depending on the clinical history and examination, other ancillary tests may be performed if systemic disease is suspected, and these studies will be discussed in the subsequent sections.

Endocrine disorders

The brain has receptors to hormones such as glucocorticoids, thyroid hormone, and estrogen. Each has been linked to cognitive difficulties, though the association can be controversial.

Thyroid disease

Thyroid disease has been associated with both encephalopathy and dementia. While the pathophysiologic association between thyroid function and cognition is unclear, thyroid receptors are located in many structures of the brain, including the limbic system [6]. Both T4 and T3 are present in relatively equal proportions in the brain and may also interact with the monoaminergic neurotransmitter systems [6].

"Hashimotos's encephalopathy"
Encephalopathy associated with antithyroid antibodies has been referred by many names, including Hashimoto's encephalitis, steroid-responsive encephalopathy associated with autoimmune thyroiditis, and nonvasculitic autoimmune inflammatory meningoencephalitis. Interestingly, no direct mechanism linking these antithyroid antibodies to a direct effect in the central nervous system, or true correlation between serum or CSF antibody titers and severity of clinical symptomatology, has been established. Due to the heterogeneity of clinical presentations, diagnosing encephalopathy associated with antithyroid antibodies can be extremely challenging, and likely represents part of the larger construct of autoimmune encephalopathy.

Patients may have a personal history of autoimmune disease [7], with clinical manifestations varying from neuropsychiatric symptoms such as psychosis and depression, to cognitive decline or seizures [8–13]. The onset is typically acute to subacute [14], though a more slowly progressive course has also been reported [15]. Other clinical signs and symptoms can include tremor, transient aphasia, myoclonus, gait ataxia, and sleep disturbances [7].

Laboratory, imaging, and EEG findings can vary in these patients. Routine thyroid studies can demonstrate hyperthyroidism, hypothyroidism, or euthyroidism. CSF studies may be normal, may show evidence of an inflammatory process or increase in protein. Brain MRI findings can also vary from no abnormalities to abnormalities such as white matter hyperintensities or changes in diffusion-weighted imaging [7,16]. EEG can show slow wave and possible sharp wave activity [17,18]. Neuropsychological testing may show global cognitive impairment [19].

Antithyroid antibodies, such as antithyroglobulin and antithyroperoxidase, may be elevated. While elevated antithyroperoxidase antibody titers are typically seen in patients with Hashimoto's encephalitis, this finding can be nonspecific, and, for example, can also be seen in those with rheumatoid arthritis [20].

Initial treatment for these patients often involves intravenous steroids, intravenous immunoglobulin, or even plasmapheresis. Treatment regimens, including the consideration for longer term immune suppression, vary among clinical reports and no standard treatment has been established to date. Improvement in clinical symptoms is encouraging, but the relapse rate can vary substantially [21].

Thyroid dysfunction and dementia

While thyroid dysfunction has been associated with encephalopathy, its association with dementia is unclear. The most consistent studies have shown that hypothyroidism is associated with impairments in general intelligence, psychomotor speed, visuospatial skills, and memory [6]. Treatment may improve cognitive function, but results can be variable [22]. The effect of hyperthyroidism and subclinical hypothyroidism on cognition has shown less consistent results [6,23–24]. The association between thyroid function and incident dementia has also been debated [25,26].

Glucose regulation and diabetes mellitus

Glucose is an essential energy source for the brain, and dysregulation of its metabolism can result in a variety of neurological symptoms, including cognitive dysfunction. Acute hypoglycemia or hyperglycemia can cause encephalopathy that typically (but not always) resolves after normalization of glucose levels, and is discussed further in Chapter 3. More chronic cognitive impairment and dementia can occur in patients with diabetes mellitus due to the effects of persistent hyperglycemia [27–32].

Systemic symptoms suggesting a diagnosis of diabetes include polydipsia, polyphagia, and polyuria, with laboratory support, such as fasting glucose $\geq$ 126 mg/dl or a hemoglobin A1c $\geqq$ 6.0% [33]. The pathophysiologic link between diabetes mellitus and cognitive decline may involve both metabolic and vascular changes in the central nervous system [34], including insulin resistance, production of advanced glycation end products, and microangiopathy. Insulin resistance may lead to oxidative stress, neuroinflammation, and cell death in the brain due to permeability of toxic lipids through the blood–brain barrier [35]. Hyperglycemia may also hinder communication between astrocytes [36]. Interestingly, several of these

mechanisms have been implicated in the pathophysiology of AD, and experimental compounds targeting the receptor for advanced glycation end products, insulin resistance, and neuroinflammation have been studied in that disease to varying degrees.

In those with longer-standing diabetes, end-organ damage includes nephropathy, retinopathy, and peripheral neuropathy. Brain MRI frequently identifies white matter hyperintensities and/or cortical atrophy [34]. Neuropsychological testing can be normal, but may show impairments in memory, processing speed, and visuospatial skills, even in the absence of frank dementia [37–39].

Several longitudinal studies have shown that diabetes mellitus is associated with an increased risk for incident dementia [28,32], an accelerated progression from MCI to dementia [40], and increased rates of brain atrophy [41]. However, another study reported an association between diabetes and a *slower* rate of cognitive decline in people already diagnosed with AD [42], and diabetes may not increase the risk of dementia when other risk factors for AD are considered, such as hypertension, apolipoprotein E4, or elevated plasma homocysteine [43,44]. While diabetes mellitus may increase the risk for both AD and vascular dementia (VaD) [45], more research needs to be performed in order to clarify the magnitude of this risk, the duration and nature of exposure required to have an effect on risk, and to better characterize the complex relationship between diabetes and cognitive decline.

Treatment for diabetes mellitus includes oral medications and insulin injections. While a hemoglobin A1c greater than 7.0% has been associated with cognitive impairment, it is unclear whether maintaining a hemoglobin A1c level less than 7.0% ameliorates this risk. In addition, hypoglycemic episodes may also increase the risk for dementia in older diabetic patients [46]. As a result, normoglycemia remains the fundamental goal for patients with diabetes mellitus.

Estrogen

Menopause can result from natural aging or from oophorectomy. Decline of estrogen levels during menopause can lead to symptoms of hot flashes, fatigue, depression, and sleep disruptions.

The role estrogen plays in relation to cognition is complex and has been hypothesized to involve neurogenesis, synaptic plasticity, and long-term potentiation in the brain [35,47]. Decreased beta amyloid production, improved endothelial function, and increased cerebral blood flow have also shown associations with estrogen. The hormone also effects inflammatory, thrombotic, and coagulation processes, and estrogens appear to interact directly with several neurotransmitter systems.

While estrogen deficiency has not been associated with encephalopathy, menopause has been associated with increased report of subjective cognitive complaints. Although perimenopausal women with estrogen deficiency may have concerns about memory, natural menopause is not typically associated with cognitive difficulties. Many of the systemic symptoms listed above, and particularly disruption of the normal sleep cycle, may lead to cognitive inefficiency.

However, estrogen replacement has not been shown to improve cognition in women who experience natural menopause, and it is not considered to modulate cognition in those already diagnosed with AD. Beginning estrogen replacement after the age of 65 years appears to increase the risk for AD, though the mechanism for this association is unknown. Due to its prothrombotic properties and the associated increased stroke risk, estrogen replacement is not recommended for patients having vascular dementia [48,49]. Unopposed estrogen increases the risk for endometrial cancer, while adding progesterone to estrogen replacement therapy may worsen performance in cognitive tasks.

Clearly, the relationship of estrogen, and more specifically estrogen replacement, to cognition is complex and incompletely understood. The association between oophorectomy and cognition also needs to be more clearly defined [48,50,51]. Extensive epidemiologic data have been collected, sometimes producing conflicting results or unexpected associations. The summation of this data does not appear to show a clear benefit for cognitive performance, and clearly this will remain an active area of research.

Electrolyte and other metabolic disorders

Electrolyte disorders

The acute encephalopathy (delirium) that occurs from electrolyte and metabolic disorders is discussed in Chapter 3.

The metabolic syndrome

The metabolic syndrome is defined by the presence of three of the following: truncal obesity, hypertriglyceridemia, a low high-density lipoprotein cholesterol level, hypertension, and fasting hyperglycemia [45]. There is increasing evidence that the metabolic syndrome and its individual components are associated with increased rates of incident dementia, although the magnitude of effect has varied between studies [52–56]. The prevalence of AD is higher in patients with the metabolic syndrome [57].

Although the pathophysiologic relationship between the metabolic syndrome and dementia is complex, some have proposed insulin resistance as a putative mechanism [45]. Insulin is produced both in the brain and transported into the brain from the peripheral circulation. Among its many functions, it may be important in clearance and degradation of amyloid, a protein implicated in the pathogenesis of AD [58]. Those carrying the apolipoprotein E4 allele may be predisposed to accelerated neuritic plaque formation in states of hyperinsulinemia and hyperglycemia [59]. Vascular dysfunction associated with dyslipidemia and hypertension may be another contributing factor in cognitive decline [45].

It is less clear whether treatment of the metabolic syndrome prevents cognitive decline [60], and, if so, at what age treatment should be instituted to provide this desired effect. While insufficient evidence supports the use of statins to prevent cognitive decline (see "Atherosclerosis and coronary artery disease" section), several studies suggest that management of hypertension may provide a protective effect from cognitive decline [61].

Systemic autoimmune disorders

Systemic immune disorders are chronic multisystem conditions associated with autoimmunity and inflammation. In addition to general medical signs and symptoms, peripheral and central nervous manifestations can occur. Patients typically present with subacute progression of cognitive symptoms, and focal neurological signs may be seen, in addition to systemic signs of the specific disorders.

These disorders may be associated with identifiable antigens or antibodies, or they may be associated with cellular inflammation only. Conditions with identifiable antigenic or antibody associations include paraneoplastic syndromes, autoimmune-mediated channelopathies, Hashimoto's encephalopathy, gluten-sensitive dementia, systemic lupus erythematosis, and Sjögren's syndrome. Conditions associated with primarily cellular immune response include Behçet's disease, sarcoidosis, and primary angiitis of the central nervous system [62].

In the evaluation of patients with suspected immune-mediated cognitive decline, laboratory tests should include pathologic antibodies or other causes for inflammation. Markers of cellular inflammation include erythrocyte sedimentation rate (ESR) and C-reactive protein (CRP) in blood tests, and investigation for lymphocytic pleocytosis, increased protein, increased IgG index, and oligoclonal bands on cerebrospinal fluid analysis. Pathologic antibodies include anti-double stranded DNA, anti-Ro (SSA), anti-La (SSB) antibodies, and antineutrophil cytoplasmic antibodies such as p-ANCA and c-ANCA. Neuroimaging may show nonspecific T2 hyperintensities, and EEG findings vary from normal to diffuse slowing to focal epileptiform activity. Additional workup for specific disorders will be discussed below. Treatment typically involves immunomodulating agents, such as intravenous methylprednisolone, intravenous immunoglobulin, or plasmapheresis. While some studies suggest that treatment may improve cognitive outcomes [63, 63a], further studies need to be performed.

Systemic lupus erythematosis

Systemic lupus erythematosis (SLE) is a chronic, multi-systemic inflammatory disease. Systemic signs and symptoms include malar rash, joint pain, myalgias, photosensitivity, and fatigue. Cognitive impairment is a common neurological manifestation, affecting 12–87% of SLE patients [64–66]. Other neuropsychiatric manifestations include headache, mood disorder, and seizures [67]. These neuropsychiatric symptoms can occur at the time of disease onset or may develop in the years following the initial diagnosis. Risk factors for neuropsychiatric SLE include quantity of SLE activity, prior neuropsychiatric SLE events such as seizure or stroke, and positive antiphospholipid (aPL) antibodies. Age and hypertension are also associated with increased risk of neuropsychiatric lupus. Both inflammatory and thrombotic processes can contribute to the pathophysiology of the disease [68].

The diagnosis of cerebral involvement in SLE is challenging, in part because symptoms may be due to, or exacerbated by, concomitant systemic disease such as renal failure or infection. If cognitive symptoms related to SLE are present, formal neuropsychological testing most likely will reveal psychomotor slowing and executive dysfunction, though memory and word-finding difficulties may be seen [64]. MRI may show nonspecific abnormalities, such as cerebral atrophy [68] or T2-weighted hyperintensities [69]. Blood work may show positive antinuclear antibodies. Patients with thromboses and/or symptoms of cerebrovascular disease should be screened for aPL antibodies. It is important to exclude other diagnoses, including glycemic dysfunction, uremia, and hypo/hypernatremia [70].

Treatment of neuropsychiatric SLE includes high-dose steroids and immunosuppression. If antiphospholipid antibodies are present, then aspirin can be considered. Risk-factor modification, including control of cardiovascular risk factors, may also be beneficial. However, more research needs to be performed, given the dearth of randomized controlled trials in this area.

Rheumatoid arthritis

While rheumatoid arthritis is a common systemic immune disorder, its association with cognitive impairment has not been as robust. However, case studies have shown an association between rheumatoid arthritis and normal pressure hydrocephalus [71–73a]. Cases of cerebral vasculitis have also been reported [74,75]. More studies should be performed in order to determine if a more definitive link with cognitive decline exists.

Nonparaneoplastic autoimmune channelopathies

Although clinical presentations of nonparaneoplastic autoimmune channelopathies can vary substantially, a common presentation is limbic encephalitis. In addition to antiglutamic acid decarboxylase, previous studies have suggested that antibodies to voltage-gated potassium channels were associated with limbic encephalitis [76,77]. However, more recent studies have shown that the pathogenic antibodies are not directed towards the channel pores themselves, but rather antigens associated in complexes that include the voltage-gated potassium channels [78,79]. Leucine-rich glioma inactivated 1 (LGI-1) is the most common of these antigens to present with limbic encephalitis, though cases with antibodies to contactin associated protein-like 2 (CASPR2) have also been reported. In addition to limbic encephalitis, antibodies to LGI-1 and glutamic acid decarboxylase can also present with rapid progression of cognitive changes, neuropsychiatric symptoms, seizures, and myoclonus mimicking Creutzfeldt–Jakob disease [78,80]. Other clinical manifestations include stiff person syndrome and cerebellar ataxia, more commonly associated with the antiglutamic acid decarboxylase antibody (also called the GAD-65 antibody) [80]. The presence of these antibodies may suggest a potentially treatable autoimmune process, with treatment focusing on immunosuppression with steroids, IVIg, and/or plasmapheresis [78,81]. Although often not associated with underlying malignancy, age- and gender-appropriate cancer screening is important, as some patients harboring these autoantibodies may be found to have an underlying malignancy.

Sjögren's syndrome

Sjögren's syndrome is a chronic inflammatory autoimmune condition associated with exocrine gland dysfunction, usually presenting clinical complaints of dry eyes and dry mouth. Involvement of the airways and extraglandular viscera may occur. While sensory polyneuropathies are the most common neurological manifestation [82], autonomic neuropathy or cranial-nerve involvement are also well-known peripheral nervous system manifestations of this disorder [83]. If present, cognitive difficulties are typically subtle, with neuropsychological testing showing impairment in attention-executive function and visuospatial skills [84,85]. A lip biopsy as well as positive anti-SSA or anti-SSB antibodies may aid in confirming this diagnosis. Cerebral MRI may show nonspecific white-matter abnormalities in some patients.

Neurosarcoidosis

Sarcoidosis is a multisystem disorder that is associated with noncaseating granulomas. While patients may also have pulmonary, cardiac, cutaneous, gastrointestinal, and ocular involvement [86–91], neurosarcoidosis can occur in isolation [92–97]. When present, neurosarcoidosis typically has a preference for the base of the brain [98]. Reported neurological manifestations vary widely, including cranial neuropathies, aseptic meningitis, hydrocephalus, seizures, spinal cord lesions, peripheral neuropathy, cerebral lesions, and vasculitis [99]. Cognitive decline and dementia can also be seen [95,96,99–102]. Although the neuropsychological profile in these patients is not adequately described, the cognitive difficulties typically affect the attention-executive function domain, and other symptoms such as fatigue may contribute to the observed severity.

Diagnosis of sarcoidosis is clinically challenging, due in part to the ability of sarcoid to mimic other disease processes such as lymphoma, tuberculosis, and metastatic disease [87]. Serum ACE levels may be abnormal, but this finding tends to be nonspecific and nonsensitive [99]. Radiographic studies can be useful. In addition to T2 hyperintensities on brain MRI, leptomeningeal thickening, parenchymal, bone, and dural lesions may exhibit gadolinium enhancement [103–105]. Chest radiography can range from normal findings to bilateral hilar lymphadenopathy and pulmonary fibrosis [98]. Chest CT or PET imaging may reveal lymph node inflammation [87]. Routine CSF shows nonspecific inflammatory markers, including mild pleocytosis, increased protein, and mildly decreased glucose. Oligoclonal bands, ACE, and elevated IgG index may be seen. However, other inflammatory disorders affecting the central nervous system, such as SLE, MS, and Behçet's can have similar CSF profiles, and CSF analysis is normal in one-third of neurosarcoid patients. For the definite diagnosis of systemic sarcoidosis, there must be histopathological confirmation of a noncaseating granuloma in one or more organs, such as the conjunctiva, lung, skin, lip, or lymph nodes [98,99]. Even if not symptomatic, muscle biopsy may identify noncaseating granulomas in patients.

Treatment includes long-term immune suppression with corticosteroids and cytotoxic agents such as methotrexate, azathioprine, cyclosporine, and cyclophosphamide. Immunomodulators that suppress TNF-alpha, and radiation treatments, may also be tried on medically refractory patients [99]. The effects of these regimens on cognition are unclear.

Behçet's disease

Behçet's disease is a multiphasic inflammatory disorder that affects the eyes, skin, mucosa, vessels, joints, lungs, GI tract, and nervous system. Symptoms include oral ulcers, genital ulcers, uveitis, and erythema nodosum. Neurological involvement occurs in 5% of cases. If present, cognitive impairment primarily affects memory, although attention/executive function may also be impaired. MRI in acute neuro-Behçet's can show regions of T2-weighted signal abnormality in the basal ganglia or brainstem and diencephalon. Diagnosis requires recurrent oral aphthae plus any two of the following: genital ulcers, skin lesions, eye involvement, or skin hyperreactivity to pinprick. Treatment includes corticosteroids and immunosuppressants, though it is unclear whether treatment improves long-term cognitive outcomes [85,106].

Central nervous system vasculitis

Vasculitis is inflammation that results in narrowing or necrosis of the blood vessels. Systemic vasculitis can affect large-, medium-, or small-sized vessels. Small vessel vasculitides include antineutrophil cytoplasmic antibody (ANCA)-positive disorders, such as Churg–Strauss syndrome and Wegener's granulomatosis, which may also affect the CNS [107]. CNS vasculitis can be part of a more widespread systemic or infectious disease process, such as SLE, hepatitis C, or drug abuse [108]. When a vasculitis is isolated in the central nervous system, it is typically referred to as a primary angiitis of the central nervous system (PACNS). PACNS generally affects the medium- and small-vessels of the brain. Clinical manifestations vary and can be nonspecific, leading to difficulty in making the diagnosis. In addition to encephalopathy, patients may have headache, strokes, seizures, cranial nerve palsies, and peripheral neuropathies [106,109]. Patients with Churg–Strauss syndrome may have asthma and allergies with cANCA-positivity, while those with Wegener's granulomatosis may have renal involvement and pANCA positivity.

When there is systemic involvement, acute phase reactants such as erythrocyte sedimentation rate and C-reactive protein are more likely to be elevated. Patients may also have anemia, elevated liver enzymes, or low complement. In the absence of systemic involvement, serologic markers of inflammation may be normal. CSF analysis may show nonspecific lymphocytic pleocytosis and elevated protein. Neuroimaging may suggest the diagnosis when ischemic or hemorrhagic lesions are visualized. Cerebral angiogram may show focal or diffuse arterial stenoses. Definitive diagnosis for PACNS requires brain and leptomeningeal biopsy that demonstrates angiitis with granulomatous inflammation and fibrinoid necrosis of the vessels [106]. Treatment regimens include steroids, cyclophosphamide, and other immunosuppressants.

Organ dysfunction and failure

Chronic kidney disease, hepatic disease, gastrointestinal disease, and cardiac abnormalities have been associated with cognitive decline.

Chronic kidney disease

Cognitive impairment in chronic kidney disease (CKD) is common, affecting 16–38% of those with end-stage renal disease [110] and up to 70% of hemodialysis patients over the age of 55 years [111]. Cognitive impairment can occur acutely during hemodialysis, and this may be a risk factor for incident dementia. While the pathophysiology by which CKD affects cognition is unclear, both acute encephalopathy and dementia have been seen. Acute effects of hemodialysis on cognition are thought to be due to recurrent episodes of cerebral ischemia, with those who have underlying dementia at higher risk for developing encephalopathy.

In addition to the acute cognitive changes associated with hemodialysis, patients with CKD on hemodialysis are at higher risk of developing dementia, even in those not experiencing episodes of encephalopathy. These patients tend to have concomitant vascular risk factors often associated with cognitive impairment, such as hypertension, diabetes mellitus, stroke, and cardiovascular disease. The processes involved with CKD may also contribute. Again, the pathophysiology is unknown, but may involve disruption of neural transmission due to leakage of uremic products such as urea, creatinine, parathyroid hormone, myoinsoitol, and beta-2 microglobulin across the blood–brain barrier [111].

In the workup for these patients, it is important to evaluate for inadequate dialysis, severe anemia, and aluminum toxicity, which may contribute to the cognitive impairment [110]. Neuroimaging may show white matter hyperintensities, although these are non-specific in appearance. On neuropsychological testing, memory and executive dysfunction may be seen; impaired general intellectual functioning may also be present [24,112,113].

To date, no studies have investigated the use of cholinesterase inhibitors specifically in end-stage renal patients. However, patients with uremic encephalopathy may improve with hemodialysis, and erythropoietin may improve cognition in those with severe anemia [110]. It is unclear if changing the frequency of hemodialysis will improve cognition in these patients. Management must be individualized and should include modification of vascular risk factors, as well as physical and cognitive activity [113].

Cardiac disease

Atherosclerosis and coronary artery disease
The presence of atherosclerosis and coronary artery disease is associated with cognitive impairment and dementia [114]. Atherosclerosis and those with lower cardiac indices have been associated with lower volumes of total brain tissue [114,115], lower white and gray matter volumes, as well as cerebral infarcts and microbleeds [114]. Other surrogate markers for heart failure, such as elevated B natriuretic peptide, have also been associated with cognitive decline. When cognitive changes occur, dysfunction tends to be in the attention-executive function domain [114,115].

The pathophysiology of these cognitive changes may involve arterial calcium deposition, leading to small vessel disease, decreased cerebral blood flow, and white matter lesions [116]. Treatment with lipid-lowering agents theoretically decreases the lipid accumulation in atherosclerosis. However, one Cochrane review suggested that the use of statins in patients at risk for vascular disease did not prevent AD or dementia late in life [117]. There is insufficient evidence that statin use is a useful treatment for dementia once cognitive decline has already occurred [118].

Blood pressure dysregulation
Mid-life hypertension has been associated with dementia, primarily due to endothelial dysfunction and atherosclerosis [116]. If hypertension persists, regional cerebral hypoperfusion and hypoxemia can occur, which may explain the findings of some studies showing a decrease in blood pressure prior to the onset for AD [60]. In addition, those with untreated, chronic hypertension in mid-life tend to develop other health conditions that may cause hypotension in later life, including coronary artery disease, congestive heart failure, and atrial fibrillation [60]. When cognitive changes occur, dysfunction primarily is seen in the attention-executive function domains [60].

Early treatment of hypertension may reduce the risk for subsequent dementia, though further studies need to be performed [119]. A Cochrane Group analysis in 2006 found inconclusive evidence that decreasing blood pressure in late life prevents the development of cognitive impairment or dementia in hypertensive patients without overt cerebrovascular disease, but the analysis was limited by methodological issues with the individual studies reviewed [120].

Atrial fibrillation and other arrhythmias
Atrial fibrillation is a risk factor for embolic stroke, and several studies suggest that the arrhythmia may also be associated with an increased risk for dementia and cognitive dysfunction [121–126]. The pathophysiology responsible for this relationship is unclear, but most likely involves cerebrovascular injury. In addition, other studies have found that atrial fibrillation was not associated with cognitive decline in those over 80 years [127,128]. Suboptimal control of atrial fibrillation is associated with cognitive dysfunction; however, if a person has dementia, this association may be due more to one's inability to manage an anticoagulation regimen rather than the arrhythmia itself [126,129]. While a relationship between atrial fibrillation and cognitive dysfunction intuitively makes sense, more studies need to be performed in order to clarify this relationship.

Liver disease

Chronic liver disease
Encephalopathy associated with chronic liver disease is discussed in Chapter 3.

Wilson's disease
Wilson's disease is an autosomal recessive disorder of copper metabolism caused by mutation in the ATP7B gene. Copper accumulates in various organs, including the liver, eyes, and central nervous system. Cognitive

symptoms may manifest as a frontal-behavioral syndrome, with disinhibition, socially inappropriate behavior, impaired social judgment, as well as difficulties with attention and executive functioning. Patients may present with jaundice from hepatic failure, and slit-lamp examination may reveal sunflower cataracts and Kayser–Fleischer rings. Neurological examination may show dysarthria, dystonia, tremor, and choreoathetosis. Laboratory testing may reveal hypoalbuminemia, anemia, coagulopathy, elevated liver enzymes, and even renal failure. Low ceruloplasmin levels and elevated 24-h urinary copper excretion may be seen. Neuroimaging can show T2 hyperintensities in the lentiform and caudate nucleus, thalamus, brain stem, and white matter [130].

Treatment aims to reduce serum free copper, which is toxic to the organs. Chelation treatments initially utilized penicillamine, though there is concern that penicillamine may actually worsen neurological symptoms. Other chelation agents include tetrathiomolybdate and trientine. Once copper levels have normalized, zinc acetate may be used for maintenance therapy. However, the effects of these treatments on neurological symptoms—particularly in improving cognitive difficulties—are unclear.

Gastrointestinal disease

Among the gastrointestinal disorders, gluten sensitivity has been associated with cognitive changes. Gluten sensitivity is a systemic autoimmune disease [131] and is most commonly associated with celiac disease. Systemically, celiac disease is associated with nonspecific symptoms such as abdominal pain, diarrhea, and bloating. If cognitive dysfunction is present, a subacute course of memory impairment may be seen. Other neurological symptoms may include gait ataxia, peripheral neuropathy, myoclonus, seizures, and headache [132]. On laboratory workup, nutritional deficiencies in folate, vitamin B12, and vitamin E may be seen, and patients may have antigliadin, antitransglutaminase, or antiendomysial antibodies. If antibody screening is negative and the diagnosis is strongly suspected, endoscopic small-bowel biopsy may be necessary to confirm the diagnosis. The effect of celiac disease on cognition is thought to be immune-mediated, and patients may respond to a gluten-free diet. However, treatment effects on long-term cognition remain unclear.

Systemic cancer and paraneoplastic disorders

Paraneoplastic syndromes of the central nervous system

Paraneoplastic disorders are immunologically mediated syndromes associated with identifiable antigens and antibodies. While it is estimated that over 80% of patients with cancer experience one or more paraneoplastic disorders, the number suffering central nervous system effects is much smaller. Although malignancy is frequently associated with paraneoplastic syndromes, neurological symptoms can be the first manifestations of an occult cancer in some patients. Patients can have a plethora of neurological manifestations; if cognitive dysfunction is present, the best-described presentation is limbic encephalitis.

Clinically, limbic encephalitis is associated with altered mental status, mood changes, hallucinations, seizures, and memory difficulties that can be acute or subacute in duration. Due to involvement of the hypothalamus, hypersomnolence and endocrine abnormalities may be seen. Neurological examination reveals a variety of findings, including parkinsonism, myoclonus, cranial nerve abnormalities, and focal sensorimotor deficits. Neuroimaging may reveal T2 hyperintensities of the mesial temporal lobes. EEG may show epileptiform discharges in the temporal region in addition to generalized or focal slowing. CSF analysis is often normal, but may show pleocytosis, elevated protein, elevated IgG levels, and oligoclonal bands. The cancers most commonly associated with limbic encephalitis include small-cell lung cancer, testicular germ cell cancer, breast cancer, thymoma, teratoma, and Hodgkin lymphoma.

While limbic encephalitis may be due to nonparaneoplastic autoimmune causes such as voltage-gated potassium channel antibodies, paraneoplastic causes should also be strongly considered in the differential diagnosis. Other considerations in the differential diagnosis include viral encephalitis, temporal lobe tumor or stroke, brain metastasis, as well as herpesvirus-6 infection in patients who have had bone marrow transplantation [133]. Limbic encephalitis has also been described in the graft-versus-host disease among patients who underwent hematopoietic stem-cell transplantation [133]. If limbic encephalitis is due to a paraneoplastic disorder, those with anti-Hu, anti-AMPA receptor, and GABAb receptor antibodies should have further workup for small-cell lung cancer, and those with anti-Ma2 antibodies should be evaluated for an occult testicular cancer. Antibodies to the AMPA receptor have also been associated with breast cancer and thymoma. As discussed in a previous section, antibodies to the region of the voltage-gated potassium channel (including LGI1 antibodies) have been associated with nonparaneoplastic autoimmune encephalopathy, but they have also been associated with paraneoplastic limbic encephalitis, especially with small-cell lung cancer and thymomas. Anti-CRMP5 or anti-CV2 antibodies have also been associated with limbic encephalitis.

While limbic encephalitis is a common presentation associated with paraneoplastic encephalopathies, extra-limbic presentations have also been seen [134]. If extra-limbic paraneoplastic encephalopathy is suspected, antineuronal antibodies may suggest an underlying thymoma [135], antineuronal nuclear autoantibody type 1 (ANNA-1 or anti-Hu) again may indicate the presence of small-cell lung cancer [136,137], and ANNA-2 (or anti-Ri) has been associated with both small-cell and breast cancer [138].

N-methy-D-aspartate receptor (NMDAR) antibodies may be associated with an occult ovarian teratoma, but may also not be associated with cancer [139,140]. Patients with anti-NMDAR encephalitis initially present with a prodrome of nonspecific symptoms such as headache, fever, nausea, or upper respiratory tract symptoms, quickly followed by psychiatric disturbances and language deterioration. Memory may also be affected but may be challenging to assess due to language difficulties. Following this intial stage, patients may develop alterations in responsiveness associated with seizures, dysautonomia, abnormal movements, and catatonia. Neuroimaging findings can be unremarkable or show nonspecific T2 hyperintensities, and EEG may show generalized slowing. The CSF findings may also be nonspecific, with lymphocytic pleocytosis, mildly increased protein concentration, and occasionally oligoclonal bands; however, NMDAR antibodies can be seen in many patients. Serum NMDAR antibodies may be normal, and a brain biopsy typically will not yield a diagnosis. Treatment involves removal of a teratoma (if present) and immunotherapy. The majority of patients recover or will have mild residual deficits. Recovery from anti-NMDA encephalitis tends to occur in reverse order of the initial presentation [140].

Similar to anti-NMDAR encephalitis, treatment of paraneoplastic encephalopathy first focuses on identification and treatment of the cancer. A variety of treatments aimed to suppress the immune system have been employed, including intravenous immunoglobulin, oral or intravenous corticosteroids, plasma-exchange, cyclophosphamide, and rituximab. There are no head-to-head studies investigating the superiority of one regimen versus another. Some studies suggest that treatment may improve neuroimaging abnormalities in extralimbic paraneoplastic encephalopathies [134] as well as clinical outcomes in anti-NMDAR encephalitis; however, further studies need to be performed to determine if treatment improves cognitive function long-term in other paraneoplastic syndromes.

Systemic cancer and dementia

Systemic cancers can be associated with dementia, both with and without brain metastases [141]. Cancers associated with cognitive impairment include colorectal and prostate cancer, as well as lymphoma [142]; however, it is unclear whether the cognitive impairment is due to the effects of chemotherapy or the cancer itself.

At least one longitudinal study has shown the opposite effect, where a history of cancer was associated with a reduced risk for AD [143]. Researchers have speculated that both cancer and AD have different effects on cell-survival mechanisms [144,145]. AD, for example, may be associated with cell death, due to loss of the Wnt signaling pathway and increases in the tumor suppressor gene p53. On the other hand, upregulation of the Wnt signaling pathway may lead to abnormal cell growth and cancer in the skin, lung, colon, prostate, and breast. Clearly, more research needs to be performed in order to clarify this possible common biological mechanism.

There are no studies that indicate whether treatment of systemic cancer can improve cognition in the absence of a paraneoplastic disorder. However, both systemic chemotherapeutic treatments and irradiation have been associated with cognitive changes.

Lymphoma

Both primary CNS lymphoma (PCNSL), a form of non-Hodgkin's lymphoma, and intravascular lymphoma (IVL) can present as rapidly progressive dementia.

In PCNSL, symptoms such as seizures and headaches can predominate, with T2-weighted hyperintensities and/or ring-enhancing lesions on brain MRI. Typically, this is a B-cell lymphoma. Since both CSF and EEG studies may be nonspecific, a brain biopsy is important in order to make a definitive diagnosis. Prognosis is poor and treatment protocols typically include systemic chemotherapy with methotrexate with or without whole brain radiation treatment.

Patients who develop dementia due to IVL can have an acute to subacute course of cognitive decline. Patients tend to be middle aged, and may have cerebrovascular symptoms such as transient ischemic attacks and strokes, as well as nonspecific systemic symptoms. The diagnosis of IVL or PCNSL is challenging, especially since laboratory findings may be nonspecific, showing an elevated lactate dehydrogenase, CSF pleocytosis, an elevated ESR, or patchy white matter changes. Definitive diagnosis requires biopsy. Systemic chemotherapy and radiation are treatment options, though prognosis remains poor [146,147].

Lymphomatosis cerebri is a rare form of lymphoma that can present in a rapidly progressive fashion, associated with gait difficulties [146,148]. MRI can show patchy T2-weighted hyperintensities that usually are not contrast enhancing [146–149].

Effects of treatment for systemic cancer

Chemotherapy-induced central nervous system toxicity

Cognitive difficulties described as an encephalopathy or dementia have been associated with many systemic chemotherapeutic regimens. Although the pathophysiology of chemotherapy-induced cognitive impairment is unclear, contributing factors may include inflammatory mechanisms, alterations in the blood–brain barrier, and changes in the small cerebral vessels. The development of cognitive symptoms can occur days to weeks after chemotherapy and tends to be dose-dependent [150].

Specific chemotherapeutic agents associated with cognitive changes include interferons, methotrexate, vincristine, ifosfamide, cyclosporine/tacrolimus, fludarabine, cytarabine (Ara-C), 5-fluorouracil, and cisplatin. In addition to cognitive difficulties, other neurological symptoms such as ataxia, parkinsonism, and cranial neuropathies can be seen. For example, both ataxia and cranial neuropathies have been associated with cytarabine and cyclosporine/tacrolimus; patients with vincristine neurotoxicity may present with an abducens nerve palsy. In addition, the posterior reversible encephalopathy syndrome (PRES) has been associated with cytarabine, cisplatin, tacrolimus, and several other medications. Taxanes may be associated with encephalopathy after whole-brain radiation or neurosurgery. Seizures and visual changes may also occur with any of these agents [150].

Neuroimaging may reveal white-matter abnormalities, and neuropsychological testing may reveal impairments in memory and attention-executive function domains [150]. Since the effects of these chemotherapeutic agents on cognition tend to be dose-dependent, early recognition of neurotoxicity is critical. Termination of treatment may allow reversal of cognitive difficulties if performed early, with more severe damage occurring with continued use [151].

Radiation-induced leukoencephalopathy

Whole-brain irradiation may be used for prophylaxis or treatment of brain metastasis in those with systemic cancers such as small-cell and non-small-cell lung cancer [150]. Both acute and delayed changes in cognition can occur. During irradiation, acute effects include headache, somnolence, and fever that may not be as severe if steroids are given prior to treatment [152].

Delayed changes in cognition can occur at least 6 months after treatment and are thought to be due to radiation-induced leukoencephalopathy. The pathophysiology of radiation-induced leukoencephalopathy may be associated with small vessel damage, permeability of the blood–brain barrier, and direct damage to the cerebral parenchymal cells. Patients may present with memory and attention-executive dysfunction of variable severity, and neuroimaging may show white-matter hyperintensities. While there are no specific treatments for radiation-induced leukoencephalopathy, stimulants such as methylphenidate may improve attention. Acetylcholinesterase inhibitors can also be tried to see if they can improve memory dysfunction.

Systemic infectious diseases

Numerous infectious diseases can cause cognitive impairment. The association of cognitive dysfunction and viral, bacterial, fungal, and prion diseases will be discussed.

Viruses

Human immunodeficiency virus (HIV)

HIV affects multiple organ systems, including the nervous system. HIV-associated neurocognitive disorder (HAND) is a common cause of subacute and chronic progressive cognitive decline [153]. HAND tends to follow the cognitive spectrum, with asymptomatic cognitive impairment, minor neurocognitive disorder, and HIV-associated dementia (HAD) [154]. The success of highly active anti-retroviral therapy (HAART) at controlling HIV infection has increased the survival of HIV infection and as more people live longer with the disease, the effects of chronic infection are becoming increasingly evident. Current estimates suggest that minor neurocognitive disorder affects 20–30% and HAD affects 2–8% of HIV-positive patients.

The cognitive decline in those with HAD is usually slowly progressive, associated with short-term memory loss, psychomotor slowing, apathy, and comprehension difficulties. In addition, patients may have motor abnormalities. Risk factors for HAD include a high HIV viral load early in the course of HIV infection, age, low CD4 counts, anemia, low body mass index, systemic symptoms, intravenous drug use, and female sex.

Opportunistic infections such as cryptococcus, tuberculosis, PCNSL, and progressive multifocal leukoencephalopathy may mimic HAND, and neuroimaging is used to exclude these other possibilities. MRI findings such as cortical and subcortical atrophy or white-matter hyperintensities can be helpful in suggesting other etiologies for cognitive symptoms. Other entities contributing to cognitive decline in HIV-positive patients include cardiovascular risk factors such as coronary artery disease, stroke, congestive heart failure, or peripheral vascular disease. Concomitant substance abuse with drugs such as alcohol, cannabis, stimulants, nicotine, or a combination thereof, may also be considered [155]. Hepatitis C infection and neurosyphilis may also occur in these patients and may also contribute to cognitive difficulties in HIV-positive patients.

HAART, especially those regimens with good cerebral penetration effectiveness, may improve cognitive symptoms [154,156], though it should be noted that cognitive recovery could be incomplete.

Hepatitis C virus (HCV)

HCV coinfection with HIV may contribute to cognitive impairment, particularly in intravenous drug users [155]. However, HCV monoinfection has been associated with cognitive impairment, even among patients with only mild liver disease. The proposed implication is that this represents a direct effect of the virus which has crossed the blood–brain barrier [157]. While the specific target of HCV on the brain is unclear, chronic monoinfection has been associated with changes in the frontal white matter on magnetic resonance spectroscopy. Neuropsychological testing can show impairments with psychomotor speed, attention, as well as working and verbal memory [158,159]. Treatment effects on cognition have not been well established.

Herpes simplex virus type 1 (HSV-1)

HSV-1 is considered to be the most common cause of viral encephalitis, and is certainly the most commonly identified viral pathogen, accounting for 25–50% of cases. Clinically, patients present with fever, seizures, behavioral changes, focal neurological signs, and altered mental status. Cognitive deficits most prominently affect memory, language, and attention-executive function domains, though global cognitive decline may be present [160]. This reflects the predilection of HSV for the temporal and frontal lobes.

Polymerase chain reaction (PCR) analysis typically shows the HSV-1 virus in the cerebrospinal fluid. It should be noted that the specificity of PCR is decreased when red blood cells are present in the CSF sample, a circumstance not uncommon in herpes encephalitis. Neuroimaging may reveal hyperintensities in the mesial temporal structures (Figure 4.1), and EEG may show focal epileptogenicity in that area.

If herpes simplex virus encephalitis is suspected, immediate treatment with acyclovir is essential to prevent mortality and morbidity. Untreated, mortality exceeds 70%, and even with treatment mortality remains 20–30%. A study of outcomes of HSV encephalitis survivors found the two most important

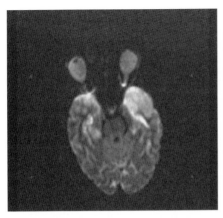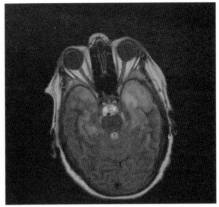

Fig 4.1 Diffusion-weighted image (DWI) and T2-weighted image in a 48-year-old man who presented with new onset of seizures, fever, headache, and behavioral disturbances. Cerebrospinal fluid analysis confirmed a diagnosis of herpes encephalitis.

predictors of poor outcome (death or institutionalization) were systemic disease severity at presentation and a delay of 2 days or more in starting antiviral therapy [161].

Even with appropriate treatment, cognitive sequelae are common [153]. These include aphasia, behavioral disinhibition, impaired learning and memory, and seizures.

Bacterial infections

Whipple's disease
Whipple's disease is an infection associated with *Tropheryma whippelii*. In addition to systemic manifestations such as arthropathy and gastrointestinal symptoms, patients can present with neurological symptoms, including oculomasticatory myorhythmias, focal neurological signs, epileptic seizures, and sleep disturbances [162]. Cognitive changes may occur, and patients may present with a frontotemporal-like dementia, with personality changes, disinhibition, and other behavioral changes [163]. Diagnosis of Whipple's disease can be confirmed with polymerase chain reaction in the serum and cerebrospinal fluid.

Treatment is sulfamethoxazole-trimethoprim. While one case report has suggested that treatment may reverse the cognitive difficulties in these patients [162], further studies need to be performed in order to determine long-term cognitive outcomes.

Neurosyphilis
Neurosyphilis, caused by *Treponema pallidum*, can occur early or late in the disease course. Early neurosyphilis is often associated with cranial neuropathies if there is meningeal involvement, or ischemic stroke if the vascular system is involved.

Late neurosyphilis can occur years after the initial infection. In addition to tabes dorsalis, patients with late neurosyphilis may have cerebral involvement, leading to syphilitic encephalitis or general paresis. Syphilitic encephalitis is characterized by a rapidly progressive dementia, often with concomitant tremor, hyperreflexia, and psychiatric symptoms. Laboratory tests such as the Venereal Disease Research Laboratory (VDRL) or rapid plasma antigen (RPR) can be used as screening measures, with confirmation on treponemal-specific tests. Rates of coinfection with HIV are high, and patients should be screened accordingly [164]. MRI may show contrast-enhancement in affected cranial nerves or associated with gummas in the brain [165].

Penicillin remains the primary treatment for neurosyphilis; however, its ability to aid recovery of long-term effects on cognition is unclear [166].

Lyme disease
Lyme disease, caused by the spirochete *Borrelia burgdorferi* is typically transmitted via the bite of the *Ixodes* family of ticks. Lyme disease can affect multiple systems, including the nervous system, skin, and

63

joints. Patients typically present with rash (characteristically erythema migrans), arthralgias, and fatigue. Neurological manifestations include cranial neuropathies, meningitis, or painful peripheral radiculopathies. An enzyme-linked immunosorbent assay test measures the concentrations of several antibodies to *B. burgdorferi*. Although useful as a screening test, interpretation of the various "bands" can be complicated.

Central nervous system involvement is rare in those with Lyme disease, but some deficits in concentration, processing speed, and memory have been reported [167–169], with case reports reporting dementia in some patients [170]. Treatment regimens have included ceftriaxone, penicillin, cefotaxime, and doxycycline, though studies have typically examined outcomes for meningitis, and cranial or peripheral neuropathies, rather than cognitive outcomes [171]. At least one study has suggested no difference between placebo and additional antibiotics on neuropsychological functioning after treating Lyme disease [172].

Fungi and parasites

Systemic fungal or parasitic infections are not typically associated with dementia or cognitive impairment. However, in opportunistic infections from toxoplasmosis, cryptococcus, or the JC virus (the cause of progressive multifocal leukoencephalopathy), cognitive decline can occur [173].

Cerebral malaria, caused by *Plasmodium falciparum*, can be associated with an encephalopathy that rapidly progresses to coma or death. Diagnosis typically requires a peripheral blood smear with Giemsa staining, and CSF studies can be unremarkable. Neuroimaging may show cerebral edema, herniation, or hemorrhages. While artesunate is the treatment of choice, its effectiveness in preventing long-term cognitive sequelae is uncertain [174].

Prion diseases

The infectious particles responsible for transmissible spongiform encephalitides (TSE) are referred to as prions. The prion protein is a normal constituent protein in the human body, although its function is uncertain. In the pathological state, the prion protein is misfolded, which induces normal copies of the prion protein to misfold, cascading and ultimately overwhelming the body's ability to clear the abnormal protein, with the clinical result of diseases such as Creutzfeldt–Jakob disease (CJD). These typically present as a rapidly progressing dementia, associated with stimulus myoclonus, behavioral changes, and parkinsonism. Cognitively, patients may present with bizarre visual complaints, including simultagnosia, hemianopia, diplopia, and hallucinations. Most CJD cases are sporadic, though hereditary and acquired forms exist. Hereditary forms may be due either to direct transmission or the result of a genetic mutation in the prion gene. The allelic makeup at codon 129 of the prion protein gene has a complex impact upon the clinical manifestations of infection, though detailed discussion is beyond the scope of this chapter [175]. TSE is felt to have a very long latent period of infection prior to emergence of clinical symptoms. However, once clinical symptoms emerge, deterioration is typically rapid.

EEG may show periodic sharp wave complexes, although these may not be present early in the clinical course and may not develop in all patients with prion disease. Cerebrospinal fluid studies can be positive for 14-3-3 or neuron specific enolase, though these results may be nonspecific and are not abnormal in all patients. False positive results can occur when the test is ordered in the incorrect clinical circumstance (e.g., viral encephalitis), as these are markers of neuronal injury, and not specifically markers of prion infection. In sporadic CJD, neuroimaging frequently reveals hyperintensities on diffusion-weighted imaging and FLAIR sequences in the basal ganglia, particularly the caudate nucleus and putamen, or so-called "cortical ribboning" in the temporal, parietal, and occipital regions [176] (Figure 4.2).

Treatment is typically symptomatic, and median survival ranges from 6 to 13 months after symptoms develop.

Complications due to transplantation

Iatrogenic complications

While rare, one iatrogenic complication associated with transplantation and dementia is CJD. Iatrogenic CJD has been associated with corneal and dura mater transplants, neurosurgical instruments, intracerebral

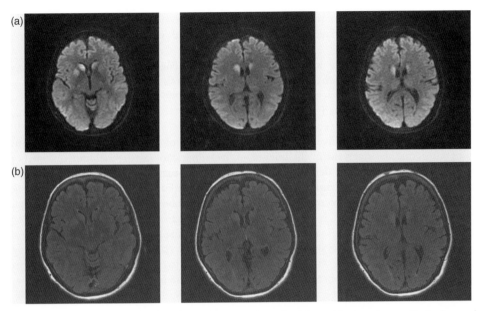

Fig 4.2 A 64-year-old woman presented with parkinsonism, apraxia, and mild cognitive impairment. She had several months of bizarre visual symptoms preceding her presentation in the hospital. Brain MRI identified symmetric thalamic hyperintensity on (a) diffusion-weighted imaging and (b) fluid-attenuated inversion recovery (FLAIR) images in a pattern consistent with Creutzfeldt–Jakob disease. The sensitivity of brain MRI depends upon the specific prion protein and the host's genetic polymorphism at codon 129 of the prion protein gene (*PRNP*).

EEG electrodes, human pituitary hormone treatment, and blood transfusion [177]. Proper sterilization and disposal of surgical tools is essential.

Complications of critical medical illness

The majority of intensive care unit admissions are adults over the age of 65 years, the same cohort that is at higher risk for developing dementia [178,179]. Common neurological manifestations associated with intensive care unit stays include polyneuropathy and encephalopathy [179]. The presence of pre-existing cognitive impairment in intensive care unit patients is under-recognized, with the best estimates around 31–37% [180]. These patients are more likely to be older, female, and residents of nursing homes.

Patients with cognitive dysfunction who have no change or improvement of their neurological status within 3 days of their ICU admission have a higher mortality rate at 30 days [179]. Having pre-existing cognitive impairment prior to an intensive care unit

admission increases the risk for developing delirium, and is associated with increased morbidity and prolonged length of hospitalization.

There is evidence of cognitive difficulties in patients who have survived critical illness [179]. In a review of patients with acute respiratory distress syndrome, acute lung injury, or respiratory failure, 25–78% of ICU survivors had neurocognitive impairments after 1 year of follow-up, with deficits in the memory and attention-executive function domains [181]. The duration of cognitive impairment after an ICU stay can be variable and can last for years [181]. There are no studies that indicate whether medical treatments such as acetylcholinesterase inhibitors are beneficial in these patients.

Drugs, toxins (including alcohol), and vitamin and mineral deficiencies

Heavy metals

Lead, mercury, and aluminum are the heavy metals that have been most clearly associated with cognitive difficulties [182]. Other heavy metals more variably associated with cognitive changes include manganese, tin, and arsenic.

Symptoms of lead encephalopathy include headaches, tremor, seizures, encephalopathy, and coma. Mercury has been associated with psychiatric/behavioral presentations, though there have been case studies that have reported subjective memory impairment and attention/executive dysfunction [183]. Key to suspecting the diagnosis is obtaining a history of (usually chronic) exposure.

Aluminum has been associated with "dialysis dementia"—the gradual development of personality changes, hallucinations, dysarthria, dysphasia, and dyspraxia associated with myoclonic jerks [184]. However, aluminum as a possible cause for "dialysis dementia" has decreased due to the elimination of aluminum from dialysate. An association between aluminum and risk for AD has been suggested, although this association is widely debated [185].

If there is concern that heavy metals may be responsible for cognitive changes, other signs on history and physical examination may provide a clue to the diagnosis. Miners and workers in manufacturing companies may be at higher risk for mercury toxicity. The presence of peripheral neuropathy may increase suspicion that lead, mercury, or arsenic toxicity is contributing to the cognitive symptoms. In evaluation of these patients, heavy-metal testing in the urine and blood may be useful. Neuropsychological testing may show impairments in the domains of memory and attention-executive function.

Treatment of heavy-metal toxicity includes chelation treatment with ethylenediaminetetraacetic acid or dimercaptosuccinic acid in lead poisoning, and dimercaprol and penicillamine with mercury poisoning. However, the efficacy of treatment for improving long-term cognitive outcomes has not been well established [186].

Solvents

A variety of solvents can lead to cognitive deficits including toluene, trichloroethylene, perchloroethylene, carbon disulfide, methyl alcohol, carbon tetrachloride, ethylene glycol, and acrylamide. Organic solvent or inhalant exposure may cause cognitive impairment due to their lipophilic properties and resulting damage to myelinated areas of the brain [182,187]. Acute effects can range from euphoria and confusion to coma and death. However, chronic use of solvents can lead to cognitive impairment and dementia, in addition to pyramidal, cerebellar, or brainstem abnormalities.

Toluene toxicity is one of the better-studied solvent exposures, and has served as the protypical pattern of "white matter dementia" [188]. Neuropsychological testing may reveal impairment in the attention-executive domain, with poor concentration and impaired insight and judgment. Fundamental language processes are typically spared. Neuroimaging in toluene toxicity shows varying degrees of leukoencephalopathy and diffuse brain atrophy, similar to the case in other solvent exposures (Figure 4.3). While treatment involves removal of the solvent exposure until symptoms resolve, cognitive effects may persist in the long-term.

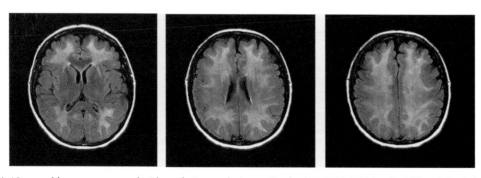

Fig 4.3 A 45-year-old woman presented with confusions and seizure. Cerebral FLAIR MRI identified T2-weighted changes consistent with a toxic leukoencephalopathy.

Carbon monoxide

Carbon monoxide poisoning is a common cause of morbidity and mortality [182] and can be due to exposure to motor exhaust fumes and faulty furnaces. It leads to cognitive changes caused by hypoxia to the brain. Carbon monoxide binds to hemoglobin with high affinity, leading to hypoxia, free radical formation, and mitochondrial damage [189]. Patients with acute or chronic carbon monoxide poisoning often present with nonspecific signs such as headache, nausea, and vomiting, as well as more severe signs such as cardiac abnormalities, altered mental status, seizures, coma, and death.

On neurological examination, parkinsonism and corticospinal tract signs may be seen. Neuropsychological testing may show dysfunction in the memory and attention-executive function domains [182]. Neuroimaging may show white-matter hyperintensities, as well as abnormalities in the basal ganglia, thalamus, and hippocampus. In addition to removing the source of the carbon monoxide poisoning, high-flow oxygen and possibly hyperbaric oxygen may be beneficial in decreasing mortality and morbidity [182,189].

However, those who survive the acute phase of carbon monoxide poisoning can have delayed sequelae, including cognitive abnormalities [182]. While gradual recovery can occur in 3–12 months, impaired attention/executive function, parkinsonism, or corticospinal tract signs may persist [190]. Patients with longer hospital admission, more sessions of hyperbaric therapy, and diffuse white-matter abnormalities on neuroimaging abnormalities are at increased risk of delayed cognitive deficits [190,191]. Hyperbaric oxygen may benefit cognition during the acute phase [189,190], though further studies need to be performed to determine if this treatment can be effective in long-term cognitive sequelae.

Vitamins

Deficiencies in B12, thiamine (B1), and niacin (B3) levels are the more common vitamin abnormalities associated with cognitive impairment [24,192].

Vitamin B12 deficiency
Vitamin B12 deficiency has been associated with cognitive impairment, as well as subacute combined degeneration, peripheral neuropathy, and other neurological manifestations. Neuropsychological testing may show abnormalities in memory, attention-executive function and visuospatial skills, with relatively preserved language [193]. Vitamin B12 levels may be decreased or in the low-normal range, and elevated methylmalonic acid levels may arguably be a better indicator of vitamin B12 insufficiency [194].

Causes of vitamin B12 deficiency include pernicious anemia, malnourishment, gastric bypass surgery, gastrinoma, or other gastrointestinal disorders [194]. Low dietary vitamin B12 intake is common among older individuals. In those with cognitive impairment due to vitamin B12 deficiency, neuroimaging may reveal nonspecific white-matter changes or cerebral atrophy [195,196]. Treatment involves replacement of vitamin B12 parenterally. However, while vitamin B12 deficiency has been associated with cognitive impairment, supplementation has not been shown to prevent the emergence or decrease progression of cognitive symptoms [24].

Thiamine (B1) and niacin (B3) deficiency

Wernicke's syndrome, due to thiamine deficiency, and pellagra, due to niacin deficiency, are discussed in Chapter 3 (Encephalopathy due to Systemic Disease).

Homocysteine

Hyperhomocysteinemia has also been associated with cognitive impairment, though the data is less robust. Those with folate abnormalities tend to present with fatigue, diarrhea, ulcers, and anemia. Levels of homocysteine are determined by dietary intake, and impaired kidney function increases the risk of having hyperhomocysteinemia [24]. However, while cross-sectional studies have indicated an association between hyperhomocysteinemia and dementia, longitudinal studies have shown variable results.

Vitamin D

Vitamin D deficiency has also emerged as a possible contributing factor to cognitive impairment [197,198], though more studies need to be performed in order to determine the exact mechanism of this possible association.

Alcohol

Alcohol consumption has been associated with cognitive impairments, possibly due to direct excitotoxic effects and indirect effects such as hypoglycemia, nutritional deficiencies (such as thiamine and niacin deficiency), and Marchiafava–Bignami syndrome [199].

Dementia due to alcohol use is gradually progressive and involves multiple domains [199]. Proposed criteria for these patients include dementia for at least 60 days after last exposure to ethanol, a minimum 35 standard drinks/week for males and 28 per week for females for more than 5 years, and significant ethanol use within 3 years of the onset of impaired cognition [199]. The glutamate excitotoxicity and oxidative stress caused by alcohol tend to primarily affect the prefrontal cortex, leading to disinhibition and attention-executive dysfunction. Other commonly affected regions are the cerebellum, hypothalamus, and superior frontal cortex. Neuroimaging may demonstrate atrophy in those areas. Brainstem involvement may also be seen due to an osmotic demyelination syndrome from metabolic dysfunction (Figure 4.4).

Although direct neurotoxic effects of alcohol to the brain may lead to dementia, light to moderate use appears to be associated with a decreased risk for cognitive difficulties or a slower progression from MCI to dementia [199–202]. Proposed mechanisms for this effect includes inhibition of platelet aggregation, increased acetylcholine in the hippocampus, decreased apolipoprotein E binding to beta-amyloid, or improvement of the lipid profile in ApoE4 carriers [203]. However, other studies show no association with cognition, and it should be noted that the definition of "light" to "moderate" alcohol consumptions tends to vary among these studies (and among cultures).

Marchiafava–Bignami is an alcohol-related disorder characterized by demyelination and necrosis of the corpus callosum. Two subtypes have been described: one associated with major impairment of consciousness and another associated with no or minor impairment of consciousness. Other symptoms include seizures, cognitive impairment, gait difficulties, and dysarthria. Treatment and management includes cessation of alcohol use and supplementation with B1 and B6.

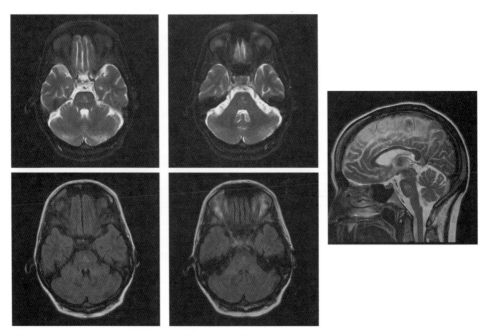

Fig 4.4 A 47-year-old woman presented with confusion and mild parkinsonism on examination. Her social history was notable for chronic alcoholism. T2-weighted and FLAIR cerebral imaging revealed T2-weighted hyperintensity in the brainstem consistent with central pontine myelinolysis.

Conclusion

There are a plethora of systemic conditions that may lead to cognitive changes, encephalopathy, and dementia. Taking a careful history and physical examination with appropriate laboratory workup is essential. While complete resolution of cognitive symptoms is not always possible, appropriate treatment of the underlying condition(s) can lead to improvement of cognitive symptoms. More research should be performed to determine the long-term effects of these treatments on cognitive outcomes.

 Five things to remember about dementia and systemic disease

1. A plethora of systemic diseases can be associated with dementia, requiring a careful history and physical examination of patients with cognitive symptoms.
2. The minimum workup for those with cognitive symptoms includes a complete blood count, complete metabolic profile, thyroid function tests, vitamin B12 levels, as well as neuroimaging with magnetic resonance imaging or computerized tomography of the brain. Further workup may be required if sequelae from a systemic disease is suspected as a contributing factor to symptoms.
3. The efficacy of anticholinergic inhibitors in dementias associated with systemic disease has not been well established.
4. Optimal treatment of systemic disease may improve cognitive symptoms, though some systemic disease may lead to irreversible change.
5. Further studies about the effect of treatments for systemic disease on long-term cognitive outcomes need to be performed.

References

1 Petersen RC, Smith GE, Waring SC, et al. Mild cognitive impairment: clinical characterization and outcome. *Arch. Neurol.* 1999;56(3):303–308.

2 Nasreddine ZS, Phillips NA, Bedirian, V, et al. The Montreal Cognitive Assessment, MoCA: a brief screening tool for mild cognitive impairment. *J. Am. Geriatr. Soc.* 2005;53(4):695–699.

3 Folstein M, Folstein S, McHugh P. "Mini-mental state". A practical method for grading the cognitive state of patients for the clinician. *J. Psychiatr. Res.* 1975;12:189–198.

4 Kokmen E, Smith GE, Petersen RC, et al. The short test of mental status. Correlations with standardized psychometric testing. *Arch. Neurol.* 1991;48(7):725–728.

5 Knopman DS, DeKosky ST, Cummings J.L, et al. Practice parameter: diagnosis of dementia (an evidence-based review). Report of the Quality Standards Subcommittee of the American Academy of Neurology. *Neurology* 2001;56(9):1143–1153.

6 Bauer M, Goetz T, Glenn T, et al. The thyroid–brain interaction in thyroid disorders and mood disorders. *J. Neuroendocrinol.* 2008;20(10):1101–1114.

7 Castillo P, Woodruff B, Caselli R, et al. Steroid-responsive encephalopathy associated with autoimmune thyroiditis. *Arch. Neurol.* 2006;63(2):175–176.

8 Canelo-Aybar C, Loja-Oropeza D, Cuadra-Urteaga J, et al. Hashimoto's encephalopathy presenting with neurocognitive symptoms: a case report. *J. Med. Case Rep.* 2010;4:33.

9 Babtain FA. Steroid responsive encephalopathy associated with autoimmune thyroiditis presenting with late onset depression. *Neurosciences (Riyadh)* 2010; 15(3):196–199.

10 Bocchetta A, Tamburini G, Cavolina P, et al. Affective psychosis, Hashimoto's thyroiditis, and brain perfusion abnormalities: case report. *Clin. Pract. Epidemiol. Ment. Health* 2007;3:31.

11 Cheriyath P, Nookala V, Srivastava A, et al. Acute confusional state caused by Hashimoto's encephalopathy in a patient with hypothyroidism: a case report. *Cases J.* 2009;2:7967.

12 Ferlazzo E, Raffaele M, Mazzu I, et al. Recurrent status epilepticus as the main feature of Hashimoto's encephalopathy. *Epilepsy Behav.* 2006;8(1):328–330.

13 Mocellin R, Lubman DI, Lloyd J, et al. Reversible dementia with psychosis: Hashimoto's encephalopathy. *Psychiatry Clin. Neurosci.* 2006;60(6):761–763.

14 Caselli RJ, Boeve BF, Scheithauer BW, et al. Nonvasculitis autoimmune inflammatory meningoencephalitis (NAIM): a reversible form of encephalopathy. *Neurology* 1999;53(7):1579–1581.

15 Galluzzi S, Geroldi C, Zanetti O, et al. Hashimoto's encephalopathy in the elderly: relationship to cognitive impairment. *J. Geriatr. Psychiatry Neurol.* 2002; 15(3):175–179.

16 Grommes C, Griffin C, Downes KA, et al. Steroid-responsive encephalopathy associated with autoimmune thyroiditis presenting with diffusion MR imaging changes. *Am. J. Neuroradiol.* 2008;29(8):1550–1551.

17 Rodriguez AJ, Jicha GA, Steeves TD, et al. EEG changes in a patient with steroid-responsive encephalopathy associated with antibodies to thyroperoxidase (SREAT, Hashimoto's encephalopathy). *J. Clin. Neurophysiol.* 2006;23(4):371–373.

18 Schauble B, Castillo PR, Boeve BF, et al. EEG findings in steroid-responsive encephalopathy associated with autoimmune thyroiditis. *Clin. Neurophysiol.* 2003;114(1):32–37.

19 Cummings RR, Bagley SC, Syed S, et al. Hashimoto's encephalopathy: a case report with neuropsychological testing. *Gen. Hosp. Psychiatry* 2007;29(3):267–269.

20 Atzeni F, Doria A, Ghiradello A, et al. Anti-thyroid antibodies and thyroid dysfunction in rheumatoid arthritis: prevalence and diagnostic value. *Autoimmunity* 2008;41(1):111–115.

21 Schiess N, Pardo CA. Hashimotos' encephalopathy. *Ann. NY Acad. Sci.* 2008;1142:254–265.

22 Begin ME, Langlois MF, Lorrain D, et al. Thyroid function and cognition during aging. *Curr. Gerontol. Geriatr. Res.* 2008;2008:1–11. doi:10.1155/2008/474868.

23 Patterson M, Lonie J, Starr JM. Thyroid function, cognition, functional independence and behavioural and psychological symptoms of dementia in Alzheimer's disease. *Int. J. Geriatr. Psychiatry* 2010;25(11): 1196–1197.

24 Etgen T, Bickel H, Forstl H. Metabolic and endocrine factors in mild cognitive impairment. *Ageing Res. Rev.* 2010;9(3):280–288.

25 Tan ZS, Beiser A, Vasan RS, et al. Thyroid function and the risk of Alzheimer's disease: the Framingham Study. *Arch. Intern. Med.* 2008;168(14):1514–1520.

26 deJong FJ, Masaki K, Chen H, et al. Thyroid function, the risk of dementia and neuropathologic changes: the Honolulu–Asia aging study. *Neurobiol. Aging* 2009; 30(4):600–606.

27 Kopf D, Frolich L. Risk of incident Alzheimer's disease in diabetic patients: a systematic review of prospective trials. *J. Alzheimers Dis.* 2009;16(4):677–685.

28 Korf ES, White LR, Scheltens P, et al. Brain aging in very old men with type 2 diabetes: the Honolulu–Asia Aging Study. *Diabetes Care* 2006;29(10):2268–2274.

29 Luchsinger JA, Reitz C, Honig LS, et al. Aggregation of vascular risk factors and risk of incident Alzheimer's disease. *Neurology* 2005;65(4):545–551.

30 Ott A, Stolk RP, van Harskamp F, et al. Diabetes mellitus and the risk of dementia: the Rotterdam Study. *Neurology* 1999;53(9):1937–1942.

31 Peila R, Rodriguez BL, Launer LJ, et al. Type 2 diabetes, APOE gene, and the risk for dementia and related pathologies: the Honolulu–Asia Aging Study. *Diabetes* 2002;51(4):1256–1262.

32 Rastas S, Pirttila T, Mattila K, et al. Vascular risk factors and dementia in the general population aged >85 years: prospective population-based study. *Neurobiol. Aging* 2010;31(1):1–6.

33 American Diabetes Association. Diagnosis and classification of diabetes mellitus. *Diab. Care* 2010;33(Suppl 1):S62–S69.

34 Selvarajah D, Tesfaye S. Central nervous system involvement in diabetes mellitus. *Curr. Diab. Rep.* 2006; 6(6):431–438.

35 Bassil N, Morley JE. Endocrine aspects of healthy brain aging. *Clin. Geriatr. Med.* 2010;26(1):57–74.

36 Gandhi GK, Ball KK, Cruz NF, et al. Hyperglycaemia and diabetes impair gap junctional communication among astrocytes. *ASN Neuro* 2010;2(2):e00030.

37 Shimada H, Miki T, Tamura A, et al. Neuropsychological status of elderly patients with diabetes mellitus. *Diab. Res. Clin. Pract.* 2010;87(2):224–227.

38 Zihl J, Schaaf L, Zillmer EA. The relationship between adult neuropsychological profiles and diabetic patients' glycemic control. *Appl. Neuropsychol.* 2010;17(1): 44–51.

39 Brands AM, Van den Berg E, Manschot SM, et al. A detailed profile of cognitive dysfunction and its relation to psychological distress in patients with type 2 diabetes mellitus. *J. Int. Neuropsychol. Soc.* 2007;13(2): 288–289.

40 Xu W, Caracciolo B, Wang HX, et al. Accelerated progression from mild cognitive impairment to dementia in people with diabetes. *Diabetes* 2010;59(11): 2928–2935.

41 van Elderen SG, de Roos A, de Craen AJ, et al. Progression of brain atrophy and cognitive decline in diabetes mellitus: a 3-year follow-up. *Neurology* 2010;75 (11):997–1002.

42 Sanz C, Andrieu S, Sinclair A, et al. Diabetes is associated with a slower rate of cognitive decline in Alzheimer disease. *Neurology* 2009;73(17):1359–1366.

43 Peters R, Poulter R, Beckett N, et al. Cardiovascular and biochemical risk factors for incident dementia in the hypertension in the very elderly trial. *J. Hypertens.* 2009;27(10):2055–2062.

44 Akomolafe A, Beiser A, Meigs JB, et al. Diabetes mellitus and risk of developing Alzheimer disease: results from the Framingham Study. *Arch. Neurol.* 2006; 63(11):1551–1555.

45 Craft S. The role of metabolic disorders in Alzheimer disease and vascular dementia: two roads converged. *Arch. Neurol.* 2009;66(3):300–305.

46 Whitmer RA, Karter AJ, Yaffe K, et al. Hypoglycemic episodes and risk of dementia in older patients with type 2 diabetes mellitus. *J. Am. Med. Assoc.* 2009;301(15): 1565–1572.

47 Henderson V. Dementia. *Continuum Lifelong Learning Neurol.* 2009;15(2):91–107.

48 Rocca WA, Grossardt BR, Shuster LT. Oophorectomy, menopause, estrogen, and cognitive aging: the timing hypothesis. *Neurodegener. Dis.* 2010;7(1–3):163–166.

49 Phung TK, Waltoft BL, Laursen TM, et al. Hysterectomy, oophorectomy and risk of dementia: a nationwide historical cohort study. *Dement. Geriatr. Cogn. Disord.* 2010;30(1):43–50.

50 Rocca WA, Grossardt BR, Shuster LT. Oophorectomy, menopause, estrogen treatment and cognitive aging: clinical evidence for a window of opportunity. *Brain Res.* 2011;1379:188–198.

51 Rocca WA, Bower JH, Maraganore DM, et al. Increased risk of cognitive impairment or dementia in women who underwent oophorectomy before menopause. *Neurology* 2007;69(11):1074–1078.

52 Forti P, Pisacane N, Rietti E, et al. Metabolic syndrome and risk of dementia in older adults. *J. Am. Geriatr. Soc.* 2010;58(3):487–492.

53 Muller M, Tang MX, Schupf N, et al. Metabolic syndrome and dementia risk in a multiethnic cohort. *Dement. Geriatr. Cogn. Disord.* 2007;24(3):185–192.

54 Raffaitin C, Gin H, Empana JP, et al. Metabolic syndrome and risk for incident Alzheimer's disease or vascular dementia: the Three-City Study. *Diab. Care* 2009;32(1):169–174.

55 Solfrizzi V, Scafato E, Capurso C, et al. Metabolic syndrome, mild cognitive impairment, and progression to dementia. The Italian Longitudinal Study on Aging. *Neurobiol. Aging* 2011;32(11):1932–1941.

56 Yaffe K, Weston AL, Blackwell T, et al. The metabolic syndrome and development of cognitive impairment among older women. *Arch. Neurol.* 2009;66(3): 324–328.

57 Panza F, Firsardi V, Seripa D, et al. Metabolic syndrome, mild cognitive impairment, and dementia. *Curr. Alzheimer Res.* 2011;8(5):492–509.

58 Strachan MW. Insulin and cognitive function. *Lancet* 2003;362(9392):1253.

59 Matsuzaki T, Sasaki K, Tanizaki Y, et al. Insulin resistance is associated with the pathology of Alzheimer disease: the Hisayama study. *Neurology* 2010; 75(9):764–770.

60 Kerola T, Kettunen R, Nieminen T. The complex interplay of cardiovascular system and cognition: How to predict dementia in the elderly *Int. J. Cardiol.* 2011;150 (2):123–129.

61 Shah K, Qurershi SU, Johnson M, et al. Does the use of antihypertensive drugs affect the incidence of progression of dementia A systematic review. *Am. J. Geriatr. Pharmacother.* 2009;7(5):250–261.

62 Rosenbloom MH, Smith S, Akdal G, et al. Immunologically mediated dementias. *Curr. Neurol. Neurosci. Rep.* 2009;9(5):359–367.

63 Wong SH, Saunders MD, Larner AJ, et al. An effective immunotherapy regimen for VGKC antibody-positive limbic encephalitis. *J. Neurol. Neurosurg. Psychiatry* 2010;81(10):1167–1169.

63a Flanagan EP, McKeon A, Lennon VA, et al. Autoimmune dementia: clinical course and predictors of immunotherapy response. *Mayo Clin. Proc.* 2010; 85(10):881–897.

64 ACR Ad Hoc Committee on Neuropscyhiatric Lupus Nomenclature. The American College of Rheumatology nomenclature and case definitions for neuropsychiatric lupus syndromes. *Arthritis Rheum.* 1999;42:599–608.

65 Schofield P. Dementia associated with toxic causes and autoimmune disease. *Int. Psychogeriatr.* 2005; (Suppl): S129–S147.

66 Ainiala H, Hietaharju A, Loukkola J, et al. Validity of the New American College of Rheumatology criteria for neuropsychiatric lupus syndromes: a population-based evaluation. *Arthritis Care Res.* 2001;45:419–423.

67 Unterman A, Nolte JE, Boaz M, et al. Neuropsychiatric syndromes in systemic lupus erythematosus: a meta-analysis. *Semin. Arthritis Rheum.* 2011;41 (1):1–11.

68 Bertsias GK, Boumpas DR. Pathogenesis, diagnosis and management of neuropsychiatric SLE manifestations. *Nat. Rev. Rheumatol.* 2010;6(6):358–367.

69 Luyendijk J, Steens SC, Ouwendijk WJ, et al. Neuropsychiatric systemic lupus erythematosus: lessons learned from magnetic resonance imaging. *Arthritis Rheum.* 2011;63(3):722–732.

70 Liberato B, Levy RA. Antiphospholipid syndrome and cognition. *Clin. Rev. Allerg. Immunol.* 2007;32: 188–191.

71 Markusse HM, Hilkens PH, van den Bent MJ, et al. Normal pressure hydrocephalus associated with rheumatoid arthritis responding to prednisone. *J. Rheumatol.* 1995;22(2):342–343.

72 Fishman RA. Normal pressure hydrocephalus and arthritis. *N. Engl. J. Med.* 1985;312(19):1255–1256.

73 Rasker JJ, Jansen EN, Haan J, et al. Normal pressure hydrocephalus in rheumatic patients. A diagnostic pitfall. *N. Engl. J. Med.* 1985;312(19):1239–1241.

73a Cantananti C, Mastropaolo S, Calabrese C, et al. A case of normal-pressure hydrocephalus associated with rheumatoid arthritis. *Aging Clin. Exp. Res.* 2010;22(2): 189–191.

74 Caballol Pons N, Montala N, Valverde J, et al. Isolated cerebral vasculitis associated with rheumatoid arthritis. *Joint Bone Spine* 2010;77(4):361–363.

75 Mrabet D, Meddeb N, Ajlani H, et al. Cerebral vasculitis in a patient with rheumatoid arthritis. *Joint Bone Spine* 2007;74(2):201–204.

76 Somers KJ, Sola CL. Voltage-gated potassium channel complex antibody associated limbic encephalitis. *Psychosomatics* 2011;52(1):78–81.

77 Malter MP, Helmstaedter C, Urbach H, et al. Antibodies to glutamic acid decarboxylase define a form of limbic encephalitis. *Ann. Neurol.* 2010;67(4):470–478.

78 Lancaster E, Martinez-Hernandez E, Dalmau J. Encephalitis and antibodies to synaptic and neuronal cell surface proteins. *Neurology* 2011;77:179–189.

79 Vincent A, Bien CG, Irani SR, et al. Autoantibodies associated with diseases of the CNS: new developments and future challenges. *Lancet Neurol.* 2011;10:759–772.

80 Chang CC, Eggers SD, Johnson JK, et al. Anti-GAD antibody cerebellar ataxia mimicking Creutzfeldt–Jakob disease. *Clin. Neurol. Neurosurg.* 2007;109(1):54–57.

81 Geschwind MD, Shu H, Haman A, et al. Rapidly progressive dementia. *Ann. Neurol.* 2008;64(1):97–108.

82 Chai J, Herrmann DN, Stanton M, et al. Painful small-fiber neuropathy in Sjogren syndrome. *Neurology* 2005;65(6):925–927.

83 Chai J, Lagigian EL. Neurological manifestations of primary Sjogren's syndrome. *Curr. Opin. Neurol.* 2010;23(5):509–513.

84 LeGuern V, Belin C, Henegar C, et al. Cognitive function and 99mRc-ECD brain SPECT are significantly correlated in patients with primary Sjogren syndrome: a case-control study. *Ann. Rheum. Dis.* 2010;69 (10):132–137.

85 Berlit P. Neuropsychiatric disease in collagen vascular diseases and vasculitis. *J. Neurol.* 2007;254(Suppl 2):1187–1189.

86 Baughman RP, Culver DA, Costabel U. Sarcoidosis. *Semin. Respir. Crit. Care. Med.* 2010;31(4):373–374.

87 Hawtin KE, Roddie ME, Mauri FA, et al. Pulmonary sarcoidosis: the 'Great Pretender.' *Clin. Radiol.* 2010; 65(8):642–650.

88 Lagana SM, Parwani AV, Nichols LG. Cardiac sarcoidosis: a pathology-focused review. *Arch. Pathol. Lab. Med.* 2010;134(7):1039–1046.

89 MacArthur KL, Forouhar F, Wu GY. Intra-abdomnial complications of sarcoidosis. *J. Formos. Med. Assoc.* 2010;109(7):484–492.

90 Marchell RM, Judson MA. Cutaneous sarcoidosis. *Semin. Respir. Crit. Care Med.* 2010;31(4):442–451.

91 Nunes H, Freynet O, Naggara N, et al. Cardiac sarcoidosis. *Semin. Respir.Crit. Care Med.* 2010;31(4):428–441.

92 Brinar VV, Habek M. Isolated central nervous system sarcoidosis: a great mimicker. *Clin. Neurol. Neurosurg.* 2008;110(9):939–942.

93 Caneparo D, Lucetti C, Nuti A, et al. A case of sarcoidosis presenting as a non-specific intramedullary lesion. *Eur. J. Neurol.* 2007;14(3):346–349.

94 Giovinale M, Fonnesu C, Soriano A, et al. Atypical sarcoidosis: case reports and review of the literature. *Eur. Rev. Med. Pharmacol. Sci.* 2009;13(Suppl 1):37–44.

95 Mariani M, Shammi P. Neurosarcoidosis and associated neuropsychological sequelae: a rare case of isolated intracranial involvement. *Clin. Neuropsychol.* 2010;24(2):286–304.

96 Oh J, Stokes K, Tyndel F, et al. Progressive cognitive decline in a patient with isolated chronic neurosarcoidosis. *Neurologist* 2010;16(1):50–53.

97 Tsao CY, Lo WD, Rusin JA, et al. Isolated neurosarcoidosis presenting as headache and multiple brain and spinal cord lesions mimicking central nervous system metastases. *Brain Dev.* 2007;29(8):514–518.

98 Statement on sarcoidosis. Joint statement of the American Thoracic Society (ATS), the European Respiratory Society (ERS) and the World Association of Sarcoidosis and Other Granulomatous Disorders (WASOG) adopted by the ATS Board of Directors and by the ERS Executive Committee. *Am. J. Respir. Crit. Care Med.* 1999;160(20):736–755.

99 Hoitsma E, Drent M, Sharma OP. A pragmatic approach to diagnosing and treating neurosarcoidosis in the 21st century. *Curr. Opin. Pulm. Med.* 2010; 16(5):472–479.

100 Friedman SH, Gould DJ. Neurosarcoidosis presenting as psychosis and dementia: a case report. *Int. J. Psychiatry Med.* 2002;32(4):401–403.

101 Pruter C, Kunert HJ, Hoff P. ICD-10 mild cognitive disorder following meningitis due to neurosarcoidosis. *Psychopathology* 2001;34(6):326–327.

102 Ruocco AC, Lacy M. Neuropsychological findings in a case of neurosarcoidosis. *J. Neuropsychiatry Clin. Neurosci.* 2010;22(1):123.E36.

103 Terushkin V, Stern BJ, Judson MA, et al. Neurosarcoidosis: presentations and management. *Neurologist* 2010;16(1):2–15.

104 Lury KM, Smith JK, Matheus MG, et al. Neurosarcoidosis—review of imaging findings. *Semin. Roentgenol.* 2004;39(4):495–504.

105 Smith JK, Matheus MG, Castillo M. Imaging manifestations of neurosarcoidosis. *Am. J. Roentgenol.* 2004;182(2):289–295.

106 Berlit P. Diagnosis and treatment of cerebral vasculitis. *Ther. Adv. Neurol. Disord.* 2010;3(1):29–42.

107 Kraemer M, Berlit P. Systemic, secondary and infectious causes for cerebral vasculitis: clinical experience with 16 new European cases. *Rheumatol. Int.* 2010; 30(11):1471–1476.

108 Haj-Ali R, Calabrese LH. Central nervous system vasculitis. *Curr. Opin. Rheumatol.* 2009;21(1):10–18.

109 Birnbaum J, Hellman DB. Primary angiitis of the central nervous system. *Arch. Neurol.* 2009;66(6):704–709.

110 Tamura M, Yaffe K. Dementia and cognitive impairment in ESRD: diagnostic and therapeutic strategies. *Kidney Int.* 2011;79(1):14–22.

111 Murray AM. Cognitive impairment in the aging dialysis and chronic kidney disease populations: an occult burden. *Adv. Chronic Kidney Dis.* 2008;15(2):123–132.

112 Yaffe K, Ackerson L, Tamura MK, et al. Chronic kidney disease and cognitive function in older adults: Findings from the Chronic Renal Insufficiency Cohort Cognitive Study. *JAGS* 2010;58(2):338–345.

113 Kurella TM, Wadley V, Yaffe K, et al. Kidney function and cognitive impairment in US adults: the Reasons for Geographic and Racial Differences in Stroke (REGARDS) study. *Am. J. Kidney Dis.* 2008; 52(2):227–234.

114 Vidal JS, Sigurdsson S, Jonsdottir MK, et al. Coronary artery calcium, brain function, and structure: the AGES-Reykjavik Study. *Stroke* 2010;41(5):891–897.

115 Jefferson AL, Himali JJ, Beiser AS, et al. Cardiac index is associated with brain aging. *Circulation* 2010; 122:690–697.

116 Staessen JA, Richart T, Birkenhager WH. Less atherosclerosis and lower blood pressure for a meaningful life perspective with more brain. *Hypertension* 2007; 49(3):389–400.

117 McGuinness B, Craig D, Bullock R, et al. Statins for the prevention of dementia. *Cochrane Database Syst. Rev.* 2009;15(2):CD003160.

118 McGuinness B, O'Hare J, Craig D, et al. Statins for the treatment of dementia. *Cochrane Database Syst. Rev.* 2010;4(8):CD007514.

119 Ligthart SA, Moll van Charante EP, Van Gool WA, et al. Treatment of cardiovascular risk factors to prevent cognitive decline and dementia: a systematic review. *Vasc. Health Risk Manag.* 2010;6:775–785.

120 McGuinness B, Todd S, Passmore P, et al. Blood pressure lowering in patients without prior cerebrovascular disease for prevention of cognitive impairment and dementia. *Cochrane Database Syst. Rev.* 2009;7(4):CD004034.

121 Bunch TJ, Weiss JP, Crandall BG, et al. Atrial fibrillation is independently associated with senile, vascular, and Alzheimer's dementia. *Heart Rhythm* 2010;7:433–437.

122 Kilander L, Andren B, Nyman H, Lind L, et al. Atrial fibrillation is an independent determinant of low cognitive function: a cross-sectional study in elderly men. *Stroke* 1988;29(9):1816–1820.

123 Ott A, Breteler MM, de Bruyne MC, et al. Atrial fibrillation and dementia in a population-based study. The Rotterdam Study. *Stroke* 1997;28(2):315–321.

124 Forti P, Maioli F, Pisacane N, Rietti E, et al. Atrial fibrillation and risk of dementia in non-demented elderly subjects with and without mild cognitive impairment. *Arch. Gerontol. Geriatr.* 2007;44(Suppl 1):155–165.

125 Flaker GC, Pogue J, Yusuf S, et al. Cognitive function and anticoagulation control in patients with atrial fibrillation. *Circ. Cardiovasc. Qual. Outcomes* 2010; 3(3):277–283.

126 van Deelan BA, van den Bemt PM, Egberts TC, et al. Cognitive impairment as determinant for sub-optimal control of oral anticoagulation treatment in elderly patients with atrial fibrillation. *Drugs Aging* 2005; 22(4):353–360.

127 Peters R, Poulter R, Beckett N, et al. Cardiovascular and biochemical risk factors for incident dementia in the Hypertension in the Very Elderly Trial. 2009; 27(10):2055–2062.

128 Marengoni A, Qiu C, Winblad B, et al. Atrial fibrillation, stroke and dementia in the very old: a population-based study. *Neurobiol. Aging* 2011;32(7):1336–1337.

129 Flaker GC, Poque J, Yusuf, et al. Cognitive function and anticoagulation control in patients with atrial fibrillation. *Circ. Cardiovasc. Qual. Outcomes* 2010;3(3):277–283.

130 Lorincz MT. Neurologic Wilson's disease. *Ann. NY Acad. Sci.* 2010;1184:173–187.

131 Hadjivassiliou M, Sanders DS, Grunewald R.A. et al. Gluten sensitivity: from gut to brain. *Lancet Neurol.* 2010;9:318–330.

132 Hu WT, Murray JA, Greenaway MC, et al. Cognitive impairment and celiac disease. *Arch. Neurol.* 2006; 63(10):1440–1446.

133 Rosenfeld M, Dalmau J. Update on paraneoplastic and autoimmune disorders of the central nervous system. *Semin. Neurol.* 2010;30(3):320–331.

134 McKeon A, Ahlskog JE, Britton JA, et al. Reversible extralimbic paraneoplastic encephalopathies with large abnormalities on magnetic resonance images. *Arch. Neurol.* 2009;66(2):268–271.

135 Vernino S, Lennon VA. Autoantibody profiles and neurological correlations of thymoma. *Clin. Cancer Res.* 2004;10(21):7270–7275.

136 Graus F, Keime-Guibert F, Rene R, et al. Anti-Hu associated paraneoplastic encephalomyelitis: analysis of 200 patients. *Brain* 2001;124(pt 6):1138–1148.

137 Porta-Ettesam J, Ruiz-Morales J, Millan JM, et al. Epilepsia partialis continua and frontal features as a debut of anti-Hu paraneoplastic encephalomyelitis with focal frontal encephalitis. *Eur. J. Neurol.* 2001; 8(4):359–360.

138 Pittock SJ, Lucchinetti CF, Lennon VA. Anti-neuronal nuclear autoantibody type 2: paraneoplastic accompaniments. *Ann. Neurol.* 2003;53(5):580–587.

139 Dalmau J, Tuzun E, Wu HY, et al. Paraneoplastic anti-N-methyl-D-aspartate receptor encephalitis associated with ovarian teratoma. *Ann. Neurol.* 2007;61(1):25–36.

140 Dalmau J, Lancaster E, Martinez-Hernandez E, et al. Clinical experience and laboratory investigations in patients with anti-NMDAR encephalitis. *Lancet Neurol.* 2011;10:63–74.

141 Knopman DS, Petersen RC, Cha RH, et al. Incidence and causes of nondegenerative nonvascular dementia: a population-based study. *Arch. Neurol.* 2006;63(2): 218–221.

142 Ricard D, Taillia H, Renard JL. Brain damage from anticancer treatments in adults. *Curr. Opin. Oncol.* 2009;21(6):559–565.

143 Roe CM, Fitzpatrick AL, Xiong C, et al. Cancer linked to Alzheimer disease but not vascular dementia. *Neurology* 2010;74(2):106–112.

144 Roe CM, Behrens MI, Xiong C, et al. Alzheimer disease and cancer. *Neurology* 2005;64(5):895–898.

145 Behrens MI, Lendon C, Roe CM. A common biological mechanism in cancer and Alzheimer's disease *Curr. Alzheimer Res.* 2009;6(3):196–204.

146 Geschwind M. Rapidly progressive dementia: prion diseases and other rapid dementias. *Continuum: Lifelong Learning Neurol.* 2010;16(2):31–56.

147 McCoyd M, Gruener G. Neurologic aspects of lymphoma and leukemias. *Continuum: Lifelong Learning Neurol.* 2010;17(1):73–94.

148 Bakshi R, Mazziotta JC, Mischel PS, et al. Lymphomatosis cerebri presenting as a rapidly progressive dementia: clinical neuroimaging and pathologic findings. *Dement. Geriatr. Cogn. Disord.* 1999;10(2):152–157.

149 Kanai R, Shibuya M, Hata T, et al. A case of 'lymphamatosis cerebri' diagnosed in an early phase and treated by whole brain radiation: case report and literature review. *J. Neurooncol.* 2008;86(1):83–88.

150 Ricard D, Taillia H, Renard JL. Brain damage from anticancer treatments in adults. *Curr. Opin. Oncol.* 2009;21(6):559–565.

151 Sioka C, Kyritsis AP. Central and peripheral nervous system toxicity of common chemotherapeutic agents. *Cancer Chemother. Pharmacol.* 2009;63(5):761–767.

152 Soussain C, Ricard D, Fike JR, et al. CNS Complications of radiotherapy and chemotherapy. *Lancet* 2009; 374(9701):1639–1651.

153 Arciniegas DB, Anderson CA. Viral encephalitis: Neuropsychiatric and neurobehavioral aspects. *Curr. Psychiatry Rep.* 2004;6(5):372–379.

154 McArthur JC, Steiner J, Sacktor N, et al. Human immunodeficiency virus-associated neurocognitive disorders: mind the gap. *Ann. Neurol.* 2010;67(6):699–714.

155 Martin-Thormeyer EM, Paul RH. Drug abuse and hepatitis C infection as comorbid features of HIV associated neurocognitive disorder: neurocognitive and neuroimaging features. *Neuropsychol. Rev.* 2009;19(2): 215–231.

156 Linger KJ, II, Hall CD, Robertson KR. Effects of antiretroviral therapy on cognitive impairment. *Curr HIV/AIDS Rep.* 2008;5(2):64–71.

157 Forton DM, Taylor-Robinson SD, Thomas HC. Cerebral dysfunction in chronic hepatitis C infection. *J. Viral Hepatitis* 2003;10:81–86.

158 Perry W, Hilsabeck RC, Hassanein TI. Cognitive dysfunction in chronic hepatitis C: a review. *Dig. Dis. Sci.* 2008;53(2):307–321.

159 Hilsabeck RC, Hassanein TI, Carlson MD, et al. Cognitive function and psychiatric symptomatology in patients with chronic hepatitis C. *J. Int. Neuropsychol. Soc.* 2003;9(6):847–854.

160 Hokkanen L, Poutianen E, Valanne L, et al. Cognitive impairment after acute encephalitis: comparison of herpes simplex and other aetiologies. *J. Neurol. Neurosurg. Psychiatry* 1996;61(5):478–484.

161 Rachilas S, Wolff M, Delatour F, et al. Outcome of and prognostic factors for herpes simplex encephalitis in adult patients: results of a multicenter study. *Clin. Infect. Dis.* 2002;35(3):254–260.

162 Rossi T, Haghighipour R, Haghighi M, et al. Cerebral Whipple's disease as a cause of reversible dementia. *Clin. Neurol. Neurosurg.* 2005;107(3):258–261.

163 Benito-Leon J, Sedano LF, Louis ED. Isolated central nervous system Whipple's disease causing reversible frontotemporal-like dementia. *Clin. Neurol. Neurosurg.* 2008;110(7):747–749.

164 Kent ME, Romanelli F. Reexamining syphilis: an update on epidemiology, clinical manifestations, and management. *Ann. Pharmacother.* 2008;42(2):226–236.

165 Fargen KM, Alvernia JE, Lin CS, et al. Cerebral syphilitic gummata: a case presentation and analysis of 156 reported cases. *Neurosurgery* 2009;64(3):568–575.

166 Jay CA. Treatment of neurosyphilis. *Curr. Treat. Options Neurol.* 2007;8(3):185–192.

167 Kaplan RF, Jones-Woodward L. Lyme encephalopathy: a neuropsychological perspective. *Semin. Neurol.* 1997;17(1):31–37.

168 Keilp JG, Corbera K, Slavov I, et al. WAIS-III and WMS-III performance in chronic Lyme disease. *J. Int. Neuropsychol. Soc.* 2006;12(1):119–129.

169 Fallon BA, Levin ES, Schweitzer PJ, et al. Inflammation and central nervous system Lyme disease. *Neurobiol. Dis.* 2010;37(3):534–541.

170 Westervelt HJ, McCaffrey RJ. Neuropsychological functioning in chronic Lyme disease. *Neuropsychol. Rev.* 2002;12(3):153–177.

171 Halperin JJ, Shapiro ED, Logigian E, et al. Practice parameter: treatment of nervous system Lyme disease (an evidence-based review): report of the Quality Standards Subcommittee of the American Academy of Neurology. *Neurology* 2007;69(1);91–102.

172 Kaplan RF, Trevino RP, Johnson GM, et al. Cognitive function in post-treatment Lyme disease: do additional antibiotics help *Neurology* 2003;60(12):1916–1922.

173 Almeida OP, Lautenschlager NT. Dementia associated with infectious diseases. *Int. Psychogeriatr.* 2005; 17(Suppl 1):S65–S77.

174 Roman G. The neurology of parasitic diseases and malaria. *Continuum: Lifelong Learning Neurol.* 2011;17(1):113–133.

175 Parchi P, Giese A, Capellari S, et al. Classification of sporadic Creutzfeldt–Jakob disease based on molecular and phenotypic analysis of 300 subjects. *Ann. Neurol.* 1999;46(2):224–233.

176 Meissner B, Kallenberg K, Sanchez-Juan P, et al. MRI lesion profiles in sporadic Creutzfeldt–Jakob disease. *Neurology* 2009;72(23):1994–2001.

177 Hamaguchi T, Noguchi-Shinohara M, Nozaki I, et al. The risk of iatrogenic Creutzfeldt–Jakob disease through medical and surgical procedures. *Neuropathology* 2009;29(5):625–631.

178 Lee HB, DeLoatch CJ, Cho S, et al. Detection and management of pre-existing cognitive impairment and associated behavioral symptoms in the intensive care unit. *Crit. Care Clin.* 2008;24(4):723–736.

179 Hopkins RO, Jackson JC. Short- and long-term cognitive outcomes in intensive care unit survivors. *Clin. Chest Med.* 2009;30(1):143–153.

180 Pisani MA, McNicoll L, Inouye SK. Underrecognition of preexisting cognitive impairment by physicians in older ICU patients. *Chest* 2003;124(6):2267–2274.

181 Hopkins RO, Jackson JC. Long-term neurocognitive function after critical illness. *Chest* 2006;130(3):869–878.

182 Schofield P. Dementia associated with toxic causes and autoimmune disease. *Int. Psychogeriatr.* 2005; 17(Suppl):S129–S147.

183 O'Carroll RE, Masterton G, Dougall N, et al. The neuropsychiatric sequelae of mercury poisoning. The Mad Hatter's disease revisited. *Br. J. Psychiatry* 1995;167(1):95–98.

184 Dunea G, Mahurkar SD, Mamdani B, et al. Role of aluminum in dialysis dementia. *Ann. Intern. Med.* 1978;88(4):502–504.

185 Tomljenovic L. Aluminum and Alzheimer's disease: after a century of controversy, is there a plausible link *J. Alzheimers Dis.* 2011;23(4):567–598.

186 Ibrahim D, Froberg B, Wolf A, et al. Heavy metal poisoning: clinical presentations and pathophysiology. *Clin. Lab. Med.* 2006;26(1):67–97.

187 Yucel M, Takagi M, Walterfang M, et al. Toluene misuse and long-term harms: A systematic review of the neuropsychological and neuroimaging literature. *Neurosci. Biobehav. Rev.* 2008;32(2008):910–926.

188 Filley CM, Heaton RK, Rosenberg NL. White matter dementia in chronic toluene abuse. *Neurology* 1990;40 (3):532–534.

189 Greer DM. Mechanisms of injury in hypoxic-ischemic encephalopathy: implications to therapy. *Semin. Neurol.* 2006;26(4):373–379.

190 Shprecher D, Metha L. The syndrome of delayed posthypoxic leukoencephalopathy. *Neurorehabilitation* 2010;26(1):65–72.

191 Ku H-L, Yang K-C, Lee Y-C, et al. Predictors of carbon monoxide poisoning-induced delayed neuropsychological sequelae. *General Hospital Psychiatry* 2010;32:310–314.

192 Flicker L, Ames D. Metabolic and endocrinological causes of dementia. *Int. Psychogeriatr.* 2005;17(Suppl): S79–S92.

193 Osimani A, Berger A, Friedman J, et al. Neuropsychology of vitamin B12 deficiency in elderly dementia patients and control subjects. *J. Geriatr. Psychiatry Neurol.* 2005;18(1):33–38.

194 Langan RC, Zawitoski KJ. Update on vitamin B12 deficiency. *Am. Fam. Physician* 2011;83(12):1425–1430.

195 Chatterjee A, Yapundich R, Palmer CA, et al. Leukoencephalopathy associated with cobalamin deficiency. *Neurology* 1996;46(3) 832–834.

196 Vogiatzoglou A, Refsum H, Johnston C, et al. Vitamin B12 status and rate of brain volume loss in community-dwelling elderly. *Neurology* 2008;71(11):826–832.

197 Llewellyn DJ, Lang IA, Langa KM, et al. Vitamin D and risk of cognitive decline in elderly persons. *Arch. Intern. Med.* 2010;170(13):1135–1141.

198 Buell JS, Dawson-Hughes B, Scott TM, et al. 25-Hydroxyvitamin D, dementia, and cerebrovascular pathology in elders receiving home services. *Neurology* 2010;74(1):18–26.

199 Brust JCM. Ethanol and cognition: Indirect effects, neurotoxicity, and neuroprotection: A review. *Int. J. Environ. Res. Public Health* 2010;7:1540–1557.

200 Anttila T, Helkala E-L, Viitanen M, et al. Alcohol drinking in middle age and subsequent risk of mild cognitive impairment and dementia in old age: a prospective population based study. *Br. Med. J.* 2004;329 (7465):539.

201 Mukamal KJ, Kuller LH, Fitzpatrick AL, et al. Prospective study of alcohol consumption and risk of dementia in older adults. *J. Am. Med. Assoc.* 2003;289: 1405–1413.

202 Solfrizzi, V, D'Intono A, Colacicco AM, et al. Alcohol consumption, mild cognitive impairment, and progression to dementia. *Neurology* 2007;68:1790–1799.

203 Hulse GK, Lautenschlager NT, Tait RJ, et al. Dementia associated with alcohol and other drug use. *Int. Psychgeriatr.* 2005;17(Suppl 1):S109–S127.

5

Stroke due to systemic diseases

Sarkis Morales-Vidal & José Biller
Loyola University Chicago, Stritch School of Medicine, Maywood, IL, USA

Introduction

Strokes can be ischemic or hemorrhagic. Ischemic strokes include arterial ischemic stroke (AIS) and cerebral venous sinus thrombosis (CVST). CVST may result in bland or hemorrhagic venous infarctions. Hemorrhagic strokes include intracerebral hemorrhage (ICH) and subarachnoid hemorrhage (SAH). We review all types of strokes associated with systemic diseases.

Endocrine disorders

Pituitary gland

Pituitary apoplexy is a neuroendocrinologic emergency. Pituitary apoplexy refers to acute infarction, hemorrhage, or hemorrhagic infarction of the pituitary gland, most commonly due to an acute expansion of a preexisting pituitary tumor, usually a macroadenoma (Figure 5.1). Causes of pituitary apoplexy are shown in Table 5.1. Clinical presentation is characterized by acute or subacute onset of severe retroorbital headaches (thunderclap), meningismus, visual loss due to chiasmatic compression, ophthalmoplegia, altered level of consciousness, and hypopituitarism [1]. The oculomotor (CNIII) is the most commonly involved cranial nerve. Cerebral ischemia may result from arterial compression or vasospasm [2,3]. Neurological deficits as a result of internal carotid artery occlusion may be the initial clinical presentation of pituitary apoplexy [3]. Pituitary apoplexy may also be

the initial presentation of a carotid-cavernous aneurysm [4].

Cranial computed tomography (CT) or magnetic resonance imaging (MRI) may show hemorrhage within the pituitary gland. MRI is more sensitive and specific. Cerebral angiography may be indicated if cerebral vasospasm is suspected [5,6]. Prompt administration of corticosteroids is needed. Surgical decompression is required in the setting of rapid deterioration of visual acuity or worsening visual-field deficits.

Thyroid disorders

Stroke has been associated with hyperthyroidism and hypothyroidism (Table 5.2).

Hyperthyroidism
Atrial fibrillation (AFib) may be the initial presentation of hyperthyroidism [11]. Approximately 15% of patients with hyperthyroidism have AFib [12]. Hyperthyroidism without cardiac arrhythmias does not increase stroke risks. While there is no increased risk of stroke from subclinical hyperthyroidism, low thyrotrophic (thyroid stimulating hormone (TSH)) levels in diabetic patients are associated with an increased risk of cardiovascular mortality [13]. Strokes among hyperthyroid patients may also result from secondary antiphospholipid antibody syndrome (APAS) [14–18], large vessel arteritis [18], or compression of the brachiocephalic vessels by a large goiter [19]. Graves' disease has been associated with Moyamoya syndrome [20–29] and CVST [30–33].

Neurological Disorders due to Systemic Disease, First Edition. Edited by Steven L. Lewis.
© 2013 Blackwell Publishing Ltd. Published 2013 by Blackwell Publishing Ltd.

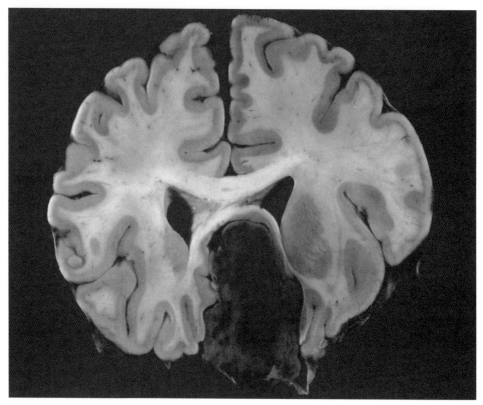

Fig 5.1 Coronal section of the brain demonstrates pituitary apoplexy in a patient with an underlying pituitary macroadenoma. (See also Plate 5.1).

Prevention of stroke recurrences in hyperthyroid patients must be individualized. Thromboembolic risk in thyrotoxic AFib is probably similar to non-valvular AFib [34]. Amongst randomized controlled clinical trials of stroke prevention with warfarin, only the Copenhagen AFASAK Study included patients

Table 5.1 Causes of pituitary apoplexy

Pituitary adenoma
Nelson Syndrome
Sheehan syndrome
Anticoagulant therapy
Intrasellar cavernous carotid aneurysms
Endocrine stimulation tests
Dopamine agonists
Head trauma
Pituitary irradiation
Induction chemotherapy for acute myelogenous leukemia
Following coronary artery bypass graft
Following catheter cerebral angiography

Table 5.2 Strokes associated with hyperthyroidism and hypothyroidism

Hyperthyroidism	Hypothyroidism
Cardioembolism associated with atrial fibrillation	Cerebrovascular atherosclerosis of large and small vessels
Antiphospholipid antibody syndrome	Arterial compression by goiter
Cerebral Vasculitis	Vasculitic variant of Hashimoto's encephalopathy [7–10]
Giant Cell Arteritis	
Moyamoya	Hypertensive intracranial hemorrhage
Internal carotid artery compression by goiter	
Cerebral venous sinus thrombosis	

Table 5.3 Putative mechanisms of atherosclerosis in hypothyroidism

Low thyroxin levels
Elevated LDL cholesterol
Increase diastolic blood pressure
Endothelial dysfunction
High homocysteine levels
Elevated CRP

Note: LDL, low-density lipoprotein cholesterol; CRP, C-reactive protein.

with hyperthyroidism [35]. Choice of antithrombotic therapy is based on other clinical variables, such as the CHADS2 score, a strong predictor of poor outcome independent of stroke severity [36]. The CHADS2 score includes congestive heart failure, hypertension, age > 75 years, diabetes mellitus, and prior stroke or transient ischemic attack (TIA). The CHADS2 score gives one point for each item, and two points for TIA or stroke.

Hypothyroidism
Large and small-vessel atherosclerotic cerebrovascular disease are the most common causes of stroke in hypothyroid patients. Hypothyroidism may be associated with progression of atherosclerosis. Low T4 levels in euthyroid hyperlipidemic patients may be a risk factor for atherosclerosis [37]. Increased cardiovascular morbidity is mostly attributed to elevated serum LDL levels, and increase in diastolic blood pressure [38]. Hypothyroidism may also cause endothelial dysfunction independent of LDL levels [39]. Moreover, low freeT4 levels raise homocysteine concentrations [40], and elevated CRP levels are observed with subclinical hypothyroidism [41]. Coronary artery disease is also common among hypothyroid patients, and women with elevated TSH may be at risk for peripheral arterial disease [42,43]. Mechanisms leading to atherosclerosis in hypothyroid patients are listed in Table 5.3.

Thyroid-replacement therapy may decrease progression of atherosclerosis [44,45]. However, cardiovascular outcomes following thyroid-replacement therapy have not been studied in large randomized controlled clinical trials.

Hyperparathyroidism

Hyperparathyroidism may be primary or secondary. Table 5.4 summarizes stroke subtypes among patients

Table 5.4 Cerebrovascular diseases associated with hyperparathyroidism

Ischemic strokes due to large or small vessel atherosclerotic cerebrovascular disease
Reversible Cerebral Vasoconstriction Syndrome
Intracerebral hemorrhage

with primary or secondary hyperparathyroidism. Excessive secretion of parathyroid hormone (PTH) causes hypercalcemia. Hypercalcemia may also cause arterial hypertension [46]. Elevated PTH levels may also accelerate atherosclerosis and arterial-wall calcification [47]. Vasoconstriction unrelated to arterial hypertension may result in the reversible cerebral vasoconstriction syndrome (RCVS)[48]. Moreover, ischemic stroke may be the initial presentation of primary hyperparathyroidism associated with the multiple endocrine neoplasia syndrome type 1 [49].

Diabetes mellitus

Diabetes mellitus (DM), an independent stroke risk factor, particularly for lacunar infarctions, is currently considered a "stroke risk equivalent" [50,51]. Diabetes mellitus increases stroke morbidity and mortality [52–55]. Strokes are often caused by cerebrovascular atherosclerosis, cardiac embolism, or rheological abnormalities [56] (Table 5.5). Serum glucose concentration and clinical outcomes reflect stress related to

Table 5.5 Strokes in diabetes mellitus

Atherosclerosis	Large-artery thromboembolism
	Small-vessel cerebrovascular disease
	Hemodynamic changes
	Elevated osteoprotegerin (OPG) levels in women
Cardioembolism	Diabetic cardiomyopathy
	Myocardial infarction
	Increased risk of left atrial thrombosis in patients with Afib [60,61]
Rheological	↑ Fibrinogen, factor V, and factor VII
	↑ Platelet adhesiveness and aggregation
	↓ Red blood cell deformability
	↓ Fibrinolytic activity

Note: Modified from ref. [56].

stroke severity, rather than a glucose effect on damaged neurons [57]. Osteoprotegerin (OPG) may be involved in the regulation of vascular calcification [58]. However, a nested case-control study showed no evidence that elevated serum OPG concentrations increased ischemic stroke risk [59].

Diabetes also influences stroke-related outcomes including risk of stroke recurrence. In the Insulin Resistance Atherosclerosis Study (IRAS), DM was associated with increased common carotid artery intimal medial thickness ($P<0.05$) [62]. Quality of stroke care and outcomes among hospitalized diabetic patients were similar to those without diabetes except for rate of r-tPA administration and cholesterol treatment [63]. Diabetic patients of African American ancestry were also less likely to have tighter BP control than whites [64]. Moreover, diabetic patients with history of previous stroke were excluded for intravenous r-tPA in the ECASS-3 study [65].

Diabetic patients with a predicted exercise capacity of >85% have a lower likelihood of stroke, myocardial infarction, or death compared to patients with a predicted exercise capacity of $\leq$85% [66]. Diabetes, homocysteine levels, and HDL levels also predict poorer cognitive function and greater disability following stroke [67]. The metabolic syndrome, a common comorbidity associated with diabetes, is an independent risk factor for stroke among patients without diabetes [68]. Long-term glycemic control prevents the microvascular complications of diabetes, but not the macrovascular complications.

Aldosterone

Ischemic or hemorrhagic strokes may result from primary hyperaldosteronism. Primary aldosteronism may cause arterial hypertension, left ventricular hypertrophy, myocardial infarction, atrial fibrillation, the metabolic syndrome, and glucose impairment. The hypokalemic variant of aldosteronism is associated with a higher cardiovascular morbidity [69]. Moreover, the aldosterone synthase gene (CYP11B2) promoter polymorphism has been found to be a risk factor for ischemic stroke among Tunisian Arabs [70–72].

Hypercortisolism

Cortisol levels increase following acute stroke [73], and an increased hypothalamic–pituitary–adrenal

(HPA) axis activity is common early after stroke [74–76]. Table 5.6 lists the mechanisms leading to stroke in patients with hypercortisolism.

Cortisol also potentiates the vasoconstrictive effects of catecholamines and causes insulin resistance. Hypercortisolism also results in hyperglycemia, obesity, dyslipidemia, and arterial hypertension. Decreased midwall systolic performance and diastolic dysfunction may also increase the risk of cardioembolic stroke [78]. Moreover, increased cortisol levels have been associated with delayed cerebral ischemia following aneurysmal subarachnoid hemorrhage [79].

Although hypercortisolism secondary to Cushing disease is associated with increased cardiovascular risk, adrenalectomy does not decrease the risk of atherosclerotic vascular complications [80].

Adrenal insufficiency

Profound hypotension from acute adrenal insufficiency may result in watershed infarctions. Arterial and venous cerebral infarctions may also be associated with Addison's disease due to a secondary APAS [81].

Testosterone

Low testosterone levels among middle-aged and older men have been associated with insulin resistance, the metabolic syndrome, and diabetes mellitus [82,83]. Low testosterone levels also predict cardiovascular events including TIAs and stroke [84]. Testosterone supplementation may be protective of myocardial ischemia in men with underlying coronary artery disease [85]. Conversely, testosterone supplementation may increase the risk of cardiovascular adverse events among older men with limitations in mobility and high prevalence of chronic disease [86].

Table 5.6 Types of strokes associated with hypercortisolism

Ischemic stroke
Large-vessel atherosclerotic cerebrovascular disease
Small-vessel atherosclerotic cerebrovascular disease
Cardioembolic stroke
Reversible Cerebral Vasoconstriction Syndrome [77].
Hypertensive Intracerebral Hemorrhage
Delayed cerebral ischemia following SAH

Estrogen and hormonal contraceptives

Oral contraceptive (OCP) use is associated with a modest increased risk of ischemic stroke [87–89]. Low estrogen (<50 mcg) OCPs have a lower risk compared to high estrogen (> 50 mcg) OCPs. Progesterone-only OCPs do not increase stroke risk. There is a weak association between OCP use and risk of subarachnoid hemorrhage.

High and low estradiol levels are associated with an increased risk of cardiovascular disease [90]. Hormone-replacement therapy with estrogen only or combined with progesterone increases stroke risk by 40% [91–93].

Arterial and cerebral venous thromboses may also be associated with the ovarian hyperstimulation syndrome. Moreover, ischemic stroke may result from ovarian induction without ovarian hyperstimulation [94–96].

Epinephrine

Arterial hypertension associated with pheochromocytomas and catecholamine-secreting paragangliomas may result in ischemic or hemorrhagic strokes (Figure 5.2a,b,c). Pheochromocytomas may also cause a RCVS and a posterior reversible encephalopathy syndrome (PRES) [97,98].

Electrolyte and other metabolic disorders

Electrolyte and metabolic disorders are commonly found among stroke patients.

Hyponatremia

Hyponatremia is the most common electrolyte disorder among critically ill neurological patients. True hyponatremia may be hypervolemic, euvolemic, or hypovolemic. Hyponatremia complicating aneurysmal SAH is most commonly due to the syndrome of inappropriate secretion of antidiuretic hormone (SIADH) [99,100]. Rarely, hyponatremia may mimic an acute stroke or be associated with subdural hemorrhage [101]. Management decisions depend on the underlying symptomatology and require careful assessment of volume status, discontinuation of any drugs potentially responsible for hyponatremia (e.g., carbamazepine, NSAIDS, SSRIs), symptom relief, prevention of progression of neurologic deficits, and avoidance of excessive correction with subsequent risk of osmotic demyelination syndrome [102,103]. Table 5.7 lists cerebrovascular diseases associated with SIADH and CSWS.

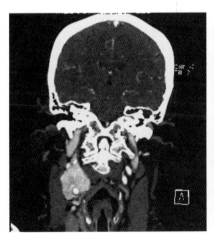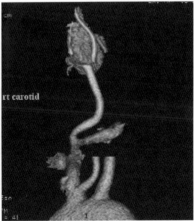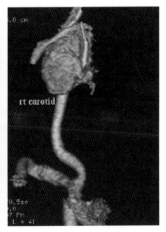

Fig 5.2 A 75-year-old woman with hemispheric TIAs. CT angiogram showed a 3 × 2 × 3.8 cm mass centered at the bifurcation of the right common carotid artery, consistent with a carotid body tumor (paraganglioma). (See also Plate 5.2).

Table 5.7 SIADH and CSWS in cerebrovascular diseases

Ischemic stroke
Intracerebral hemorrhage
Subarachnoid hemorrhage
Cerebral venous sinus thrombosis
Arteriovenous malformation
Subdural hemorrhage
Epidural hemorrhage

Note: SIADH, syndrome of inappropriate secretion of antidiuretic hormone; CSWS, cerebral salt wasting syndrome.

Hypernatremia

Ischemic and hemorrhagic strokes may result from hypernatremic dehydration [104,105]. Hypernatremia in stroke patients may also result from diabetes insipidus. Hypernatremia is often iatrogenic and frequently associated with poor prognosis [106]. Following aneurysmal SAH, hypernatremia correlates with low left ventricular ejection fraction (LVEF), elevated cardiac troponin levels, and pulmonary edema [107,108]. Management requires proper calculation of water deficits, adequate free water replacement, and limitation of sodium intake.

Calcium

Hypercalcemia induces vasoconstriction, enhances platelet adhesion and aggregation, and may cause arterial hypertension. Rarely, cerebral embolization from calcific aortic or mitral valves is due to underlying hypercalcemia [109].

Magnesium

Magnesium is a noncompetitive antagonist of voltage-dependent calcium channels. Hypomagnesemia may result in delayed cerebral ischemia and worse clinical outcomes following aneurysmal SAH and ischemic strokes. During the acute stroke period, hypomagnesemia correlates with the degree of ischemic injury. Magnesium deficiency may also promote the development and progression of large vessel atherosclerotic cerebrovascular disease. The efficacy of intravenous magnesium in acute ischemic stroke has not yet been established [110–113].

Bone metabolism and stroke

Decreased bone mineral density (BMD) and osteoporosis of the femoral neck correlates with risk of stroke and death [114]. Reduced levels of vitamin D have also been proposed as a potential stroke risk [115,116]. Moreover, among post-menopausal women, carotid artery atherosclerosis plaque scores correlated with low total BMD [117]. Furthermore, elderly disabled patients with stroke with serum 25-OH vitamin D concentrations of < 12 nmol/L had an increased risk of hip fractures. Supplemental vitamin D and elemental calcium may reduce the risk of hip fractures and prevent further decrease in BMD among patients with longstanding hemiparetic strokes [118].

Systemic autoimmune disorders

Strokes in systemic autoimmune disorders may result from vasculitis or cardioembolism. Vasculitis affecting the brain may be infectious or noninfectious, and may be complicated by ischemic or hemorrhagic strokes. Cerebral vasculitis may involve small, medium, or large caliber blood vessels. Figure 5.3 illustrates an approach to noninfectious vasculitis. Table 5.8 lists subtypes of cerebrovascular disorders associated with a selected group of autoimmune disorders. Detailed description of each entity is beyond the scope of this review.

Wegener's granulomatosis

Wegener's granulomatosis (WG) is a multisystem small-vessel vasculitis [119] WG involves small arteries, arterioles, and venules, and is characterized by necrotizing granulomas of the upper and lower respiratory tract, and glomerulonephritis. The paranasal sinuses and lungs are most commonly affected. Peripheral nervous system (mononeuropathy, mononeuropathy multiplex, or polyneuropathy) involvement is more common. Ischemic and hemorrhagic strokes, cerebral venous thrombosis, retinal and optic nerve ischemia, and a vasculitic encephalopathy have been reported [120–122]. Cardioembolic strokes may result from non-bacterial thrombotic endocarditis (NBTE) [123]. Orbital pseudotumor, hypertrophic pachymeningitis,

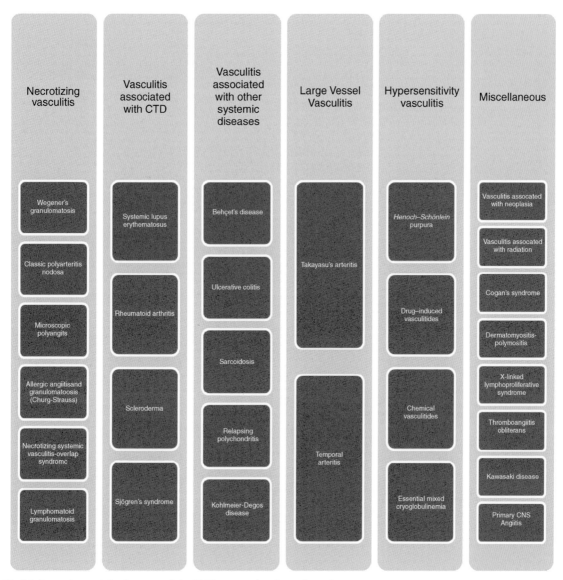

Fig 5.3 Systemic, noninfectious vasculitis. (CTD: connective tissue disease).

and myelopathies may be observed as well. Most affected persons have elevated antineutrophil cytoplasmic antibodies (cANCA). Lower cANCA levels may be seen in inactive or localized forms of the disease. CT of the sinuses and orbits may show opacification of the sinuses or bony destruction. MRI may demonstrate focal granulomas or strokes. Treatment is with a combination of corticosteroids and cyclophosphamide. Other options include methotrexate, azathioprine, mycophenolate mofetil, or rituximab.

Polyarteritis nodosa

Polyarteritis nodosa (PAN) is a focal, segmental, necrotizing vasculitis with a predilection for small and medium caliber blood vessels [119,124,125]. PAN is often associated with chronic hepatitis B infection. The kidneys are preferentially involved. Coronary artery involvement may cause myocardial infarction or heart failure. Mononeuropathies, mononeuropathy multiplex, and polyneuropathy are the most common neurological manifestations. Ischemic stroke subtypes are most often

Table 5.8 Stroke types of selected systemic autoimmune disorders and vasculitides

Autoimmune disorder	Cerebrovascular disease
Wegener's granulomatosis	Ischemic stroke
	SVD
	LVD
	Cardioembolic
	ICH
	SAH
	CVST
	Vasculitic encephalopathy
Polyarteritis nodosa	Ischemic stroke
	LVD
	Cardioembolism
	ICH
	SAH
Microscopic polyangiitis	Ischemic stroke
	Hemorrhagic stroke
	Spinal SAH
Churg Strauss syndrome	Ischemic stroke
	Vasculitis
	CRAO
	Cardioembolic
	ICH
	CVST
Rheumatic fever	Cardioembolic stroke
	Rheumatic AFib
	Prosthetic heart valve
	Hemorrhagic stroke from anticoagulant use
SLE and APAS	Prothrombotic states
	Cardioembolism
	Valvulopathy
	Atrial fibrillation
	Atherosclerosis
	CVST
	Vascular cognitive impairment
	AION
Rheumatoid arthritis	Vessel compression
	Accelerated atherosclerosis
	CNS vasculitis
	Focal ischemia
	Diffuse cerebritis
	ICH
	SAH
Sjögren syndrome	Hypercoagulable states
	APAS
	CNS vasculitis
	Vasculitic encephalopathy

Table 5.8 (*Continued*)

Autoimmune disorder	Cerebrovascular disease
Temporal arteritis	AION/PION/CRAO/BRAO/Choroidal ischemia
	Ischemic stroke
	Spinal cord ischemia
Takayasu disease	Ischemic stroke
	Hemorrhagic stroke
	Aneurysmal SAH
	Subclavian Steal Syndrome
Ankylosing Spondylitis	Arterial compression
	Spinal cord ischemia

Note: Afib, atrial fibrillation; AION: anterior ischemic optic neuropathy; PION, posterior ischemic optic neuropathy; CRAO, central retinal artery occlusion; BRAO, branch retinal artery occlusion; ICH, intracerebral hemorrhage; SVD, small-vessel disease; LVD, large-vessel disease; SAH, subarachnoid hemorrhage.

lacunar, but large artery involvement and cardioembolic strokes may be observed. Strokes may also be secondary to the APAS [126]. Intracerebral hemorrhage results from underlying arterial hypertension secondary to renal involvement [127–129]. SAH results from intracranial aneurysm rupture [130–132]. Retinal vasculitis may account for ocular ischemia or hemorrhages [133]. Angiography may demonstrate arterial beading or microaneurysms. Diagnosis requires tissue (kidney, skin, muscle/peripheral nerve) biopsy. Treatment is with corticosteroids and cyclophosphamide. Antivirals are used in hepatitis B positive patients.

Microscopic polyangiitis

Microscopic polyangiitis (MPA), is a small vessel necrotizing and nongranulomatous vasculitis with preferential involvement for the kidneys and lungs (Goodpasture syndrome) [134]. The most common presentation of MPA is with alveolitis associated with a nephritic or nephrotic syndrome secondary to crescentic glomerulonephritis. Mononeuropathy multiplex or polyneuropathy are the most common neurological manifestations. Ischemic and hemorrhagic strokes, and spinal SAH are seldom observed [135–138]. Acute phase reactants in serum are usually elevated. More specific markers are the ANCA with perinuclear immune-fluorescent distribution (p-ANCA) and the proteinase-3 ANCA (PR3-ANCA). Diagnosis is confirmed with biopsy (renal, lung, muscle/nerve). Treatment is with corticosteroids and cyclophosphamide. Plasmapheresis is useful in selected patients.

Churg strauss syndrome

Churg Strauss syndrome (CSS), also known as allergic granulomatosis, is a rare, idiopathic, eosinophilic, necrotizing granulomatous small-vessel vasculitis. Asthma is the usual initial clinical manifestation. The skin, heart, and gastrointestinal tract are also frequently involved. Cranial neuropathies, mononeuropathies, mononeuropathy multiplex, and polyneuropathies, are the most common neurological complications. Albeit rare, ischemic and hemorrhagic strokes, cerebral venous sinus thrombosis, and central retinal artery occlusion have been reported [139–145]. Marked eosinophilia is evident, P-ANCA may be positive, and antimyeloperoxidase activity may be elevated. Patients with negative P-ANCA have a higher risk of cardiomyopathy. Treatment is with corticosteroids and cyclophosphamide. Unresponsive patients may require other immunosuppressive agents or plasma exchange.

Connective tissue diseases (CTD)

Systemic lupus erythematosus (SLE) and rheumatic fever (RF) are often associated with mitral and/or aortic valvular heart involvement. Atrial fibrillation is a common complication of rheumatic mitral stenosis. The cardiac inflammatory response may eventually lead to thromboembolism.

Ischemic strokes among patients with SLE may result from accelerated atherosclerosis, hypercoagulability (e.g., APAS), endothelial dysfunction,

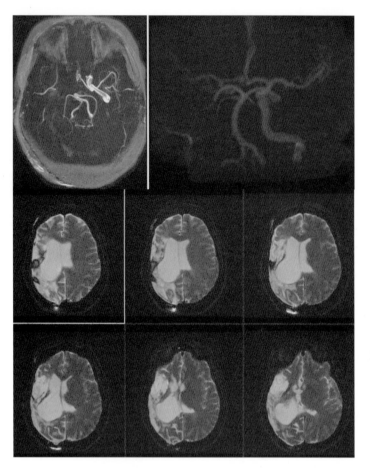

Fig 5.4 A 25-year-old woman with history of SLE, APAS, immune thrombocytopenic purpura, and hereditary spherocytosis (status post splenectomy), had sudden onset of left hemiparesis. T2-weighted MRI of the brain showed a right middle cerebral artery territory infarction. MRA showed absent flow of the right internal carotid artery.

mitral/aortic valvulopathy (Libman–Sacks endocarditis), or arterial hypertension. True immune-mediated CNS vasculitis is uncommon. SAH is rarely seen. Focal seizures may result from local vasculopathy, due to circulating immune complexes. Transverse myelopathy may result from thrombosis or vasculitis. True vasculitis is treated with high-dose intravenous methylprednisolone. The use of cyclophosphamide, azathioprine, or IVIG remains anecdotal.

Antiphospholipid antibodies (aPLs) are acquired antibodies against anionic phospholipid-containing moieties in cell membrane [146]. The IgG isotypes of anticardiolipin (aCL) and lupus anticoagulant (LA) are the aPLs mostly associated with risk for first ischemic stroke (Figure 5.4a,b,c) [147]. Their presence is often associated with the APAS, an acquired auto-immune prothrombotic syndrome associated with arterial and venous thrombosis, recurrent unexplained

fetal loss, and thrombocytopenia. Diagnosis of APAS is based on clinical and laboratory criteria [148]. Specific therapy and duration of treatment must be determined on an individual basis [147]. Positivity of aPLs in healthy individuals may not confer increased vascular thrombo-occlusive risk; therefore, prophylactic use of antiaggregants in those individuals may not be necessary. Antiplatelet is preferred over anticoagulation therapy in patients with arterial strokes without evidence of venous thrombosis [147].

Rheumatoid arthritis (RA) may predispose to stroke [149–154]. Use of selective cyclo-oxygenase-2 (COX-2) inhibitors has been linked with an increased risk of cardiovascular events including strokes [155]. A small and medium caliber panarteritis may complicate longstanding erosive, nodular RA associated with positive rheumatoid factor. Albeit rare, rheumatoid cerebral vasculitis may present with focal brain ischemia or intracranial hemorrhage.

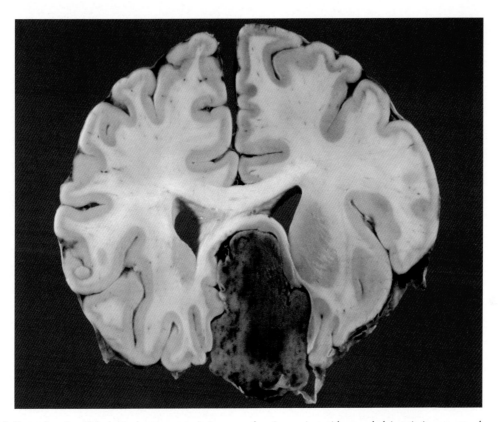

Plate 5.1 Coronal section of the brain demonstrates pituitary apoplexy in a patient with an underlying pituitary macroadenoma

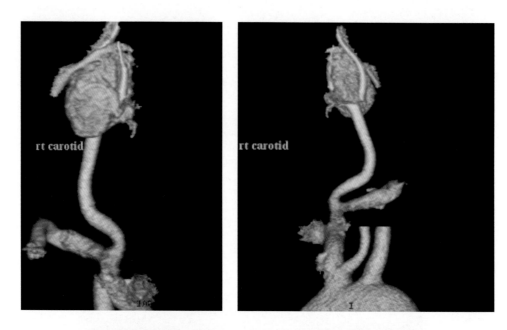

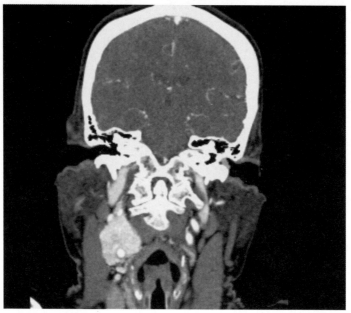

Plate 5.2 A 75-year-old woman with hemispheric TIAs. CT angiogram showed a 3 × 2 × 3.8 cm mass centered at the bifurcation of the right common carotid artery, consistent with a carotid body tumor (paraganglioma).

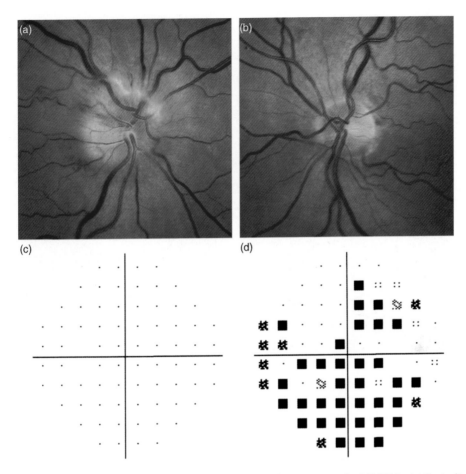

Plate 7.1 Typical examination findings in non-arteritic anterior ischemic optic neuropathy (NAION). (a) Optic-disc edema with associated hemorrhages in the affected right eye, as seen within several days of the onset of visual loss. Note that the disc edema is more severe at the superior aspect of the disc. (b) The optic disc in the unaffected left eye is structurally congested with a small cup (that is, a "disc at risk"). (c) Pattern deviation from the Humphrey visual field of the unaffected left eye is normal. (d) Pattern deviation of the affected right eye shows inferior altitudinal and central visual-field defects.

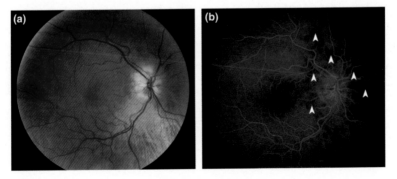

Plate 7.5 Typical examination and fluorescein angiogram findings in arteritic anterior ischemic optic neuropathy secondary to giant cell arteritis. (a) Pallid optic-disc edema in the right eye, as seen within several days of the onset of visual loss. (b) Fluorescein angiogram of the right eye shows areas of choroidal nonperfusion (arrowheads), which are not evident on funduscopic examination, but are highly suggestive of giant cell arteritis.

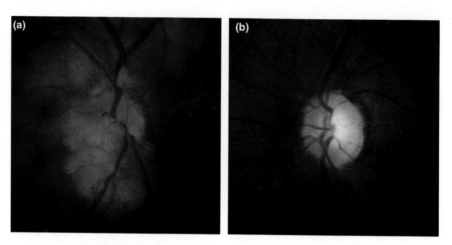

Plate 7.6 Optic-disc granuloma secondary to sarcoidosis. (a) The optic disc in the affected right eye is partially obscured by a large granuloma. The granuloma disappeared following several months of corticosteroid treatment. (b) The optic disc in the unaffected left eye is normal.

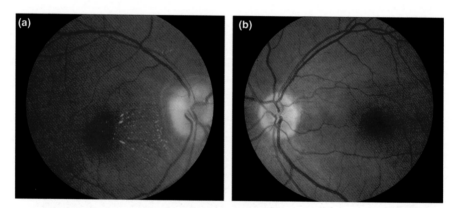

Plate 7.10 Neuroretinitis due to cat scratch disease. The patient had a history of exposure to cats and positive *Bartonella henselae* titers. (a) Optic-disc edema and a partial macular star figure are present in the affected right eye. (b) Normal optic disc and macula in the unaffected left eye.

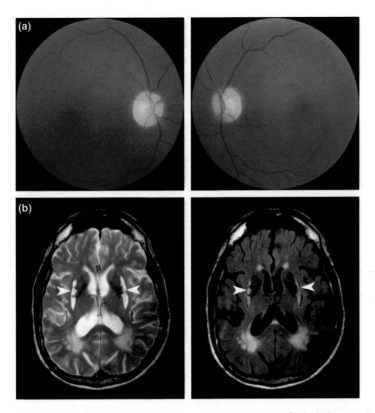

Plate 7.11 Bilateral toxic optic neuropathies due to methanol ingestion in a patient with alcoholism. (a) Diffuse optic atrophy is present in both eyes several months after the visual loss developed. (b) Axial T2-weighted and FLAIR MRI show periventricular white-matter signal changes and putaminal necrosis (arrowheads), a highly characteristic finding in patients with methanol poisoning.

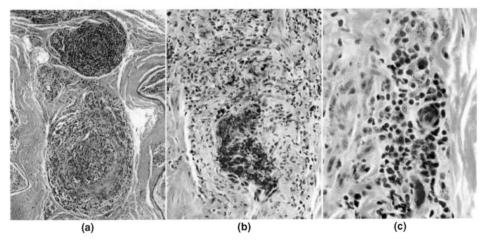

Plate 11.2 Sural nerve biopsy. (a) Transverse H&E section demonstrating epineurial perivascular inflammation with disruption of the vessel wall. (b) Longitudinal Masson-Trichrome section demonstrating fibrinoid necrosis. (c) Longitudinal Masson-Trichome preparation demonstrating hemosiderin-laden macrophages. Findings were diagnostic for necrotizing vasculitis

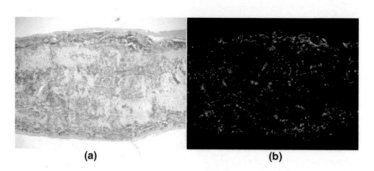

(a)   **(b)**

Plate 11.4 Targeted fascicular sciatic nerve biopsy. (a) Transverse paraffin section demonstrating amorphous congophilic material throughout the endoneurium and (b) apple-green birefringence with polarized light, diagnostic of amyloid

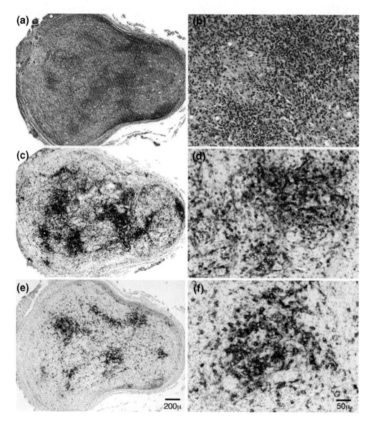

Plate 11.5 Targeted fascicular sciatic nerve biopsy. Transverse paraffin sections demonstrating immature mononuclear cells extensively infiltrating the endoneurium of a nerve fascicle (a, b) with reactivity for CD45 (lymphocytes) (c, d) and CD20 (B-cells) (e, f) diagnostic of B-cell neurolymphomatosis

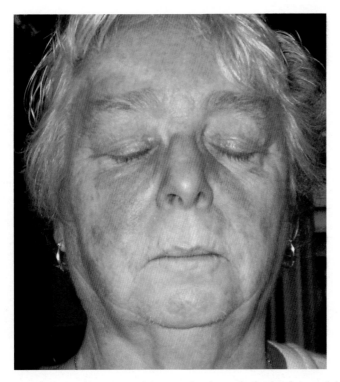

Plate 13.3 Dermatomyositis. Moderate erythematous rash is appreciated over the forehead, around the eyes, and across the malar region of the face.

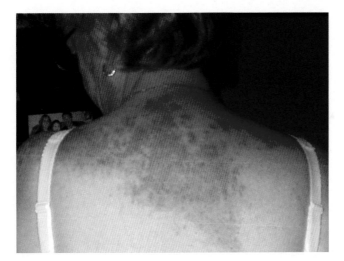

Plate 13.4 Dermatomyositis. Maculopapular erythematous rash across the upper back and posterior neck (shawl sign).

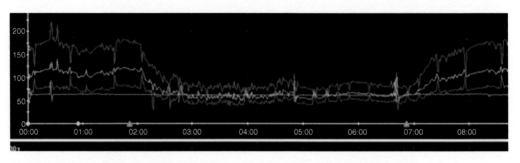

Plate 14.1 Tilt-table testing in familial amyloidosis. This figure demonstrates orthostatic hypotension on head-up tilt-table testing in a patient with transthyretin (Phe64Leu) amyloidosis, due to severe autonomic neuropathy.

Treatment is with corticosteroids; cyclophosphamide may be required. Rheumatoid involvement of the cervical spine may rarely compromise vertebral artery blood flow.

A few patients with scleroderma have a focal cerebral arteritis. Treatment is with corticosteroids [156,157]. Central nervous system (CNS) involvement in Sjögren syndrome may present with encephalopathy or strokes [158]. Arterial compression associated with ankylosing spondylitis is a rare cause of stroke [159]. Spinal cord infarction is an unusual complication of ankylosing spondylitis.

Vasculitis associated with other systemic diseases

Behçet's disease, more prevalent among Middle Eastern and Mediterranean populations, is a multisystem small-vessel vasculitis characterized by relapsing, painful orogenital ulcerations, iritis, uveitis, polyarthritis, synovitis, erythema nodosum, and cutaneous vasculitis [160–163]. Arterial and venous involvements are frequent. Systemic and pulmonary circulation aneurysms may develop. Meningoencephalitis, CNS white-matter involvement, and cerebral venous thrombosis are the most frequent manifestations of neuro-Behçet's. Other neurological manifestations include cerebral and retinal vasculitis. Treatment is with corticosteroids. Other options include cyclophosphamide, azathioprine, chlorambucil, infliximab, or etanercept. Cerebral venous thrombosis is treated with a combination of anticoagulants and corticosteroids.

Strokes associated with ulcerative colitis may result from an underlying hypercoagulable state or cerebral vasculitis [164,165]. Common manifestations of neurosarcoidosis include cranial neuropathies (CN VII), meningoencephalitis, hydrocephalus, peripheral neuropathy, or myopathy. The exceptional vasculitic form of sarcoidosis primarily affects the eyes, meninges, cerebral arteries, and veins [166].

Cerebral arteritis can also complicate relapsing polychondritis [167,168] a rare disorder of cartilage, characterized by auricular, nasal, and laryngotracheal chondritis. Aortic regurgitation is a frequent complication. Neurovascular complications include ischemic and hemorrhagic strokes.

Kohlmeier–Degos disease, also known as malignant atrophic papulosis, is an unusual vaso-occlusive disease of unknown etiology. Necrotizing arteritic skin lesions often antedate neurological manifestations.

Cerebrovascular complications include ischemic and hemorrhagic strokes [169].

Large-vessel arteritidies

Giant cell arteritis (temporal arteritis) is a large vessel arteritis most commonly found among people of Northern European ancestry, particularly Scandinavians, who have the highest incidence [170]. The disease is rare among African Americans. The disease is observed among patients older than 50 years of age. Typical presentation includes unilateral temporal headaches, jaw claudication, polymyalgia rheumatica, visual loss, and elevation of inflammatory markers (ESR and CRP). Tongue numbness may result from lingual ischemia [171]. Blindness most often results from anterior ischemic optic neuropathy (arteritic anterior ischemic neuropathy). Other neuro-ophthalmological complications include posterior ischemic optic neuropathy (PION), central and branch retinal artery occlusion, choroidal ischemia, diplopia, eyelid ptosis, pupillary abnormalities, nystagmus, and internuclear ophthalmoplegia [172–175]. Diagnosis is confirmed with temporal artery biopsy. If clinical suspicion is high and unilateral biopsy is negative, the contralateral superficial temporal artery is biopsied. Treatment is with high-dose corticosteroids.

Takayasu disease is an idiopathic granulomatous large-vessel arteritis affecting mostly the aortic arch and its branches. Involvement of the media and elastic lamina eventually leads to fibrosis with consequent hardening of the vessel wall and luminal narrowing. Takayasu disease is more common among young women (usually 15–40 years of age). Patients of Asian ancestry have a higher risk. Constitutional symptoms are common. Limb ischemia causes claudication. Proximal subclavian artery stenosis may lead to a subclavian steal syndrome [176]. Intracerebral hemorrhage may result from secondary hypertension or ruptured intracranial aneurysms [177–179]. Ischemic strokes result from arterial steno-occlusive disease or artery to artery embolism [180]. Elevated antiphospholipid antibodies have been associated with Takayasu arteritis [181]. Management of intracerebral hemorrhage requires tight blood pressure control. Antithrombotics are used in cases of ischemic stroke. Corticosteroids are used to decrease disease progression.

Hypersensitivity vasculitis

Hypersensitivity vasculitides or angiitis are also known as leukocytoclastic vasculitis (LCV) [182]. Patients with LCV develop skin lesions, particularly on the legs. The disease may be localized to the skin or may involve other organs. The joints, gastrointestinal tract, and kidneys are most commonly affected. Examples of LCV are Henoch–Schönlein purpura (HSP), drug-induced LCV, and cryoglobulinemia.

HSP, a systemic small-vessel vasculitis characterized by immunoglobulin A (IgA), C3, and immune complex deposition, usually affects children. Most common clinical manifestations are purpura, arthralgias, abdominal pain, and hematuria. Involvement of the cerebral vessels can cause brain infarction and intracerebral or subarachnoid hemorrhage [183–189]. Some patients present with PRES. Treatment is often supportive. Most patients with cerebral involvement are treated with corticosteroids.

A variety of drugs associated with CNS vasculitides can result in reversible cerebral vasonstriction syndrome (RCVS) [190–192]. Table 5.9 list drugs associated with RCVS and CNS vasculitis.

Table 5.9 Drugs associated with reversible cerebral vasoconstriction syndrome

Selective serotonin reuptake inhibitors (SSRIs)
Cannabis
Cocaine
Ecstasy
Amphetamines
Lysergic acid diethylamide (LSD)
Alcohol (binge drinking)
Tacrolimus (FK-506)
Cyclophosphamide
Intravenous immunoglobulin (IVIG)
Interferon alpha
Ephedrine
Pseudoephedrine
Phenylpropanolamine
Bromocriptine
Lisuride
Triptans
Ergotamine tartrate
Isometheptene
Ginseng
Methergine
Nicotine patches

Cryoglobulinemia most commonly affects the kidneys and skin. Cryoglobulin-containing immune complexes may cause vasculitis. The Brouet classification of cryoglobulinemia includes simple (type I or monoclonal) and mixed (type II and type III). Mixed cryoglobulinemia is often associated with hepatitis C virus infection. A vasculitic neuropathy is the most common neurologic manifestation. Central nervous system involvement may be responsible for ischemic or hemorrhagic strokes and cerebral venous thrombosis [193]. Treatment is with immunosuppressants.

Organ dysfunction and failure

Heart failure

In the Survival and Ventricular Enlargement study (SAVE), for every 5% reduction in the LVEF there was an 18% increase risk of stroke [194]. The multicenter Studies of Left Ventricular Dysfunction (SOLVD) showed that for every 10% decrease in EF, there was a 58% increase risk of stroke among women but not in men [195]. However, in another multicenter cohort study, LVEF < 50% was independently associated with an increased stroke risk in both men and women [196]. Takotsubo disease or "neurogenic stunned cardiomyopathy" is often observed after subarachnoid hemorrhage and may be a potential cause of cardioembolic stroke [197].

Respiratory failure

Stroke patients are at an increased risk of aspiration pneumonia, pulmonary embolism, neurogenic pulmonary edema, or acute respiratory distress syndrome. Pulmonary embolism remains the most preventable cause of hospital death [198]. Stroke patients have an increased risk of deep vein thrombosis. Paradoxical embolism may be a cause of ischemic stroke in patients with pulmonary embolism [199,200]. An ongoing prospective study is evaluating "silent cerebral infarcts" diagnosed by restricted diffusion on MRI among patients with pulmonary embolism and a patent foramen ovale [201].

Gastrointestinal disorders and liver failure

Gastrointestinal bleeding (GIB) is a rare occurrence after stroke [202]. In the Registry of the Canadian

Stroke Network, GIB was independently associated with death or severe dependence at discharge and mortality at 6 months [203]. Patients with cardioembolic stroke are at an increased risk of visceral thromboembolism. Subdiaphragmatic visceral infarction is a rare occurrence among patients with fatal stroke [204].

Impaired cerebral autoregulation, cerebral hyperemia, and altered reactivity to carbon dioxide have been found among patients with liver failure [205]. Cerebral hyperemia plays an important role in the development of cerebral edema, and recovery of cerebral hemodynamics and metabolic stability have been observed after orthotopic liver transplantation in patients with fulminant liver failure [205,206]. Impaired coagulation and platelet function may result in intracranial hemorrhage.

Renal failure

Low effective glomerular filtration rate (eGFR) on admission is an independent predictor of stroke mortality [207]. Hypertension is an independent and treatable factor leading to ischemic or hemorrhagic stroke. Secondary hypertension must always be suspected in stroke patients, particularly in those with a history of refractory hypertension or hypertension at a young age [208]. Renal dysfunction is also an independent predictor of adverse outcome in aneurysmal subarachnoid hemorrhage [209].

Arterial and venous strokes may be associated with nephrotic and nephritic syndromes [210]. Arterial thrombosis is more common in cases of membranous glomerulonephritis whereas cerebral venous thrombosis is more common in cases of minimal-change disease [211–213].

Cancer and paraneoplastic disorders

Ischemic and hemorrhagic strokes often complicate a variety of neoplastic disorders. Ischemic strokes may result from NBTE, tumoral embolism, underlying hypercoagulability, hyperviscosity associated with paraproteinemic or myeloproliferative disorders, adverse effects of chemotherapy, radiation-induced accelerated atherosclerosis, tumoral encasement of intracranial blood vessels, or neoplastic angioendotheliomatosis (angiotropic lymphoma). Hemorrhagic strokes result from underlying bleeding diatheses,

disseminated intravascular coagulation (DIC), hemorrhagic metastases, ruptured neoplastic intracranial aneurysms, radiation vasculopathy, or cerebral sinovenous thrombosis. Table 5.10 illustrates mechanisms of stroke associated with cancer [214,215]. Proposed mechanisms of thrombosis associated with malignancies are shown in Table 5.11.

Chemotherapy and stroke

Chemotherapeutic agents associated with stroke or "stroke like syndromes" include L-asparaginase, BCNU, bevacizumab, bleomycin, carboplatin, cisplatin, danazol, doxorubicin, erlotinib, erythropoietin, estramustine, 5-fluorouracil, interleukin, imatinib mesylate, methotrexate, mitomycin, nelarabine, and tamoxifen [216].

Systemic infectious diseases

Cerebral vasculitis may also be secondary to a variety of bacterial, viral, fungal, rickettsial, spirochetal, or parasitic organisms [217,218]. *Chlamydia pneumoniae*, *Helicobacter pylori*, and cytomegalovirus have been associated with progression of atherosclerosis [219,220]. Furthermore, ischemic strokes may follow systemic infections, particularly those involving the respiratory tract [221].

Bacterial meningitis

Arterial ischemic strokes among patients with purulent acute bacterial meningitis may result from arterial encroachment by purulent exudates in the subarachnoid space, infective cerebral arteritis, or cerebral vasospasm [222]. Intracranial hemorrhage may be secondary to ruptured infectious (mycotic) aneurysms or cerebral sino-venous thrombosis [223].

Infective endocarditis

Strokes may be the initial presentation of infective endocarditis (IE). Most strokes are ischemic and often the result of embolism of infected material. Intracranial hemorrhage may be secondary to ruptured mycotic aneurysms or septic arteritis. Prodromal symptoms may occur prior to mycotic aneurysmal rupture [224]. Most mycotic aneurysms regress with

Table 5.10 Stroke in patients with cancer

Ischemic stroke	Hemorrhagic stroke

• Cardioembolism
  ○ NBTE
  ○ Atrial myxoma
• Large and small-vessel cerebrovascular disease
  ○ Accelerated atherosclerosis
• Hypoperfusion
  ○ Arterial compression
  ○ Arterial hypotension
• Hypercoagulable states
  ○ Cancer-associated thrombosis
  ○ Hyperviscosity
• Blood-vessel encasement
  ○ Meningioma
• Cancer-therapy related
  ○ Radiation vasculopathy
  ○ Chemotherapy
    ■ L-asparaginase
    ■ Platinum compounds
    ■ Fluorouracil
    ■ Mitomycin
    ■ Tamoxifen
    ■ Growth factors
    ■ Erythropoietin
  ○ Central venous catheters
    ■ Thrombosis with right to left shunt
	• Hemorrhagic metastases
	• Blood dyscrasias
	• Cerebral venous sinus thrombosis
	• Atrial fibrillation
	  ○ Postoperative AFib
	  ○ Compression of left atrium or pulmonary veins by esophageal cancer

Table 5.11 Possible mechanisms of thrombosis associated with cancer

	Pathophysiology
Macrophage or monocyte interaction with cancer cells	Release of IL-1, IL-6, TNF-alpha Activation of platelets, factor X, and factor XII Release of tissue factor
Endothelial dysfunction	L-1, IL-6, and TNF-alpha-induced endothelial dysfunction Chemotherapy-induced endothelial dysfunction
Substances in tumor cells	Cysteine proteases Tissue factor

Note: IL, interleukin; TNF, tumor necrosis factor.

the use of antibiotics alone. Ruptured mycotic aneurysm require surgical or endovascular treatment.

Tuberculosis

Strokes are a frequent complication of tuberculous (TB) meningitis. Most commonly involving lenticulostriate branches of the middle or anterior cerebral arteries, strokes due to TB meningitis carry a high mortality and morbidity [225].

Septic cerebral venous sinus thrombosis

Infections spreading from the sphenoid and ethmoid sinuses may cause septic cavernous sinus venous thrombosis. Cavernous sinus thrombosis can cause ischemic stroke due to carotid artery occlusion [226].

Leptospirosis

Leptospirosis may be complicated by hemorrhagic strokes. Ischemic stroke may result from infectious vasculitis or moyamoya like syndrome [227].

Meningovascular syphilis

Meningovascular syphilis is observed in the late stages of the disease. Pathologic studies demonstrate a lymphomonocellular proliferative endarteritis with transmural and perivascular infiltration as well as subintimal fibroblastic proliferation. Heubner's arteritis describes the predominant involvement of medium and large size arteries. Nissl–Alzheimer's arteritis describes the predominant involvement of arterioles. Angiitis results in luminal narrowing leading to ischemic stroke or aneurymal formation leading to intracerebral or subarachnoid hemorrhage. Meningovascular syphilis as a cause of stroke should be suspected among young patients with history of sexually transmitted disease or HIV [228,229].

Fungal infections

Most common fungal organisms associated with stroke are Aspergillus, Cryptococcus, Phycomycetes (Mucor, Rhizopus, Absidia), Histoplasma, Candida, and Coccidioides. The most common *Aspergillus* species associated with stroke is *Aspergillus fumigatus*. Frequently observed among cardiac transplant patients, *Aspergillus fumigatus* is angioinvasive leading to vasculitis and weakening of the arterial wall. Intracerebral and SAH may occur either from rupture of a vessel or a mycotic aneurysm. Ischemic stroke is often due to intravascular thrombosis or embolization of fungal vegetations. Ischemic strokes carry a high risk for hemorrhagic transformation [230].

Human immunodeficiency virus

HIV infection increases the risk of ischemic stroke and ICH [231]. Among HIV-infected patients, cerebral infarctions are uncommon in the absence of cerebral non-HIV infection, lymphoma, or embolic sources [232]. HIV cerebral vasculopathy is associated with cerebral aneurysms [233,234],. Polymorphisms in the SDF1 and CX3CR1 gene and the CD4 cell count influence the course of atherosclerosis in patients with HIV

[235]. Combination antiretroviral therapy is an independent predictor of subclinical atherosclerosis in HIV-infected patients [236]. Cytomegalovirus can infect endothelial cells, possibly contributing to CNS vasculopathy [237]. Use of illicit drugs is an important comorbidity in cases of HIV associated stroke [238].

Ischemic stroke may also be the initial presentation of cryptococcal meningitis in AIDS [239] A brain abscess due to toxoplasma may have a stroke-like presentation [240]. The immune reconstitution inflammatory syndrome may manifest with extensive leukoaraiosis [241].

Cerebrospinal fluid (CSF) is abnormal in more than half of patients with stroke associated with HIV [242]. Hypercoagulable studies must be interpreted carefully when evaluating HIV-associated stroke, since false positive results may occur [243].

Infections in the international traveler

Several endemic tropical diseases may account for strokes in the international traveler [244]. Examples include Dengue fever, cerebral malaria, arbovirus-related encephalitis, and Chagas disease. Dengue fever, transmitted by the bite of the *Aedes aeypti* or *Aedes albopictus* mosquito, may present as ischemic stroke [245]. Patients with dengue hemorrhagic fever (DHF) complicated by acute renal failure are more likely to have a prior history of stroke [246]. Ischemic stroke, with or without cerebral edema, may also be the initial presentation of cerebral malaria due to *Plasmodium falciparum* [247,248]. Japanese encephalitis has been reported to cause stroke [249]. Strokes may also be the initial presentation of neurocysticercosis [250–252]. Cardiomyopathy is an independent risk factor of stroke in Chagas disease [253].

Complications due to organ transplantation

Cerebrovascular disease in organ transplant recipients includes ischemic stroke, intracranial hemorrhage, and CVST (Table 5.12) [254–265]. Since most neurological and neurovascular complications overlap with various types of organ transplantation, we will focus our discussion focus on heart, lung, and kidney transplantation.

Table 5.12 Neurological complications in organ-transplant recipients

Ischemic stroke	Intracranial hemorrhage	CVST
Cardioembolism	Hemorrhagic conversion of ischemic stroke	Dehydration
Intracardiac thrombosis		Opportunistic infections
Infective endocarditis	Blood dyscrasias	
Atherosclerosis of large or small vessels	Coagulopathy	Hypercoagulable states
Global hypoperfusion	Thrombocytopathy	
Anoxic encephalopathy	Angioinvasive fungal infection	
Watershed infarctions	Aneurymal SAH	
Hypercoagulable states		
Polycythemia (kidney transplantation)		
Angioinvasive fungal infection		
Cerebral vasculitis associated with GVHD		
Spinal cord ischemia due to iliac arteries for allograft blood supply in kidney-transplant recipients		

Note: GVHD, graft versus host disease; SAH, subarachnoid hemorrhage; CVST, cerebral venous sinus thrombosis.

Heart transplantation

During the immediate post-transplantation period, mechanisms involved in neurologic dysfunction include arterial hypotension, cardioembolism from postoperative arrhythmias, left-ventricular thrombus, and intracerebral hemorrhage. Air embolism may occur at the time of implantation of mechanical circulatory support systems. Atherosclerotic aortic arch plaque and carotid atherosclerosis are other sources of emboli. Neurologic complications developing months following heart transplantation are frequently due to opportunistic infections, immunosuppressant side effects, or lymphoproliferative disorders [266,267].

Lung transplantation

Neurological complications are quite frequent following lung transplantation (Figure 5.5). Encephalopathy is the most common neurological complication; perioperative stroke and encephalopathy are the most common severe neurological complications. Bilateral lung transplantation increases the risk for severe neurological complications. Cerebrovascular events include ischemic infarctions, subarachnoid hemorrhage, intraventricular hemorrhage, and intracerebral hemorrhage. Intracerebral hemorrhage may result from invasive aspergillosis. Cerebrovascular complications often occur during the first year post-lung transplantation [268].

Renal transplantation

Neurological complications, including stroke, are a major contributor to morbidity and mortality among renal-transplant patients. Hypertension, diabetes, and accelerated atherosclerosis may be acquired during dialysis or following renal transplantation. Calcineurin-inhibitors may cause PRES [269]. Severe neurological syndromes may also be caused by the monoclonal antibody OKT3 with associated dysfunction of the blood–brain barrier [270]. CNS infections are among the most common neurological complication. Meningitis, either acute or chronic, may be due to *Listeria monocytogenes*, *Cryptococcus neoformans*, or other organisms. *Aspergillus fumigatus* may cause hemorrhagic cerebral infarctions or frank intracerebral hemorrhage.

Complications of critical medical illness

Cardiac arrest

Neurons are more vulnerable to ischemia than other cells. The Sommer sector (CA1), the folium (CA3, CA4), neocortical layers 3 and 5, and Purkinje cells of the cerebellum are most susceptible to ischemia. Neurons of the basal ganglia and brainstem are more resistant [271].

Global cerebral ischemia has a rostro-caudal pattern with the midbrain more prone to permanent damage than the lower brainstem [272]. Duration

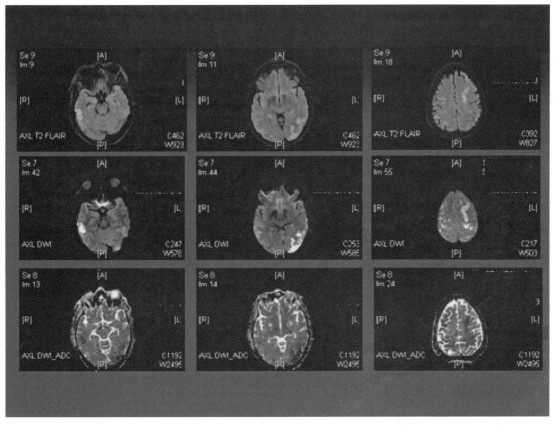

Fig 5.5 A 36-year-old woman with history of cystic fibrosis, status post lung transplantation (2 weeks prior), on cyclosporine, was found unresponsive. On examination she was drowsy, had reduced verbal output, gaze paresis to the left, and left upper extremity paresis. She had hyponatremia of 131 mEq/L and thrombocytopenia of 59 K/uL. Cyclosporine level was 497 ng/mL (reference range: 150–250 ng/mL). Troponin level was 2.71 ng/mL (reference range: 0–0.1 ng/mL). EKG showed changes suggestive of anterior wall myocardial ischemia. She had an emergent cardiac catheterization that showed no evidence of coronary artery disease. The Stroke Team was then called while the patient was in the cardiac angiography suite. Brain MRI showed bilateral hyperintensities on FLAIR (top images) and restricted diffusion (middle and bottom images) not limited to cerebrovascular territories, consistent with posterior reversible encephalopathy syndrome (PRES).

of brain ischemia influences the degree of brain damage. Cardiac arrest may lead to complete (no flow) or incomplete (low flow) cerebral ischemia. Ventricular fibrillation and asystole usually lead to complete cerebral ischemia, whereas pulseless electrical activity leads to incomplete cerebral ischemia [273]. Coronary artery disease is the most common culprit of cardiac arrest [274]. Ischemic or hemorrhagic strokes can result in cardiac arrest, usually preceded by respiratory arrest [274]. A frontal–hypothalamic–brainstem pathway is probably involved in focal brain insult induced cardiac arrest. Duration of cardiac arrest correlates with neurological prognosis [275]. Immediately after cardiac arrest, patients may lack all evidence of brain function [275]. In cases of short-duration cardiac arrest, only selective cognitive functions are affected [275]. Memory impairment could be the only noticeable deficit after cardiac arrest [275].

Sepsis and stroke

Stroke may be the initial manifestation of sepsis [276]. Infectious cerebral vasculitis may cause ischemic strokes. Mycotic aneurysms may cause either subarachnoid (SAH) or intracerebral hemorrhage. SAH may complicate meningococcal sepsis [277]. SAH may also be the initial manifestation of *Bacillus cereus* sepsis complicating chemotherapy for acute myelogenous leukemia [278]. The cerebral veins or sinuses may also become infected [279].

Drugs, toxins, alcohol, and vitamin and mineral deficiencies

Examination of vital signs provides useful clues to a possible overdose or poisoning. Decreased blood pressure, heart rate, and temperature are commonly observed with overdose of narcotics and sedative-hypnotics. Conversely, increased blood pressure, heart rate, and temperature are observed with overdose of cocaine, amphetamines, sympathomimetics, and anticholinergics.

Opiates

Heroin is an illicit drug used intravenously, subcutaneously, sniffed, or smoked. Ischemic strokes associated with heroin abuse may result from infective endocarditis, cerebral vasculitis without septic embolization, bacterial meningitis (particularly among HIV infected patients), global hypoperfusion, or embolization of foreign material. Intracranial hemorrhage may result from ruptured mycotic aneurysms, vasculitis, or coagulopathies associated with liver disease (e.g., hepatitis C). Ischemic strokes have also been reported immediately following sniffing heroin. Embolization of foreign material has been reported with parenteral paregoric, oral meperidine, hydromorphone suppositories and "Ts and Blues" (Pentazocine-tripelennamine) [280–283].

Amphetamines, amphetamine-like products, and cocaine

Amphetamines and amphetamine-like products may cause ischemic and hemorrhagic stroke [284]. Examples of amphetamine-like products include phenylpropanolamine [PPA], ephedrine, pseudoephedrine, methylphenidate, dextroamphetamine, methamphetamine, and ecstasy. Putative mechanisms include acute and chronic hypertension, small-vessel vasculitis, vasospam including RCVS, microembolization of talc (with "ecstasy"), and valvular heart disease (with fenfluramine and dexfenfluramine).

Cocaine blocks the reuptake of norepinephrine and other catecholamines, as well as the blockage of sodium channels. Impaired platelet aggregation has

been described in vitro. Cocaine causes ischemic or hemorrhagic strokes by similar mechanisms described for amphetamines. Cardioembolic strokes may follow acute myocardial infarction from cocaine-induced coronary artery vasospasm. Furthermore, cognitive impairment with associated cocaine use may result from cerebrovascular changes.

Other drugs of abuse

Phencyclidine, an NMDA receptor blocker, may cause arterial hypertension. Transient monocular blindness and hemorrhagic strokes may follow PCP use. Lysergic acid diethylamide (LSD) may result in severe hypertension and cerebral vasospasm. Hypotension and cerebral vasospasm represent possible mechanisms leading to strokes among marijuana users. Sedative-hypnotic drugs cause depression of respiratory centers leading to possible hypoperfusion-related stroke [284].

Ethanol

Hemorrhagic stroke may result from hypertension or blood dyscrasias. Heavy alcohol drinking is a cardiovascular risk factor. Activation of the hypothalamic–pituitary–adrenal axis may be a contributing factor. Alcohol raises blood pressure, may cause heart failure, increases triglycerides, increases cancer risk, and can lead to or precipitate cardiac arrhythmias. Conversely, moderate alcohol consumption may lower ischemic stroke risk, but not hemorrhagic stroke risk [285].

Vitamin B6, B12, and folate

Homocysteine promotes atherosclerosis and is an independent risk factor for stroke [286]. Causes of hyperhomocysteinemia include genetic, dietary, advanced age, high protein intake, low intake of fruits and vegetables, drugs (e.g., L-Dopa, antiepileptic drugs, fibrates, folic acid antagonists, methotrexate), cigarette smoking, alcohol, and certain disease states (e.g., leukemia, renal disease, sickle cell disease). Mutations in methylenetetrahydrofolate reductase (C677T), methionine synthase (D919G), and cystathionine β-synthetase lead to mild, moderate (200–400 μmol/L), and severe (up to fortyfold) elevations of homycysteine levels respectively. Supplementation of folate, vitamin B12, and vitamin B6 with normalization of homocysteine levels have not been shown to decrease stroke risk [287].

Lipid-soluble vitamins

Vitamin D deficiency has been associated with hypertension, diabetes mellitus, increased intimal media thickness, coronary artery calcification, myocardial infarction, heart failure, and stroke. Vitamin D receptors in the cardiovascular system include heart myocytes, endothelial cells, and vascular smooth muscle. Vitamin D affects inflammation and cell proliferation and differentiation, with anti-atherosclerotic effects. Vitamin D deficiency is easy to screen and treat but so far no randomized control trials support this intervention in the general population [288].

Minerals deficiencies and stroke

Normalization of zinc intake in stroke patients with zinc deficiency may enhance neurological recovery [289]. Reactive thrombocytosis causing ischemic stroke has been reported in patients with iron deficiency, splenectomy, and infection [290]. In animals, copper deficiency has been associated with anemia and cardiac hypertrophy [291]. Ischemic stroke has been reported during infancy in patients with Menkes' disease [292]. High magnesium intake has been associated with lower risk of ischemic stroke among male smokers [293]. Magnesium supplementation in women did not reduce the development of cardiovascular disease, although an inverse association with stroke could not be discarded [294]. Magnesium infusion after coronary artery bypass graft surgery reduced the incidence of postoperative atrial fibrillation. Magnesium given within 12 h of acute stroke has not been proven to favorably benefit outcomes [295,296].

Five things to remember about stroke due to systemic disease

1. Strokes associated with systemic diseases can be challenging and a high index of suspicion is necessary.
2. Numerous systemic disorders can be associated with stroke.
3. Diagnosis of these conditions is often inferential, and requires systematic investigative efforts.
4. Differential diagnosis of systemic causes of stroke includes an array of metabolic, infectious, demyelinating, and genetic disorders.
5. Early diagnosis and appropriate management of underlying systemic causes of stroke may reduce morbidity and mortality and improve outcomes.

References

1 Bills DC, Meyer FB, Laws ERJr, Davis DH, Ebersold MJ, Scheithauer BW, Ilstrup DM, Abboud CF. A retrospective analysis of pituitary apoplexy. *Neurosurgery* 1993;33(4):602–608.
2 Ahmed SK, Semple PL. Cerebral ischaemia in pituitary apoplexy. *Acta Neurochir. (Wien)* 2008;150(11):1193–1196. Epub 2008 Oct 29.
3 Rosenbaum TJ, Houser OW, Laws ER. Pituitary apoplexy producing internal carotid artery occlusion. Case report. *J. Neurosurg.* 1977;47(4):599–604.
4 Romano A, Chibbaro S, Marsella M, Ippolito S, Benericetti E. Carotid cavernous aneurysm presenting as pituitary apoplexy. *J. Clin. Neurosci.* 2006;13(4):476–479.
5 Cardoso ER, Peterson EW. Pituitary apoplexy and vasospasm. *Surg. Neurol.* 1983;20(5):391–395.
6 Pozzati E, Frank G, Nasi MT, Giuliani G. Pituitary apoplexy, bilateral carotid vasospasm, and cerebral infarction in a 15-year-old boy. *Neurosurgery* 1987;20(1):56–59.
7 Zipper SG. Circumscribed vasculitis with posterior artery infarct in Hashimoto encephalopathy. *Nervenarzt* 2002;73(12): 1205; author reply 1206.
8 Becker H, Hofmann M, von Einsiedel H, Conrad B, Sander D. Circumscribed vasculitis with posterior infarct in Hashimoto encephalopathy. *Nervenarzt* 2002;73(4):376–379. German. PubMed PMID: 12040987.
9 Nolte KW, Unbehaun A, Sieker H, Kloss TM, Paulus W. Hashimoto encephalopathy: a brainstem vasculitis? *Neurology* 2000;54(3):769–770.
10 Shein M, Apter A, Dickerman Z, Tyano S, Gadoth N. Encephalopathy in compensated Hashimoto thyroiditis:

a clinical expression of autoimmune cerebral vasculitis. *Brain Dev.* 1986;8(1):60–64.

11 Klein I, Ojamaa K. Thyroid hormone and the cardiovascular system. *N. Engl. J. Med.* 2001;344:501–509.

12 Petersen P. Thromboembolic complications in atrial fibrillation. *Stroke* 1990;21:4–13.

13 Seghieri G, Bardini G, Fascetti S, Moruzzo D, Franconi F. Stroke is related to lower serum thyrotropin levels in patients with diabetes mellitus. *Diab. Res. Clin. Pract.* 2003;62(3):203–209.

14 Marongiu F, Conti M, Murtas ML, Sorano GG, Mameli G, Salis G, Mathieu A, Martino E. Anticardiolipin antibodies in Graves' disease: relationship with thrombin activity in vivo. *Thromb. Res.* 1991;64:745–749.

15 Mayaudon H, Crozes P, Riveline JP, Boyer B, Simon P, Bauduceau B. Anticorps antiphospholipides au cours d'une maladie de Basedow. *Presse Med.* 1994;23:1496.

16 Hofbauer LC, Spitzweg C, Heufelder AE. Graves' disease associated with the primary antiphospholipid syndrome. *J. Rheumatol.* 1996;23:1435–1437.

17 Squizzato A, MD; Gerdes VEA, MD, PhD; Brandjes DPM, MD, PhD; Büller HR, MD, PhD; Stam J, MD, PhD. Thyroid diseases and cerebrovascular disease. *Stroke* 2005;36:2302–2310.

18 Hofbauer LC, Heufelder AE. Coagulation disorders in thyroid diseases. *Eur. J. Endocrinol.* 1997;136:1–7.

19 Silvestri R, De Domenico P, Raffaele M, Lombardo N, Casella C, Gugliotta MA, Meduri M. Vascular compression from goiter as an unusual cause of cerebrovascular accident. *Ital. J. Neurol. Sci.* 1990;11(3):307–308.

20 Lee R, Sung K, Park YM, Yu JJ, Koh YC, Chung S. A case of Moyamoya disease in a girl with thyrotoxicosis. *Yonsei Med. J.* 2009;50(4):594–598.

21 Ni J, Gao S, Cui LY, Li SW. Intracranial arterial occlusive lesion in patients with Graves' disease. *Chin. Med. Sci. J.* 2006;21(3):140–144.

22 Shen AL, Ryu SJ, Lin SK. Concurrent moyamoya disease and Graves' thyrotoxicosis: case report and literature review. *Acta Neurol. Taiwan* 2006;15(2):114–119.

23 Sasaki T, Nogawa S, Amano T. Co-morbidity of moyamoya disease with Graves' disease. Report of three cases and a review of the literature. *Intern. Med.* 2006;45 (9):649–653. Epub 2006 Jun 1.

24 Hsu SW, Chaloupka JC, Fattal D. Rapidly progressive fatal bihemispheric infarction secondary to Moyamoya syndrome in association with Graves thyrotoxicosis. *Am. J. Neuroradiol.* 2006;27(3):643–647.

25 Golomb MR, Biller J, Smith JL, Edwards-Brown M, Sanchez JC, Nebesio TD, Garg BP. A 10-year-old girl with coexistent moyamoya disease and Graves' disease. *J. Child. Neurol.* 2005;20(7):620–624.

26 Im SH, Oh CW, Kwon OK, Kim JE, Han DH. Moyamoya disease associated with Graves disease: special considerations regarding clinical significance and management. *J. Neurosurg.* 2005;102(6):1013–1017.

27 Nakamura K, Yanaka K, Ihara S, Nose T. Multiple intracranial arterial stenosis around the circle of Willis in association with Graves' disease: report of two cases. *Neurosurgery* 2003;53(5):1210–1214.

28 Kim JY, Kim BS, Kang JH. Dilated cardiomyopathy in thyrotoxicosis and Moyamoya disease. *Int. J. Cardiol.* 2001;80(1):101–103.

29 Kushima K, Satoh Y, Ban Y, Taniyama M, Ito K, Sugita K. Graves' thyrotoxicosis and Moyamoya disease. *Can. J. Neurol. Sci.* 1991;18(2):140–142.

30 Siegert CEH, Smelt AHM, de Bruin TWA. Superior sagittal sinus thrombosis and thyrotoxicosis. Possible association in two cases. *Stroke.* 1995;26:496–497.

31 O'Hare AJ, Molloy E. Cerebral venous sinus thrombosis precipitated by Graves' disease and factor V Leiden mutation. *Ir. Med. J.* 2003;96:46–47.

32 Silburn PA, Sandstrom PA, Staples C, Mowat P, Boyle RS. Deep cerebral venous thrombosis presenting as an encephalitic illness. *Postgrad. Med. J.* 1996;72:355–368.

33 Karouache A, Mounach J, Bouraza A, Ouahabi H, Reda R, Boutaleb N, Mossadaq R. Cerebral thrombophlebitis revealing hyperthyroidism: two cases report and literature review. *Rev. Med. Interne.* 2004;25:920–923.

34 Petersen P. Thromboembolic complications in atrial fibrillation. *Stroke* 1990;21:4–13.

35 Petersen P, Boysen G, Godtfredsen J, Andersen ED, Andersen B. Placebo-controlled, randomised trial of warfarin and aspirin for prevention of thromboembolic complications in chronic atrial fibrillation. The Copenhagen AFASAK study. *Lancet* 1989;1(8631):175–179.

36 Lip GY. Anticoagulation therapy and the risk of stroke in patients with atrial fibrillation at 'moderate risk' [CHADS2 score=1]: simplifying stroke risk assessment and thromboprophylaxis in real-life clinical practice. *Thromb. Haemost.* 2010;103(4):683–685.

37 Bruckert E, Giral P, Chadarevian R, Turpin G. Low free-thyroxine are a risk factor for subclinical atherosclerosis in euthyroid hyperlipidemic patients. *J. Cardiovasc. Risk* 1999;6:327–331.

38 Tagami T, Tamanaha T, Shimazu S, Honda K, Nanba K, Nomura H, Yoriko SU, Usui T, Shimatsu A, Naruse M. Lipid profiles in the untreated patients with Hashimoto thyroiditis and the effects of thyroxine treatment on subclinical hypothyroidism with Hashimoto thyroiditis. *Endocr. J.* 2010;57(3):253–258.

39 Ichiki T. Thyroid hormone and atherosclerosis. *Vascul. Pharmacol.* 2010;52(3–4):151–156.

40 Orzechowska-Pawilojc A, Sworczak K, Lewczuk A, Babinska A. Homocysteine, folate and cobalamin levels

in hypothyroid women before and after treatment. *Endocr. J.* 2007;54(3):471–476.

41 Christ-Crain M, Meier C, Guglielmetti M, Huber PR, Riesen W, Staub JJ, Muller B. Elevated C-reactive protein and homocysteine values: cardiovascular risk factors in hypothyroidism? A cross-sectional and a double-blind, placebo-controlled trial. *Atherosclerosis* 2003;166:379–386.

42 Perk M, O'Neill BJ. The effect of thyroid hormone therapy on angiographic coronary artery disease progression. *Can. J. Cardiol.* 1997;13:273–276.

43 Powell J, Zadeh JA, Carter G, Greenhalgh RM, Fowler PB. Raised serum thyrotrophin in women with peripheral arterial disease. *Br. J. Surg.* 1987;74:1139–1141.

44 Nagasaki T, Inaba M, Henmi Y, Kumeda Y, Ueda M, Tahara H, Sugiguchi S, Fujiwara S, Emoto M, Ishimura E, Onoda N, Ishikawa T, Nishizawa Y. Decrease in carotid intima-media thickness in hypothyroid patients after normalization of thyroid function. *Clin. Endocrinol. (Oxf).* 2003;59(5):607–612.

45 Perk M, O'Neill BJ. The effect of thyroid hormone therapy on angiographic coronary artery disease progression. *Can. J. Cardiol.* 1997;13(3):273–276.

46 Resnick LM. Calcium, parathyroid disease, and hypertension. *Cardiovasc. Rev. Rep.* 1982;3:1341.

47 Perkovic V, Hewitson TD, Kelynack KJ, Matic M, Tait MG, Becker GJ. Parathyroid hormone has a prosclerotic effect on the vascular smooth muscle cells. *Kidney Blood Press Res.* 2003;26:27–33.

48 Yarnell RR, Caplan LR. Basilar artery narrowing and hyperparathyroidism: illustrative case. *Stroke* 1986;17:1022–1024.

49 Mitre K, Mack D, Babovic-Vuksanovic G, Thompson S, Kumar. Ischemic stroke as the presenting symptom of primary hyperparathyroidism due to multiple endocrine neoplasia type 1. *J. Pediatr.* 153(4):582–585 N.

50 Arboix A. Stroke prognosis in diabetes mellitus: new insights but questions remain. *Exp. Rev. Cardiovasc. Ther.* 2009;7(10):1181–1185.

51 Ho JE, Paultre F, Mosca L. Women's Pooling Project. Is diabetes mellitus a cardiovascular disease risk equivalent for fatal stroke in women? Data from the Women's Pooling Project. *Stroke* 2003;34(12):2812–2816.

52 Kamalesh M, Shen J, Eckert GJ. Long term postischemic stroke mortality in diabetes: a veteran cohort analysis. *Stroke* 2008;39(10):2727–2731.

53 Marso SP, Kennedy KF, House JA, McGuire DK. The effect of intensive glucose control on all-cause and cardiovascular mortality, myocardial infarction and stroke in persons with type 2 diabetes mellitus: a systematic review and meta-analysis. *Diab. Vasc. Dis. Res.* 2010;7(2):119–130.

54 Smith SA. Etiology. Higher "normal" glycated hemoglobin levels were associated with increased risk for diabetes, CVD, stroke, and mortality in adults. *Ann. Intern. Med.* 2010;153(2):JC1–J13.

55 Heidemann C, Boeing H, Pischon T, Nöthlings U, Joost HG, Schulze MB. Association of a diabetes risk score with risk of myocardial infarction, stroke, specific types of cancer, and mortality: a prospective study in the European Prospective Investigation into Cancer and Nutrition (EPIC)-Potsdam cohort. *Eur. J. Epidemiol.* 2009;24(6):281–288.

56 Biller J, Love BB. Diabetes and stroke. *Med. Clin. N. Am.* 1993;77(1):95–110.

57 Woo J, Lam CW, Kay R, Wong AH, Teoh R, Nicholls MG. The influence of hyperglycemia and diabetes mellitus on immediate and 3-month morbidity and mortality after acute stroke. *Arch. Neurol.* 1990;47(11):1174–1177.

58 Browner WS, Lui LY, CummingsSR. Associations of serum osteoprotegerin levels with diabetes, stroke, bone density, fractures, and mortality in elderly women. *J. Clin. Endocrinol. Metab.* 2001;86(2):631–637.

59 Nybo M, Johnsen SP, Dethlefsen C, Overvad K, Tjønneland A, Jørgensen JO, Rasmussen LM. Lack of observed association between high plasma osteoprotegerin concentrations and ischemic stroke risk in a healthy population. *Clin. Chem.* 2008;54(12):1969–1974.

60 Dublin S, Glazer NL, Smith NL, Psaty BM, Lumley T, Wiggins KL, Page RL, Heckbert SR Diabetes mellitus, glycemic control, and risk of atrial fibrillation. *J. Gen. Intern. Med.* 2010;25(8):853–858.

61 Wysokinski WE, Ammash N, Sobande F, Kalsi H, Hodge D, McBane RD. Predicting left atrial thrombi in atrial fibrillation. *Am. Heart J.* 2010;159(4):665–671.

62 Singh TP, Groehn H, Kazmers A. Vascular function and carotid intimal-medial thickness in children with insulin-dependent diabetes mellitus. *J. Am. Coll. Cardiol.* 2003;41(4):661–665.

63 Reeves MJ, Vaidya RS, Fonarow GC, Liang L, Smith EE, Matulonis R, Olson DM, Schwamm LH. for the Get With The Guidelines Steering Committee and Hospitals. Quality of care and outcomes in patients with diabetes hospitalized with ischemic stroke. Findings from Get With the Guidelines-Stroke. *Stroke* 2010.

64 Cummings DM, Doherty L, Howard G, Howard VJ, Safford MM, Prince V, Kissela B, Lackland DT. Blood pressure control in diabetes mellitus—temporal progress yet persistent racial disparities: National results from the REasons for Geographic and Racial Differences in Stroke (REGARDS) Study. *Diab. Care.* 2010.

65 Gonzalez-Hernandez AN, Fabre-Pi O, Lopez-Fernandez JC, Diaz-Nicolas S. Intravenous tissue plasminogen activator thrombolysis in patients with diabetes mellitus

and previous stroke. *Stroke* 2009;40(12):e707; author reply e708.

66 Pierre-Louis B, Aronow WS, Yoon JH, Ahn C, DeLuca AJ, Weiss MB, Kalapatapu K, Pucillo AL, Monsen CE. Incidence of myocardial infarction or stroke or death at 47-month follow-up in patients with diabetes and a predicted exercise capacity ≤ 85% vs >85% during an exercise treadmill sestamibi stress test. *Prev. Cardiol.* 2010;13(1):14–17.

67 Gazzaruso C, Garzaniti A, Giordanetti S, Falcone C, Fratino P. Silent coronary artery disease in type 2 diabetes mellitus: the role of lipoprotein(a), homocysteine and apo(a) polymorphism. *Cardiovasc. Diabetol.* 2002;1:5.

68 Gupta AK, Dahlof B, Sever PS, Poulter NR. Anglo-Scandinavian Cardiac Outcomes Trial-Blood Pressure Lowering Arm Investigators. Metabolic syndrome, independent of its components, is a risk factor for stroke and death but not for coronary heart disease among hypertensive patients in the ASCOT-BPLA. *Diab. Care* 2010;33(7):1647–1651.

69 Born-Frontsberg E, Reincke M, Rump LC, Hahner S, Diederich S, Lorenz R, Allolio B, Seufert J, Schirpenbach C, Beuschlein F, Bidlingmaier M, Endres S, Quinkler M. Participants of the German Conn's Registry. Cardiovascular and cerebrovascular comorbidities of hypokalemic and normokalemic primary aldosteronism: results of the German Conn's Registry. *J. Clin. Endocrinol. Metab.* 2009;94(4):1125–1130.

70 Saidi S, Mahjoub T, Almawi WY. Aldosterone synthase gene (CYP11B2) promoter polymorphism as a risk factor for ischaemic stroke in Tunisian Arabs. *J. Renin Angiotensin Aldosterone Syst.* 2010.

71 Saidi S, Mallat SG, Almawi WY, Mahjoub T. Association between renin–angiotensin–aldosterone system genotypes and haplotypes and risk of ischemic stroke of atherosclerotic etiology. *Acta Neurol. Scand.* 2009;119(6):356–363.

72 Catena C, Colussi G, Nadalini E, Chiuch A, Baroselli S, Lapenna R, Sechi LA. Cardiovascular outcomes in patients with primary aldosteronism after treatment. *Arch. Intern. Med.* 2008;168(1):80–85.

73 Selaković VM, Jovanović MD, Jovicić A. Changes of cortisol levels and index of lipid peroxidation in cerebrospinal fluid of patients in the acute phase of completed stroke. *Vojnosanit Pregl.* 2002;59(5): 485–491.

74 Craft TK, Devries AC. Vulnerability to stroke: implications of perinatal programming of the hypothalamic–pituitary–adrenal axis. *Front. Behav. Neurosci.* 2009;3:54.

75 Rosmond R, Björntorp P. The hypothalamic–pituitary–adrenal axis activity as a predictor of cardiovascular

disease, type 2 diabetes and stroke. *J. Intern. Med.* 2000;247(2):188–197.

76 Fassbender K, Schmidt R, Mössner R, Daffertshofer M, Hennerici M. Pattern of activation of the hypothalamic–pituitary–adrenal axis in acute stroke. Relation to acute confusional state, extent of brain damage, and clinical outcome. *Stroke* 1994;25(6):1105–1108.

77 Nguyen JH, Lodish MB, Patronas NJ, Ugrasbul F, Keil MF, Roberts MD, Popovic J, Stratakis CA. Extensive and largely reversible ischemic cerebral infarctions in a prepubertal child with hypertension and Cushing disease. *J. Clin. Endocrinol. Metab.* 2009;94(1):1–2.

78 Muiesan ML, Lupia M, Salvetti M, Grigoletto C, Sonino N, Boscaro M, Rosei EA, Mantero F, Fallo F. Left ventricular structural and functional characteristics in Cushing's syndrome. *J. Am. Coll. Cardiol.* 2003;41 (12):2275–2279.

79 Vergouwen MD, van Geloven N, de Haan RJ, Kruyt ND, Vermeulen M, Roos YB. Increased cortisol levels are associated with delayed cerebral ischemia after aneurysmal subarachnoid hemorrhage. *Neurocrit. Care* 2010;12(3):342–345.

80 Sereg M, Szappanos A, Toke J, Karlinger K, Feldman K, Kaszper E, Varga I, Gláz E, Rácz K, Tóth M. Atherosclerotic risk factors and complications in patients with non-functioning adrenal adenomas treated with or without adrenalectomy: a long-term follow-up study. *Eur. J. Endocrinol.* 2009;160(4):647–655.

81 von Scheven E, Athreya BH, Rose CD, Goldsmith DP, Morton L. Clinical characteristics of antiphospholipid antibody syndrome in children. *J. Pediatr.* 1996;129 (3):339–345.

82 Li C, Ford ES, Li B, Giles WH, Liu S. Association of testosterone and sex hormone-binding globulin with metabolic syndrome and insulin resistance in men. *Diab. Care* 2010.

83 Yeap BB. Androgens and cardiovascular disease. *Curr. Opin. Endocrinol. Diab. Obes.* 2010.

84 Yeap BB, Hyde Z, Almeida OP, Norman PE, Chubb SA, Jamrozik K, Flicker L, Hankey GJ. Lower testosterone levels predict incident stroke and transient ischemic attack in older men. *J. Clin. Endocrinol. Metab.* 2009;94(7):2353–2359.

85 Yeap BB. Androgens and cardiovascular disease. *Curr. Opin. Endocrinol. Diab. Obes.* 2010.

86 Basaria S, Coviello AD, Travison TG, Storer TW, Farwell WR, Jette AM, Eder R, Tennstedt S, Ulloor J, Zhang A, Choong K, Lakshman KM, Mazer NA, Miciek R, Krasnoff J, Elmi A, Knapp PE, Brooks B, Appleman E, Aggarwal S, Bhasin G, Hede-Brierley L, Bhatia A, Collins L, LeBrasseur N, Fiore LD, Bhasin S. Adverse events associated with testosterone administration. *N. Engl. J. Med.* 2010;363(2):109–122.

87 Vitale C, Fini M, Speziale G, Chierchia S. Gender differences in the cardiovascular effects of sex hormones. *Fundam. Clin. Pharmacol.* 2010.

88 Victory R, Diamond MP. Oral contraceptives and cardiovascular disease: emerging evidence on potential associations with angina, myocardial infarction and stroke. *Womens Health (Lond Engl).* 2005;1(1):133–145.

89 Carwile E, Wagner AK, Crago E, Alexander SA. Estrogen and stroke: a review of the current literature. *J. Neurosci. Nurs.* 2009;41(1):18–25; quiz 26–27.

90 Renoux C, Dell'aniello S, Garbe E, Suissa S. Hormone replacement therapy use and the risk of stroke. *Maturitas* 2008;61(4):305–309.

91 Billeci AM, Paciaroni M, Caso V, Agnelli G. Hormone replacement therapy and stroke. *Curr. Vasc. Pharmacol.* 2008;6(2):112–123.

92 Billeci A, Caso V, Paciaroni M, Palmerini F, Agnelli G. Hormone-replacement therapy, dementia and stroke. *Womens Health (Lond. Engl).* 2007;3(6):699–710.

93 Inoue N, Hashiguchi A, Ichimura H, Yoshioka S, Goto S, Ushio Y. Stroke in women during long-term hormone replacement therapy influencing coagulation systems. *Stroke* 2007;38(5):e10; author reply e11. Erratum in: *Stroke* 2007; 38 (6): e36. Ushio, Yukitake [corrected to Ushio, Yukitaka].

94 Qazi A, Ahmed AN, Qazi MP, Usman F, Ahmad A. Ischaemic stroke with ovarian hyperstimulation syndrome. *J. Pak. Med. Assoc.* 2008;58(7):411–413.

95 Togay-Isikay C, Celik T, Ustuner I, Yigit A. Ischaemic stroke associated with ovarian hyperstimulation syndrome and factor V Leiden mutation. *Aust. N. Z. J. Obstet. Gynaecol.* 2004;44(3):264–266.

96 Di Micco P, D'Uva M, Romano M, Di Marco B, Niglio A. Stroke due to left carotid thrombosis in moderate ovarian hyperstimulation syndrome. *Thromb. Haemost.* 2003;90(5):957–960.

97 Majic T, Aiyagari V. Cerebrovascular manifestations of pheochromocytoma and the implications of a missed diagnosis. *Neurocrit. Care* 2008;9(3):378–381. PubMed PMID: 18509763.

98 Petramala L, Cavallaro G, Polistena A, Cotesta D, Verrienti A, Ciardi A, Lucia P, Filetti S, D'Erasmo E, De Toma G, Letizia C. Multiple catecholamine-secreting paragangliomas: diagnosis after hemorrhagic stroke in a young woman. *Endocr. Pract.* 2008;14(3):340–346. PubMed PMID: 18463041.

99 Isotani E, Suzuki R, Tomita K, et al. Alterations in plasma concentrations of natriuretic peptides and antidiuretic hormone after subarachnoid hemorrhage. *Stroke* 1994;25(11):2198–2203.

100 Sherlock M, O'Sullivan E, Agha A, Behan LA, Rawluk D, Brennan P, Tormey W, Thompson CJ. The incidence and pathophysiology of hyponatraemia after subarachnoid haemorrhage. *Clin. Endocrinol. (Oxf.)* 2006;64(3):250–254.

101 Huff JS. Stroke mimics and chameleons. *Emerg. Med. Clin. N. Am.* 2002;20(3):583–595.

102 Wright WL, Asbury WH, Gilmore JL, Samuels OB. Conivaptan for hyponatremia in the neurocritical care unit. *Neurocrit. Care* 2009;11(1):6–13.

103 Nakamura T, Okuchi K, Matsuyama T, Fukushima H, Seki T, Konobu T, Nishio K. Performance characteristics of a sliding-scale hypertonic saline infusion protocol for the treatment of acute neurologic hyponatremia. *Neurol. Med. Chir. (Tokyo)* 2009;49(5):185–191; discussion 191–192.

104 AlOrainy IA, O'Gorman AM, Decell MK. Cerebral bleeding, infarcts, and presumed extrapontine myelinolysis in hypernatraemic dehydration. *Neuroradiology* 1999;41(2):144–146.

105 Adrogue HJ, Madias NE. Hypernatremia. *N. Engl. J. Med.* 2000;342(20):1493–1499.

106 Qureshi AI, Suri MF, Sung GY, Straw RN, Yahia AM, Saad M, Guterman LR, Hopkins LN. Prognostic significance of hypernatremia and hyponatremia among patients with aneurysmal subarachnoid hemorrhage. *Neurosurgery* 2002;50(4):749–755.

107 Fisher LA, Ko N, Miss J, Tung PP, Kopelnik A, Banki NM, Gardner D, Smith WS, Lawton MT, Zaroff JG. Hypernatremia predicts adverse cardiovascular and neurological outcomes after SAH. *Neurocrit. Care* 2006;5 (3):180–185.

108 Li M, Li W, Wang L, Hu Y, Chen G. Relationship between serum sodium level and brain ventricle size after aneurysmal subarachnoid hemorrhage. *Acta Neurochir. Suppl.* 2008;105:229–232.

109 Gorelick PB, Sloan MA, Caplan LR. Chapter 48. *Uncommon Causes of Stroke.* In: Louis R Caplan, editor, 2nd ed. Cambridge University Press, 2008.

110 van den Bergh WM, Algra A, van der Sprenkel JW, Tulleken CA, Rinkel GJ. Hypomagnesemia after aneurysmal subarachnoid hemorrhage. *Neurosurgery* 2003;52(2):276–281.

111 van den Bergh WM, Algra A, van der Sprenkel JW, Tulleken CA, Rinkel GJ. Hypomagnesemia after aneurysmal subarachnoid hemorrhage. *Neurosurgery* 2003;52(2):276–281.

112 Barbagallo M, Belvedere M, Dominguez LJ. Magnesium homeostasis and aging. *Magnes. Res.* 2009;22(4):235–246.

113 Cojocaru IM, Cojocaru M, Burcin C, Atanasiu NA. Serum magnesium in patients with acute ischemic stroke. *Rom. J. Intern. Med.* 2007;45(3):269–273.

114 Nordström A, Eriksson M, Stegmayr B, Gustafson Y, Nordström P. Low bone mineral density is an independent risk factor for stroke and death. *Cerebrovasc. Dis.* 2010;29(2):130–136.

115 Sato Y, Asoh T, Kondo I, Satoh K. Vitamin D deficiency and risk of hip fractures among disabled elderly stroke patients. *Stroke* 2001;32:1673–1677.

116 Sato Y, Maruoka H, Oizumi K. Amelioration of hemiplegia-associated osteopenia more than 4 years after stroke by 1-hydroxyvitamin D3 and calcium supplementation. *Stroke* 1997;28:736–739.

117 Uyama O, Yoshimoto Y, Yamamoto Y, Kawai A. Bone changes and carotid atherosclerosis in postmenopausal women. *Stroke* 1997;28:1730–1732.

118 Poole KES, Loveridge N, Barker PJ, Halsall DJ, Rose C, Reeve J, Warburton EA. Reduced vitamin D in acute stroke. *Stroke* 2006;37:243–245.

119 Arbusow V, Samtleben W. Neurologic complications in ANCA-associated vasculitis. *Dtsch. Med. Wochenschr.* 1999;124(27):835–841.

120 Savitz JM, Young MA, Ratan RR. Basilar artery occlusion in a young patient with Wegener's granulomatosis. *Stroke* 1994;25(1):214–216.

121 Takei H, Komaba Y, Kitamura H, Hayama N, Osawa H, Furukawa T, Hasegawa O, Iino Y, Katayama Y. Aneurysmal subarachnoid hemorrhage in a patient with Wegener's granulomatosis. *Clin. Exp. Nephrol.* 2004;8 (3):274–278.

122 Nardone R, Lochner P, Tezzon F. Wegener's granulomatosis presenting with intracerebral hemorrhages.

123 Jiménez Caballero PE, Segura Martín T. Cardioembolic stroke secondary to non-bacterial endocarditis in Wegener disease. *Eur. J. Neurol.* 2007;14(6): 683–685.

124 Fourcade G, Lequellec A, Blard JM, Pagès M. Cerebral angiitis caused by periarteritis nodosa. *Rev. Neurol. (Paris)* 2005;161(3):323–325. French.

125 Boddaert J, Verny M. Central nervous system vasculitis and of the peripheral nerves in the elderly. *Ann. Med. Interne. (Paris)* 2002;153(7):450–458.

126 Kirdianov SIu, Baranov AA, Nasonov EL, Salozhin KV, Gur'eva MS, Abaïtova NE, Bazhina OV. Antibodies to phospholipids and the vascular endothelium in nodular polyarteritis. *Klin. Med. (Mosk.)* 2001;79(5):32–36. Russian.

127 Fourcade G, Lequellec A, Blard JM, Pagès M. Cerebral angiitis caused by periarteritis nodosa. *Rev. Neurol. (Paris)* 2005;161(3):323–325.

128 Reichart MD, Bogousslavsky J, Janzer RC. Early lacunar strokes complicating polyarteritis nodosa: thrombotic microangiopathy. *Neurology* 2000;54(4):883–889. PubMed PMID: 10690981.

129 Sharma S, Kumar S, Mishra NK, Gaikwad SB. Cerebral miliary micro aneurysms in polyarteritis nodosa: report of two cases. *Neurol. India* 2010;58(3):457–459.

130 Topaloglu R, Kazik M, Saatci I, Kalyoncu M, Cil BE, Akalan N. An unusual presentation of classic

131 De Reuck J. Dorsal thalamic haemorrhage complicating polyarteritis nodosa: a clinico-pathologic case report. *Acta Neurol. Belg.* 2003;103(1):40–42.

132 Shimizu M, Honma M, Endo K, Hoshi A, Matsuura Y, Watanabe A, Saito N, Yamamoto T. Recurrent multiple cerebral hemorrhages complicated with polyarteritis nodosa. *Rinsho Shinkeigaku* 2002;42(7):603–607.

133 Takahashi JC, Sakai N, Iihara K, Sakai H, Higashi T, Kogure S, Taniguchi A, Ueda HI, Nagata I. Subarachnoid hemorrhage from a ruptured anterior cerebral artery aneurysm caused by polyarteritis nodosa. *Case report. J. Neurosurg.* 2002;96(1):132–134.

134 Honda H, Hasegawa T, Morokawa N, Kato N, Inoue K. A case of MPO-ANCA related vasculitis with transient leukoencephalopathy and multiple cerebral hemorrhage. *Rinsho Shinkeigaku* 1996;36(9):1089–1094.

135 Isoda K, Nuri K, Shoda T, Kotani T, Satoh T, Ishida S, Takeuchi T, Makino S, Hanafusa T. Microscopic polyangiitis complicated with cerebral infarction and hemorrhage: a case report and review of literature. *Nihon Rinsho Meneki Gakkai Kaishi* 2010;33(2):111–115.

136 Han S, Rehman HU, Jayaratne PS, Carty JE. Microscopic polyangiitis complicated by cerebral haemorrhage. *Rheumatol. Int.* 2006;26(11):1057–1060.

137 Ito Y, Suzuki K, Yamazaki T, Yoshizawa T, Ohkoshi N, Matsumura A. ANCA-associated vasculitis (AAV) causing bilateral cerebral infarction and subsequent intracerebral hemorrhage without renal and respiratory dysfunction. *J. Neurol. Sci.* 2006;240(1–2):99–101.

138 Deshpande PV, Gilbert R, Alton H, Milford DV. Microscopic polyarteritis with renal and cerebral involvement. *Pediatr. Nephrol.* 2000;15(1–2):134–135.

139 Sonneville R, Lagrange M, Guidoux C, Michel M, Khellaf M, Russel S, Hosseini H. The association of cardiac involvement and ischemic stroke in Churg Strauss syndrome. *Rev. Neurol. (Paris)* 2006;162 (2):229–232.

140 Hoffman PM, Godfrey T, Stawell RJ. A case of Churg–Strauss syndrome with visual loss following central retinal artery occlusion. *Lupus* 2005;14(2):174–175.

141 Udono T, Abe T, Sato H, Tamai M. Bilateral central retinal artery occlusion in Churg–Strauss syndrome. *Am. J. Ophthalmol.* 2003;136(6):1181–1183.

142 Chang Y, Kargas SA, Goates JJ, Horoupian DS. Intraventricular and subarachnoid hemorrhage resulting from necrotizing vasculitis of the choroid plexus in a patient with Churg–Strauss syndrome. *Clin. Neuropathol.* 1993;12(2):84–87.

143 Nishino R, Murata Y, Oiwa H, Arakawa T, Sunakawa M, Tsuge M, Miyanaka Y, Harada T, Katayama S, Umemura T, Shimomura T, Nakamura S. A case of

polyarteritis nodosa in a child. *Pediatr. Nephrol.* 2005;20(7):1011–1015.

Churg–Strauss syndrome presented as right thalamic hemorrhage. *No To Shinkei* 1999;51(10):891–894.

144 Sonneville R, Lagrange M, Guidoux C, Michel M, Khellaf M, Russel S, Hosseini H. The association of cardiac involvement and ischemic stroke in Churg Strauss syndrome. *Rev. Neurol. (Paris).* 2006;162(2):229–232.

145 Teresa Sartori M, Briani C, Munari M, Amistà P, Pagnan A, Zampieri P. Cerebral venous thrombosis as a rare onset of Churg–Strauss syndrome. *Thromb. Haemost.* 2006;96(1):90–92. PubMed PMID: 16807658.

146 Chavari AE, Harris EN, Asherson RA, et al. Anticardiolipin antibodies: isotype distribution and phospholipid specificity. *Ann. Rheum. Dis.* 1987;46(1):1–6.

147 Dafer RM, Biller J. Antiphospholipid syndrome: role of antiphospholipid antibodies in neurology. *Hematol. Oncol. Clin. N. Am.* 2008;22(1):95–105, vii. Review.

148 Miyakis S, Lockshin MD, Atsumi T, et al. International consensus statement on an update of the classification criteria for definite antiphospholipid syndrome (APS). *J. Thromb. Haemostasis* 2006;4(2):295–306.

149 Leker RR, MD. Stroke complicating systemic immune mediated disorders. Semin. *Cerebrovasc. Dis. Stroke* 5:21–27.

150 Caballol Pons N, Montalà N, Valverde J, Brell M, Ferrer I, Martínez-Yélamos S. Isolated cerebral vasculitis associated with rheumatoid arthritis. *Joint Bone Spine* 2010;77(4):361–363.

151 Turesson C, Matteson EL. Vasculitis in rheumatoid arthritis. *Curr. Opin. Rheumatol.* 2009;21(1):35–40.

152 Webb FW, Hickman JA, Brew DS. Death from vertebral artery thrombosis in rheumatoid arthritis. *Br. Med. J.* 1968;2(5604):537–538.

153 Loeb M, Bookman A, Mikulis D. Rheumatoid arthritis and vertebral artery occlusion: a case report with angiographic and magnetic resonance demonstration. *J. Rheumatol.* 1993;20(8):1402–1405.

154 Zenmyo M, Ijiri K, Sasaki H, Sakakima H, Taketomi E, Nagayoshi R, Yamamoto T, Komiya S. Magnetic resonance angiography for vertebral artery evaluation in rheumatoid arthritis patients. *Neurosurgery* 2010;66(6):1174–1180.

155 Lenzer J. FDA advisers warn: COX 2 inhibitors increase risk of heart attack and stroke. *Br. Med. J.* 2005;330(7489):440. PubMed PMID: 15731142.

156 Estey E, Lieberman A, Pinto R, et al. Cerebral arteritis in scleroderma. *Stroke* 1979;10:595–597.

157 Oddis CV, Eisenbis CHJr, Reidbord HE, et al. Vasculitis in systemic sclerosis: association with Sjogren's syndrome and CREST syndrome variant. *J. Rheumatol.* 1987;14:942–948.

158 Delalande S, De Seze J, Ferriby D, Vermersch P. Neurological manifestations in Sjögren syndrome. *Rev. Med. Interne.* 2010;31(Suppl 1):S8–S15.

159 McCarey D, Sturrock RD. Comparison of cardiovascular risk in ankylosing spondylitis and rheumatoid arthritis. *Clin. Exp. Rheumatol.* 2009;27(4 Suppl 55):S124–S126.

160 Vivante A, Bujanover Y, Jacobson J, Padeh S, Berkun Y. Intracardiac thrombus and pulmonary aneurysms in an adolescent with Behçet disease. *Rheumatol. Int.* 2009;29(5):575–577.

161 Denecke T, Staeck O, Amthauer H, Hänninen EL. PET/CT visualises inflammatory activity of pulmonary artery aneurysms in Behçet disease. *Eur. J. Nucl. Med. Mol. Imaging* 2007;34(6):970.

162 Akman-Demir G, Serdaroglu P, Taşçi B. Clinical patterns of neurological involvement in Behçet's disease: evaluation of 200 patients. *The Neuro-Behçet Study Group. Brain* 1999;122(Pt 11):2171–2182.

163 Tabbara KF, Al-Hemidan AI. Infliximab effects compared to conventional therapy in the management of retinal vasculitis in Behçet disease. *Am. J. Ophthalmol.* 2008;146(6):845–850. e1.

164 Druschky A, Heckmann JG, Druschky K, Huk WJ, Erbguth F, Neundörfer B. Severe neurological complications of ulcerative colitis. *J. Clin. Neurosci.* 2002;9(1):84–86.

165 Monge Argiles JA, Bautista Prados J, Ortega Ortega MD, Pérez Vicente JA, Morales Ortiz A. Megadolicobasilar, ulcerative colitis and ischemic stroke. *Neurologia* 2003;18(4):221–224.

166 Titlic M, Bradic-Hammoud M, Miric L, Punda A. Clinical manifestations of neurosarcoidosis. *Bratisl Lek Listy* 2009;110(9):576–579.

167 Stewart SS, Ashizawa T, Dudley AWJr, Goldberg JW, Lidsky MD. Cerebral vasculitis in relapsing polychondritis. *Neurology* 1988;38(1):150–152.

168 Massry GG, Chung SM, Selhorst JB. Optic neuropathy, headache, and diplopia with MRI suggestive of cerebral arteritis in relapsing polychondritis. *J. Neuroophthalmol.* 1995;15(3):171–175.

169 Burrow JN, Blumbergs PC, Iyer PV, Hallpike JF. Kohlmeier–Degos disease: a multisystem vasculopathy with progressive cerebral infarction. *Aust. N. Z. J. Med.* 1991;21(1):49–51.

170 Carolei A, Sacco S. Headache attributed to arteritis, cerebral venous thrombosis, and other vascular intracranial disturbances. *Handb. Clin. Neurol.* 2010;97C:529–540.

171 Zimmermann AT, Brown M. Tongue infarction in giant cell (temporal) arteritis. *Intern. Med. J.* 2008;38(5):376.

172 DelMonte DW, Bhatti MT. Ischemic optic neuropathy. *Int. Ophthalmol. Clin.* 2009;49(3):35–62.

173 Hall JK. Giant-cell arteritis. *Curr. Opin. Ophthalmol.* 2008;19(6):454–460.

174 Belenguer-Benavides A, Vilar-Cambies C, Geffner-Sclarsky D. [Stroke as the first manifestation of temporal

arteritis: three case reports and a review of its patho-genesis and treatment]. *Rev. Neurol.* 2004;39(3): 227–232.

175 Mohan N, Kerr G. Spectrum of giant cell vasculitis. *Curr. Rheumatol. Rep.* 2000;2(5):390–395.

176 Georgios T, Heliopoulos I, Vadikolias K, Birbilis T, Piperidou C. Subclavian steal syndrome secondary to Takayasu Arteritis in a young female Caucasian patient. *J. Neurol. Sci.* 2010.

177 Magge SN, Chen HI, Stiefel MF, Ernst L, Cahill AM, Hurst R, Storm PB. Multiple ruptured cerebral aneur-ysms in a child with Takayasu arteritis. *J. Neurosurg. Pediatr.* 2008;1(1):83–87.

178 Kanda M, Shinoda S, Masuzawa T. Ruptured vertebral artery–posterior inferior cerebellar artery aneurysm associated with pulseless disease—case report. *Neurol. Med. Chir. (Tokyo).* 2004;44(7):363–367.

179 Kim DS, Kim JK, Yoo DS, Huh PW, Cho KS, Kang JK. Takayasu's arteritis presented with subarachnoid hem-orrhage: report of two cases. *J. Kor. Med. Sci.* 2002;17 (5):695–698.

180 Wang ZG, Gu YQ, Zhang J, Li JX, Yu HX, Luo T, Guo LR, Chen B, Li XF, Qi LX. Challenges in management of cerebral ischemia due to Takayasu's arteritis. *Zhonghua Wai Ke Za Zhi* 2006;44(1):14–17.

181 Morović-Vergles J. Takayasu's arteritis associated with antiphospholipid antibodies. *Rheumatol. Int.* 2006;26(8):773–774.

182 Nadeau SE. Neurologic manifestations of systemic vas-culitis. *Neurol. Clin.* 2002;20(1):123–50, vi.

183 Murakami H, Takahashi S, Kawakubo Y, Kinukawa N, Funaki S, Harada K. Adolescent with Henoch–Schönlein purpura glomerulonephritis and intracranial hemorrhage possibly secondary to the reactivation of latent CMV. *Pediatr. Int.* 2008;50(1):112–115.

184 Misra AK, Biswas A, Das SK, Gharai PK, Roy T. Henoch–Schonlein purpura with intracerebral haemorrhage. *J. Assoc. Phys. India* 2004;52: 833–834.

185 Wen YK, Yang Y, Chang CC. Cerebral vasculitis and intracerebral hemorrhage in Henoch–Schönlein purpura treated with plasmapheresis. *Pediatr. Nephrol.* 2005; 20(2):223–225.

186 Paolini S, Ciappetta P, Piattella MC, Domenicucci M. Henoch–Schönlein syndrome and cerebellar hemor-rhage: report of an adolescent case and literature review. *Surg. Neurol.* 2003;60(4):339–342.

187 Imai T, Okada H, Nanba M, Kawada K, Kusaka T, Itoh S. Henoch–Schönlein purpura with intracerebral hem-orrhage. *Brain Dev.* 2002;24(2):115–117.

188 Ng CC, Huang SC, Huang LT. Henoch–Schönlein pur-pura with intracerebral hemorrhage: case report. *Pediatr. Radiol.*

189 Altinörs N, Cepoğlu C. Surgically treated intracerebral hematoma in a child with Henoch Schönlein purpura. *J. Neurosurg. Sci.* 1991;35(1):47–49.

190 Pettersson T, Karjalainen A. Diagnosis and management of small vessel vasculitides. *Duodecim* 2010;126 (12):1496–1507.

191 Iglesias-Gamarra A, Restrepo JF, Matteson EL. Small-vessel vasculitis. *Curr. Rheumatol. Rep.* 2007; 9(4):304–311.

192 Ducros A. Reversible cerebral vasoconstriction syn-drome. *Rev. Neurol. (Paris)* 2010;166(4):365–376.

193 Ballouch L, Hommadi A, Karouach A, Bamou Y. [Cry-oglobulinemia type I and ischemic strokes]. *Ann. Biol. Clin. (Paris)* 2007;65(5):563–568. French.

194 Loh E, Sutton MS, Wun CC, Rouleau JL, Flaker GC, Gottlieb SS, Lamas GA, Moye LA, Goldhaber SZ, Pfeffer MA. Ventricular dysfunction and the risk of stroke after myocardial infarction. *N. Engl. J. Med.* 1997;336:251–257.

195 Dries DL, Rosenberg YD, Waclawiw MA, Domanski MJ. Ejection fraction and risk of thromboembolic events in patients with systolic dysfunction and sinus rhythm: evidence for gender differences in the studies of left ventricular dysfunction trials. *J. Am. Coll. Cardiol.* 1997;29(5):1074–1080.

196 Hays AG, Sacco RL, Rundek T, Sciacca RR, Jin Z, Liu R, Homma S, Di Tullio MR. Left ventricular systolic dysfunction and the risk of ischemic stroke in a multi-ethnic population. *Stroke* 2006;37:1715–1719.

197 Banning AP, Cuculi F, Lim CC. Takotsubo cardio-myopathy. *Br. Med. J.* 2010;340:c1272. doi: 10.1136/bmj.c1272.

198 Park B, Messina L, Dargon P, Huang W, Ciocca R, Anderson FA. Recent trends in clinical outcomes and resource utilization for pulmonary embolism in the United States: findings from the nationwide inpatient sample. *Chest* 2009;136(4):983–990.

199 apostolle F, Borron SW, Surget V, Sordelet D, Lapandry C, Adnet F. Stroke associated with pulmonary embolism after air travel. *Neurology* 2003;60(12):1983–1985.

200 Biller J, Adams HPJr, Johnson MR, Kerber RE, Toffol GJ. Paradoxical cerebral embolism: eight cases. *Neurol-ogy* 1986;36(10):1356–1360.

201 Allendörfer J, Tanislav C, Puille M, Grebe M, Stolz E, Jauss M. Risk factors for pulmonary embolism in patients with stroke and patent foramen ovale. *Cere-brovasc. Dis.* 2007;24(1):138–139.

202 Misra UK, Kalita J, O'Donnell MJ, Kapral M, Silver F. Gastrointestinal bleeding after acute ischemic stroke. *Neurology* 2009;73(2):160–161.

203 O'Donnell MJ, Kapral MK, Fang J, Saposnik G, Eikel-boom JW, Oczkowski W, Silva J, Gould L, D'Uva C, Silver FL. On behalf of the Investigators of the Registry

of the Canadian Stroke Network. Gastrointestinal bleeding after acute ischemic stroke. *Neurology* 2008;71:650–655.

204 Abboud H, Labreuche J, Gongora-Riverra F, Jaramillo A, Duyckaerts C, Steg PG, Hauw J-J, Amarenco P. Prevalence and determinants of subdiaphragmatic visceral infarction in patients with fatal stroke. *Stroke* 2007;38:1442–1446.

205 Vaquero J, Chung C, Blei AT. Cerebral blood flow in acute liver failure: a finding in search of a mechanism. *Metab. Brain Dis.* 2004;19(3–4):177–194.

206 Ardizzone G, Arrigo A, Panaro F, Ornis S, Colombi R, Distefano S, Jarzembowski TM, Cerruti E. Cerebral hemodynamic and metabolic changes in patients with fulminant hepatic failure during liver transplantation. *Transpl. Proc.* 2004;36(10):3060–3064.

207 Tsagalis G, Akrivos T, Alevizaki M, Manios E, Stamatellopoulos K, Laggouranis A, Vemmos KN. Renal dysfunction in acute stroke: an independent predictor of long-term all combined vascular events and overall mortality. *Nephrol. Dial. Transpl.* 2009;24(1):194–200.

208 Kuroda S, Nishida N, Uzu T, Takeji M, Nishimura M, Fujii T, Nakamura S, Inenaga T, Yutani C, Kimura G. Prevalence of renal artery stenosis in autopsy patients with stroke. *Stroke* 2000;31:61–65.

209 Zacharia BE, Ducruet AF, Hickman ZL, Grobelny BT, Fernandez L, Schmidt JM, Narula R, Ko LN, Cohen ME, Mayer SA, Connolly ES. Renal dysfunction as an independent predictor of outcome after aneurysmal subarachnoid hemorrhage. *Stroke* 2009;40:2375–2381.

210 Leno C, Pascual J, Polo JM, Berciano J, Sedano C. Nephrotic syndrome, accelerated atherosclerosis, and stroke. *Stroke* 1992;23(6):921–922.

211 Burns A, Wilson E, et al. Cerebral venous sinus thrombosis in minimal change nephritic syndrome. *Nephrol. Dial. Transpl.* 1995;10:30–34.

212 Cameron JS. The nephritic syndrome and its complications. *Am. J. Kidney Dis.* 1987;10:157–171.

213 Llin CC. et al. Thalamic stroke secondary to straight sinus thrombosis in a nephritic child. *Pediatr. Nephrol.* 2002;17:184–1866. J-J Sheu, H-Y Chiou, J-H Kang, Y-H Chen, H-C Lin. Tuberculosis and the risk of ischemic stroke. A 3-year follow-up study. *Stroke* 2010; 41:244.

214 Bick RL. Cancer-associated thrombosis. *N. Engl. J. Med.* 2003;349(2):109–111. PubMed PMID: 12853582.

215 Winters J, Garcia D. Cancer-associated thrombosis. *Hematol. Oncol. Clin. N. Am.* 2010;24(4):695–707.

216 Dietrich J, Wen PY. Neurologic complications of chemotherapy. Medlink. Publications dates: Originally released December 10 1996; last updated May 25 2009; expires May 25, 2012.

217 Chen M. Stroke as a complication of medical disease. *Semin. Neurol.* 2009;29(2):154–162.

218 Ionita CC, Siddiqui AH, Levy EI, Hopkins LN, Snyder KV, Gibbons KJ. Acute ischemic stroke and infections. *J. Stroke Cerebrovasc. Dis.* 2010.

219 Chen M. Stroke as a complication of medical disease. *Semin. Neurol.* 2009;29(2):154–162.

220 Stassen FR, Vainas T, Bruggeman CA. Infection and atherosclerosis. An alternative view on an outdated hypothesis. *Pharmacol. Rep.* 2008;60(1):85–92.

221 Emsley HC, Hopkins SJ. Acute ischaemic stroke and infection: recent and emerging concepts. *Lancet Neurol.* 2008;7(4):341–353.

222 Sanchetee P. Stroke and central nervous system infections. *J. Indian Med. Assoc.* 2009;107(6): 372–377.

223 Gironell A, Domingo P, Mancebo J, Coll P, Martí-Vilalta JL. Hemorrhagic stroke as a complication of bacterial meningitis in adults: report of three cases and review. *Clin. Infect. Dis.* 1995;21(6):1488–1491.

224 Peters PJ, Harrison T, Lennox JL. A dangerous dilemma: management of infectious intracranial aneurysms complicating endocarditis. *Lancet Infect. Dis.* 2006;6 (11):742–748.

225 Lammie GA, Hewlett RH, Schoeman JF, Donald PR. Tuberculous cerebrovascular disease: a review. *J. Infect.* 2009;59(3):156–166.

226 Bousser MG, Ferro JM. Cerebral venous thrombosis: an update. *Lancet Neurol.* 2007;6(2):162–170.

227 del Brutto OH. Cerebrovascular disease in the tropics. *Rev. Neurol.* 2001;33(8):750–762.

228 Adeva Bartolomé MT, Zurdo Hernández JM, Hernández Bayo JM. Meningovascular neurosyphilis. *Rev. Clin. Esp.* 2007;207(8):405–407.

229 Ghanem KG. Neurosyphilis: A historical perspective and review. *CNS Neurosci. Ther.* 2010.

230 Del Brutto OH. Central nervous system mycotic infections. *Rev. Neurol.* 2000;30(5):447–459.

231 Dobbs MR, BergerJR, Stroke in HIV infection and AIDS. *Expert Rev. Cardiovasc. Ther.* 2009;7 (10):1263–1271.

232 Connor MD, Lammie GA, Bell JE, Warlow CP, Simmonds P, Brettle RD. Cerebral infarction in adult AIDS patients. *Stroke* 2000;31:2117–2126.

233 Kossorotoff M, Touzé E, Godon-Hardy S, Serre I, Mateus C, Mas JL, Zuber M. Cerebral vasculopathy with aneurysm formation in HIV-infected young adults. *Neurology* 2006;66(7):1121–1122.

234 Bulsara KR, Raja A, Owen J. HIV and cerebral aneurysms. *Neurosurg. Rev.* 2005;28(2):92–95.

235 Coll B, Parra S, Alonso-Villaverde C, Aragonés G, Montero M, Camps J, Joven J, Masana L. The role of immunity and inflammation in the progression of

atherosclerosis in patients with HIV infection. *Stroke* 2007;38:2477–2484.

236 Jericó C, Knobel H, Calvo N, Sorli ML, Guelar A, Gimeno-Bayón JL, Saballs P, López-Colomés JL, Pedro-Botet J. Subclinical carotid atherosclerosis in HIV-infected patients. Role of combination antiretroviral therapy. *Stroke* 2006;37:812–817.

237 Saul RF, Gallagher JG, Mateer JE. Sudden hemiparesis as the presenting sign in cryptococcal meningoencephalitis. *Stroke* 1986;17:753–754.

238 Malouf R, Jacquette G, Dobkin J, Brust JC. Neurologic disease in human immunodeficiency virus-infected drug abusers. *Arch. Neurol.* 1990;47:1002–1007.

239 Rodríguez-Quiñónez A, Schneck MJ, Biller J, Brown HG. AIDS, stroke, and cryptococcus infection. *Seminars in cerebrovascular disease and stroke* 2004;4(4):234–237.

240 Ramachandran PV, Alappat Jacob P, Madhusudan KS, Vijayan VP, Kumar Sanal P. Cerebral toxoplasmosis in a patient with AIDS. *Ind. J. Radiol. Imag.* 1999;9(4):202–203.

241 A Case of Leukoareosis in Immune Reconstitution Inflammatory Syndrome; First Annual Stroke Conference Poster Presentation, September 26, 2008, Waterfront Place, Morgantown, WV.

242 McArthur JC, Sipos E, Cornblath DR, et al. Identification of mononuclear cells in CSF of patients with HIV infection. *Neurology* 1989;39:66–70.

243 Restrepo L, McArthur J. Stroke and HIV infection. *Stroke* 2003;34:e176–e177.

244 Carod-Artal FJ. Strokes caused by infection in the tropics. *Rev. Neurol.* 2007;44(12):755–763.

245 Liou LM, Lan SH, Lai CL. Dengue fever with ischemic stroke: a case report. *Neurologist* 2008;14(1):40–42. PubMed PMID: 18195656.

246 Lee IK, Liu JW, Yang KD. Clinical characteristics, risk factors, and outcomes in adults experiencing dengue hemorrhagic fever complicated with acute renal failure. *Am. J. Trop. Med. Hyg.* 2009;80(4):651–655. PubMed PMID: 19346394.

247 Kaushik RM, Kaushik R, Varma A, Chandra H, Gaur KJ. *Plasmodium falciparum* malaria presenting with vertebrobasilar stroke. *Int. J. Infect. Dis.* 2009;13(5):e292–e294.

248 Leopoldino JF, Fukujima MM, Gabbai AA. Malaria and stroke. Case report. *Arq. Neuropsiquiatr.* 1999;57(4):1024–1026. PubMed PMID: 10683697.

249 Shoji H, Hiraki Y, Kuwasaki N, Toyomasu T, Kaji M, Okudera T. Japanese encephalitis in the Kurume region of Japan: CT and MRI findings. *J. Neurol.* 1989;236(5):255–259. PubMed PMID: 2547914.

250 Castro-Lima H, Raicher I, Lee HW, Marchiori PE. Neurocysticercosis presenting with stroke. *Arq. Neuropsiquiatr.* 2010;68(1):146.

251 Tellez-Zenteno JF, Negrete-Pulido O, Cantú C, Márquez C, Vega-Boada F, García Ramos G. Hemorrhagic stroke associated to neurocysticercosis. *Neurologia* 2003;18(5):272–275. Spanish. PubMed PMID: 12768515.

252 Rocha MS, Brucki SM, Ferraz AC, Piccolo AC. Cerebrovascular disease and neurocysticercosis. *Arq. Neuropsiquiatr.* 2001;59(3-B):778–783.

253 Carod-Artal FJ, Gascon J. Chagas disease and stroke. *Lancet Neurol.* 2010;9(5):533–542.

254 Lee J, Raps E. Neurologic complications of transplantation. *Neurol. Clin.* 16(1):21–33.

255 Oliveras A, Roquer J, Puig JM, Rodríguez A, Mir M, Orfila MA, Masramon J, Lloveras J. Stroke in renal transplant recipients: epidemiology, predictive risk factors and outcome. *Clin. Transpl.* 2003;17(1):1–8.

256 Senzolo M, Ferronato C, Burra P. Neurologic complications after solid organ transplantation. *Transpl. Int.* 2009;22(3):269–278.

257 Ponticelli C, Campise MR. Neurological complications in kidney transplant recipients. *J. Nephrol.* 2005;18(5):521–528.

258 Saner FH, Nadalin S, Radtke A, Sotiropoulos GC, Kaiser GM, Paul A. Liver transplantation and neurological side effects. *Metab. Brain Dis.* 2009;24(1):183–187.

259 Martínez-Hernández E, Rosenfeld MR, Pruitt A, Dalmau J. Neurological complications of transplantation. *Neurologia* 2008;23(6):373–386.

260 Ardizzone G, Arrigo A, Schellino MM, Stratta C, Valzan S, Skurzak S, Andruetto P, Panio A, Ballaris MA, Lavezzo B, Salizzoni M, Cerutti E. Neurological complications of liver cirrhosis and orthotopic liver transplant. *Transpl. Proc.* 2006;38(3):789–792.

261 Cemillán CA, Alonso-Pulpón L, Burgos-Lázaro R, Millán-Hernández I, del Ser T, Liaño-Martínez H. Neurological complications in a series of 205 orthotopic heart transplant patients. *Rev. Neurol.* 2004;38(10):906–912.

262 Torre-Cisneros J, Lopez OL, Kusne S, Martinez AJ, Starzl TE, Simmons RL, Martin M. CNS aspergillosis in organ transplantation: a clinicopathological study. *J. Neurol. Neurosurg. Psychiatr.* 1993;56(2):188–193.

263 Martínez AJ. The neuropathology of organ transplantation: comparison and contrast in 500 patients. *Pathol. Res. Pract.* 1998;194(7):473–486.

264 Hotson JR, Enzmann DR. Neurologic complications of cardiac transplantation. *Neurol. Clin.* 1988;6(2):349–365.

265 Kato T, Nakatani T, Kitamura S. Posttransplant complications in cardiac transplant recipients at National

Cardiovascular Center. *Kyobu Geka.* 2007;60(11): 963–968.

266 Pérez-Miralles F, Sánchez-Manso JC, Almenar-Bonet L, Sevilla-Mantecón T, Martínez-Dolz L, Vílchez-Padilla JJ. Incidence of and risk factors for neurologic complications after heart transplantation. *Transpl. Proc.* 2005;37(9):4067–4070.

267 Lazar RM, Shapiro PA, Jaski BE, Parides MK, Bourge RC, Watson JT, Damme L, Dembitsky W, Hosenpud JD, Gupta L, Tierney A, Kraus T, Naka Y. Neurological events during long-term mechanical circulatory support for heart failure. The Randomized Evaluation of Mechanical Assistance for the Treatment of Congestive Heart Failure (REMATCH) Experience. *Circulation* 2004;109:2423–2427.

268 Mateen FJ, Dierkhising RA, Rabinstein AA, van de Beek D, Wijdicks EF. Neurological complications following adult lung transplantation. *Am. J. Transpl.* 2010; 10(4):908–914.

269 Bechstein WO. Neurotoxicity of calcineurin inhibitors: impact and clinical management. *Transpl. Int.* 2000; 13(5):313–326.

270 Parizel PM, Snoeck HW, van den Hauwe L, Boven K, Bosmans JL, Van Goethem JW, Van Marck EA, Cras P, De Schepper AM, De Broe ME. Cerebral complications of murine monoclonal CD3 antibody (OKT3): CT and MR findings. *Am. J. Neuroradiol.* 1997;18(10): 1935–1938.

271 Taoufik E, Probert L. Ischemic neuronal damage. *Curr. Pharm. Des.* 2008;14(33):3565–3573. Review.

272 Leech RW, Alvord ECJr., Anoxic–ischemic encephalopathy in the human neonatal period. The significance of brain stem involvement. *Arch. Neurol.* 1977;34(2): 109–113.

273 Harukuni I, Bhardwaj A. Mechanisms of brain injury after global cerebral ischemia. *Neurol. Clin.* 2006; 24(1):1–21. Review.

274 Ghosh R, Pepe P. The critical care cascade: a systems approach. *Curr. Opin. Crit. Care* 2009;15(4):279–283. Review.

275 Rittenberger JC, Sangl J, Wheeler M, Guyette FX, Callaway CW. Association between clinical examination and outcome after cardiac arrest. *Resuscitation* 2010;81(9):1128–1132.

276 Hess B, Hitzenberger P, Grisold JW, Finsterer J. Stroke as initial manifestation of a fulminant *C. perfringens* sepsis. *Can. J. Neurol. Sci.* 2008;35(2): 260–261.

277 Michieletto P, Summonti D. [On a case of subarachnoid hemorrhage in the course of hyperacute meningococcic sepsis]. *G. Mal. Infett. Parassit.* 1971;23(3):142–143. Italian.

278 Kawatani E, Kishikawa Y, Sankoda C, Kuwahara N, Mori D, Osoegawa K, Matsuishi E, Gondo H. [*Bacillus cereus* sepsis and subarachnoid hemorrhage following consolidation chemotherapy for acute myelogenous leukemia]. *Rinsho Ketsueki* 2009;50(4): 300–303.

279 Ferro JM, Canhâo P. Complications of cerebral vein and sinus thrombosis. *Front. Neurol. Neurosci.* 2008; 23: 161–171. Review

280 Bartolomei F, Nicoli F, Swiader L, Gastaut JL. [Ischemic cerebral vascular stroke after heroin sniffing. A new case]. *Presse. Med.* 1992;21(21):983–986. French

281 Brust JC, Richter RW. Stroke associated with addiction to heroin. *J. Neurol. Neurosurg. Psychiatr.* 1976; 39(2):194–199.

282 Neiman J, Haapaniemi HM, Hillbom M. Neurological complications of drug abuse: pathophysiological mechanisms. *Eur. J. Neurol.* 2000;7(6):595–606. Review.

283 Büttner A, Mall G, Penning R, Weis S. The neuropathology of heroin abuse. *Forensic Sci. Int.* 2000;113 (1–3):435–442. Review

284 Kelly MA, Gorelick PB, Mirza D. The role of drugs in the etiology of stroke. *Clin. Neuropharmacol.* 1992;15 (4):249–275. Review.

285 Schuckit MA. Alcohol-use disorders. *Lancet* 2009;373 (9662):492–501.

286 Boysen G, Brander T, Christensen H, Gideon R, Truelsen T. Homocysteine and risk of recurrent stroke. *Stroke* 2003;34(5):1258–1261.

287 Ntaios G, Savopoulos C, Grekas D, Hatzitolios A. The controversial role of B-vitamins in cardiovascular risk: an update. 2009; 102 (12): 847–854.

288 Berthold G, Krone W, Heiner K. Vitamin D and cardiovascular disease. 2009; 7 (3): 414–422.

289 Aquilani R, Baiardi P, Scocchi M, Ladarola P, Verri M, Sessarego P, Boschi F, Pasini E, Pastoris O., Vigilio S. Normalization of zinc intake enhances neurological retrieval of patients suffering from ischemic strokes. *Nutr. Neurosci.* 2009;12(5):219–225.

290 Williams B, Morton C. Cerebral vascular accident in a patient with reactive thrombocytosis: a rare cause of stroke. *Am. J. Med. Sci.* 2008;336(3):279–281.

291 Saari JT, Stinnett Ho, Dahlen GM. Cardiovascular measurements relevant to heart size in copper-deficient rats. *J. Trace Med. Med. Biol.* 1999;13(1–2):27–33.

292 Hsich GE, Robertson RL, Irons M, Soul JS, du Plessis AJ. Cerebral infarction in Menkes' disease. *Pediatr. Neurol.* 2000;23(5):425–428.

293 Larsson SC, Virtanen MJ, Mars M, et al. Magnesium, calcium, potassium, and sodium intakes and risk of stroke in male smokers. *Arch. Intern. Med.* 2008; 168(5):459–465.

294 Song Y, Manson JE, ZCook NR, Albert CM, Buring JE, Liu S. Dietary magnesium intake and risk of cardiovascular disease among women. *Am. J. Cardiol.* 2005; 96(8):1135–1141.

295 Kohno H, Koyanagi T, Kasegawa H, Miyazaki M. Three-day magnesium administration prevents atrial fibrillation after coronary arty bypass grafting. *Ann. Thorac. Surg.* 2005;79(1):117–126.

296 Muir KW, Leek KR, Ford I, Davis S. Intravenous magnesium efficacy in stroke (IMAGES) study investigators. Magnesium for acute stroke (intravenous Magnesium Efficacy in Stroke trial): randomized controlled trial. *Lancet* 2004;363(9407):439–445.

6 Seizures due to systemic disease

Matthew T. Hoerth and Joseph I. Sirven
Mayo Clinic, Phoenix, AZ, USA

Introduction

According to the International League Against Epilepsy (ILAE) a seizure is defined as "a transient occurrence of signs and/or symptoms due to abnormal excessive or synchronous neuronal activity in the brain [1]." A seizure should be considered a symptom, not a diagnosis. The diagnosis of epilepsy is made when repetitive seizures occur without provocation. As described in this chapter, a diverse variety of systemic disorders can provoke a seizure. Epilepsy is defined as a propensity for having recurrent unprovoked seizures. It should be noted that although all of the diseases described below cause seizures, only a relative few of them result in epilepsy. Many diseases cause an alteration significant enough for the normal brain to have a seizure. By definition these types of seizures would be "provoked."

Seizures are thought to result from an imbalance in the excitatory and inhibitory postsynaptic potentials in the brain. When enough neurons synchronize, the clinical presentation of a seizure occurs [2]. There are two basic types of seizures: focal and generalized. Focal seizures have a signature electroencephalogram (EEG) finding that appears to come from a discrete area of the brain. This implies that there is some sort of focal derangement in a specific area of the neuronal infrastructure. Generalized seizures appear to occur in all areas of the brain at once. Traditionally, this implies a diffuse alteration of excitatory/inhibitory mechanisms [1]. For many of the conditions discussed in this chapter, seizures appear generalized as is the case for any metabolic derangement. Conditions that cause focal seizures are noted, suggesting focal insults to specific areas in the brain. These conditions may be more likely to lead to comorbid epilepsy.

Endocrine disorders

It is well established that hormones influence the potential for seizures [3]. Table 6.1 lists hormones and their impact on raising or lowering seizure potential. It should be noted that in the case of patients who do not have an underlying potential for seizures, extreme deviations from normal are required to cause a seizure. On the other hand, for those with a predisposition for seizures (i.e., patients with epilepsy) much smaller hormonal imbalances can lead to a clinical effect. Much of the knowledge of how hormones influence seizures arises from studies in patients with epilepsy.

Thyroid conditions

Grave's disease is the prototypical example of a hyperthyroid state. Seizures secondary to hyperthyroidism without other cause is rare. Less than 20 cases have been published in the literature [4]. These seizures have presented as generalized tonic–clonic convulsions and have been noted to be associated with diffuse slow (2–2.5 Hz) spike and wave activity on the EEG and activated by hyperventilation [5].

Autoimmune antibodies to thyroperoxidase is a well-established cause of seizures. This condition is most often referred to as steroid-responsive

Neurological Disorders due to Systemic Disease, First Edition. Edited by Steven L. Lewis.
© 2013 Blackwell Publishing Ltd. Published 2013 by Blackwell Publishing Ltd.

Table 6.1 Hormones and their impact on raising or lowering seizure potential

Hormone	Metabolite	Potential for seizure
Estrogen		Increases
Progesterone	Allopregnanolone	Decreases
Testosterone	Estradiol	Increases
Cortisone/hydrocortisone		Decreases
Thyroid hormones		Increases

encephalopathy associated with autoimmune thyroiditis (SREAT) [6], but also goes by the name Hashimoto encephalopathy or nonvasculitic autoimmune inflammatory meningoencephalitis (NAIM) [7]. In addition to seizures, other neurologic symptoms of cognitive decline, tremor, ataxia, and aphasia can occur. These patients can have abnormal magnetic resonance imaging (MRI) scans of the brain suggestive of inflammation. The presence of antibodies to thyroperoxidase does not require the presence of alterations in thyroid hormone and can be easily overlooked [6].

Parathyroid conditions

Several case reports suggest that hypoparathyroidism can result in seizures [8,9]. The mechanism of this is felt to be as a result of hypocalcemia. Parathyroid hormone serves to maintain serum calcium levels by acting on bone and kidney resorption of calcium. Also, it aids in the conversion of vitamin D to its active form. Hypoparathyroidism can be congenital or acquired, the acquired form typically being either postsurgical or autoimmune. Other symptoms besides seizures that suggest a hypoparathyroid state with hypocalcemia are distal paresthesias, irritability, fatigue, neuromuscular irritability, and alterations in mood [8]. Seizures in these cases are relatively rare and should be alleviated by correcting serum calcium levels.

Diabetes mellitus

Both diabetes mellitus type 1 and type 2 imply an inability to properly regulate serum glucose levels.

Elevations in serum glucose have been well established to cause neurologic symptoms, the most prominent being coma and seizures. Hyperglycemia manifests clinically in two ways, as nonketotic hyperosmolar coma and as diabetic ketoacidosis [10]. Seizures in diabetic ketoacidosis are relatively rare, since the brain's metabolic requirements can be satisfied by ketones. In contrast, seizures in nonketotic hyperosmolar coma are relatively frequent, occurring in up to one-fourth of patients [11]. This condition is seen most typically with serum glucose levels above 600 mg/dL. Glucose is a major contributor to serum osmolarity. With hyperglycemia focal or multifocal brain lesions can be seen. Subsequently, seizures in hyperosmolar coma appear focal in both clinical presentation and on EEG [11]. These seizures have been described in the occipital head regions, potentially relating to a similar mechanism to that seen in posterior reversible encephalopathy syndrome (PRES) (see Transplant section below) [12]. In addition in nonketotic hyperosmolar coma, lower levels of γ-amino butyric acid (GABA) are reported leading to a higher potential for seizures to occur [10].

Hypoglycemia can also directly lead to seizures. Diabetes mellitus itself is not a cause of hypoglycemic episodes; rather, it is the treatment with either oral hypoglycemics or insulin therapy that causes the problem. Besides iatrogenic reasons, hypoglycemia is also seen with insulinoma, sepsis, alcoholism, and neoplasms. The mechanism of seizures with low blood glucose relates to the rate at which the glucose level falls and not to the absolute glucose concentration. The more rapid a reduction, the more likely a seizure will occur. Typically, blood glucose levels are below 40 mg/dL before a seizure is precipitated [11]. Blood glucose level screening and intravenous glucose administration typifies the laboratory assessment and therapy of status epilepticus and altered level of consciousness protocols used in emergency departments, as this is an easily treatable cause of these potentially life-threatening conditions.

Pregnancy and eclampsia

Much of what is known about sex hormone interaction with seizures comes from investigations of catamenial epilepsy, delineating how estrogen and progesterone alter seizure threshold. The exact relationship of estrogen and its metabolites in epilepsy is not entirely understood but several animal models suggest the direct action of the hormone on the brain can act as a proconvulsant. In contrast, progesterone is felt to have an antiepileptic effect via its metabolite allopregnanolone, which is synthesized in the brain itself. This sex steroid has an allosteric binding site on the GABA receptor, resulting in desensitization and subsequent decreased overall excitability [13]. Overall, it may be the balance between estrogen and progesterone levels that affect seizure threshold.

One of the most concerning conditions resulting from pregnancy is eclampsia. Preeclampsia is a diagnosis that requires hypertension and proteinuria with other clinical features, including peripheral edema, headache, and visual disturbances. When generalized tonic–clonic seizures occur along with preeclampsia it is then deemed eclampsia. Transcranial Doppler studies suggest that vasoconstriction of the intracerebral arteries may be one of the mechanisms by which this condition is mediated. This mechanism is identical to that of PRES (see Transplant section below). Magnesium sulfate is the traditional treatment of choice for severe preeclampsia to prevent seizures from occurring [14]. Magnesium acts as a calcium antagonist on calcium channels of vascular smooth muscle, decreasing contraction of arterioles. In addition, decreased N-methyl-D-aspartate (NMDA) receptor binding occurs in the presence of magnesium, theoretically decreasing potential for seizure activity. No matter the mechanism of action, magnesium sulfate has been shown effective in decreasing the incidence of seizures in preeclampsia [15].

Electrolyte and other metabolic disorders

Electrolytes play an important role in maintaining the homeostasis in all body tissues, including the brain. Neural signal transmission by neurons depends on electrical potential differences that are created by shunting of ions either into (potassium) or out of (sodium) the cell. In addition, other ions (calcium) are also used in second messenger systems and for release of neurotransmitters. Therefore, electrolyte and metabolic derangements can have significant impact on neuronal function and in turn, lead to seizures.

As discussed with blood sugar above, electrolyte abnormalities need to be evaluated as they are an easily treatable cause of seizures. Table 6.2 provides a suggested

list of laboratory parameters to check in a patient who presents with a seizure. Often, metabolic-induced seizures are difficult to treat with antiepileptic drugs without correction of the underlying metabolic abnormality.

Hyponatremia

Sodium is the main constituent in establishing serum osmolarity. As serum sodium decreases, fluid leaves the vasculature and enters the extracellular space. Organ systems have processes in which this extracellular fluid is managed. The brain has such a system, however depending on the rate at which the sodium concentration changes, this regulation system may not be able to compensate for the excessive extracellular fluid volume. Clinically, this is manifested by cerebral edema. The larger the rate of change, the more likely it is to produce clinical symptoms.

Typically, neurologic symptoms of hyponatremia depend on the severity of cerebral edema. Seizures have been noted when serum concentrations drop below 115 mEq/L [16]. This is dependent on the rate of sodium-level decrement rather than the absolute serum sodium concentration. Patients with chronic hyponatremia can have low sodium concentrations and be asymptomatic. Seizures related to hyponatremia have been associated with a relatively

Table 6.2 Suggested laboratory evaluation for evaluation of acute seizure

Finger-stick and/or serum blood glucose
Complete blood count
Electrolyte panel
  Sodium
  Potassium
  Calcium
  Magnesium
Phosphorus
Creatinine and blood urea nitrogen
Liver function tests
Ammonia
Urinalysis
Urine drug screen (also serum if high suspicion)
Blood alcohol level
Antiepileptic drug levels (if patient is taking)
Coagulation panel (if intracerebral hemorrhage is suspected)
Arterial blood gas

high mortality and can be treated by the infusion of normal or hypertonic saline depending on the acuity of the patient [16]. Caution, however, should be taken in the rate of sodium correction so as to not worsen cerebral edema, as this may lead to cerebral herniation and death, as well as to avoid demyelination. Sodium should not be corrected at a rate faster than 0.5–0.7 mEq/L/h [16].

Hypernatremia

Increased sodium concentrations have also been noted to cause seizures. Similar to hyponatremia, the rate of increase in sodium concentration correlates more closely with symptomatology than the absolute level. Hypernatremia causes loss of extracellular fluid to the vasculature, ultimately leading to cerebral shrinkage. This shrinkage can be severe enough to cause rupture of bridging veins leading to intracranial hemorrhage. Hemorrhage can then provoke seizures. Seizures can also occur outside of hemorrhage related to the shifts of intracellular and extracellular fluid [16]. If patients have coexisting acidemia or uremia, convulsions tend to be more frequent [11]. Neurologic symptoms improve with treatment of the high sodium levels.

Hypomagnesemia

As with calcium (see hypoparathyroidism above), magnesium is a divalent cation that is necessary in several biological mechanisms. Also, similar to calcium, magnesium acts to decrease NMDA receptor excitability and stabilize neuronal membranes [15]. With low levels of magnesium, symptoms of membrane hyperexcitability can also occur. These symptoms include seizures, tetany, cramping, and cardiac conduction abnormalities. Treatment can be effective in alleviating these symptoms with intravenous magnesium sulfate, similar to what is done for severe preeclampsia [16].

Hypophosphatemia

Of the electrolyte abnormalities, hypophosphatemia is a less common cause of seizures. When it does occur, it may cause generalized tonic–clonic seizures. Other symptoms of low phosphorous levels are paresthesias, myalgias, myoclonus, tremors, and altered consciousness [11]. When hypophosphatemia is identified and

treated, levels of calcium, potassium, and magnesium should also be checked since replacement of these electrolytes may also be necessary.

Inborn errors of metabolism

Inborn errors of metabolism are rare and the conditions are numerous. An abbreviated list of inborn errors of metabolism that present with seizures is listed in Table 6.3 [17]. A detailed description of these conditions is beyond the scope of this chapter. Please refer to the review article by Burton for further details [18]. Several of these conditions are evaluated during routine neonatal screening. In some, dietary modifications are sufficient to decrease the severity of illness or prevent symptoms. In others, no well-established treatment for the underlying disease process exists. Symptomatic treatment with antiepileptic medications and supportive care is warranted in such cases. Symptoms which

Table 6.3 Inborn errors of metabolism presenting with seizures

Urea cycle defects
Organic acidurias
Disorders of biotin metabolism
Peroxisomal disorders
Molybendum cofactor deficiency
Pyridoxine dependency
Disorders of fructose metabolism
Nonketotic hyperglycinemia
Propionic acidemia
d-Glyceric acidemia
Leigh disease
GM1 gangliosidosis
GM2 gangliosidosis
Infantile neuroaxonal dystrophy
Neuronal ceroid lipofuscinosis
Glucose transporter defect 1 deficiency
Multiple carboxylase deficiency
Aminoacidurias
Urea cycle deficits
Disorders of folate metabolism
Tyrosinemia type 1
Phenylketonuria
Pyruvate dehydrogenase deficiency
Pyruvate carboxylase deficiency
Carbohydrate-deficient glycoprotein syndrome
Organic acidurias

suggest an inborn error of metabolism are early-onset myoclonic seizures, tonic seizures, or infantile spasms without any other cause identified. Although genetic in nature, not all cases have an identifiable positive family history. The EEG can be helpful in some cases, since several inborn errors of metabolism may have a characteristic pattern [17].

Systemic autoimmune disorders

The broad category of systemic autoimmune disorders is unified by the simple premise that the body's own immune system recognizes itself as foreign and ultimately attacks itself. The disorders reviewed here have all been associated with seizures. Although most autoimmune disorders seem to affect one body system primarily, there is often a diffuse involvement of many organ systems, including the central nervous system (CNS).

Systemic lupus erythematosis

Within the diagnostic criteria for systemic lupus erythematosis are neuropsychiatric symptoms. These symptoms include psychosis and seizures [19]. Seizures in lupus are often not discussed as a major impact on the patient's overall quality of life. Typically, symptoms of arthritis and renal dysfunction predominate. Isolated seizures do occur. In one series, 60 of 519 patients (12%) had at least one seizure; however, recurrence was relatively rare, occurring in only 7 (1.3%) [20]. Seizures in lupus tend to have characteristics consistent with partial seizures. Several different mechanisms have been proposed with regard to the pathogenesis. Possibilities of antibodies to neuronal structures, or local vascular inflammation causing focal neurologic damage have been suggested. Perhaps the most compelling evidence relates to positive antiphospholipid antibodies (see below) seen more frequently in lupus patients who have seizures. No matter the mechanism, patients with lupus who have a higher activity of disease tend to have a higher risk of developing seizures [21]. The treatment of seizures in the setting of lupus has not been well established. Lupus patients should be screened for metabolic derangements or focal neurologic processes (i.e., stroke) as appropriate. If the risk for recurrent seizures is apparent, treatment with antiepileptic medications should be undertaken.

Antiphospholipid syndrome

The major neurologic complication of antiphospholipid syndrome is ischemic stroke. However, several other neurologic symptoms including epilepsy, migraine, dementia, and chorea have been described [22]. Relatively few cases of seizures secondary to positive antiphospholipid antibodies or anticardiolipin antibodies have been reported. One case of status epilepticus in a postpartum patient revealed focal seizures on EEG. Postmortem examination in this case demonstrated thrombotic microangiopathy suggesting microvascular ischemia as a mechanism of epileptogenesis [23].

Sjögren's syndrome

The classic clinical triad in Sjögren's syndrome is dry eyes, dry mouth, and arthritis. In about half of patients these are the only manifestations of their illness. The presence of endonuclear autoantibodies anti-Ro (SSA) and anti-La (SSB) provide serologic support for the diagnosis. However when neurologic involvement exists, the most common symptom is neuropathy. The incidence of seizures in Sjögren's Syndrome is low and estimated to occur in approximately 1.5% of patients [24]. Similar to patients with systemic lupus erythematosis, a vascular pathology may lead to the development of seizures.

Sarcoidosis

Sarcoidosis is a multisystem granulomatous disorder primarily affecting the lungs, skin, eyes, and liver. Neurologic involvement occurs in only approximately 5% of patients with sarcoidosis. A 2005 literature review of cases of seizures in patients with sarcoidosis discovered a total of 30 cases. Only one third of these patients did well, while nearly half of these patients died. The presence of seizures in the setting of sarcoidosis suggests a poor prognosis. Patients who passed away seemed to have a more aggressive relapsing or progressive course [25].

Primary systemic vasculitis

The category of primary systemic vasculitis is a spectrum of diseases that include an immune-mediated attack on the various-sized blood vessels. This includes disorders such as Wegener's granulomatosis, Takayasu's arteritis, lymphomatoid granulomatosis,

Behçet's disease, and serum sickness, which have all been associated with seizures as late complications of these illnesses. Necrotizing types of vasculitis include polyarteritis nodosa, Churg–Strauss syndrome, and overlap syndrome, which can have more aggressive CNS pathology. In these instances, seizures are seen when the disease is acute and active. Other associated neurologic symptoms include headache, confusion, and focal neurologic deficits [11]. Primary CNS vasculitis can also cause seizures, likely in similar mechanisms to the systemic causes of vasculitis [24]. Treatment of all of these conditions is immunosuppression. The type of immunosuppression varies depending on the patient and specific type of vasculitis. If focal damage resulting from vascular inflammation is evident suggesting a potential for seizure recurrence, long-term treatment with antiepileptic drugs may be warranted even if the vasculitis is well controlled.

Crohn's disease

Crohn's disease is an immune-mediated inflammatory condition primarily affecting the small intestine. Systemic involvement outside of the nervous system includes arthritis, ankylosing spondylitis, iritis, erythema nodosum, and pyoderma gangrenosum [26]. Seizures are the most common neurologic manifestation of this primarily gastrointestinal disorder [26]. Seizures in Crohn's disease patients tend to occur with exacerbation of their autoimmune disorder. The cause of a high incidence of seizures in Crohn's disease is unknown but has been noted to be much higher than that in patients with ulcerative colitis, another inflammatory bowel disease.

Celiac disease

Although the pathogenesis of this disorder is not completely understood, celiac disease appears to involve an immune-mediated reaction to the epithelium of the small bowel, presumably related to exposure to dietary gluten [27]. This disorder is treated primarily with a gluten-free diet whereby gastrointestinal symptoms improve. Various neurologic symptoms have been described in association with celiac disease. Seizures are relatively rare in this disorder and have been estimated to occur in about 6% of patients. The mechanism of neurologic involvement is not entirely clear. It has been noted, however, that the gluten-free diet may not be as effective for the neurologic symptoms as it is for the intestinal ones [27].

Organ dysfunction and failure

The ability of neurons to normally propagate signals depends on multiple factors including a balance between inhibitory and excitatory influences. This balance depends on neuronal functioning and the microenvironment that it exists in. Supporting glial cells help regulate this microenvironment allowing for signal propagation. Several other organ systems in the body act to regulate the homeostasis of the body's internal systems. This overall regulation of homeostasis has effects on the microenvironment surrounding neurons. If this homeostasis is disrupted, then seizures can be a result. Two major organ systems regulate the homeostasis of the body; the hepatic and renal systems.

Liver failure

One of the hallmarks of end-stage liver disease is the development of hepatic encephalopathy. Altered level of consciousness is typically the main presenting symptom, and asterixis and myoclonus may be seen. At times the encephalopathy may not be overt, but when formally tested, difficulties with concentration and attention are discovered. With worsening disease, this can progress to obtundation and coma. Seizures occur with hepatic encephalopathy as well especially as encephalopathy worsens [28]. However, seizures are more frequent in fulminant liver failure. This may be related to the development of cerebral edema in acute, as opposed to chronic, hepatic dysfunction. If cerebral edema develops, it can progress to cerebral herniation and is associated with high mortality rates. Other symptoms suggesting cerebral edema are hypertension, bradycardia, and increased muscle tone, progressing to the development of papilledema, decerebrate posturing, sluggish pupillary reflexes, and ultimately herniation and cessation of respiration [28].

The treatment of hepatic encephalopathy due to chronic liver dysfunction (cirrhosis) primarily centers around reducing serum ammonia via decreased intestinal absorption or production of ammonia; treatment of acute hepatic encephalopathy due to fulminant hepatic failure additionally includes aggressive management of any associated increased intracranial pressure.

Kidney failure

The mechanism of seizures in kidney failure is similar to that of liver failure. Seizures are related to the ensuing encephalopathy. Various mechanisms cause encephalopathy. Obviously, uremic encephalopathy is one of the most common causes, but Wernicke's encephalopathy, dialysis dementia, hypertensive encephalopathy, disequilibrium syndrome, electrolyte abnormalities, or drug toxicity can occur. The pathophysiology of uremic encephalopathy is not entirely clear. Presumptively, there is an accumulation of multiple organic toxins which then exert toxic effects on the CNS. Treatment is typically with dialysis or renal transplantation [29].

The symptomatic treatment of seizures in both kidney and liver failure should be undertaken in a similar manner to seizures in other patients. However, special attention should be taken regarding the mechanism of elimination of the medication used. Most antiepileptic medications are hepatically metabolized. Exceptions include gabapentin, pregabalin, levetiracetam, and lacosamide which are renally excreted. Of note, renally excreted antiepileptic medications are not contraindicated in kidney failure and can be cleared with dialysis. Alternatively, some hepatically metabolized antiepileptic medications can be used in the setting of liver failure with caution. Modified

dosing schedules would be necessary, expecting a prolonged duration of action. Appropriate rational selection of antiepileptic medications should be individualized for each patient.

Systemic cancer and paraneoplastic disorders

Patients with cancer are often medically complicated. The complications of cancer can be related to the malignancy itself or related to its treatment. There are innumerable systemic and neurologic cancer-related complications, seizures being only one of them. Table 6.4 summarizes mechanisms in which seizures can be related to cancer and its treatment [30]. Seizures in these conditions can be either focal or generalized, depending on the mechanism. Evaluation of a seizure in a cancer patient should be identical to the evaluation in any other patient. However, special attention should be made to imaging studies, cerebrospinal fluid (CSF) examination, and concurrent medications.

Solid-organ malignancies

Identifying a seizure in a patient either with an active solid-organ tumor or history of one should raise concern for metastasis to the brain. As outlined in Table 6.4, there are many other potential causes for seizures in these patients. However, the identification of a metastatic lesion to the brain can dramatically alter patient prognosis. A detailed history and neurologic examination is important to help delineate a

Table 6.4 Possible mechanisms of seizures in cancer patients

Seizures related to cancer	Seizures related to cancer treatment
Brain metastasis	Meningoencephalitis (immunosuppression)
Ischemic stroke (hypercoagulable state)	Medication toxicity
Hemorrhagic stroke (coagulopathy)	Brain radiation
Leptomeningeal carcinomatosis	Organ failure (liver or kidney)
Organ failure (liver or kidney)	Electrolyte abnormalities (medication side effects)
Electrolyte abnormalities	Chemotherapy (intravenous or intrathecal)
Paraneoplastic (limbic encephalitis)	Posterior reversible encephalopathy syndrome (PRES)
Hypoxia (lung disease or pulmonary embolism)	Symptom management (analgesics, antiemetics, antibiotics)

focal lesion. When questioning the patient and observers about the seizure event, special attention should be made to the way in which the seizure begins. Features that suggest a partial onset include head turning to one side, unilateral automatisms, asymmetric/unilateral motor activity, or any other symptom to suggest focality. The presence of a partial onset seizure suggests the likelihood of a focal structural lesion. EEG can help aid in determination of a focal versus a generalized process. Even interictal EEG can demonstrate focal slowing or epileptiform discharges in metastatic disease. However, the diagnostic modality of choice is MRI scan of the brain with gadolinium contrast. MRI can help determine the presence and extent of metastatic disease, including detecting the seizure focus as well as clinically silent lesions [30].

Hematologic malignancies

Hematologic malignancies and seizures should be approached in a similar manner to solid-organ tumors. Seizures give rise to concern for CNS involvement. If imaging is unremarkable and no other cause of seizures is determined, lumbar puncture is necessary. Microscopic CSF identification of malignant cells can be present in the setting of negative MRI. Furthermore, a single CSF examination may not be adequate, with repeated lumbar punctures increasing the diagnostic yield of observing abnormal cells. Treatment of hematologic malignancies can differ greatly from solid-organ tumors in chemotherapeutic agents as well as the use of stem-cell transplantation [31]. Please see section of stem-cell transplantation and seizures below.

Cancer treatment

Surgery, chemotherapy, and radiation therapy are the mainstays of treatment for most solid-organ malignancies. Several chemotherapeutic agents have been associated with the development of seizures. Table 6.5 lists these agents and some mechanisms of development of seizures [30]. Many of these agents are able to cross the blood–brain barrier and achieve levels detectable in the CSF. The use of intrathecal chemotherapy used in some cases for CNS involvement of certain malignancies increases the likelihood of seizures to develop.

Radiation therapy is delivered to a tumor or tumor bed. Effects of radiation can be seen for months after therapy has been completed. Radiation to the brain

Table 6.5 Chemotherapeutic agents associated with seizures

Anthracyclines (via tumor lysis syndrome)
Bevacizumab (via PRES)
Cisplatinum (via electrolyte abnormalities or PRES)
Cyclophosphamide (via tumor lysis syndrome)
Cytarabine (high-dose or intrathecal via tumor lysis syndrome)
Etoposide (via PRES)
Ifosfamide (via SIADH)
Interferon-α (via PRES)
Interleukin-2 (via thrombotic thrombocytopenic purpura)
L-asparaginase (via tumor lysis syndrome)
Methotrexate (high-dose or intrathecal via tumor lysis syndrome)
Nitrosoureas (when given intra-arterially)
Vincristine (via SIADH or tumor lysis syndrome)

Abbreviations: PRES, posterior reversible encephalopathy syndrome; SIADH, syndrome of inappropriate ADH secretion.

has been associated with seizures. Typically, radiation to the brain is done in the setting of primary or metastatic brain tumors. However, prophylactic whole-brain radiation has been used in some types of malignancy including some lung cancers [30].

Paraneoplastic syndromes

Paraneoplastic neurologic syndromes have been noted to occur prior to the diagnosis of cancer. When malignancies are identified in this manner, the potential for early treatment of the cancer may lead to a better overall prognosis. The treatment of choice for neurological symptoms associated with paraneoplastic syndromes is a definitive treatment of the underlying cancer. Diagnosis is based upon identification of an autoimmune antibody in the setting of neurological symptoms and a malignancy. When antibodies are present but no malignancy is identified, periodic appropriate cancer screening should be highly considered.

These syndromes are relatively rare and can present with a diversity of neurologic symptoms including seizures. Table 6.6 lists paraneoplastic antibodies, associated malignancies, and most frequent symptoms [32–40]. How these types of autoantibodies cause seizures and other neurologic symptoms is an emerging

Table 6.6 Autoantibodies associated with paraneoplastic seizures

Antibody	Cancer	Other neurologic symptoms
Anti-Hu (ANNA-1)	Lung, kidney, breast, prostate	Neuropathy, ataxia, cognitive impairment, neuromuscular junction disorder, myelopathy, aphasia
ANNA-2	Breast, cervical, lung, bladder, ovarian	Brainstem symptoms, spasticity, extrapyramidal, autonomic dysfunction, cognitive impairment
ANNA-3	SCLC, esophagus	Ataxia, neuropathy, autonomic dysfunction, brainstem symptoms, cognitive impairment, myelopathy
Anti-Ta	Testicular	Cognitive impairment, ataxia, neuropathy, motor neuron disease
Anti-Ma	Breast, parotid, lung, testicular	Cognitive impairment, headache, brainstem symptoms, ataxia, extrapyramidal, dyssomnia
Anti-CRMP5	SCLC, thymoma	Cognitive impairment, psychosis, extrapyramidal, ataxia, brainstem symptoms, neuropathy, autonomic dysfunction, neuromuscular junction disorder
Voltage-gated potassium channel (VGKC)	SCLC, thymoma, breast, hematologic	Cognitive impairment, hallucinations, dyssomnia, extrapyramidal, myoclonus, autonomic dysfunction, neuropathy
N-Methyl-D-Aspartate (NMDA) receptor	Ovarian, testicular, SCLC	Psychiatric, extrapyramidal, autonomic dysfunction
Glutamic acid decarboxylase (GAD)-65	SCLC, pancreatic, thymoma, diabetes mellitus	Stiff-person syndrome, ataxia

Abbreviation: SCLC, small cell lung cancer.

field. In the future, better understanding of these antibodies and their interaction with the nervous system may lead to improved treatments for these patients.

Systemic infectious diseases

One of the ways in which infectious diseases of the nervous system present in the CNS is seizures. In addition, the development of epilepsy can be a result of previous brain infections, even from several years back. Ultimately, infectious agents in the nervous system can cause focal disruption of the cerebral cortex, leading to a focus where seizures can emanate. This section describes systemic infections that may lead to the development of seizures. Primary CNS infections are excluded from the scope of this chapter.

Sepsis

In addition to cardiovascular complications of a bacterial infection identified in the blood stream, nervous system complications are often present. The most common symptom is encephalopathy. The encephalopathy related to sepsis is multifactorial. Factors such as hemodynamic dysfunction, metabolic derangements, hypoxemia, and inflammatory mediators all likely to contribute to the CNS dysfunction. All of these factors contribute to the inability of the brain to regulate neuronal transmission leading to encephalopathy and potential seizures. Inflammation may be one of the most important contributors to cerebral dysfunction in sepsis. Proinflammatory cytokines trigger endothelial activation. This cascade leads to disruption of the blood–brain barrier. With the breakdown of the blood–brain barrier, exogenous toxins, inflammatory mediators, and infectious agents are able to enter the CNS. The ensuing inflammatory process attempting to eliminate the infectious agents itself may lead to neuronal circuit damage causing seizures [41].

The sepsis patient with altered mental status must be examined carefully for focal signs or for evidence of status epilepticus. Evaluation for nuchal rigidity,

115

cranial neuropathy, abnormal muscle tone or posturing, and abnormal reflexes should be conducted. If any suggestion of focality is detected or there is uncertainty, neuroimaging may be warranted. Obviously, overt motor seizures should be addressed. Nonconvulsive status epilepticus may be underrecognized in this clinical situation. Careful observation of the patient for subtle myoclonus, eye fluttering, or nystagmus may be helpful clues to lead to the diagnosis of nonconvulsive status epilepticus. The diagnostic test of choice is EEG [41]. Once seizures are identified in patients with sepsis, treatment may offer some challenges. Since these patients are often in the intensive care unit with hemodynamic instability this may limit the types of antiepileptic medications that can be used. If unable to take oral medications, many of the intravenous agents including benzodiazepines, barbiturates, and phenytoin can decrease heart rate and blood pressure, worsening hemodynamic instability. Presuming ongoing treatment is necessary, intravenous valproate, levetiracetam, and lacosamide may be reasonable alternatives if other agents cannot be used.

Cerebral abscess from systemic infections

Similar to embolic stroke and malignant brain metastasis, infections from elsewhere in the body can be hematologically spread from one area in the body to the brain. The prototypical example of this is infective endocarditis. As in cardioembolism, infection on valves of the left side of the heart can break free and seed other areas of the body. More than any other organ system, there is a relatively higher proportion of blood flow to the brain as well as a direct hemodynamic flow. In approximately 30% of cases of infective endocarditis the brain is involved [42]. The most common neurologic complication in this disorder is ischemic stroke; however, mycotic aneurysms leading to intracerebral hemorrhages and cerebral abcesses can also occur. In the latter two complications, seizures can occur as a result as focal irritation of the cerebral cortex. Embolic events are more common with *Staphylococcus aureus* and *Enterobacteriaceae* infections since they tend to be more virulent organisms [42].

Special note should be made for neurocysticercosis and the development of seizures. Neurocysticercosis is the most common cause of epilepsy worldwide. It is

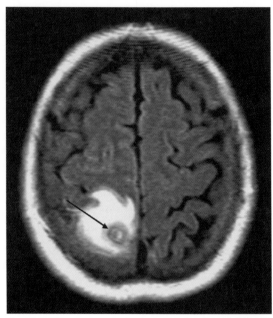

Fig 6.1 MRI appearance of neurocystercicosis. Axial FLAIR (fluid attenuation inversion recovery) MRI demonstrating a cerebral cystercicosis lesion. The cyst wall of the *Taenia solium* organism in the larval stage is indicated by the arrow. The hyperintensity surrounding this lesion represents vasogenic edema.

caused by infection by the larval form of the pork tapeworm *Taenia solium* and is more common in South America, Central America, Asia, and sub-Saharan Africa. Humans typically contract cysticercosis via the fecal–oral route by ingesting eggs released by *Taenia solium* tapeworm carriers, such as can occur through eating vegetables that were in contact with sewage-contaminated irrigation water. The eggs eventually move into various areas in the body, including the brain. The larval cysts that result in the brain can evolve over years, later calcifying [43] (Figure 6.1). These lesions can be highly epileptogenic. If solitary, resection can be considered, but may be risky. More often in third-world countries, the burden of cysts in the brain are too numerous to consider surgical options. Antihelmintic therapy with albendazole can be considered for patients with viable lesions [43]. However, the natural course is that the parasite dies spontaneously leaving a lesion that still has epileptogenic potential. Long-term antiepileptic medications are often indicated for these patients.

Table 6.7 Antimicrobials associated with seizures

Beta-lactams
Carbapenems
Quinolones
Isoniazid (depletion of vitamin B6)
Metronidazole

Antimicrobial treatment

Certain antimicrobial medications have been associated with increasing the propensity for seizures. A list of the classes of medications that have been associated with seizures is listed in Table 6.7 [11]. Risk of seizures with these medications is increased in those with known epilepsy. However, new-onset seizures can be seen associated with antimicrobials, and can also be considered provoked seizures under the correct circumstances. The mechanism of seizure provocation is likely unique to each class of medications. They may exert their effect on either neurotransmitter synthesis or on activation of neuronal receptors. Drug–drug interactions with antiepileptic medications may also play a role in those with epilepsy [44]. As discussed further below (Section on Drugs, toxins (including alcohol), and vitamin and mineral deficiencies) an accurate medication history is necessary in patients presenting with seizures.

Seizures as a complication due to transplantation and its medicines

Patients who are undergoing evaluation for transplantation have complex medical conditions. Organ-system failure compounded with major surgical intervention and immunosuppression provide many different mechanisms that can precipitate seizures. Table 6.8 lists many of these potential causes of seizures in these individuals [45]. Treatment of seizures in these patients should be individualized with regards to their underlying disease process, potential for seizure recurrence, and the stage of evaluation for transplantation.

Solid-organ transplantation

About one-third of all patients who undergo solid-organ transplantation experience a neurologic complication. Neurologic complications may vary somewhat depending upon the type of transplant, but commonly include seizure, ischemic stroke, intracerebral

Table 6.8 Mechanisms for seizures in transplant patients

Cerebrovascular insult
  Ischemic stroke
  Intracerebral hemorrhage
  Venous thrombosis
Hypoxic-ischemic encephalopathy
Central nervous system infection
Metabolic derangement
Rejection encephalopathy
Hepatic/uremic encephalopathy
Immunosuppression toxicity
Posterior reversible encephalopathy syndrome
  Medication-related
  Related to hypertensive emergency
Drug toxicity/withdrawal
  Antimicrobials
  Immunosuppressants
  Analgesics
Antiemetics
  Antidepressants
  Sedative/hypnotics

hemorrhage, CNS infection, and encephalopathy. Seizures in these patients occur more frequently in patients who are experiencing immunosuppressant toxicity, electrolyte imbalance, CNS infection, or have focal brain lesions. Neuroimaging is indicated for patients with focal presentations and EEG is helpful for those who have altered mental status. If CNS infection is suspected, then CSF analysis is useful and indicated; however, in some cases empiric treatment may be necessary [46].

Stem-cell transplantation

The purpose of stem-cell transplantation is to destroy native dysfunctional or neoplastic hematopoietic progenitor cells with chemotherapy and replace them with those from a normal matched donor. This process puts patients at risk for seizures not only related to the transplant surgery and severe immunosuppression, but also related to malignancy and chemotherapy. Seizures are more common during the initial stages of bone marrow depletion, where medication toxicity, and metabolic and hematologic derangements are more likely. During later stages of chronic immunosuppression, seizures are still possible, related to recurrent disease or toxicity from immunosuppressants

117

[31]. These patients should be closely monitored, especially during the initial phases of their treatment. Attempts to avoid drug toxicity and metabolic derangements should be taken.

Posterior reversible encephalopathy syndrome

PRES is also known as reversible posterior leukoencephalopathy syndrome (RPLS). This is a clinical syndrome resulting from multiple different etiologies, with the clinical triad of acute or subacute onset of headaches, seizures, and visual disturbance. Other neurologic symptoms can include a decreased level of consciousness including progression to stupor and coma. PRES is discussed here due to the association between this syndrome and immunosuppressant medications. However, the more frequent and classical presentation of PRES is in the setting of hypertensive emergency and encephalopathy. The immunosuppressant medications listed in Table 6.9 have a potential to cause this syndrome. In addition to immunosuppressants, chemotherapeutics have been implicated and have been noted in Table 6.5. Toxicity of these medications may increase the potential for developing PRES.

Seizures in PRES are typically noted to be secondarily generalized tonic–clonic seizures. Long-term antiepileptic drug therapy may not be necessary in all cases, and may depend on clinical course and whether stroke occurs concomitantly with PRES, which has been noted to occur. The pathogenesis of this disease is not entirely clear. Current theory suggests that normal autoregulation of cerebral blood flow is altered preferentially in the posterior cerebral circulation. This leads to extravasation of fluid to the extracellular space and symptoms described above [47]. Neuroimaging is helpful in establishing the diagnosis and yields a typical radiographic appearance as demonstrated in Figure 6.2.

Table 6.9 Some medications related to posterior reversible encephalopathy syndrome

Tacrolimus (FK-506)
Cyclosporine
High-dose steroids
Muromonab-CD3 (OKT3)
Busulfan

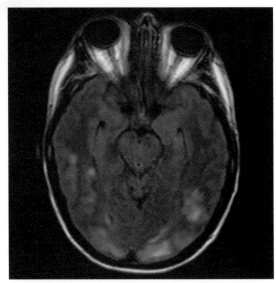

Fig 6.2 MRI appearance of posterior reversible encephalopathy syndrome. Axial FLAIR (fluid attenuation inversion recovery) MRI demonstrating vasogenic edema predominately located in the distribution of the posterior cerebral circulation.

Seizures as a complication of critical medical illness—status epilepticus

As discussed in the Section "Organ dysfunction and failure" above, patients with organ failure can develop seizures. In the intensive care unit, critically ill patients can develop the complication of status epilepticus. Essentially this type of ongoing seizure activity can be conceptually thought of as an "organ system failure" of the CNS. The development of status epilepticus in critically ill patients suggests a poor prognosis. Mortality rates exceed 20% if seizures last longer than 60 min [48].

A practical working definition of status epilepticus is "a condition characterized by an epileptic seizure which is so frequently repeated or so prolonged as to create a fixed and lasting epileptic condition [49]." Other definitions include continuous or repetitive seizures lasting greater than 10 min [48]. No matter how it is defined, ongoing seizure activity is felt to be detrimental to patients and should be considered a neurologic emergency. Figure 6.3 provides an example of a treatment and evaluation algorithm for adult patients in status epilepticus [50,51]. As stated in the introduction,

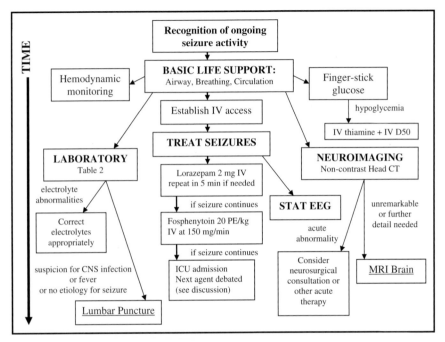

Fig 6.3 Example treatment algorithm for status epilepticus. IV, intravenous; D50, 50% dextrose solution; CT, computerized tomography; EEG, electroencephalogram; MRI, magnetic resonance imaging; ICU, intensive care unit; PE, phenytoin equivalents; min, minutes.

seizures (including status epilepticus) should be considered a symptom and not a diagnosis. The differential diagnosis of status epilepticus for critically ill patients is broad, but contains many etiologies covered elsewhere in this chapter (Table 6.10). The most common cause is subtherapeutic antiepileptic drug levels in patients with epilepsy, followed by alcohol withdrawal. A thorough evaluation for the cause of status epilepticus should be undertaken concurrently with treatment utilizing antiepileptic drugs.

The basis for the initial treatment of status epilepticus comes from the 1998 VA cooperative study [52]. This pivotal trial established that the use of benzodiazepines, most specifically lorazepam or diazepam, were most effective in halting continuous seizure activity. Lorazepam was favored due to its ease of use. After this, the use of phenytoin or fosphenytoin is second-line therapy. Fosphenytoin is a derivative of phenytoin, converted to its parent compound in the liver allowing for faster and safer administration of the medication [51]. If seizures continue after the administration of two medications, it is considered refractory status epilepticus. Optimal treatment at this point

Table 6.10 Differential diagnosis of status epilepticus in the critically ill

Preexisting epilepsy (with or without subtherapeutic drug level)
Ischemic stroke
Intracerebral hemorrhage
CNS infection (including meningitis, encephalitis, brain abscess)
Acute head trauma
Anoxic brain injury
Brain tumors
CNS demyelination
Electrolyte disorder
Alcohol withdrawal
Drug intoxication or toxicity (illicit or prescription)
Glucose imbalance (hyperglycemia, hypoglycemia)
Vitamin B6 deficiency
Posterior reversible encephalopathy syndrome
Hepatic failure
Renal failure
Inflammatory disorders
Systemic infection (sepsis)

119

is debated. Midazolam, propofol, phenobarbital, and pentobarbital infusions have all been suggested, but no evidence suggests which therapy is superior. Even less is established about fourth-line therapy. Other intravenous agents available that could be considered include valproic acid, levetiracetam, and lacosamide; however, there is little to no evidence to support their use in status epilepticus [50].

Status epilepticus has two types of clinical presentations, convulsive and nonconvulsive, the difference being in the presence or absence of overt motor activity. There is no current evidence to suggest that these different presentations should have different treatment approaches. In the nonresponsive critically ill patient, nonconvulsive status epilepticus can be easily overlooked. The best way to establish this diagnosis is to obtain an EEG demonstrating a pattern consistent with status epilepticus [48]. A high clinical suspicion for nonconvulsive status epilepticus in any patient who is unresponsive without clear cause is essential.

Drugs, toxins (including alcohol), and vitamin and mineral deficiencies

Ingested exogenous substances should always be considered in patients who present with seizures. When evaluating a patient who had just experienced a seizure for an unknown reason, an extensive substance history should be taken. If the patient is unable or unwilling to provide this history, family or friends can be an invaluable resource. A list of commonly abused substances is summarized in Table 6.11. In addition to illicit drugs, discussion should include both prescription and nonprescription medications. Many patients do not realize that vitamin and mineral supplements need to be disclosed to their physician (see Dietary Supplements section below). A detailed history and laboratory examination can be helpful in discerning the difference between a cryptogenic seizure and a provoked seizure due to an ingested substance.

Alcohol

The pharmacologic properties of ethanol include inhibition of glutamate transmission (decrease in excitation) and a facilitation of GABA transmission (increase in inhibition). With chronic ingestion of ethanol, the effects of this substance cause an upregulation of glutamate receptors and a downregulation of GABA receptors [53]. In a steady state where ethanol is present, the system is able to keep a normal homeostasis between excitation and inhibition with the altered number of receptors. However, when alcohol is withdrawn from the system, homeostasis ceases to exist. This is the mechanism by which alcohol withdrawal seizures are produced. It is the abrupt discontinuation of chronic alcohol which puts a patient at the most risk for seizures.

Delirium tremens is the term that has been given to the alcohol-withdrawal state. From the mechanism described above, it is no surprise that other symptoms include tremor, hallucinations, and autonomic dysfunction. Alcohol-related seizures usually occur within 7–30 h after the last drink the patient ingested. However, seizures have occurred up to 2 or more weeks after cessation of medication [54]. Seizures related to alcohol are the leading cause of status epilepticus in patients without previously diagnosed epilepsy. This is likely due to the prevalence of alcohol use, since only 3% of alcohol-withdrawal seizures result in status epilepticus [54]. Alcohol-related seizures present as a generalized tonic–clonic convulsion. Seizures may cluster. If focal onset to a seizure is noted, further investigation may be warranted.

Intravenous benzodiazepines have been determined to be effective in the treatment of alcohol-related seizures. After a single seizure, 2 mg of lorazepam demonstrated a significant benefit over placebo in preventing a subsequent seizure in the next 6 h [55]. Many hospitals have protocols for treatment of the alcohol-withdrawal state. An example of an alcohol-withdrawal protocol is outlined in Table 6.12 [56]. Typically, this includes a scoring system for various patient-care parameters including presence of tremors, level of confusion, and hemodynamics. Increasing doses of benzodiazepines are given for increasing symptoms. Usually, this type of protocol needs to be conducted in an intensive care setting due to the risk of hemodynamic instability, seizures, and need for frequent monitoring.

Sedative/hypnotics

The sedative/hypnotic class of medications includes substances such as benzodiazepines, barbiturates, and γ-hydroxybutyric acid (GHB). In general, these

Table 6.11 Commonly abused substances (and mechanism of seizure)

Substance	Mechanism of seizure
Ethanol	Withdrawal
Opiates	Intoxication or overdose
Morphine	
Heroin	
Fentanyl	
Meperidine (metabolite normeperidine)	
Oxymorphone	
Hydromorphone	
Codeine	
Oxycodone	
Hydrocodone	
Sedative/hypnotics	Withdrawal
Benzodiazepines	
Barbiturates	
γ-Hydroxybutyric acid (GHB)	
Stimulants	Intoxication or overdose
Cocaine	
Methamphetamine	
Methylenedioxymethamphetamine (MDMA, ecstasy)	
Hallucinogens	Intoxication or overdose
D-Lysergic acid diethylamide (LSD)	
Mescaline (peyote)	
Psilocybin (mushrooms)	
Phencyclidine	Intoxication or overdose
Marijuana	Unclear
Inhalants	Intoxication or overdose

medications act on the GABA receptor. They exert their action on an allosteric binding site acting to allow for the influx of chloride ions into the cell. This inhibits depolarization of the neuron, decreasing overall excitability. Benzodiazepines and barbiturates are effective in the treatment of acute seizures as well as epilepsy. Short-acting formulations of these prescription medications are most popular and have the most potential for abuse. The substance GHB is more commonly known as the "date rape" drug. It likely acts on other neuronal receptors in addition to GABA, and has been given its nickname for its amnestic effects [54]. Both myoclonus and seizures have been reported in association with intoxication with GHB [55].

Seizures in the setting of sedative/hypnotic use occur in the withdrawal state, much like ethanol (discussed above). With chronic stimulation, there is an upregulation of GABA receptors in the brain. When stimulation of the inhibitory receptor is taken away, the balance between excitation and inhibition then favors excitation and a seizure occurs. Similar to alcohol, the withdrawal state can be accompanied by tremor, agitation, and autonomic instability [54]. Flumazenil is an antagonist to the benzodiazepine binding site on the GABA receptor, and can reverse the effects of medication overdose. Caution should be taken however, since acutely reversing the benzodiazepine effect can quickly precipitate a withdrawal state.

Treatment of sedative/hypnotic withdrawal seizures is identical to that of alcohol withdrawal. The major difference is the half-life of the dependent medication. This may change the length of treatment. Special

Table 6.12 Example alcohol withdrawal protocol

Step 1—Rate each of the following symptoms on a scale
from 0 to 7: 0 = absent symptoms, 7 = most severe
symptoms

Nausea and vomiting

Tremor

Sweating

Anxiety

Agitation

Tactile disturbances

Auditory disturbances

Headaches

Orientation and confusion (0–4 rating only)

Step 2—Tabulate total score and administer medication
accordingly

Score	Lorazepam dose	Chlordiazepoxide dose
0–9	None	None
10–12	1 mg PO/0.5 mg IV	25 mg PO
13–14	2 mg PO/1 mg IV	50 mg PO
15–17	3 mg PO/1.5 mg IV	75 mg PO
18 or more	4 mg PO/2 mg IV	100 mg PO

Step 3—Repeat hourly administering medication as
appropriate

attention should always be taken when discontinuing
the patient's chronic sedative/hypnotic use. A general
rule of thumb is that the longer the patient has been on
the medication the slower the titration. When prescribing these types of medications for chronic use,
patients need to be counseled to not discontinue the
medication abruptly.

Marijuana

Marijuana contains numerous cannabinoid compounds, but the most psychoactive component is
Δ-9-tetrahydrocannabinol (Δ-9-THC). It is created
from the leaves of the *Cannabis sativa* plant. Typically
marijuana is smoked, but can also be taken orally.
Δ-9-THC acts on endocannabinoid receptors in the
brain, which act to release both glutamate (excitatory)
and GABA (inhibitory) [54]. The effect on seizures is
not entirely clear. One small placebo-controlled study
of epilepsy patients showed increased rates of seizure
freedom in those who were given cannabaniods [57].
On the contrary, other reports have noted worsening
seizures with marijuana use [55].

Stimulants

Stimulants act on the CNS releasing dopamine, norepinephrine, and serotonin. Cocaine has been well
described to cause seizures and even status epilepticus
without other signs of toxicity. It can be ingested in
multiple different ways including intranasal, parenteral,
or inhaled as "crack." Seizures typically occur several
hours after exposure and may be related to the drug's
metabolites. It has been reported to occur in up to 9% of
cocaine users [54]. Methamphetamines ("speed") can
be taken enterally, parenterally, or inhaled. It has been
demonstrated in animal models that seizures attributed
to these substances relate to a breakdown of the blood–
brain barrier from hyperthermia. This leads to neuronal
degeneration in the mesial temporal structures of the
brain, contributing to seizures [58]. Methylenedioxy-
methamphetamine (MDMA), also called ecstasy, has
properties of both a stimulant and a hallucinogen.
Overdose of MDMA can cause seizures, malignant
hyperthermia, delirium, coma, and death [59].

Seizures secondary to stimulant overdose are often
refractory to antiepileptic medications. Presumably, as
the offending agent is cleared from the system, the
patient's symptoms, including seizures, should
improve. Nonetheless even if refractory, seizures
should be treated in the typical manner, including
status epilepticus [55].

Hallucinogens

Hallucinogens can either be from natural substances
such as peyote and mushrooms, or synthetic agents such
as D-lysergic acid diethylamide (LSD) and phencyclidine
(PCP). Use of these substances causes an altered senso-
rium in which the user perceives sensations that are not
actually true. It has been reported that the clinical
effects of these substances can last weeks or even years
as "flashbacks" when levels of the substance are
undetectable. Very high doses of the hallucinogens
can case seizures and coma. If seizures occur and
PCP toxicity is suspected, other symptoms including
fever, hypertension, nystagmus, psychosis, delirium,
and coma may also suggest the diagnosis [54].

Inhalants

Inhalants are volatile substances that are used recrea-
tionally in order to have clinical effects. They tend to
be popular in younger populations because of their

wide availability. Substances in this category include glues, solvents, marker pens, aerosols, bottled fuel gas, and anesthetics. Related seizures are typically seen in overdose rather than a withdrawal state [54].

Vitamin B6 (pyridoxine) dependency

Pyridoxine-dependent seizures are rare, but can present during infancy with repetitive seizures or status epilepticus [17]. Vitamin B6 is a cofactor in amino acid and neurotransmitter metabolism. Four different enzyme decencies have been identified leading to this genetic cause of epilepsy. This syndrome presents in the neonatal period with myoclonic seizures. Typically, these seizures are resistant to traditional antiepileptic medications and are only responsive to pyridoxine supplementation. Empiric administration of pyridoxine in neonates presenting with ongoing seizure activity should be strongly considered, as lack of supplementation can lead to irreversible neurologic damage [60].

Dietary supplements

Establishing a connection between seizures and dietary supplements can be difficult. Dietary supplements are not regulated by the U.S. Food and Drug Administration, in contrast to prescription medications. There are a wide variety of supplements available and many do not have strong clinical evidence to support their use for the condition they are taken for. Furthermore, since rigorous safety trials are not conducted on these products, the side effect profile is unclear. Also, patients often do not realize that they need to disclose this information to their treating physicians, since they do not need a prescription for them. Table 6.13 lists several dietary supplements that have a possible association with seizures [61]. The evidence for the association between these supplements and seizures has only been established through case reports. Further systematic study into the clinical effects and side effects of dietary supplements may be

Table 6.13 Supplements with possible association with seizures

Ephedrine
Pseudoephedrine
Phenylpropanolamine
Creatine
Ginkgo biloba
St. John's wort

difficult, but necessary to further understand the association between these substances and seizures.

Conclusion

Seizures can occur in a wide variety of general medical conditions. Seizures in these disorders can be understood by one of two mechanisms. The first cause results from a diffuse disruption of homeostasis in the body disrupting the brain's ability to balance excitatory and inhibitory potentials. The second is a result of a focal insult to the brain itself, whether it be through breakdown of the blood–brain barrier, inflammation, or otherwise. Discovering which of these two final pathways is leading to seizures can help lead to the cause of a patient's presentation. The first cause results in generalized onset seizures, while the second results in focal onset seizures.

As discussed in this chapter, when any patient presents with a seizure, a detailed history and physical exam is essential in order to establish the cause. Many comorbid conditions should be considered as potential etiologies for the patient's event. Many of the conditions described here are easily screened for during initial history taking. If not revealed or no history is available, routine laboratory testing or neuroimaging can be very helpful. If a systemic disorder is identified, in many cases treating the underlying cause can alleviate the seizures. This may avoid the need for using antiepileptic medications in some patients.

Five things to remember about seizures due to systemic disease

1. Seizures are a result of imbalance of excitatory and inhibitory influence on neuronal circuits.
2. Seizures should be considered a symptom of an underlying process and not a diagnosis. An investigation into the etiology is warranted, especially in the setting of systemic disease.
3. Careful history and physical examination should be conducted and if focal signs or symptoms are discovered, neuroimaging is especially indicated.
4. In patients with altered mental status, especially without known cause, an EEG should be considered.
5. Antiepileptic drug therapy may not be needed in all patients who have a seizure. If indicated, individualized selection should be based on the patient's unique clinical situation.

References

1 Berg AT, Berkovic SF, Brodie MJ, Buchhalter J, Cross JH, van Emde Boas W, Engel J, French J, Glauser TA, Mathern GW, Moshé SL, Nordli D, Plouin P, Scheffer IE. Revised terminology and concepts for organization of seizures and epilepsies: report of the ILAE Commission on Classification and Terminology, 2005–2009. *Epilepsia* 2010;51(4):676–685. Epub 2010 Feb 26.

2 Benardo LS. Chapter 27: Pathophysiology of the Epilepsies. *Neurological Therapeutics: Principles and Practice Editor-in-chief, John H. Noseworthy.* London, New York: Martin Dunitz, 2003.

3 Hamed SA. Neuroendocrine hormonal conditions in epilepsy: relationship to reproductive and sexual functions. *Neurologist* 2008;14(3):157–169.

4 Vergely N, Garnier P, Guy C, Khalfallah Y, Estour B. Seizure during Graves' disease. *Epileptic Disord.* 2009; 11(2):136–137. Epub 2009 Mar 9.

5 Maeda T, Izumi T. Generalized convulsions with diffuse spike and wave bursts emerging with Graves' disease. 2006;37(5):305–307.

6 Castillo P, Woodruff B, Caselli R, Vernino S, Lucchinetti C, Swanson J, Noseworthy J, Aksamit A, Carter J, Sirven J, Hunder G, Fatourechi V, Mokri B, Drubach D, Pittock S, Lennon V, Boeve B. Steroid-responsive encephalopathy associated with autoimmune thyroiditis. *Arch. Neurol.* 2006;63(2):197–202.

7 Caselli RJ, Boeve BF, Scheithauer BW, O'Duffy JD, Hunder GG. Nonvasculitic autoimmune inflammatory meningoencephalitis (NAIM): a reversible form of encephalopathy. *Neurology* 1999;53(7):1579–1581. Department of Neurology, Mayo Clinic Scottsdale, AZ 85259, USA.

8 Bindu M, Harinarayana CV. Hypoparathyroidism: a rare treatable cause of epilepsy—report of two cases. *Eur. J. Neurol.* 2006;13(7):786–788.

9 Su YC, Lin YM, Hou SW, Chen CC, Chong CF, Wang TL. Hypoparathyroidism-induced epilepsy: an overlooked cause. *Am. J. Emerg. Med.* 2006;24(5):617–618.

10 Guisado R, Arieff AI. Neurologic manifestations of diabetic comas: correlation with biochemical alterations in the brain. *Metabolism* 1975;24(5):665–679.

11 Messing RO, Simon RP. Seizures as a manifestation of systemic disease. *Neurol. Clin.* 1986;4(3):563–584.

12 Moien-Afshari F, Téllez-Zenteno JF. Occipital seizures induced by hyperglycemia: a case report and review of literature. *Seizure* 2009;18(5):382–385. Epub 2009 Jan 9.

13 Steinhoff BJ. Optimizing therapy of seizures in patients with endocrine disorders. *Neurology* 2006;67(12 Suppl 4):S23–S27.

14 Belfort MA, Anthony J, Saade GR, Allen JC Jr., Nimodipine Study Group. A comparison of magnesium sulfate and nimodipine for the prevention of eclampsia. *N. Engl. J. Med.* 2003;348(4):304–311.

15 Euser AG, Cipolla MJ. Magnesium sulfate for the treatment of eclampsia: a brief review. *Stroke* 2009; 40(4):1169–1175. Epub 2009 Feb 10.

16 Castilla-Guerra L, del Carmen Fernández-Moreno M, López-Chozas JM, Fernández-Bolaños R. Electrolytes disturbances and seizures. *Epilepsia* 2006;47(12):1990–1998. Review.

17 Nordli DRJr, De Vivo DC. Classification of infantile seizures: implications for identification and treatment of inborn errors of metabolism. *J. Child. Neurol.* 2002;17(Suppl 3):3S3–3S7; discussion 3S8.

18 Burton BK. Inborn errors of metabolism in infancy: a guide to diagnosis. *Pediatrics* 1998;102(6):E69. Review.

19 Hochberg MC. Updating the American College of Rheumatology Revised criteria for the classification of systemic lupus erythematosus. *Arthritis Rheum.* 1997;40:1725.

20 Appenzeller S, Cendes F, Costallat LT. Epileptic seizures in systemic lupus erythematosus. *Neurology* 2004; 63:1808–1812.

21 Cimaz R, Guerrini R. Epilepsy in lupus. *Lupus* 2008; 17(9):777–779.

22 Katzav A, Chapman J, Shoenfeld Y. CNS dysfunction in the antiphospholipid syndrome. *Lupus* 2003;12(12):903–907. Review.

23 Coward LJ, Kullmann DM, Hirsch NP, Howard RS, Lucas SB. Catastrophic primary antiphospholipid syndrome presenting as status epilepticus. *J. Neurol. Neurosurg. Psychiatry* 2005;76(11):1607–1608.

24 Najjar S, Bernbaum M, Lai G, Devinsky O. Immunology and epilepsy. *Rev. Neurol. Dis.* 2008;5(3):109–116.

25 Sponsler JL, Werz MA, Maciunas R, Cohen M. Neurosarcoidosis presenting with simple partial seizures and solitary enhancing mass: case reports and review of the literature. *Epilepsy Behav.* 2005;6(4):623–630. Epub 2005 Apr 26. Review.

26 Elsehety A, Bertorini TE. Neurologic and neuropsychiatric complications of Crohn's disease. *South Med. J.* 1997;90(6):606–610.

27 Bürk K, Farecki ML, Lamprecht G, Roth G, Decker P, Weller M, Rammensee HG, Oertel W. Neurological symptoms in patients with biopsy proven celiac disease. *Mov. Disord.* 2009;24(16):2358–2362.

28 Menon KVN, Kamath PS. Chapter 117: Hepatic encephalopathy—diagnosis and management. *Neurological Therapeutics: Principles and Practice Editor-in-chief, John H. Noseworthy.* London, New York: Martin Dunitz, 2003.

29 Brouns R, De Deyn P.P. Neurological complications in renal failure: a review. *Clin. Neurol. Neurosurg.* 2004;107(1):1–16.

30 Grewal J, Grewal HK, Forman AD. Seizures and epilepsy in cancer: etiologies, evaluation, and management. *Curr. Oncol. Rep.* 2008;10(1):63–71. Review.

31 Saiz A, Graus F. Neurological complications of hematopoietic cell transplantation. *Semin. Neurol.* 2004;24 (4):427–434. Review.

32 Voltz R. Paraneoplastic neurological syndromes: an update on diagnosis, pathogenesis, and therapy. *Lancet Neurol.* 2002;1(5):294–305. Review.

33 Lucchinetti CF, Kimmel DW, Lennon VA. Paraneoplastic and oncologic profiles of patients seropositive for type 1 antineuronal nuclear autoantibodies. *Neurology* 1998;50 (3):652–657.

34 Rosenfeld MR, Eichen JG, Wade DF, Posner JB, Dalmau J. Molecular and clinical diversity in paraneoplastic immunity to Ma proteins. *Ann. Neurol.* 2001;50:339–348.

35 Hoffmann LA, Jarius S, Pellkofer HL, Schueller M, Krumbholz M, Koenig F, Johannis W, la Fougere C, Newman T, Vincent A, Voltz R. Anti-Ma and anti-Ta associated paraneoplastic neurological syndromes: 22 newly diagnosed patients and review of previous cases.

J. Neurol. Neurosurg. Psychiatry 2008;79(7):767–773. Epub 2008 Jan 25. Review.

36 Chan KH, Vernino S, Lennon VA. ANNA-3 anti-neuronal nuclear antibody: marker of lung cancer-related autoimmunity. *Ann. Neurol.* 2001;50(3):301–311.

37 Yu Z, Kryzer TJ, Griesmann GE, Kim K, Benarroch EE, Lennon VA. CRMP-5 neuronal autoantibody: marker of lung cancer and thymoma-related autoimmunity. *Ann. Neurol.* 2001;49(2):146–154.

38 Dalmau J, Gleichman AJ, Hughes EG, Rossi JE, Peng X, Lai M, Dessain SK, Rosenfeld MR, Balice-Gordon R, Lynch DR. Anti-NMDA-receptor encephalitis: case series and analysis of the effects of antibodies. *Lancet Neurol.* 2008;7(12):1091–1098. Epub 2008 Oct 11.

39 Saiz A, Blanco Y, Sabater L, González F, Bataller L, Casamitjana R, Ramió-Torrentà L, Graus F. Spectrum of neurological syndromes associated with glutamic acid decarboxylase antibodies: diagnostic clues for this association. *Brain* 2008;131(Pt 10):2553–2563. Epub 2008 Aug 7.

40 Tan KM, Lennon VA, Klein CJ, Boeve BF, Pittock SJ. Clinical spectrum of voltage-gated potassium channel autoimmunity. *Neurology* 2008;70(20):1883–1890.

41 Iacobone E, Bailly-Salin J, Polito A, Friedman D, Stevens RD, Sharshar T. Sepsis-associated encephalopathy and its differential diagnosis. *Crit. Care Med.* 2009;37 (10 Suppl):S331–S336. Review.

42 Tunkel AR, Kaye D. Neurologic complications of infective endocarditis. *Neurol. Clin.* 1993;11(2):419–440.

43 Abba K, Ramaratnam S, Ranganathan LN. Antihelmintics for people with neurocysticercosis. *Cochrane Database Syst. Rev.* 2010;3:CD000215.

44 Sander JW, Perucca E. Epilepsy and comorbidity: infections and antimicrobials usage in relation to epilepsy management. *Acta Neurol. Scand. Suppl.* 2003;180:16–22. Review.

45 Chabolla DR, Wszolek ZK. Pharmacologic management of seizures in organ transplant. *Neurology* 2006;67(12 Suppl 4):S34–S38. Review.

46 Senzolo M, Ferronato C, Burra P. Neurologic complications after solid organ transplantation. *Transpl. Int.* 2009;22(3):269–278. Epub 2008 Dec 6. Review.

47 Vaughn C, Zhang L, Schiff D. Reversible posterior leukoencephalopathy syndrome in cancer. *Curr. Oncol. Rep.* 2008;10(1):86–91. Review.

48 Abou Khaled KJ, Hirsch LJ. Updates in the management of seizures and status epilepticus in critically ill patients. *Neurol. Clin.* 2008;26(2):385–408, viii.

49 Gastaut H. Classification of status epilepticus. *Adv. Neurol.* 1983;34:15–35.

50 Hoerth MT, Drazkowski JF. Seizure emergencies in older adults. *Aging Health* 2010;6(1):97–110.

51 Manno EM. New management strategies in the treatment of status epilepticus. *Mayo Clin. Proc.* 2003;78(4): 508–518. Review.

52 Treiman DM, Meyers PD, Walton NY, Collins JF, Colling C, Rowan AJ, Handforth A, Faught E, Calabrese VP, Uthman BM, Ramsay RE, Mamdani MB. A comparison of four treatments for generalized convulsive status epilepticus. Veterans Affairs Status Epilepticus Cooperative Study Group. *N. Engl. J. Med.* 1998;339(12):792–798.

53 Roberto M, Madamba SG, Moore SD, et al. Ethanol increases GABAergic transmission at both pre- and postsynaptic sites in rat central amygdala neurons. *Proc. Natl. Acad. Sci. USA* 2003;100:2053–2058.

54 Brust JC. Seizures, illicit drugs, and ethanol. *Curr. Neurol. Neurosci. Rep.* 2008;8(4):333–338.

55 Brust JC. Seizures and substance abuse: treatment considerations. *Neurology* 2006;67(12 Suppl 4):S45–S48.

56 Sullivan JT, Sykora K, Schneiderman J, Naranjo CA, Sellers EM. Assessment of alcohol withdrawal: the revised Clinical Institute Withdrawal Assessment for Alcohol scale (CIWA-Ar). *Br. J. Addict.* 1989;84:1353–1357.

57 Cunha JM, Carlini EA, Pereira AE, et al. Chronic administration of cannabidiol to healthy volunteers and epileptic patients. *Pharmacology* 1980;21:175–185.

58 Bowyer JF, Ali S. High doses of methamphetamine that cause disruption of the blood–brain barrier in limbic regions produce extensive neuronal degeneration in mouse hippocampus. *Synapse* 2006;60:521–532.

59 Kalant H. The pharmacology and toxicology of "ecstasy" (MDMA) and related drugs. *Can. Med. Assoc. J.* 2001;165:917–928.

60 Plecko B, Stöckler S. Vitamin B6 dependent seizures. *Can. J. Neurol. Sci.* 2009;36(Suppl 2):S73–S77. Review.

61 Haller CA, Meier KH, Olson KR. Seizures reported in association with use of dietary supplements. *Clin. Toxicol. (Phila.)* 2005;43(1):23–30. Review.

7 Neuro-ophthalmology of systemic disease

Matthew J. Thurtell[1] and Janet C. Rucker[2]
[1]University of Iowa, Iowa City, IA, USA
[2]Mount Sinai Medical Center, New York, NY, USA

Systemic disease and its treatments can produce a number of neuro-ophthalmic manifestations. Ischemic optic neuropathies often occur in patients with vascular risk factors, such as diabetes and hypertension, and in giant cell arteritis. Characteristic neuro-ophthalmic deficits can occur with other endocrine disorders, including Graves' disease and pituitary adenomas. Several autoimmune, rheumatologic, and infectious conditions can cause optic neuropathies. Neoplastic disease involving the optic nerves, extraocular muscles, cranial nerves, and brain can cause visual loss, eye-movement dysfunction, or pupillary abnormalities, as can paraneoplastic disorders. Certain surgical procedures carry a risk of specific neuro-ophthalmic complications, such as posterior ischemic optic neuropathy. Numerous drugs, including antibiotic, antiarrhythmic, chemotherapeutic, sedative, and anticonvulsant agents, can produce specific neuro-ophthalmic abnormalities, such as papilledema, optic neuropathies, or eye-movement disorders. While not intended to review all possible neuro-ophthalmic manifestations of systemic disease, we discuss those that are important or commonly encountered in clinical practice. We refer the reader to more comprehensive texts for a detailed account [1,2].

Endocrine disorders

Diabetes mellitus

Patients with *nonarteritic anterior ischemic optic neuropathy* (NAION) often have diabetes. Ischemic optic neuropathies are the most common cause of an acute optic neuropathy in patients over 50 years of age. Ischemic optic neuropathies are subdivided into anterior and posterior variants, depending on the segment of optic nerve affected. Ischemia to the optic nerve head results in anterior ischemic optic neuropathy (AION) and, by definition, optic-disc edema is present acutely. In contrast, ischemia to the retrobulbar portion of the optic nerve results in posterior ischemic optic neuropathy (PION), in which there is a normal-appearing optic nerve acutely. AION is subdivided into non-arteritic (NAION) and arteritic variants. Over 90% of cases of AION are due to NAION. The arteritic variant, classically due to giant cell arteritis, is discussed below (in the section on systemic autoimmune disorders).

NAION is thought to be due to hypoperfusion of the optic nerve head, which receives its arterial supply from the short posterior ciliary arteries. NAION is characterized by sudden onset of painless monocular visual loss that progresses over hours to days. Examination reveals diffuse or segmental (often

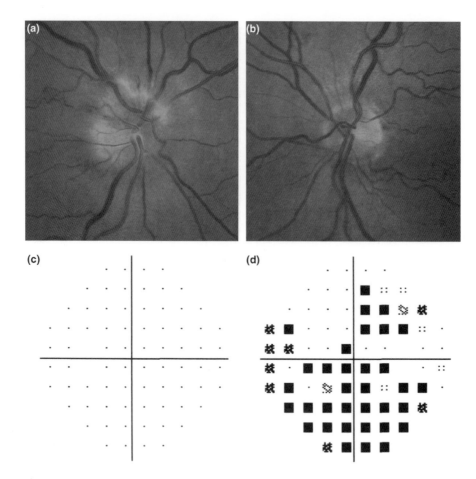

Fig 7.1 Typical examination findings in non-arteritic anterior ischemic optic neuropathy (NAION). (a) Optic-disc edema with associated hemorrhages in the affected right eye, as seen within several days of the onset of visual loss. Note that the disc edema is more severe at the superior aspect of the disc. (b) The optic disc in the unaffected left eye is structurally congested with a small cup (that is, a "disc at risk"). (c) Pattern deviation from the Humphrey visual field of the unaffected left eye is normal. (d) Pattern deviation of the affected right eye shows inferior altitudinal and central visual-field defects. (See also Plate 7.1).

superior) optic-disc edema (Figure 7.1a), often accompanied by an altitudinal visual-field defect affecting the inferior portion of the visual field (Figure 7.1d), although superior or diffuse field loss can occur. The visual acuity at presentation is better than or equal to 20/64 in around 50% of patients with NAION, while it is worse than or equal to 20/200 in about 34% [3]. An important funduscopic sign, and probably the most important risk factor, is the presence of a small optic nerve, with a small or absent physiologic cup (termed the "disc at risk"), in the unaffected eye (Figure 7.1b) [4]. Four to six weeks after the onset of visual loss, the optic-disc edema resolves and the disc becomes pale. The visual-field defect usually persists, although there may be a mild improvement in visual acuity [5]. At present, there is no effective treatment for NAION, although aspirin is often recommended, as is treatment of vascular risk factors. Up to 25% of patients with NAION have diabetes [3]. Diabetes is more strongly associated with NAION in younger patients, and may be associated with increased risk of NAION occurring in the fellow eye [6,7].

Diabetic patients, especially those with type-1 diabetes and coexisting retinopathy, can develop *diabetic papillopathy*, which is characterized by transient unilateral or bilateral disc edema without associated visual loss. The disc edema often lasts for several months, and is thought to be a transient and benign phenomenon, possibly due to microangiopathy with reversibly decreased perfusion of the optic nerve head. However, some of these patients will develop classic NAION with vision loss and, thus, the term *incipient NAION* may be more appropriate [8].

Microvascular cranial mononeuropathies of the third (oculomotor), fourth (trochlear), and sixth (abducens) cranial nerves also occur with increased frequency in patients with diabetes [9]. In fact, these cranial mononeuropathies were referred to as diabetic cranial nerve palsies, until it was recognized that not all patients who developed them had diabetes. The cranial nerve palsy is generally very painful [10] and spontaneous resolution within 8–12 weeks is the rule. A classic clinical hallmark of microvascular ischemic third-nerve palsy is lack of pupil involvement. Mild pupil involvement, with an average of 0.8 mm of anisocoria, may be seen in up to one-third of patients with microvascular third-nerve palsies, but the pupil generally remains reactive [11]. When there is significant pupil involvement in a patient with a complete third-nerve palsy, urgent imaging with CT or MR angiography is mandatory to exclude a posterior communicating (PCOM) artery aneurysm. However, sparing of the pupil does not exclude a PCOM aneurysm when the third-nerve palsy is incomplete and, thus, urgent vascular imaging is also indicated in this setting. A percentage of patients with presumed microvascular cranial mononeuropathies will eventually be found to have a structural lesion and neuroimaging should be considered [12]. In the absence of complete spontaneous resolution within 8–12 weeks, imaging is essential to exclude a structural lesion.

Thyroid disorders

Thyroid disease, in particular *Graves' disease*, can be accompanied by *thyroid eye disease* (TED), which is the most common orbital disease encountered in clinical practice. TED is typically painless and bilateral, although it can be asymmetric. The inferior and medial recti are the muscles most commonly affected, resulting in restriction of eye elevation and abduction. Other signs of orbital disease are often present, including proptosis, periorbital edema, conjunctival injection and chemosis, eyelid retraction, lagophthalmos (inability to close the eye),

lid lag (higher eyelid position than normal in downgaze), and von Graefe's sign (slowed descent of the eyelid during movement from upgaze to downgaze) [13]. An optic neuropathy can result from optic nerve compression at the orbital apex by the enlarged extraocular muscles. Although TED is a clinical diagnosis, patients may be hyperthyroid, hypothyroid, or euthyroid and, thus, thyroid function tests (thyroid-stimulating hormone, T3, and T4 levels) should be obtained. While thyroid-stimulating antibodies are often present in patients with TED and can be an important disease marker in euthyroid patients [14], extraocular muscle antibodies might be a more specific serologic marker of both disease presence and activity [15,16]. At present, testing for extraocular muscle antibodies is not commercially available. Imaging of the orbit is the most useful investigation when the diagnosis is uncertain and typically reveals enlargement of the extraocular muscle bellies with relative sparing of the muscle tendons (Figure 7.2); axial and coronal CT or MR imaging could be obtained, although MRI is preferable as there is no radiation dose to the lens [17].

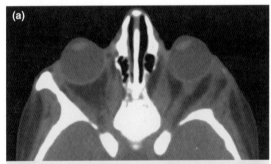
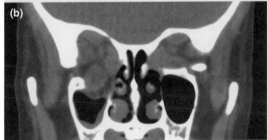

Fig 7.2 Typical radiologic findings in thyroid eye disease. (a) Axial CT of the orbits shows enlargement of extraocular muscle bellies with sparing of muscle tendons. (b) Coronal CT of the orbits shows enlargement of the extraocular muscle bellies with crowding at the orbital apex. The patient had bilateral compressive optic neuropathies and underwent orbital decompression surgery.

Most patients have only mild disease and do not require specific treatment, although supportive interventions, such as prism lenses for diplopia, can be helpful. In those with more severe disease, treatment options include immunosuppression with systemic corticosteroids, radiation therapy, and orbital decompression surgery [18]. Strabismus and eyelid surgery may be required to improve ocular misalignment and eyelid position when the disease has stabilized or following orbital decompression surgery [18]. Radioactive iodine therapy, often given to those patients with hyperthyroidism, can worsen TED and should be avoided in these patients [19,20]. Discontinuation of smoking should also be strongly advised, since smoking can worsen TED and decrease the effects of treatment [21].

Pituitary disorders

Pituitary adenomas often produce neuro-ophthalmic manifestations, such as bitemporal visual-field defects due to chiasmal compression, and cranial nerve palsies due to cavernous sinus invasion (Figure 7.3). When there is long-standing visual loss, funduscopic examination may reveal a characteristic form of optic atrophy known as *bow-tie* atrophy. While functioning pituitary adenomas often cause endocrine manifestations, nonfunctioning adenomas do not and, consequently, the patient may be asymptomatic or have only neuro-ophthalmic manifestations. As these tumors are usually slow-growing, visual loss is often insidious and can go unnoticed until severe or incidentally discovered at the time of an ophthalmic examination. Automated static perimetry is thus essential to determine the extent and severity of visual-field loss (Figure 7.3), which varies depending on the exact site of visual pathway compression (Figure 7.4). MR imaging defines the extent of the lesion (Figure 7.3) and is important for treatment planning. When there is visual loss due to visual pathway compression, or diplopia due to cranial nerve compression, surgical decompression is usually required, although medical treatment with dopamine agonists can be effective for prolactinomas. Observation or medical treatment may be advocated in patients who do not have neuro-ophthalmic complications. The prognosis for visual recovery after decompression is variable, depending on the degree of optic atrophy, severity of visual-field loss, and tumor size [22].

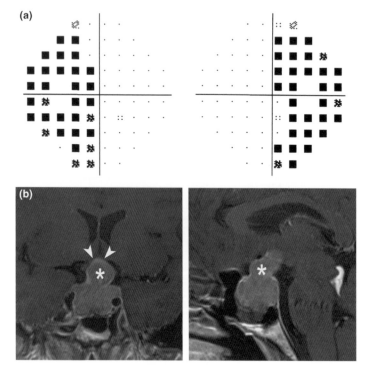

Fig 7.3 Bitemporal hemianopia secondary to nonfunctioning pituitary macroadenoma. (a) Pattern deviation from the Humphrey visual fields reveals an incomplete bitemporal hemianopia. (b) Coronal and sagittal MRI shows a large enhancing lesion (asterisk) extending from the pituitary fossa into the suprasellar cistern to compress the optic chiasm (arrowheads).

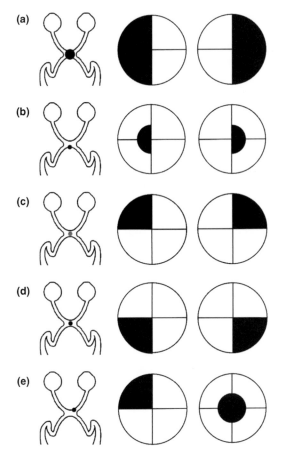

Fig 7.4 Visual-field defects secondary to chiasmal lesions.
(a) Large lesions of the chiasm produce a complete
bitemporal hemianopia. (b) Lesions of the posterior chiasm
produce a macular bitemporal hemianopia. (c) Lesions of the
inferior chiasm produce an upper bitemporal hemianopia.
(d) Lesions of the superior chiasm produce an inferior
bitemporal hemianopia. (e) Lesions at the junction of the
chiasm and optic nerve produce a junctional scotoma, which
is characterized by a central field defect on the side of the
lesion (due to optic nerve involvement) and a contralateral
temporal defect (due to chiasmal involvement).

Pituitary apoplexy is a rare and life-threatening
clinical syndrome that results from infarction of, or
hemorrhage into, a pituitary adenoma. Subsequently,
the tumor rapidly increases in size, leading to the sudden
onset of a variable constellation of symptoms and signs,
including headache, meningism, visual loss, diplopia,
stupor, and cardiovascular collapse due to acute adrenal failure [23,24]. There may be a precipitating factor,

such as anticoagulation or major surgery, in a minority
of patients [25]. The diagnosis can be confirmed with
CT or MR imaging, but is often delayed because most
patients have undiagnosed adenomas [25]. Urgent
treatment with parenteral corticosteroids is required
if there is acute adrenal failure, but the timing of surgical
decompression, which is often indicated in those
patients with neuro-ophthalmic deficits, especially
visual loss, remains controversial [26,27].

Electrolyte and other metabolic disorders

Electrolyte disorders

Electrolyte disorders do not commonly produce neuro-
ophthalmic manifestations. However, rapid correction
of hyponatremia can produce an *osmotic demyelination syndrome*, rarely with associated eye-movement
abnormalities, such as fascicular third nerve palsy,
nystagmus, or ocular bobbing (in which there are intermittent rapid downward eye movements, followed by a
slow drift back to central position) [28,29]. In other
metabolic conditions, such as in *non-ketotic hyperglycemia*, there can be transient reversible homonymous visual-field defects [30], or tonic conjugate eye
deviation due to associated seizures [31]. A variety of
abnormal spontaneous eye movements, such as ocular
bobbing and its variants, can be associated with metabolic disorders causing coma [2].

Lipid storage disorders

Although rarely encountered in clinical practice, several
of the lipid storage disorders can produce neuro-ophthalmic manifestations. *Niemann-Pick disease* (type C)
[32] and *Tay-Sachs disease* [33] can both produce a
vertical saccadic palsy, with relative sparing of other
eye movements. The infantile form of Tay-Sachs disease
produces a *cherry red spot* in the fundus, where the red
color of the normal fovea is accentuated due to the
accumulation of gangliosides in the surrounding retinal
ganglion cells [34]. While funduscopic abnormalities are
not present in late-onset Tay-Sachs disease, eye movement recordings show characteristic "multistep" hypometric saccades, with reduced smooth pursuit and
optokinetic nystagmus gain [35]. *Gaucher's disease* produces a horizontal saccadic palsy, which can improve
with enzyme replacement therapy [36]. *DAF syndrome*

(downgaze palsy, ataxia, and foam cells) produces a downgaze palsy, with a subsequent loss of upgaze, horizontal gaze, and, eventually, a complete supranuclear ophthalmoplegia [37].

Abetalipoproteinemia

Abetalipoproteinemia can produce bilateral ptosis and a progressive ophthalmoplegia that resembles a reversed bilateral internuclear ophthalmoplegia, with slowing of abducting saccades and dissociated nystagmus in the adducting eye [38,39]. It is likely that these eye-movement abnormalities are due to vitamin E deficiency, since similar deficits are seen in patients with other causes of vitamin E deficiency [40].

Wilson's disease

Wilson's disease is a copper storage disease that classically causes an akinetic-rigid syndrome, with associated psychiatric symptoms and liver failure. The *Kayser-Fleischer ring*, a brown discoloration to the peripheral cornea, is a characteristic sign of the disease and may be present prior to the onset of symptoms from the disease [41]. Several eye-movement abnormalities have been described in patients with Wilson's disease, including slow vertical saccades [42], eyelid-opening apraxia [43], and "distractibility of gaze", where the patient is unable to voluntarily fixate on a target unless other competing visual stimuli are removed [44].

Systemic autoimmune disorders

Vasculitis

Some forms of vasculitis produce neuro-ophthalmic manifestations, mostly due to their ischemic complications. *Arteritic anterior ischemic optic neuropathy* (AAION) is classically caused by *giant cell (temporal) arteritis* (GCA), a granulomatous vasculitis that affects medium and large arteries, especially the cranial branches of the aortic arch (superficial temporal, posterior ciliary, ophthalmic, and extracranial vertebral arteries). Timely diagnosis and differentiation from the nonarteritic variant (discussed above in the section on endocrine disorders) is crucial, so treatment can be initiated to prevent visual loss in the fellow eye. Up to 50% of patients with GCA present with visual symptoms, with 70–80% of those presenting with arteritic AION [45]. Arteritic AION presents with sudden unilateral visual loss, with the optic-disc edema often being pallid rather than hyperemic, as is usually seen in NAION (Figure 7.5). Visual acuity at presentation is between count fingers and no light perception in half of patients, compared to a quarter of patients with NAION [45]. There is often visual loss in the other eye within days to weeks if treatment is not initiated in a timely fashion. Other symptoms, including headache, jaw claudication, scalp tenderness, proximal muscle pain, malaise, weight loss, and fever, can precede the visual loss by months, but over 20% of patients with a positive temporal artery biopsy deny having any other symptoms [46]. *Transient monocular visual loss*, which is often induced by postural changes and is thought to be due to transient ischemia of the optic nerve head, precedes permanent visual loss in up to 30% of patients. *PION* (in which there is no optic-disc edema) and *central retinal artery occlusion* are less frequent causes of visual loss from GCA. *Transient diplopia*, thought to be due to ischemia of the extraocular muscles or cranial nerves, occurs in about 5–10% of patients [47]. *Homonymous* and *cortical visual-field loss* can occur due to posterior circulation ischemia from vertebral artery inflammation. The

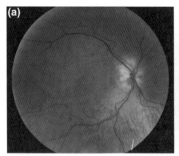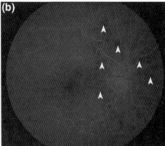

Fig 7.5 Typical examination and fluorescein angiogram findings in arteritic anterior ischemic optic neuropathy secondary to giant cell arteritis. (a) Pallid optic-disc edema in the right eye, as seen within several days of the onset of visual loss. (b) Fluorescein angiogram of the right eye shows areas of choroidal nonperfusion (arrowheads), which are not evident on funduscopic examination, but are highly suggestive of giant cell arteritis. (See also Plate 7.5).

erythrocyte sedimentation rate (ESR) is often highly elevated, but a normal ESR does not exclude the diagnosis. The C-reactive protein (CRP) is a helpful adjunct to the ESR, with the two providing a combined sensitivity of 99% for the diagnosis, as determined from a series of patients with positive temporal artery biopsies [47,48]. However, a temporal artery biopsy is required to confirm the diagnosis; the specimen must be at least 2 cm in length to minimize false-negative results [49]. Whenever arteritic AION is suspected, empiric treatment with corticosteroids should be commenced immediately, while arranging for and awaiting the results of urgent temporal artery biopsy. Either high dose oral or intravenous corticosteroids may be used, although admission for intravenous dosing ensures that the patient is receiving the medication and allows for management of systemic side effects. When the biopsy is positive, oral corticosteroid treatment often has to be given for 18–24 months to prevent recurrent symptoms and complications [50].

Wegener's granulomatosis, a granulomatous and necrotizing vasculitis that typically involves the lungs and kidneys, has an orbital form in which patients develop diplopia due to extraocular muscle involvement [51]. Other neuro-ophthalmic manifestations, such as optic neuropathy and cranial nerve palsy, have been reported [52]. Antineutrophil cytoplasmic antibodies with cytoplasmic staining (c-ANCA) are often detected, although biopsy is required for diagnosis. Treatment is with cyclophosphamide, often given in conjunction with corticosteroids.

Neuro-ophthalmic complications can also be seen in *Churg–Strauss syndrome*, *polyarteritis nodosa*, and *Behçet's disease*, but are uncommon [52]. There is inflammation of arteries *and* veins in patients with Behçet's disease and, thus, they can develop venous sinus thrombosis with papilledema due to intracranial hypertension [53].

Other rheumatologic disorders

Optic neuritis, in which there is monocular visual loss with associated pain, as in idiopathic demyelinating optic neuritis, can occur in patients with *systemic lupus erythematosus* (SLE). *Homonymous* and *cortical visual-field loss* in SLE can result from either cerebral inflammation or ischemia related to the presence of antiphospholipid antibodies. A variety of other neuro-ophthalmic complications can occur in association with SLE, as well as in *rheumatoid arthritis*, *Sjögren's syndrome*, and *scleroderma*, but are rare [52].

Sarcoidosis

Sarcoidosis is a multisystem granulomatous disease of unknown etiology. While it most often involves the lungs, the central nervous system and eye are also commonly involved. Indeed, there are myriad ophthalmic manifestations, including uveitis, vitritis, and retinal vasculitis [54]. Visual loss can also occur due to optic neuropathy, which may be secondary to optic nerve infiltration, inflammation, or granuloma of the optic nerve head (Figure 7.6) [55]. Involvement of the chiasm or retrochiasmal visual pathways can also cause visual loss [55], while rarer causes of visual loss include neuroretinitis (inflammation of the optic disc and retina, producing disc edema and a macular star) and optic perineuritis (inflammation of the periphery of the optic nerve, producing disc edema with spared central vision) [52]. Diplopia, ptosis, and lagophthalmos are common and can be due to involvement of the third, fourth, sixth, and seventh cranial nerves [55]. Histopathologic confirmation is required to establish the diagnosis. MRI can reveal enhancement of the meninges, cranial nerves, and other neural structures, but the imaging changes are nonspecific. The serum angiotensin-converting enzyme (ACE) level is raised in the majority of patients, but is only moderately sensitive and specific for the diagnosis [56]. Chest x-ray or CT may reveal signs of pulmonary sarcoidosis, such as hilar lymphadenopathy, and help to guide subsequent trans-bronchial lymph-node biopsy. Corticosteroids remain the standard treatment, although steroid-sparing agents may be effective in some patients [55].

Organ dysfunction and failure

Hypertension

Hypertension is considered a risk factor for *NAION* (see section on endocrine disease) and is present in up to 47% of patients who develop NAION [3]. Hypertension is more strongly associated with NAION in patients who are less than 50 years old [7]. It has been suggested that NAION might be triggered by nocturnal hypotension, since many patients with NAION awaken with the visual loss [57]. Consequently,

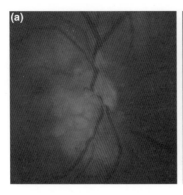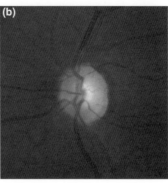

Fig 7.6 Optic-disc granuloma secondary to sarcoidosis. (a) The optic disc in the affected right eye is partially obscured by a large granuloma. The granuloma disappeared following several months of corticosteroid treatment. (b) The optic disc in the unaffected left eye is normal. (See also Plate 7.6).

elimination of night-time antihypertensive medication dosing has been suggested as a preventative measure in patients at risk for NAION [57].

Bilateral optic-disc edema can occur in patients who have *malignant hypertension* [58]. The disc edema is thought to be due to raised intracranial pressure, although lumbar puncture is not routinely performed to confirm this in such patients. Bilateral disc edema in the absence of encephalopathy or raised intracranial pressure may be due to optic nerve head ischemia (NAION), especially when there is associated visual loss, or due to severe hypertensive retinopathy.

Many patients with *microvascular cranial nerve palsies* of the third, fourth, and sixth nerves have hypertension, as well as diabetes, as a risk factor (microvascular cranial nerve palsies are discussed in detail in the section on endocrine disorders). One study suggests that hypertension alone may not be a true risk factor for microvascular sixth-nerve palsies [9], although they can occur with other causes of raised blood pressure, such as pre-eclampsia [59].

Posterior reversible encephalopathy syndrome (PRES) usually occurs in the setting of abrupt increases in blood pressure. Symptoms include headache, altered mental status, seizures, and visual loss [60]. The visual loss results from bilateral parieto-occipital involvement, with symmetrically decreased visual acuity and color vision, but normal pupillary function and a normal ophthalmoscopic examination (unless the patient also has papilledema or hypertensive retinopathy). Brain MRI classically shows symmetrically increased signal in the posterior parietal and occipital white matter on the T2-weighted images due to vasogenic edema. However, it is now known that signal change can also be seen in the frontal lobes, brainstem,

and cerebellum, occasionally as an isolated finding [61]. In most cases, vision gradually recovers with treatment of the hypertension, although visual prognosis is guarded in patients with restricted diffusion on diffusion-weighted imaging [62].

Respiratory failure

Patients with *respiratory failure* occasionally develop papilledema (optic-disc edema due to raised intracranial pressure), which, if left untreated, can produce severe irreversible visual loss [63]. In many, the respiratory failure is due to *obstructive sleep apnea* or *obesity hypoventilation syndrome*. Both of these conditions are strongly associated with obesity, which is also well known to be associated with *idiopathic intracranial hypertension* (previously known as *pseudotumor cerebri*). While it is established that there are acute rises in intracranial pressure during obstructive apneas [64], it remains unclear if those are sufficient to cause papilledema, or if the papilledema is in fact due to idiopathic intracranial hypertension (i.e., not directly related to the respiratory failure). Regardless, the underlying respiratory condition should be addressed, in addition to giving specific treatment for the raised intracranial pressure.

Hepatic failure

Hepatic encephalopathy can produce a characteristic eye-movement abnormality known as *periodic alternating gaze deviation*. As the name suggests, there are conjugate involuntary gaze deviations that change direction every 1–2 min during periods of coma

[65]. There is no structural lesion present on imaging, although there may be other focal neurologic signs, and the abnormal eye movements resolve with treatment of the hepatic encephalopathy.

Systemic cancer and paraneoplastic disorders

Systemic cancer

Visual loss can result from *optic nerve infiltration, carcinomatous,* or *lymphomatous meningitis,* or *compression of the optic nerve* by a metastatic deposit (Figure 7.7). Intracranial neoplasms and neoplastic meningitis can cause *papilledema* due to raised intracranial pressure with or without obstructive hydrocephalus, visual-field defects due to involvement of the optic chiasm or retrochiasmal visual pathways (Figure 7.8), and a variety of eye-movement abnormalities, including external ophthalmoplegia due to *cranial nerve palsies, nuclear* or *supranuclear gaze palsies* (Figure 7.9), and *nystagmus.*

Horner's syndrome results from a lesion of the sympathetic fibers passing from the hypothalamus to the orbit, and is characterized by ipsilateral eyelid ptosis and pupillary miosis with or without facial anhidrosis. It can be caused by a variety of benign and malignant neoplasms, including neoplasms of the brainstem, spinal cord, lung apex (the classic *Pancoast's tumor*), neck (such as *neuroblastoma* in young children), skull base, cavernous sinus, or orbit. Other symptoms and signs, and pharmacologic pupillary testing, might help localize the causative lesion and indicate the area of interest for imaging studies [66].

Paraneoplastic disorders

Paraneoplastic syndromes result from tissue damage mediated by autoantibodies produced in response to a remote tumor, which is often occult and undiagnosed at symptom onset. Identification of paraneoplastic antibodies in serum or cerebrospinal fluid assists with diagnosis and, despite the initial suggestion that specific antibodies correlate with specific syndromes, it is now thought that the antibody present is more tightly correlated with the cancer type than the neurological syndrome [67]. As the paraneoplastic syndrome often

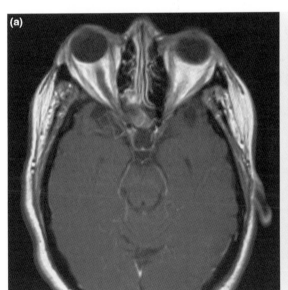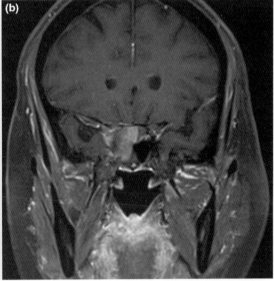

Fig 7.7 Right optic neuropathy due to compression by a breast cancer metastasis. The patient was receiving chemotherapy for metastatic breast cancer when she developed progressive visual loss in her right eye. (a) Axial postcontrast T1-weighted MRI shows an enhancing lesion compressing the intracanalicular portion of the right optic nerve. (b) Coronal postcontrast T1-weighted MRI with fat suppression shows the lesion arising from the sphenoid bone.

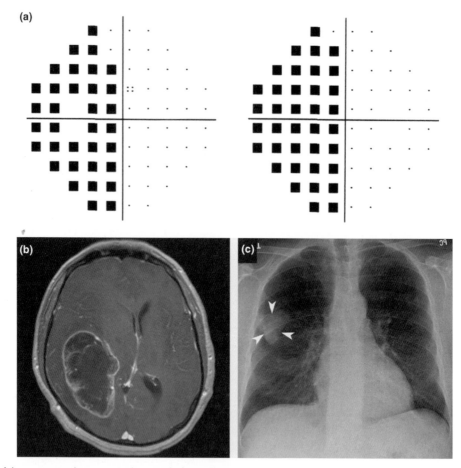

Fig 7.8 Left homonymous hemianopia due to right-hemisphere metastasis. The patient was a long-term smoker, who had a several week history of headache and difficulty seeing to the left. (a) Pattern deviation from the Humphrey visual fields shows a complete left homonymous hemianopia. (b) Axial postcontrast T1-weighted MRI shows a ring-enhancing lesion in the posterior right hemisphere that is causing mass effect and midline shift. Biopsy of the lesion revealed adenocarcinoma. (c) Chest x-ray shows the primary lesion in the periphery of the right lung (arrowheads).

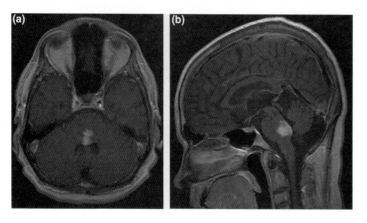

Fig 7.9 Presumed low-grade glioma in the pons in a man with neurofibromatosis type 1. The patient developed a horizontal saccadic palsy with sparing of other horizontal eye movements, likely due to isolated involvement of the paramedian pontine reticular formation (which houses the burst neurons responsible for generating horizontal saccades). (a) Axial and (b) sagittal postcontrast T1-weighted MRI shows an enhancing lesion extending into the pontine tegmentum.

precedes the diagnosis of the primary tumor, an exhaustive search for a tumor is essential, since it might be potentially curable and treatment of an underlying tumor may improve the paraneoplastic syndrome.

Paraneoplastic optic neuropathy is a rare condition that is most often associated with collapsin response-mediator protein 5 (CRMP-5) antibodies and underlying small-cell lung cancer. It typically presents with painless bilateral subacute visual loss, and examination reveals decreased visual acuity, dyschromatopsia, central scotomas, and bilateral disc edema accompanied by signs of inflammation in the vitreous and the retina [68].

Cranial nerve palsies, nuclear or *supranuclear gaze palsies*, and *nystagmus* can be caused by paraneoplastic disorders. *Paraneoplastic brainstem encephalitis* occurs most often with small-cell lung cancer and testicular cancers, and is associated with anti-Hu and anti-Ma2 antibodies; vertical gaze palsy is the most consistent ocular motor feature [69]. *Downbeat nystagmus* is a common feature of paraneoplastic cerebellar degeneration associated with anti-Hu and anti-Yo antibodies and small-cell lung, breast, and ovarian cancers. Excessive irrepressible saccadic eye movements in all directions (*opsoclonus*) or confined to the horizontal plane (*ocular flutter*) can be part of the *opsoclonus–myoclonus syndrome*; 50% of children with this syndrome will be found to have a neuroblastoma [70] and many will have anti-Ri antibodies. In adults, opsoclonus and ocular flutter can be associated with small-cell lung, breast, and ovarian cancers. Paraneoplastic antibodies are often not detected, but there may be anti-Ri and anti-Hu antibodies. Other causes of opsoclonus and ocular flutter, such as brainstem encephalitis, need to be considered if no tumor is found [2].

Systemic infectious diseases

Optic neuritis and neuroretinitis

Infections can affect the optic nerve via several mechanisms: direct anterior optic nerve inflammation with optic-disc edema (*papillitis*); direct posterior optic nerve inflammation (*retrobulbar optic neuritis*); peripheral optic nerve inflammation (*optic perineuritis*); infarction of the optic nerve or retina due to secondary vasculitis; and papilledema from meningitis or meningoencephalitis. *Lyme disease, cat scratch disease*, and *syphilis* are the most common infectious causes of optic neuropathy, although other infections, including *tuberculosis, toxoplasma, toxocara, herpes zoster, West Nile virus*, and *HIV*, can also affect the optic nerves.

Lyme disease, caused by *Borrelia burgdorferi*, is a well-known cause of *optic neuritis*, mimicking idiopathic demyelinating optic neuritis. However, screening of patients with typical idiopathic optic neuritis in Lyme endemic areas is not routinely recommended. Lyme disease testing should be pursued when optic neuritis follows a tick bite or is accompanied by *erythema migrans* or another symptom suggestive of Lyme disease [71].

Cat scratch disease, caused by *Bartonella henselae*, is a common cause of *neuroretinitis*, in which there is optic-disc edema in combination with retinal involvement, manifesting as hard exudates arranged in a star-like configuration around the macula (Figure 7.10) [72]. Lyme disease and syphilis cause neuroretinitis less frequently. It is important to recognize that the development of the macular star may lag behind development of optic-disc edema, so there should be a low threshold for obtaining *Bartonella* titers in patients with visual loss, optic-disc edema, and

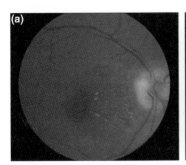 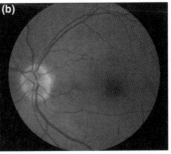

Fig 7.10 Neuroretinitis due to cat scratch disease. The patient had a history of exposure to cats and positive *Bartonella henselae* titers. (a) Optic-disc edema and a partial macular star figure are present in the affected right eye. (b) Normal optic disc and macula in the unaffected left eye. (See also Plate 7.10).

137

exposure to cats. The optic-disc edema typically resolves over several weeks, but the macular star figure may persist for 6–12 months.

Meningitis, encephalitis, and intracerebral abscess

Systemic infections producing *acute* or *chronic meningitis* can cause papilledema and sixth-nerve palsies due to raised intracranial pressure. Those producing a basilar meningitis, such as *tuberculosis*, can cause ophthalmoplegia as a result of cranial nerve palsies.

Some forms of *encephalitis* can present with isolated neuro-ophthalmic manifestations. Patients with acquired immunodeficiency syndrome (AIDS) can develop neuro-ophthalmic manifestations, including visual loss, papilledema, and eye-movement abnormalities, which may be directly related to the HIV infection or its complications [73]. *Progressive multifocal leukoencephalopathy*, a rare condition associated with AIDS and JC virus infection, often produces visual loss or cortical blindness due to retrochiasmal visual pathway involvement, but can also cause eye-movement abnormalities such as supranuclear and nuclear gaze palsies or nystagmus [74].

Systemic infections producing *intracerebral abscesses* can also give rise to neuro-ophthalmic manifestations, including papilledema due to raised intracranial pressure, visual loss, and eye-movement abnormalities. The deficit depends on the location of the abscess in the brain parenchyma.

Whipple's disease

Whipple's disease, caused by *Tropheryma whippelii*, can cause a *vertical saccadic palsy*, in which there is preservation of vertical vestibular-evoked eye movements [75]. A *global saccadic palsy* can develop over time. Whipple's disease can also produce a characteristic abnormality of eye and jaw movements, called *oculomasticatory myorhythmia*, in which there are 1 Hz pendular vergence (convergent–divergent) oscillations of the eyes with synchronized masticatory muscle contractions [76].

Complications due to transplantation

Transplantation does not commonly produce neuro-ophthalmic manifestations. However, many neuro-ophthalmic manifestations can be produced by post-transplantation immunosuppression as a result of the direct effects of treatment, as in PRES resulting from immunosuppressant toxicity (see section on drugs, toxins, and vitamin and mineral deficiencies), or the indirect effects of treatment, as in opportunistic infections (see section on systemic infectious diseases) and neoplastic conditions (see section above on systemic cancer and paraneoplastic disorders).

Complications of critical medical illness

Critical medical illness

Critical medical illnesses can occasionally produce neuro-ophthalmic manifestations, including visual loss or eye-movement abnormalities occurring in the setting of severe metabolic disturbance (see section on electrolyte and other metabolic disorders) and organ failure (see section on organ dysfunction and failure). Several relatively benign neuro-ophthalmic manifestations can result from treatments or procedures performed in the setting of critical medical illness, including pupillary abnormalities. Jugular central venous lines can occasionally be associated with a *Horner's syndrome* due to trauma to the sympathetic fibers ascending on the carotid artery, or due to secondary thrombophlebitis [77]. Use of nebulized bronchodilators, such as ipratropium, can produce an isolated fixed and dilated *pharmacologic pupil* when the nebulizer mask is loosely fitted [78]; the diagnosis can be confirmed by demonstrating a lack of pupillary response to pilocarpine drops.

Surgical procedures

Certain surgical procedures carry an increased risk of specific neuro-ophthalmic complications. *Ischemic optic neuropathy*, in the form of NAION or PION, can be precipitated by intraocular surgery (presumably via raised intraocular pressure and decreased ocular perfusion pressure), *spine surgery*, and other surgical procedures associated with severe hypotension or blood loss. Over 50% of patients with perioperative PION develop it following lumbar spinal surgery [79]. The PION is bilateral in over 70% of cases. Proposed intraoperative risk factors include hypotension, anemia, hypovolemia, hemodilution, decreased oxygenation, and blood loss, but cases have been reported in which there was no appreciated risk factor [80].

A selective *saccadic palsy* is an infrequent complication of cardiovascular surgery, especially *ascending aortic aneurysm repair*. Typically, all voluntary and reflexive saccades are impaired [81]. MRI is often normal, although a dorsal pontine lesion may be present [82]. The mechanism of injury is uncertain, although ischemia to the brainstem reticular formation, which houses the burst neurons for saccades, is likely.

Drugs, toxins (including alcohol), and vitamin and mineral deficiencies

Drugs and toxins

Toxic optic neuropathies can be caused by several drugs, including *ethambutol, chloramphenicol*, and *linezolid*. The effect is dependent on dose and duration of treatment, and may result from metabolic impairment as well as mitochondrial dysfunction. Patients typically present with subacute, progressive, bilateral visual loss. Examination reveals bilaterally decreased visual acuity, dyschromatopsia (loss of color vision), and central visual-field defects. However, there may be little or no optic-disc pallor on funduscopic examination. Management consists of removal of the offending agent and supplementation with B-complex vitamins. Visual toxicity from ethambutol, an antimycobacterial agent, is well established, and may result from involvement of the retina as well as the optic nerve [83]. Visual loss begins several months after the treatment is initiated, especially in patients with renal insufficiency. Most patients improve following discontinuation of the drug. As with ethambutol, the optic nerve toxicity from chloramphenicol and linezolid begins several months after the treatment is initiated. However, vision may fully recover with discontinuation of the drug. A severe bilateral optic neuropathy can occur as a result of methanol ingestion in patients with alcohol dependence (Figure 7.11).

Several medications have been implicated in the pathogenesis of *NAION*, including *amiodarone* and *phosphodiesterase type-5 inhibitors* for erectile

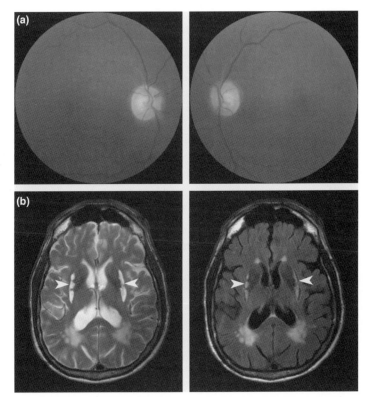

Fig 7.11 Bilateral toxic optic neuropathies due to methanol ingestion in a patient with alcoholism. (a) Diffuse optic atrophy is present in both eyes several months after the visual loss developed. (b) Axial T2-weighted and FLAIR MRI show periventricular white-matter signal changes and putaminal necrosis (arrowheads), a highly characteristic finding in patients with methanol poisoning. (See also Plate 7.11).

Table 7.1 Eye-movement disorders from drug and toxin exposure (adapted from refs. [2,89])

Eye-movement disorder	Drug/toxin
Gaze palsy	Baclofen, barbiturates, carbamazepine, phenytoin, tricyclic antidepressants
Internuclear ophthalmoplegia	Phenothiazines, tricyclic antidepressants, toluene
Divergence palsy	Benzodiazepines
Convergence spasm	Phenytoin
Bilateral vestibular palsy	Aminoglycosides (irreversible)
Oculogyric crisis	Carbamazepine, lithium, phenothiazines, butyrophenones, metoclopramide
Opsoclonus	Lithium, L-tryptophan, tricyclic antidepressants, phenytoin, benzodiazepines, metyrosine, cocaine, chlordecone, thallium, strychnine, toluene, organophosphates
Downbeat nystagmus	Carbamazepine, alcohol (reversible and irreversible), lithium (irreversible), phenytoin, felbamate, amiodarone, opioids, toluene
Primary position upbeat nystagmus	Tobacco, organophosphates
Periodic alternating nystagmus	Phenytoin, lithium
Pendular nystagmus	Toluene (irreversible)
Positional nystagmus	Alcohol
Gaze-evoked nystagmus	Marijuana, anticonvulsants

dysfunction [84,85]. Establishing a direct relationship between use of a medication and NAION is problematic, since most patients also have vascular risk factors and a "disc-at-risk." Nevertheless, the possibility should be discussed with the patient, so that an informed decision can be made regarding continuation or discontinuation of the medication.

Medications strongly associated with *increased intracranial pressure* and *papilledema* include *tetracycline antibiotics* (such as doxycycline and minocycline), *vitamin A*, and *lithium* [86]. Elimination of the offending agent will usually decrease the intracranial pressure, although other interventions may be required.

PRES can be seen with toxicity from immunosuppressive medications, including *cyclosporine, tacrolimus*, and *sirolimus* [87]. A detailed description of the syndrome and imaging findings is described above (in the section on organ dysfunction and failure). Symptoms and imaging abnormalities are often reversible with a reduction in the dose or discontinuation of the offending agent. A similar syndrome can occur following angiographic procedures, and is thought to occur due to breakdown of the blood–brain barrier by the contrast media, with consequent neurotoxic effects [88]. Once infarction has been excluded, a full recovery of vision can be expected within hours to days without specific intervention.

Many medications are known to produce eye-movement abnormalities such as nystagmus, gaze palsy, and opsoclonus (see Table 7.1). The eye-movement abnormalities are usually due to acute toxicity and are reversible, but the deficits produced by some drugs may be permanent [89].

Vitamin and mineral deficiencies

Vitamin B12 (cobalamin) deficiency is a well-known cause of optic neuropathy, although uncommon in developed countries. Other causes include vitamin B1 (thiamine), vitamin B2 (riboflavin), and folic-acid deficiencies [90]. Clinical signs are similar to those seen with toxic optic neuropathies. There is often an improvement in vision with vitamin repletion.

Wernicke's encephalopathy, from thiamine deficiency, can cause ophthalmoplegia, nystagmus, ataxia, and altered mental status. Less than 50% of patients have a classic presentation [91]. Over half of

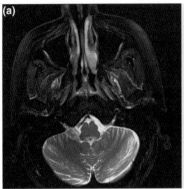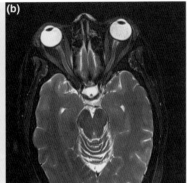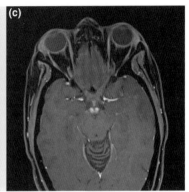

Fig 7.12 Typical radiologic findings in Wernicke's encephalopathy. The patient had gastric cancer and developed confusion, diplopia, and ataxia following several months of vomiting. Examination revealed bilateral abduction deficits with gaze-evoked and upbeat nystagmus. Axial T2-weighted MRI shows increased signal in the (a) dorsal medulla and (b) periaqueductal gray. (c) Axial postcontrast T1-weighted MRI with fat saturation shows enhancement of the mamillary bodies, which is a highly characteristic finding in Wernicke's encephalopathy.

patients have a symmetric or asymmetric horizontal ophthalmoplegia, including abduction deficits and gaze palsies, and some may have a vertical ophthalmoplegia. Gaze-evoked and upbeat nystagmus is also commonly present. Rarely, patients can develop an optic neuropathy with associated optic-disc edema [92]. MRI may reveal signal abnormalities in the floor of the fourth ventricle, peri-aqueductal gray matter, mamillary bodies, and thalamic periventricular areas on T2-weighted imaging (Figure 7.12) [91]. Parenteral administration of thiamine often results in a rapid improvement in the eye-movement abnormalities and optic neuropathy, although an incomplete recovery is not uncommon, especially if treatment is delayed.

 Five things to remember about the neuro-ophthalmology of systemic disease

1. Ischemic optic neuropathies, the most common cause of optic neuropathy in patients over the age of 50, can be classified into a nonarteritic variant (occurring in patients with vascular risk factors) and an arteritic variant (occurring in patients with giant cell arteritis).
2. Painful isolated ocular motor cranial nerve palsies in older patients with vascular risk factors are often due to microvascular ischemia.
3. Pituitary apoplexy should be considered in patients with sudden onset headache, severe vision loss, and eye-movement dysfunction, especially in the postoperative setting, because urgent neurosurgical decompression may be required.
4. Ethambutol, chloramphenicol, and linezolid can cause toxic optic neuropathies; amiodarone and phosphodiesterase type-5 inhibitors can cause anterior ischemic optic neuropathies; and tetracyclines, vitamin A derivatives, and lithium can cause raised intracranial pressure with papilledema.
5. Wernicke's encephalopathy can cause ophthalmoplegia, nystagmus, ataxia, and altered mental status, which can be reversible if thiamine replacement is given in a timely fashion.

References

1 Miller NR, Newman NJ, Biousse V, Kerrison JB (eds). *Walsh & Hoyt's Clinical Neuro-Ophthalmology*, 6th ed. Philadelphia: Lippincott Williams & Wilkins, 2005.

2 Leigh RJ, Zee DS. *The Neurology of Eye Movements*, 4th ed. New York: Oxford University Press, 2006.

3 The Ischemic Optic Neuropathy Decompression Trial Research Group. Characteristics of patients with non-arteritic anterior ischemic optic neuropathy eligible for the Ischemic Optic Neuropathy Decompression Trial. *Arch. Ophthalmol.* 1996;114:1366–1374.

4 Beck RW, Servais GE, Hayreh SS. Anterior ischemic optic neuropathy. IX. Cup-to-disc ratio and its role in pathogenesis. *Ophthalmology* 1987;94:1503–1508.

5 The Ischemic Optic Neuropathy Decompression Trial Research Group. Optic nerve decompression surgery for nonarteritic anterior ischemic optic neuropathy (NAION) is not effective and may be harmful. *J. Am. Med. Assoc.* 1995;273:625–632.

6 Preechawat P, Bruce BB, Newman NJ, Biousse V. Anterior ischemic optic neuropathy in patients younger than 50 years. *Am. J. Ophthalmol.* 2007;144:953–960.

7 Hayreh SS, Joos KM, Podhajsky PA, Long CR. Systemic diseases associated with nonarteritic anterior ischemic optic neuropathy. *Am. J. Ophthalmol.* 1994;118:766–780.

8 Hayreh SS, Zimmerman MB. Incipient nonarteritic anterior ischemic optic neuropathy. *Ophthalmology* 2007;114:1763–1772.

9 Patel SV, Holmes JM, Hodge DO, Burke JP. Diabetes and hypertension in isolated sixth nerve palsy: a population-based study. *Ophthalmology* 2005;112:760–763.

10 Wilker SC, Rucker JC, Newman NJ, Biousse V, Tomsak RL. Pain in ischaemic ocular motor cranial nerve palsies. *Br. J. Ophthalmol.* 2009;93:1657–1659.

11 Jacobson DM. Pupil involvement in patients with diabetes-associated oculomotor nerve palsy. *Arch. Ophthalmol.* 1998;116:723–727.

12 Chou KL, Galetta SL, Liu GT, et al. Acute ocular motor mononeuropathies: prospective study of the roles of neuroimaging and clinical assessment. *J. Neurol. Sci.* 2004;219:35–39.

13 Gaddipati RV, Meyer DR. Eyelid retraction, lid lag, lagophthalmos, and von Graefe's sign quantifying the eyelid features of Graves' ophthalmopathy. *Ophthalmology* 2008;115:1083–1088.

14 Goh SY, Ho SC, Seah LL, Fong KS, Khoo DH. Thyroid autoantibody profiles in ophthalmic dominant and thyroid dominant Graves' disease differ and suggest ophthalmopathy is a multiantigenic disease. *Clin. Endocrinol. (Oxf.)* 2004;60:600–607.

15 de Bellis A, Perrino S, Coronella C, et al. Extraocular muscle antibodies and the occurrence of ophthalmopathy in Graves' disease. *Clin. Endocrinol. (Oxf.)* 2004;60:694–698.

16 Gopinath B, Musselman R, Adams CL, et al. Study of serum antibodies against three eye muscle antigens and the connective tissue antigen collagen XIII in patients with Graves' disease with and without ophthalmopathy: correlation with clinical features. *Thyroid* 2006;16:967–974.

17 Kahaly GJ. Recent developments in Graves' ophthalmopathy imaging. *J. Endocrinol. Invest.* 2004;27:254–258.

18 Bartalena L, Tanda ML. Graves' ophthalmopathy. *N. Engl. J. Med.* 2009;360:994–1001.

19 Tallstedt L, Lundell G, Torring O, et al. Occurrence of ophthalmopathy after treatment for Graves' hyperthyroidism. *N. Engl. J. Med.* 1992;326:1733–1738.

20 Bartalena L, Marcocci C, Bogazzi F, et al. Relation between therapy for hyperthyroidism and the course of Graves' ophthalmopathy. *N. Engl. J. Med.* 1998;338:73–78.

21 Eckstein A, Quadbeck B, Mueller G, et al. Impact of smoking on the response to treatment of thyroid associated ophthalmopathy. *Br. J. Ophthalmol.* 2003;87:773–776.

22 Monteiro ML, Zambon BK, Cunha LP. Predictive factors for the development of visual loss in patients with pituitary macroadenomas and for visual recovery after optic pathway decompression. *Can. J. Ophthalmol.* 2010;45:404–408.

23 Sibal L, Ball SG, Connolly V, et al. Pituitary apoplexy: a review of clinical presentation, management and outcome in 45 cases. *Pituitary* 2004;7:157–163.

24 Semple PL, Webb MK, de Villiers JC, Laws ER Jr., Pituitary apoplexy. *Neurosurgery* 2005;56:65–73.

25 Biousse V, Newman NJ, Oyesiku NM. Precipitating factors in pituitary apoplexy. *J. Neurol. Neurosurg. Psychiatry* 2001;71:542–545.

26 Lubina A, Olchovsky D, Berezin M, et al. Management of pituitary apoplexy: clinical experience with 40 patients. *Acta Neurochir. (Wien)* 2005;147:151–157.

27 Agrawal D, Mahapatra AK. Visual outcome of blind eyes in pituitary apoplexy after transsphenoidal surgery: a series of 14 eyes. *Surg. Neurol.* 2005;63:42–46.

28 Hawthorne KM, Compton CJ, Vaphiades MS, et al. Ocular motor and imaging abnormalities of midbrain dysfunction in osmotic demyelination syndrome. *J. Neuroophthalmol.* 2009;29:296–299.

29 Zegers-Beyl D, Flament-Durand J, Borenstein S, Brunko E. Ocular bobbing and myoclonus in central pontine myelinolysis. *J. Neurol. Neurosurg. Psychiatry* 1983;46:564–565.

30 Freedman KA, Polepalle S. Transient homonymous hemianopia and positive visual phenomena in nonketotic hyperglycemic patients. *Am. J. Ophthalmol.* 2004;137:1122–1124.

31 Venugopal N, Ramakrishnan R, Saravanan, Eapen P. Tonic eye deviation due to nonketotic hyperglycaemia induced focal seizures: case report. *Ind. J. Ophthalmol.* 2005;53:200–201.

32 Fink JK, Filling-Katz MR, Sokol J, et al. Clinical spectrum of Niemann–Pick disease type C. *Neurology* 1989;39:1040–1049.

33 Jampel RS, Quaglio ND. Eye movements in Tay–Sachs disease. *Neurology* 1964;14:1013–1019.

34 Kivlin JD, Sanborn GE, Myers GG. The cherry-red spot in Tay–Sachs and other storage diseases. *Ann Neurol* 1985;17:356–360.

35 Rucker JC, Shapiro BE, Han YH, et al. Neuro-ophthalmology of late-onset Tay-Sachs disease (LOTS). *Neurology* 2004;63:1918–1926.

36 Pensiero S, Accardo A, Pittis MG, et al. Saccade testing in the diagnosis and treatment of type 3 Gaucher disease. *Neurology* 2005;65:1837.

37 Cogan DG, Chu FC, Bachman DM, et al. The DAF syndrome. *Neuroophthalmology* 1981;2:7.

38 Yee RD, Cogan DG, Zee DS. Ophthalmoplegia and dissociated nystagmus in abetalipoproteinemia. *Arch. Ophthalmol.* 1976;94:571–575.

39 Cohen DA, Bosley TM, Savino PJ, et al. Primary aberrant regeneration of the oculomotor nerve: occurrence in a patient with abetalipoproteinemia. *Arch. Neurol.* 1985; 42:821–823.

40 Cremer PD, Halmagyi GM. Eye movement disorders in a patient with liver disease. *Neuroophthalmology* 1996; 16:276.

41 Rodman R, Burnstine M, Esmaeli B, et al. Wilson's disease: presymptomatic patients and Kayser–Fleischer rings. *Ophthalmic Genet.* 1997;18:79–85.

42 Kirkham TH, Kamin DF. Slow saccadic eye movements in Wilson's disease. *J. Neurol. Neurosurg. Psychiatry* 1974;37:191–194.

43 Keane JR, Lid-opening apraxia in Wilson's disease. *J. Clin. Neuroophthalmol.* 1988;8:31–33.

44 Lennox G, Jones R. Gaze distractibility in Wilson's disease. *Ann. Neurol.* 1989;25:415–417.

45 Hayreh SS, Zimmerman B. Management of giant cell arteritis. Our 27-year clinical study: new light on old controversies. *Ophthalmologica* 2003;217:239–259.

46 Hayreh SS, Podhajsky PA, Zimmerman B. Occult giant cell arteritis: ocular manifestations. *Am. J. Ophthalmol.* 1998;125:521–526.

47 Hayreh SS, Podhajsky PA, Raman R, Zimmerman B. Giant cell arteritis: validity and reliability of various diagnostic criteria. *Am. J. Ophthalmol.* 1997;123:285–296.

48 Parikh M, Miller NR, Lee AG, et al. Prevalence of a normal C-reactive protein with an elevated erythrocyte sedimentation rate in biopsy-proven giant cell arteritis. *Ophthalmology* 2006;113:1842–1845.

49 Carroll SC, Gaskin BJ, Danesh-Meyer HV. Giant cell arteritis. *Clin. Exp. Ophthalmol.* 2006;34:159–173.

50 Kawasaki A, Purvin V. Giant cell arteritis: an updated review. *Acta Ophthalmol.* 2009;87:13–32.

51 Fechner FP, Faquin WC, Pilch BZ. Wegener's granulomatosis of the orbit: a clinicopathological study of 15 patients. *Laryngoscope* 2002;112:1945–1950.

52 Golnik KC. Neuro-ophthalmologic manifestations of systemic disease: rheumatologic/inflammatory. *Ophthalmol. Clin. N. Am.* 2004;17:389–396.

53 Wechsler B, Vidailhet M, Piette JC, et al. Cerebral venous thrombosis in Behçet's disease: clinical study and long-term follow-up of 25 cases. *Neurology* 1992;42:614–618.

54 Jabs DA, Johns CJ. Ocular involvement in chronic sarcoidosis. *Am. J. Ophthalmol.* 1986;102:297–301.

55 Constantino T, Digre K, Zimmerman P. Neuro-ophthalmic complications of sarcoidosis. *Semin. Neurol.* 2000;20: 123–137.

56 Power WJ, Neves RA, Rodriguez A, et al. The value of combined serum angiotensin-converting enzyme and gallium scan in diagnosing ocular sarcoidosis. *Ophthalmology* 1995;102:2007–2011.

57 Hayreh SS. Role of nocturnal arterial hypotension in the development of ocular manifestations of systemic arterial hypertension. *Curr. Opin. Ophthalmol.* 1999;10: 474–482.

58 Lip GY, Beevers M, Dodson PM, Beevers DG. Severe hypertension with lone bilateral papilloedema: a variant of malignant hypertension. *Blood Press* 1995;4:339–342.

59 Thurtell MJ, Sharp KL, Spies JM, Halmagyi GM. Isolated sixth cranial nerve palsy in preeclampsia. *J. Neuroophthalmol.* 2006;26:296–298.

60 Hinchey J, Chaves C, Appignani B, et al. A reversible posterior leukoencephalopathy syndrome. *N. Engl. J. Med.* 1996;334:494–500.

61 Lee VH, Wijdicks EF, Manno EM, Rabinstein AA. Clinical spectrum of reversible posterior leukoencephalopathy syndrome. *Arch. Neurol.* 2008;65:205–210.

62 Covarrubias DJ, Luetmer PH, Campeau NG. Posterior reversible encephalopathy syndrome: prognostic utility of quantitative diffusion-weighted MR images. *Am. J. Neuroradiol.* 2002;23:1038–1048.

63 Reeve P, Harvey G, Seaton D. Papilloedema and respiratory failure. *Br. Med. J.* 1985;291:331–332.

64 Jennum P, Borgesen SE. Intracranial pressure and obstructive sleep apnea. *Chest* 1989;95:279–283.

65 Averbuch-Heller L, Meiner Z. Reversible periodic alternating gaze deviation in hepatic encephalopathy. *Neurology* 1995;45:191–192.

66 Almog Y, Gepstein R, Kesler A. Diagnostic value of imaging in Horner syndrome in adults. *J. Neuroophthalmol.* 2010;30:7–11.

67 Pittock SJ, Kryzer TJ, Lennon VA. Paraneoplastic antibodies coexist and predict cancer, not neurological syndrome. *Ann. Neurol.* 2004;56:715–719.

68 Cross SA, Salomao DR, Parisi JE, et al. Paraneoplastic autoimmune optic neuritis with retinitis defined by CRMP-5-IgG. *Ann. Neurol.* 2003;54:38–50.

69 Dalmau J, Graus F, Villarejo A, et al. Clinical analysis of anti-Ma2-associated encephalitis. *Brain* 2004;127:1831–1844.

70 Ko MW, Dalmau J, Galetta SL. Neuro-ophthalmologic manifestations of paraneoplastic syndromes. *J. Neuro-ophthalmol.* 2008;28:58–68.

71 Jacobson DM. Lyme disease and optic neuritis: long-term follow-up of seropositive patients. *Neurology* 2003;60:881–882.

72 Bar S, Segal M, Shapira R, Savir H. Neuroretinitis associated with cat scratch disease. *Am. J. Ophthalmol.* 1990;110:703–705.

73 Mansour AM. Neuro-ophthalmic findings in acquired immunodeficiency syndrome. *J. Clin. Neuroophthalmol.* 1990;10:167–174.

74 Ormerod LD, Rhodes RH, Gross SA, et al. Ophthalmologic manifestations of acquired immune deficiency syndrome-associated progressive multifocal leukoencephalopathy. *Ophthalmology* 1996;103:899–906.

75 Averbuch-Heller L, Paulson GW, Daroff RB, Leigh RJ. Whipple's disease mimicking progressive supranuclear palsy: the diagnostic value of eye movement recording. *J. Neurol. Neurosurg. Psychiatry* 1999;66:532–535.

76 Schwartz MA, Selhorst JB, Ochs AL, et al. Oculomasticatory myorhythmia: a unique movement disorder occurring in Whipple's disease. *Ann. Neurol.* 1986;20:677–683.

77 Talks SJ, Shah P, Sinha PA. Horner's syndrome following central line insertion. *Anaesthesia* 1994;49:553.

78 Eustace N, Gardiner C, Eustace P, Marsh B. Nebulised ipratropium causing a unilateral fixed dilated pupil in the critically ill patient: a report of two cases. *Crit. Care Resusc.* 2004;6:268–270.

79 Cheng MA, Sigurdson W, Tempelhoff R, Lauryssen C. Visual loss after spine surgery: a survey. *Neurosurgery* 2000;46:625–630.

80 Newman NJ. Perioperative visual loss after nonocular surgeries. *Am. J. Ophthalmol.* 2008;145:604–610.

81 Solomon D, Ramat S, Tomsak RL, et al. Saccadic palsy after cardiac surgery: characteristics and pathogenesis. *Ann. Neurol.* 2008;63:355–365.

82 Eggers SD, Moster ML, Cranmer K. Selective saccadic palsy after cardiac surgery. *Neurology* 2008;70:318–320.

83 Vistamehr S, Walsh TJ, Adelman RA. Ethambutol neuroretinopathy. *Semin. Ophthalmol.* 2007;22:141–146.

84 Nagra PK, Foroozan R, Savino PJ, et al. Amiodarone induced optic neuropathy. *Br. J. Ophthalmol.* 2003;87:420–422.

85 Thurtell MJ, Tomsak RL. Nonarteritic anterior ischemic optic neuropathy with PDE-5 inhibitors for erectile dysfunction. *Int. J. Impot. Res.* 2008;20:537–543.

86 Friedman DI. Medication-induced intracranial hypertension in dermatology. *Am. J. Clin. Dermatol.* 2005;6:29–37.

87 Singh N, Bonham A, Fukui M. Immunosuppressive-associated leukoencephalopathy in organ transplant recipients. *Transplantation* 2000;69:467–472.

88 Lantos G. Cortical blindness due to osmotic disruption of the blood–brain barrier by angiographic contrast material: CT and MRI studies. *Neurology* 1989;39:567–571.

89 Halmagyi GM, Thurtell MJ. Central eye movement disorders. In Albert DM, Miller JW, Azar DT, Blodi BA, editors, *Albert and Jakobiec's Principles and Practice of Ophthalmology*, 3rd ed. Philadelphia: WB Saunders, 2008, pp. 4101 Philadelphia 4132.

90 Sadun AA. Metabolic optic neuropathies. *Semin. Ophthalmol.* 2002;17:29–32.

91 Zuccoli G, Gallucci M, Capellades J, et al. Wernicke encephalopathy: MR findings at clinical presentation in twenty-six alcoholic and nonalcoholic patients. *Am. J. Neuroradiol.* 2007;28:1328–1331.

92 Longmuir R, Lee AG, Rouleau J. Visual loss due to Wernicke syndrome following gastric bypass. *Semin. Ophthalmol.* 2007;22:13–19.

8 Neuro-otology of systemic disease

Terry D. Fife
Barrow Neurological Institute, Phoenix, AZ, USA

A variety of systemic illnesses affect the auditory and vestibular system and many more may lead to symptoms such as imbalance and dizziness. Table 8.1 outlines some of these disorders and their associated neuro-otological manifestations.

Among the most common mechanisms for dysfunction of the auditory and vestibular system is ototoxicity. This is especially associated with medications such as loop diuretics, aminoglycosides, and other compound exposures that can lead to vestibular damage or tinnitus over time.

Autoimmune disorders can affect the inner ear as a primary condition or as part of a more systemic rheumatologic illness. Infections may also affect the labyrinth either directly, by extension from the middle ear, or by recrudescence of latent herpes family viruses.

Infection or postinfectious dysimmune brainstem encephalitis may also lead to central vestibular dysfunction leading to myoclonus, nystagmus, and ataxia.

While neoplastic effects from metastases can certainly affect the temporal bone or central vestibular system, paraneoplastic disorders causing central vertigo, nystagmus, and cerebellar dysfunction may also occur and are more difficult to recognize.

This chapter reviews the auditory and vestibular manifestations that may be encountered in patients with systemic illnesses.

Endocrine disease

Labyrinth

Few endocrinological disorders have direct effects on the labyrinth. A large retrospective and smaller prospective study of veterans both suggest that for those under age 60, hearing loss is more prevalent among those with diabetes than among those without diabetes [1,2].

Bilateral vestibular loss, sensorineural hearing loss, and abnormal labyrinthine morphology may occur in Kallmann syndrome, a sporadic or heritable syndrome more common in males and consisting of anosmia and hypogonadotropic hypogonadism [3].

Vestibular dysfunction, a larger vestibular aqueduct or Mondini malformation of the temporal bone, and often congenital hearing loss may be associated with Pendred's syndrome, a genetic disorder associated with goiter and hypothyroidism [4].

In a recent controlled study, patients with benign paroxysmal positional vertigo have been found to have more osteopenia and osteoporosis than matched controls, and those with recurrent BPPV tended to have the lowest bone-density scores [5]. This has led to speculation that osteoporosis may predispose patients to benign paroxysmal positional vertigo.

Vestibulocochlear nerve

Several metabolic or endocrine-related disorders may cause bone remodeling leading to compression of the vestibulocochlear nerve within the temporal bone. Advanced acromegaly [6], fibrous dysplasia alone or with endocrinopathy (McCune–Albright syndrome) [7], Paget's disease of the bone [8], and osteogenesis imperfecta [9] may lead to changes in skull size and contour that can lead to circumferential compression of the vestibulocochlear nerves over time.

Dizziness or imbalance

Hypothyroidism may present with gait imbalance and poor balance. The mechanism appears to be complex

Neurological Disorders due to Systemic Disease, First Edition. Edited by Steven L. Lewis
© 2013 Blackwell Publishing Ltd. Published 2013 by Blackwell Publishing Ltd.

Table 8.1 Clinical neuro-otological conditions in systemic diseases

Systemic disease	Associated neuro-otological condition[a]
Diabetes	Bilateral hearing loss[a]
Hypothyroidism	Gait imbalance
Kallman syndrome	Bilateral hearing loss; vestibular loss
Pendred's syndrome	Bilateral hearing loss; vestibular loss; Mondini malformation
Paget's disease of bone; acromegaly	Hearing loss; vestibular loss
Fibrous dysplasia (McCune–Albright disease)	Hearing loss; vestibular loss
Hyperviscosity syndromes	Hearing loss; vestibular loss
Vitamin B12 deficiency	Gait imbalance
Alport's syndrome	Bilateral hearing loss; vestibular loss
Mitochondrial diseases	Bilateral hearing loss, vestibular symptoms
Autoimmune inner ear disorders	Bilateral hearing loss; fluctuating hearing; vestibular symptoms
Susac's syndrome	Fluctuating hearing, ataxia, vestibular symptoms
Wegener's granulomatosis	Hearing loss; vestibular loss; granulomatous parenchymal lesions
Neurosarcoidosis	Hearing loss; vestibular loss; granulomatous parenchymal lesions
Hashimoto's encephalopathy	Ataxia, tremor, nystagmus
Focal neoplasm of temporal bone	Hearing loss; vestibular loss; parenchymal lesions
Infiltrative or metastatic neoplasm	Nystagmus, ataxia, vertigo, nausea—depending on location
Leptomeningeal carcinoma, lymphoma	Ataxia, nystagmus, nausea, vertigo, +/− hearing loss
Paraneoplastic syndromes	Ataxia, nystagmus, vertigo
Varicella zoster oticus (Ramsay Hunt syndrome)	Unilateral vestibular loss, hearing loss
Bacterial meningitis	Bilateral hearing loss, +/− vestibular dysfunction
Basilar (chronic) meningitis	Gait ataxia, vertigo, nystagmus, hearing loss
Brainstem encephalitis	Gait ataxia, myoclonus/tremor, ocular flutter
Acute cerebellitis	Ataxia, nystagmus, vertigo with head movements
Aminoglycoside ototoxicity	Bilateral vestibular loss, bilateral hearing loss
Acute alcohol intoxication	Ataxia, mild gaze nystagmus, dizziness
Wernicke's encephalopathy	Ataxia, nausea, vertigo, nystagmus, gaze limitations, nausea
Radiation labyrinthopathy	Bilateral hearing loss; +/− bilateral vestibular loss

[a]Tinnitus may accompany any disorder that produces sensorineural hearing loss.

involving reduced metabolism and cerebral blood flow that influences reaction time, central postural mechanisms, and cerebellar signal processing [10–12]. Hypothyroidism should be considered one of the treatable causes of nonspecific gait imbalance.

Hyperlipidemia and hyperviscosity syndromes

Labyrinth

Vertigo and tinnitus have been reported in hyperlipidemia that was responsive to lipid-lowering agents [13]. The mechanism may be related to hyperviscosity, though this remains speculative.

There are several types of hyperviscosity syndromes that can affect blood flow through the labyrinthine venules causing tinnitus, vertigo, and fluctuating hearing [14]. The same process commonly leads to headaches, fatigue, visual disturbances, and Raynaud's phenomenon, and may also lead to stroke, venous sinus thrombosis, and renal failure. Normal serum viscosity should be <1.8 cP and hyperviscosity symptoms begin to occur when viscosity reaches 5.0 cP or so. Disorders that can lead to hyperviscosity include Waldenström's macroglobulinemia, polycythemia rubra vera, extreme leukocytosis or thrombocythemia, or gammopathy associated with multiple myeloma. Management consists of appropriate treatment of the underlying cause through plasmapheresis, administration of fluids, or chemotherapy.

Metabolic disorders

Labyrinth

Alport's syndrome is a heritable (X-linked and autosomal recessive) disorder associated with hearing loss, vestibular loss, corneal dystrophy, anterior lenticonus (a cone-shaped protrusion of the lens surface into the anterior chamber of the eye), retinal dystrophy, and progressive renal dysfunction leading to renal failure. The disorder is due to a defect in the genes mediating the formation of certain forms of type IV collagen, a constituent of the basement membranes of the glomerulus, cochlea, lung, lens capsule, and Bruch and Descemet membranes in the eye. The defective collagen chain formation results in glomerulosclerosis and sensorineural hearing loss usually starting late in the first decade of life. Although the molecular and genetic basis of this condition has greatly advanced in recent years, to date there is still no treatment.

Dizziness or imbalance

Vitamin B12 deficiency may cause imbalance. The mechanism is probably related to defects in central myelination related to the deficiency that affects the spinal cord causing subacute combined degeneration, though peripheral neuropathy may also occur and contribute to disequilibrium. Subacute combined degeneration derives its name by the involvement of two spinal cord funicles: the dorsal column that mediates vibratory and joint position sense, and the corticospinal tract that carries motor fibers. Hence, the classic finding of loss of proprioception and a Babinski sign relate to dysfunction of these tracts. Encephalopathic effects of B12 deficiency may accompany the myelopathy and neuropathy.

Most B12 deficiency results from insufficient formation of intrinsic factor, a glycoprotein secreted by the parietal cells of the stomach that is required to absorb vitamin B12. In many such cases, antiparietal cell antibodies cause atrophic gastritis preventing proper absorption of the vitamin from food. In other instances, B12 may not be absorbed due to prior gastric surgery, due to insufficient B12 in the diet, or rarely from chronic intestinal infestation by the fish tapeworm *Diphyllobothrium latum* that competes for vitamin B12 absorption. Prompt treatment of the B12 deficiency may improve the gait imbalance [15].

Mitochondrial cytopathies

In recent years, mitochondrial DNA mutations have been linked to a growing number of disorders including mitochondrial encephalomyopathy, lactic acidosis, and stroke-like episodes (MELAS), myoclonic epilepsy and ragged red fibers (MERRF), Kearns–Sayre syndrome, and maternally inherited Leigh syndrome and retinitis pigmentosa (NARP) and Leber's hereditary optic neuropathy (LHON).

Among the neuro-otological manifestations of mitochondrial disorders, hearing loss is most common. One study reported that 7.4% of the patients with sensorineural hearing loss had the A3243G MELAS mutation suggesting this is one of the more common gene defects causing hearing loss [16]. Hence, mitochondrial disease is among the more common genetic causes of hearing loss. This appears to be related to cochlear dysfunction and varies with the precise genetic defect and degree of heteroplasmy. Heteroplasmy is the presence of more than one mitochondrial genome. Even small reductions in the percentage of normal mitochondrial DNA can lead to disease.

In MELAS due to the A3243G mutation, the percentage of mutated mitochondrial DNA in skeletal muscle correlates directly with hearing loss that may present as sudden hearing loss or more commonly as gradual hearing loss [17].

The mechanism of hearing loss is likely related in part to the high metabolic activity of the stria vascularis and the hair cells. Due to the observation that some patients sustain permanent sudden hearing loss with spells, it appears that acute metabolic impairment of the stria vascularis causes irreversible cochlear hair cell loss. In addition, hearing loss may also be influenced by noise exposure or ototoxic exposure. For example, people with the mitochondrial A1555G mutation in the 12S rRNA gene are highly susceptible to hearing loss from noise exposure and also to the ototoxic effects of aminoglycosides [18]. Interestingly, the binding site of aminoglycosides is on the 12S rRNA gene.

Among mitochondriopathies, several studies have found that Kearns–Sayre syndrome (KSS) and large deletions of mitochondrial DNA resulted in slow progression of hearing loss. However, in MELAS with the A3243G mutation, 80% had experienced abrupt or stepwise hearing loss, often in association with encephalopathy or stroke-like episodes [17].

Systemic autoimmune disorders

Labyrinth and vestibulocochlear nerve

Autoimmune inner ear disease (AIED) is a primary inner-ear disorder characterized by rapidly progressive, often fluctuating, bilateral sensorineural hearing loss occurring over weeks to months. Vestibular symptoms, including vertigo and general imbalance, may also occur. AIED is a clinical diagnosis based on the clinical history and response to corticosteroids [19]. In one study, nearly one-half of patients with AIED had clinical symptoms compatible with endolymphatic hydrops or Meniere's syndrome [20]. Hence, some unknown percentage of bilateral Meniere's disease may actually be caused by AIED.

Other immune-mediated or collagen vascular diseases may also rarely produce a clinical picture similar to isolated AIED and these including Cogan's syndrome [21], Susac's syndrome, Behçet's [22], rheumatoid arthritis, systemic lupus erythematosus [23], Wegener's granulomatosis and polyarteritis nodosa, and relapsing polychondritis [24]. Sarcoidosis is discussed separately below.

Cogan's syndrome is an AIED associated with hearing loss, vertigo, nausea, and tinnitus, along with nonsyphilic interstitial keratitis, a nonsuppurative inflammation of the cornea [21].

Wegener's granulomatosis manifests in nearly half of cases with middle ear pathology but may also lead to inner ear dysfunction and rarely CNS involvement.

Susac's syndrome is a rare disorder of unknown origin characterized by the triad of encephalopathy, fluctuating hearing loss, and visual loss, resulting from microangiopathy of the brain, cochlea, and retina. The most common neuro-otologic manifestation is sensorineural hearing loss, particularly at low frequencies [25].

The work up for suspected inner ear disease related to multiorgan autoimmune disease should include antinuclear antibodies, complement levels (C3, C4), rheumatoid factor, anti-nuclear cytoplasmic antibodies (ANCA), Westergren sedimentation rate, C-reactive protein, and possibly anti-68-kDa protein antibodies.

Central vestibular function

Sarcoidosis is a chronic multisystem granulomatous disorder characterized by the epithelioid, noncaseating granulomas within the affected tissue. Neurosarcoidosis is a rare manifestation of the disease, clinically affecting only 5% of patients and may affect hearing and vestibular function [26]. Vestibular loss has been reported both in isolation and together with hearing loss. The hearing loss due to sarcoidosis is often bilateral and frequently associated with fluctuating hearing. An extensive review of the world literature of neurosarcoidosis found hearing loss in 12.2% and nystagmus in 8.6% of patients with neurosarcoidosis [27]. Vestibular function is affected bilaterally in two-thirds of cases [26].

Sarcoidosis-related vestibular loss may result from vasculitis or granulomatous inflammation of the vestibulocochlear nerves [28] or labyrinth [29]. Auditory dysfunction may result from granulomatous inflammation of the arachnoid vessels, the cochlear nuclei, vestibulocochlear nerves, the labyrinth, or temporal-bone involvement.

Vasculitis from any systemic collagen vascular disease can potentially involve the CNS and some, such as Wegener's granulomatosis, may sometimes produce parenchymal granulomatous lesions. Rheumatoid arthritis can lead to ligamentous erosion predisposing to central brainstem compression from atlanto-axial subluxation. This can manifest with headache, neck pain, nystagmus, diplopia, ataxia, and vertigo worsened by vertical head positioning.

Hashimoto's encephalopathy (see also Chapter 4) is a presumed autoimmune encephalopathy sometimes referred to as a steroid responsive encephalopathy associated with autoimmune thyroiditis (SREAT) [30]. Clinical features include ataxia, tremor, and ocular motor abnormalities ranging from increased square wave jerks and nystagmus, to ocular flutter, to opsoclonus with myoclonic jerks and confusion. Because it is found in association with elevated antithyroglobulin antibodies or antithyroid peroxidase antibodies, it has been referred to as Hashimoto's encephalitis, though its appearance seems unrelated to thyroid function at the time. Corticosteroids have been advocated but due to its relative rarity, there are no prospective trials confirming efficacy in this condition.

Systemic cancer and paraneoplastic disorders

Vestibulocochlear nerve and cerebellum

Systemic neoplasms that affect the vestibular or auditory system are limited mainly to those that have some proclivity to affect the bony labyrinth or the central nervous system. Neoplastic processes that spread to the bone include head and neck squamous cell carcinoma, breast carcinoma, lung adenocarcinoma, renal-cell carcinoma, prostate carcinoma, malignant melanoma, rhabdomyosarcoma, osteosarcoma, and non-Hodgkin's lymphoma. Rhabdomyosarcoma is the most common malignancy of the temporal bone in children. Tumors arising from nearby locations such as meningioma, chordoma, parotid malignancy, and nasopharyngeal carcinoma may spread to the temporal bone affecting auditory or vestibular function.

Leptomeningeal carcinomatosis or lymphomatosis may lead to bilateral hearing and vestibular loss [31]. The vestibulocochlear nerves within the subarachnoid space become seeded with tiny foci of tumor leading to hearing or vestibular dysfunction that may be asymmetric. Leptomeningeal neoplasia also affects the basal cisterns often leading to ataxia and nystagmus from cerebellar dysfunction. In many cases, other cranial neuropathies will also occur causing swallowing difficulty, facial weakness or numbness, diplopia, and dysarthria. Bilateral vestibular loss causes unsteadiness of gait and oscillopsia during head movements. Patients often exhibit falling on Romberg testing during eye closure or when walking on uneven ground. Examination shows bilateral abnormalities in head impulse testing and reduced dynamic visual acuity. A bithermal caloric test or rotational chair testing will confirm severely reduced vestibulo-ocular reflexes.

Paraneoplastic syndromes that may cause dizziness, vertigo, imbalance, and ataxia are mainly those that affect the vestibulocerebellum. The syndromes associated with anti-Purkinje cell antibody (anti-Yo), anti-Tr antibody, and anti-CRMP5 tend to be most strongly associated with cerebellar degeneration [32] (Table 8.2). Histologically, paraneoplastic cerebellar degeneration shows severe loss of cerebellar Purkinje cells and inflammatory infiltrates.

Clinical features of paraneoplastic cerebellar degeneration include truncal ataxia with progressive worsening, limb dysmetria, impairment of rapid alternating movements, prominent horizontal gaze evoked nystagmus, impaired pursuit tracking, saccadic dysmetria, and dysarthric speech. Patients may report dizziness, but the most prominent feature is incoordination of limbs and imbalance. Patients with known malignancies or relatively rapid onset (4 weeks to 4 months) of cerebellar dysfunction should be evaluated for possible paraneoplastic cerebellar degeneration. The paraneoplastic syndrome can predate any signs of a malignancy so those that test positive for one of the antibodies should undergo appropriate tumor screening studies [33].

Table 8.2 Selected paraneoplastic syndromes with vestibulocerebellar syndrome

Antibody	Syndrome	Associated malignancy	Reactive against
Anti-Yo	Cerebellar ataxia	Ovarian, breast carcinoma	Purkinje cells
Anti-Hu	Cerebellar ataxia, limbic encephalitis, sensory neuropathy	Lung small-cell carcinoma	Nuclear neuronal antibodies-1
Anti-Ri	Cerebellar ataxia, opsoclonus, myoclonus, brainstem encephalitis	Breast carcinoma, gynecological carcinoma, lung small-cell carcinoma	Nuclear neuronal antibodies-2
Anti-Tr	Cerebellar ataxia	Hodgkin's lymphoma	Purkinje cells
Anti-CRMP5/CV2	Neuropathy, encephalomyelitis, cerebellar ataxia, autonomic dysfunction, myelopathy	Lung small-cell carcinoma, thymoma	Collapsin response-mediator protein (CRMP)

Systemic infectious disease

Neuro-otological manifestations of systemic infections cause symptoms when they are located within the temporal bone or labyrinth, when they affect the vestibulocochlear nerves within the subarachnoid space, or when they affect brainstem and cerebellar structures that mediate vestibular function. Hearing loss localizes to the vestibulocochlear nerves or the labyrinth itself since central auditory pathways have extensive bilateral connections.

Herpes zoster oticus leads to blistering in the limited sensory distribution of the 7th cranial nerve. This sometimes leads to a small patch of painful vesicles in the external ear canal or occasionally behind the ear, though in some cases the skin eruption is not present in herpes zoster oticus. When accompanied by ipsilateral Bell's palsy the syndrome is referred to as Ramsay Hunt syndrome. This condition is caused by reactivation of latent varicella-zoster virus affecting the 7th and 8th cranial nerves. Herpes zoster oticus and Ramsay Hunt syndrome may be treated with corticosteroids (e.g., prednisone 60 mg daily for 7 days) and anti-herpes-virus therapy (acyclovir, famciclovir, or valaciclovir). Other viral syndromes such as measles and mumps can lead to hearing loss.

Luetic (syphilitic) otitis may be either congenital or acquired and may mimic immune-mediated inner ear disease as well as idiopathic AIED and should be included in the differential diagnosis along with a variety of systemic immune-mediated disorders described below. Syphilitic otitis may produce a clinical picture indistinguishable from bilateral endolymphatic hydrops (Meniere's syndrome).

Bacterial meningitis may cause suppurative and inflammatory labyrinthitis that damages the organ of Corti leading to deafness in up to 30% of survivors. Postinfectious neuronal loss in the cochlear spiral ganglion can limit the value of cochlear implantation in this patient population. Chronic basilar meningitis due to tuberculosis and fungal meningitis may lead to combined hearing and vestibular loss.

A syndrome of brainstem encephalitis characterized by the acute onset of ataxia with shuttering tremor, myoclonus, ocular flutter or outright opsoclonus, and cognitive inefficiency has been reported and appears to occur sporadically [34]. Agents known to cause brainstem encephalitis include West Nile Virus, Herpes simplex virus 1, and paraneoplastic syndrome especially associated with neuroblastoma. However, in many instances, tests for these conditions are negative hence other causes may also cause this brainstem syndrome [35]. Many such cases are most likely postinfectious dysimmune disorders. Clonazepam helps manage the tremors, and with time most patients improve over 6–12 months.

Acute cerebellar ataxia (cerebellitis) following a viral illness may also produce dizziness, ataxia, and nystagmus. While most common in children, it also occurs in adolescents and adults. Ataxia commonly develops over hours to a day or two and slowly resolves after 1–4 weeks. Clinical features include headache, truncal ataxia, impaired pursuit, ocular flutter, gaze-evoked nystagmus, limb dysmetria, and dysarthria. The most commonly associated viruses include varicella zoster virus, Epstein–Barr virus, enterovirus, adenovirus, coxsackie and echovirus, cytomegalovirus, mycoplasma, and mumps [36]. The differential diagnosis includes *Listeria rhombencephalitis*, acute disseminated encephalomyelitis (ADEM), multiple sclerosis, neuroblastoma, and CNS lymphoma. Treatment can include anti-herpes-virus antimicrobial therapy if a herpes family virus is suspected. Most cases have complete recovery within 2–4 weeks, with a worse prognosis implied if there are brainstem symptoms.

Complications of transplantation

Severe hearing loss has been observed temporally related to orthotopic liver transplantation in about 3% of patients. While the cause is not clear, patients receiving calcineurin inhibitors such as tacrolimus or cyclosporine appeared slightly more likely to develop hearing loss [37].

Drugs and toxins

Aminoglycoside ototoxicity is the most common recognized cause of bilateral vestibular loss. Bilateral peripheral vestibular loss from aminoglycosides usually presents with gait unsteadiness and dizziness aggravated by any kind of head movement. Usually, overt spinning is not present since the loss affects both ears symmetrically when aminoglycosides are given systemically. As symptoms progress, vestibular loss may become irreversible and accompanied by oscillopsia (Figure 8.1) and then by tinnitus and hearing

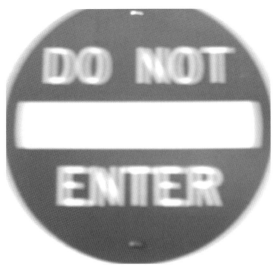

Fig. 8.1 A depiction of how oscillopsia appears to the patient in bilateral vestibular loss.

loss, depending on which aminoglycoside is used. Vestibular testing shows reduced or absent caloric nystagmus and reduced gain on rotational chair testing (Figure 8.2).

In 1947, the United States Food and Drug Administration (FDA) approved streptomycin for the treatment of tuberculosis as well as other infections. By the mid-1950s it became increasingly apparent that streptomycin could lead to peripheral vestibular loss [38–40]. The use of streptomycin continued due to its life-saving antimicrobial effects and because serious ototoxicity seemed relatively rare according to many reports at that time [41–42]. In 1967, gentamicin was approved by the FDA, and because it caused fewer adverse effects when administered intravenously, it became much more widely used than streptomycin.

The aminoglycosides selectively damage vestibular or cochlear hair cells. Streptomycin and gentamicin are the most vestibulotoxic, tobramycin is intermediate, and amikacin, neomycin, and kanamycin are more cochleotoxic [43]. It has been estimated that 3–4% of patients that receive gentamicin develop

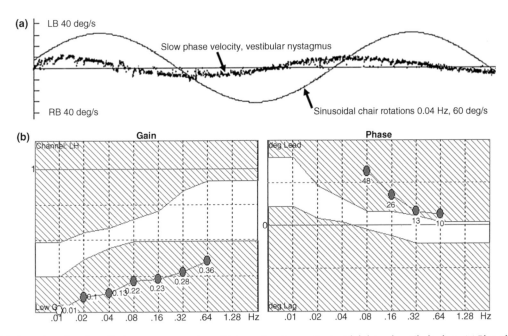

Fig. 8.2 Severely reduced vestibular responses to sinusoidal rotations in a patient with bilateral vestibular loss. (a) Plot of the slow phase velocity of nystagmus evoked by 0.04 Hz sinusoidal rotations, showing severely reduced vestibulo-ocular reflex (VOR) responses. (b) Summary of VOR gain and phase lead showing reduced gain at all frequencies tested.

vestibular loss [44]. This is probably an underestimate since only the most severely affected patients are likely to connect unsteadiness without hearing loss to an intravenous antibiotic. The likelihood of vestibulotoxicity increases in patients on renal dialysis [45,46], perhaps because there is no longer a concern for kidney damage since the patient is already receiving dialysis.

Recent studies in the mouse model of dihydrostreptomycin suggest that hair cells are targeted because aminoglycosides enter outer hair cells through large mechanically gated channels in the mechanosensory hair bundles. The aminoglycoside molecules then block the channels through which they entered. When this occurs, the aminoglycoside goes through the channel and effectively traps itself in the hair cell [47,48]. It rapidly accumulates and may eventually cause cellular injury. Increased extracellular calcium in the surrounding endolymph reduces the entry of aminoglycosides and reduces its channel-blocking affinity [49].

A number of studies have attempted to find a method of staving off aminoglycoside ototoxicity, but none so far has been found to be clinically beneficial. Susceptibility to aminoglycoside toxicity varies from person to person. Such variability has been encountered even in mice [50]. Some patients develop vestibulotoxicity even when gentamicin, for example, is given properly, though prolonged administration or doses that cause toxic drug levels increase the odds of ototoxic effects. A mutation in the human mitochondrial 12s RNA gene at nucleotide A1555G is associated with irreversible hearing loss following administration of even small amounts of aminoglycoside but does not seem to convey susceptibility to vestibular loss [51].

Ototoxicity may also occur with other drugs including cisplatin, loop diuretics, aspirin, and with chronic exposure to certain organic solvents such as jet fuel, cleaning agents, or solvents containing toluene, trichloroethylene, and xylene [52]. Quinines and aspirin can cause hearing loss and tinnitus but may also cause an intoxication syndrome referred to as cinchonism. Cinchonism includes tinnitus, hearing loss, vertigo, nausea, headache, and visual impairment. Medications that have been associated with tinnitus are outlined in Table 8.3.

Table 8.3 Medications and compounds that may cause tinnitus

Category	Drug or compound
Analgesics	Aspirin, nonsteroidal anti-inflammatory drugs
Antibiotics	Aminoglycosides, chloramphenicol, erythromycin, tetracycline, vancomycin
Chemotherapeutic agents	Bleomycin, cisplatin, methotrexate, vincristine
Loop diuretics	Bumetanide, ethacrinic acid, furosemide
Miscellaneous	Chloroquines, lead, mercury, quinine, organic solvents

Acute ethanol intoxication produces a well-known cerebro-cerebellar disturbance that produces impairment of gaze holding, gait ataxia, dysarthria, limb incoordination, and altered reaction time and judgment. Chronic alcohol ingestion as well as gastric bypass surgery may result in deficient thiamine intake or absorption that can lead to Wernicke's encephalopathy (see also Chapter 3). This disorder is characterized by ataxia, ophthalmoparesis, diplopia, confusion, and memory loss. Carbohydrate ingestion (including alcohol itself) in the absence of sufficient thiamine may exacerbate Wernicke's encephalopathy, which is treated by urgent replenishment of thiamine.

Radiation exposure to the labyrinth, vestibulocochlear nerve, or brainstem can lead to hearing and/or vestibular loss. Hearing loss may be progressive and its onset is often delayed for months to a year or two after radiation [53]. Radiation can lead to direct effects on the membranous labyrinth, regional vasculopathy, osteonecrotic changes in the temporal bone, and reduced mobility of the ossicular chain leading to otosclerosis. The late effects of radiation from fractionated, whole-brain, or radiosurgery (Gamma knife or Cyberknife) include tinnitus and hearing loss; less is known about the frequency of vestibular loss [54].

Five things to remember about vertigo/hearing loss/tinnitus due to systemic disease

1. Herpes zoster oticus alone or with facial palsy (Ramsay Hunt syndrome) represents reactivation of latent varicella zoster virus that can be effectively treated with corticosteroids and anti-herpes-virus medications.
2. Certain medications such as aminoglycosides, cisplatin, and loop diuretics are especially toxic to the inner ear but may produce imbalance and vague unsteadiness not necessarily with spinning vertigo.
3. Autoimmune inner ear disease (AIED) is a primary inner-ear disorder characterized by progressive, often fluctuating, bilateral sensorineural hearing loss occurring over weeks to months.
4. Leptomeningeal carcinomatosis or lymphomatosis may affect the vestibulocochlear nerves leading to ataxia, dizziness, and hearing loss at presentation before other cranial nerve involvement is apparent.
5. Neoplasm, granulomatous disease, or bony remodeling (e.g., Paget's disease) may affect the temporal bones resulting in direct invasion or compressive interruption of cochleovestibular function.

References

1 Kakarlapudi V, Sawyer R, Staecker H. The effect of diabetes on sensorineural hearing loss. *Otol. Neurotol.* 2003;24:382–386.

2 Vaughan N, James K, McDermott D, Griest S, Fausti S. A 5-year prospective study of diabetes and hearing loss in a veteran population. *Otol. Neurotol.* 2006;27:37–43.

3 Hill J, Elliott C, Colquhoun I. Audiological, vestibular and radiological abnormalities in Kallman's syndrome. *J. Laryngol. Otol.* 1992;106:530–534.

4 Johnsen T, Larsen C, Friis J, Hougaard-Jensen F. Pendred's syndrome. Acoustic, vestibular and radiological findings in 17 unrelated patients. *J. Laryngol. Otol.* 1987;101:1187–1192.

5 Jeong SH, Choi SH, Kim JY, Koo JW, Kim HJ, Kim JS. Osteopenia and osteoporosis in idiopathic benign positional vertigo. *Neurology* 2009;72:1069–1076.

6 Mortensen A, Bojsen-Møller M, Rasmussen P. Fibrous dysplasia of the skull with acromegaly and sarcomatous transformation. *J. Neuro-Oncol.* 1989;7:25–29.

7 Morrissey DD, Talbot JM, Schleuning, AJ. Fibrous dysplasia of the temporal bone: reversal of sensorineural hearing loss after decompression of the internal auditory canal. *Laryngoscope* 1997;107:1336–1340.

8 Monsell, EM. The mechanism of hearing loss in Paget's disease of the bone. *Larygoscope* 2004;114:598–606.

9 Hayes M, Parker G, Ell J, Sillence D. Basilar impression complicating osteogenesis imperfecta type IV: the clinical and neuroradiological findings of four cases. *J. Neurol. Neurosurg. Psychiatry* 1999;66:357–364.

10 Barnard RO, Campbell MJ, McDonald WI. Pathological findings in a case of hypothyroidism with ataxia. *J. Neurol. Neurosurg. Psychiatry* 1971;34:755–760.

11 Tanaka M, Kawarabayashi T, Okamoto K, et al. Reduction of cerebral blood flow and metabolic rate of oxygen in a case of hypothyroidism presenting cerebellar ataxia. *Rinsho Shinkeigaku* 1987;27:1262–1265.

12 Edvardsson B, Persson S. Subclinical hypothyroidism presenting with gait abnormality. *Neurologist* 2010;16:115–116.

13 Saadah HA. Vestibular vertigo associated with hyperlipidemia: response to antilipidemic therapy. *Arch. Intern. Med.* 1993;153:1846, 1849.

14 Brandt T. Hyperviscosity syndrome and vertigo. In: *Vertigo: Its Multisensory Syndromes*, 2nd ed. London: Springer-Verlag;2003: 341–342.

15 Ahmed A, Kothari MJ. Recovery of neurologic dysfunction using vitamin B12. *J. Clin. Neuromusc. Dis.* 2010;11:198–201.

16 Majamaa K, Moilanen JS, Uimonen S, Remes AM, Salmela PI, Karppa M, et al. Epidemiology of A3243G, the mutation for mitochondrial encephalomyopathy, lactic acidosis, and stroke like episodes: prevalence of the mutation in an adult population. *Am. J. Hum. Genet.* 1998;63:447–454.

17 Chinnery PF, Elliott C, Green GR, Rees A, et al. The spectrum of hearing loss due to mitochondrial DNA defects. *Brain* 2000;123:82–92.

18 Prezant TR, Agapian JV, Bohlman MC, Bu X, Oztas S, Qiu W-Q, et al. Mitochondrial ribosomal RNA mutation associated with both antibiotic-induced and non-syndromic deafness. *Nat. Genet.* 1993;4:289–294.

19 Ruckenstein MJ. Autoimmune inner ear disease. *Curr. Opin. Otolaryngol. Head Neck Surg.* 2004;12: 426–430.

20 Hughes GB, Barna BP, Calarese LH. Immunologic disorders of the inner ear. In: Bailey BJ, editor, *Head and*

Neck Surgery-Otolaryngology. Philadelphia, PA: Lippincott;1993, pp. 1833–1842.

21 Mazlumzadeh M. Matteson EL. Cogan's syndrome: an audiovestibular, ocular, and systemic autoimmune disease. *Rheum. Dis. Clin. N. Am.* 2007;33:855–874, vii–viii.

22 Mahdi B, Mehdi GM, Reza HM, Mahdieh T, Taghi SM. Hearing loss in Behcet syndrome. *Otolaryngol. Head Neck Surg.* 2007;137:439–442.

23 Karatas E, Onat AM, Durucu C, Baglam T, Kanlikama M, et al. Audiovestibular disturbance in patients with systemic lupus erythematosus. *Otolaryngol. Head Neck Surg.* 2007;136:82–86.

24 McAdam LP, O'Hanlan MA, Bluestone R, Pearson CM. Relapsing polychondritis: prospective study of 23 patients and a review of the literature. *Medicine* 1976;55:193–215.

25 Roeser MM, Driscoll CLW, Shallop JK, Gifford RH, et al. Susac syndrome: report of cochlear implantation and review of otologic manifestations in twenty-three patients. *Otol. Neurotol.* 2008;30:34–40.

26 Colvin IB. Audiovestibular manifestations of sarcoidosis: a review of the literature. *Laryngoscope* 2006;116:75–82.

27 Mende D, Suchenwirth RM. Neurosarcoidosis. Comparative analysis of the clinical profile based on 537 cases from the world literature up to 1963 and from 1976–1988. *Fortschritte Neurol. Psychiatr.* 1990;58:7–18.

28 Von Brevern M, Lempert T, Bronstein AM, Kocen R. Selective vestibular damage in neurosarcoidosis. *Ann. Neurol.* 1997;42:117–120.

29 Aviles Manoso P, Juan Ivars C, Portell Soriano M, Ramos Fernandez J. Neurosarcoidosis. Sensorineural hearing loss. *Acta Otorrinolaringol. Esp.* 1997;48:229–231.

30 Castillo P, Woodruff, B, Caselli R, Vernino S, et al. Steroid-responsive encephalopathy associated with autoimmune thyroiditis. *Arch. Neurol.* 2006;63:197–202.

31 Pollack L, Milo R, Kossych V, Rabey MJ. Bilateral vestibular failure as a unique presenting sign in carcinomatous meningitis: case report. *J. Neurol. Neurosurg. Psychiatry* 2001;70:704–705.

32 Pelosof LC, Gerber DE. Paraneoplastic syndromes: An approach to diagnosis and treatment. *Mayo Clin. Proc.* 2010;85:838–854.

33 Posner JB. Paraneoplastic cerebellar degeneration. *Can. J. Neurol. Sci.* 1993;20(Suppl 3):S117–S122.

34 Brumlik J, Means ED. Tremorine-tremor, shivering and acute cerebellar ataxia in the adult and child—a comparative study. *Brain* 1969;92:157–190.

35 Blaes FV, Fuhlhuber V, Korfei M, Tschernatsch M, et al. Surface-binding autoantibodies to cerebellar neurons in opsoclonus syndrome. *Ann. Neurol.* 2005;58: 313–317.

36 Sawaishi Y, Takada G. Acute cerebellitis. *Cerebellum* 2002;1:223–228.

37 Rifai K, Bahr MJ, Cantz T, Klempnauer J, et al. Severe hearing loss after liver transplantation. *Transplant. Proc.* 2005;37:1918–1919.

38 Northington P. Syndrome of bilateral vestibular paralysis and its occurrence from streptomycin therapy. *Arch. Otolaryngol.* 1950;52:380–396.

39 Bolletti M, De Vido G. Streptomycin toxicity in children with special reference to cochleo-vestibular damages. *Acta Paediatrica Latina* 1952;5:1–30.

40 Osterberg AC, Oleson JJ, Yuda NN, Rauh CE, Parr HG, Will LW. Cochlear, vestibular, and acute toxicity studies of streptomycin and dihydrostreptomycin pantothenate salts. *Antibiot. Annu.* 1956–1957: 564–573.

41 Wilson WR, Geraci JE. Treatment of streptococcal infective endocarditis. *Am. J. Med.* 1985;78:128–137.

42 McCracken GHJr. Aminoglycoside toxicity in infants and children. *Am. J. Med.* 1986;80(6B):172–178.

43 Selimoglu E. Aminoglycoside-induced ototoxicity. *Curr. Pharm. Des.* 2007;13:119–126.

44 Kahlmeter G, Dahlager JI. Aminoglycoside toxicity: a review of clinical studies published between 1975 and 1982. *J. Antimicrob. Chemother.* 1984;13(Suppl A): 9–22.

45 Chong TK, Piraino B, Bernardini J. Vestibular toxicity due to gentamicin in peritoneal dialysis patients. *Perit. Dial. Int.* 1991;11:152–155.

46 Gailiunas P.Jr., Dominguez-Moreno M, Lazarus M, et al. Vestibular toxicity of gentamicin: incidence in patients receiving long-term hemodialysis therapy. *Arch. Intern. Med.* 1978;138:1621–1624.

47 Marcotti W, van Netten SM, Kros CJ. The aminoglycoside antibiotic dihydrostreptomycin rapidly enters mouse outer hair cells through the mechano-electrical transducer channels. *J. Physiol.* 2005;567(Pt 2):505–521.

48 Waguespack JR, Ricci AJ. Aminoglycoside ototoxicity: permeant drugs cause permanent hair cell loss. *J. Neurophysiol.* 2005;567(Pt 2):359–360.

49 Warchol ME. Cellular mechanisms of aminoglycoside ototoxicity. *Curr. Opin. Otolaryngol. Head Neck Surg.* 2010;18:454–458.

50 Hochman J, Blakley BW, Wellman M, Blakley L. Prevention of aminoglycoside-induced sensorineural hearing loss. *J. Otolaryngol.* 2006;35:153–156.

51 Noguchi Y, Yashima T, Ito T, Sumi T, Tsuzuku T, Kitamura K. Audiovestibular findings in patients with mitochondrial A1555G mutation. *Laryngoscope* 2004; 114:344–348.

52 Steyger PS. Potentiation of chemical ototoxicity by noise. *Semin. Hear.* 2009;30:38–46.

53 Wang LF, Kuo WR, Ho KY, Lee KW, Lin CS. A long-term study on hearing status in patients with nasopharyngeal carcinoma after radiotherapy. *Otol. Neurotol.* 2004; 25:168–173.

54 Bhandare N, Jackson A, Eisbruch A, Pan CC, et al. Radiation therapy and hearing loss. *Int. J. Radiat. Oncol. Biol. Phys.* 2010;76(3 Suppl):S50–S57.

Movement disorders due to systemic disease

Brandon R. Barton & Christopher G. Goetz
Rush University Medical Center, Chicago, IL, USA

Introduction

Movement disorders may occur as a secondary complication of a broad range of medical diseases. Abnormal movements may either occur as a presenting sign of a medical illness, as a complication during the course of a progressive disease process, or as a result of medical treatments. The prognosis and treatment significantly depend on identifying the underlying pathophysiology, and in many cases early recognition and detection of the underlying causative etiology may offer the opportunity for stabilization or reversal of the movement disorder. In addition, being familiar with the most common movement disorders associated with a particular medical illness may allow the clinician to vigilantly search for their occurrence and rapidly diagnose them in their early stages, which may allow for more successful intervention. It is critical to correctly classify a given movement disorder, because the differential diagnosis changes with each disorder. As parkinsonism, other tremors, dystonia, chorea, ataxia, or myoclonus may be caused by a very diverse spectrum of underlying causes, the clinician must maintain a broad differential diagnosis, collect a detailed medical history, and perform a comprehensive neurological examination in approaching a patient with a movement disorder, particularly when multiple medical comorbidities are present.

The pathophysiology of movement disorders is complex and not clearly defined for each medical illness. In general, abnormal function of the basal ganglia or its connections may result from direct structural insults, biochemical imbalances of the several neurotransmitters involved in neuronal communication, or alterations of electrophysiological function. In order to discuss the common systemic causes of movement disorders, a brief description of the different manifestations of common movement disorder phenomenologies is necessary.

Parkinsonism

Parkinsonism is a term describing a motor syndrome with the cardinal features of bradykinesia, rest tremor, rigidity, and postural instability. Parkinsonism may occur from abnormalities in the striatonigral dopaminergic pathway, which travels from the substantia nigra to the subcortical nuclei, which include the putamen and caudate nucleus (also known as the striatum), thalamus, and their cortical connections. Other basal-ganglia nuclei and posterior fossa structures regulate these nuclei. While the most common cause of parkinsonism in the adult patient is idiopathic Parkinson's disease, there are a broad spectrum of medical conditions or treatments that are associated with signs of parkinsonism [1]. In general, secondary parkinsonism presents less commonly with rest tremor, has more rapid or subacute onset, displays more symmetric akinesia and rigidity, and commonly involves an early-onset gait disorder with postural instability and falls. Drugs that block dopamine receptors or deplete the brain of dopamine (many used for psychiatric illnesses, cancer management, and gastrointestinal disorders) cause a picture that is largely indistinguishable from Parkinson's disease, making the medication history particularly important to review.

Neurological Disorders due to Systemic Disease, First Edition. Edited by Steven L. Lewis.
© 2013 Blackwell Publishing Ltd. Published 2013 by Blackwell Publishing Ltd.

Dystonia

Dystonia is characterized by sustained, involuntary, slower, repetitive, and patterned muscle contractions leading to twisting movements or abnormal postures of the neck, trunk, face, arms, or legs [2]. It is thought to involve perturbations of the neuroanatomical circuitry that links the basal-ganglia nuclei, sensorimotor system, and posterior fossa structures (brainstem, cerebellum) [3]. Physiologically, both agonist and antagonist muscles simultaneously contract, and there is overflow of abnormal muscle contractions into adjacent muscles. This results in visible distortion of the affected body regions, and is typically more prominent during voluntary actions. Dystonia usually worsens with stress or fatigue and improves with rest or relaxation, leading not infrequently to a psychogenic misdiagnosis. Adult-onset dystonia typically starts in a focal region with minimal spread, while younger-onset cases frequency become generalized. Dystonic movements may be classified by their clinical characteristics, anatomical distribution, or by etiology. Primary dystonia, by definition, occurs in the absence of other neurologic deficits, and has been associated with several predisposing genetic mutations [4]. Secondary or symptomatic dystonia should be suspected when dystonic movements occur along with other abnormalities on the general medical or neurological examination, when there is rapid presentation, onset in a location or with a pattern atypical for patient demographics, or in the context of a medical condition or treatment associated with dystonia. Acute dystonic reactions can occur from medications sometimes prescribed in the management of non-neurological medical illnesses.

Tremor

Tremor is a frequent complication of medications and chronic medical disease, and encompasses a variety of phenomenologies. Tremor is an oscillatory, usually rhythmic, sinusoidal, to-and-fro movement affecting one or more body parts involving alternating or synchronous contractions of reciprocally innervated antagonistic muscles. The rate, location, amplitude, and constancy vary depending on tremor type [5]. Tremor induced by drugs and metabolic disorders typically causes postural and/or action tremor. Parkinsonian tremor, in contrast, usually occurs at rest. Cerebellar tremors may occur in all positions (including at rest, but are worse with action).

Chorea

Chorea is an involuntary, irregular, unpredictable, purposeless, nonrhythmic, abrupt, rapid, nonsustained movement that flows from one body part to another in a continuous, random sequence of movements. Choreic movements are unpredictable in their direction and distribution and can sometimes be partially suppressed or "camouflaged" (parakinesias). Chorea may sometimes resemble a slower "worm-like" movement called athetosis, or may present as a more proximal flinging movement called ballismus. Chorea results from a broad range of systemic or hereditary diseases, with the differential diagnosis relying on the presence of accompanying findings [6]. The primary anatomical target underlying many forms of chorea is the striatum (caudate nucleus and putamen), and many forms of chorea relate at least in part to enhanced responsiveness of this nucleus to dopaminergic stimulation.

Myoclonus

Myoclonic movements are sudden, brief, shock-like involuntary jerks caused by either muscle contractions (positive myoclonus) or by transient inhibition of muscular activity (negative myoclonus). Most myoclonus is arrhythmic, and can be generated from multiple locations in the neuraxis, although cortical localization is most common. Myoclonus may be generalized or focal, and may be symmetric or asymmetric. Symptomatic myoclonus secondary due to medical disorders is usually accompanied by ataxia and mental status changes, with a broad differential diagnosis [7]. Generalized myoclonus is seen in a large array of metabolic encephalopathies related to medical illness or medications, but there are some forms that are characteristic of specific diagnoses.

Ataxia

Dysmetria, past-pointing, excessive corrections, rebound, dysdiadochokinesis, poor precision, excessive speed or corrections, are the features of ataxic syndromes. Gait is typically wide based, with variable step length and difficulty adjusting to sudden changes. Muscle tone may be decreased. Characteristic associated dysarthria is termed "scanning speech," which is subfluent with articulation deficits. Cerebellar tremor is of low frequency, but often high amplitude with action. Oculomotor dysfunction shows saccadic smooth pursuit, dysmetric saccades, nystagmus, and square wave jerks. Ataxia has a broad differential diagnosis of an increasing number of genetic, medical, and heredodegenerative causes [8].

Tics

Tics are movements (motor tics) or vocalizations (vocal tics) that are characteristically repetitive stereotypic actions of irregular frequency, often preceded by an inner urge, followed by relief after performance. They may be simple (brief, purposeless actions) or complex (coordinated sequences of action or speech, resembling voluntary actions). Tics are usually suppressible, are less likely to interfere with normal movements or actions, and can vary in frequency, type, and severity over time, with remissions and exacerbations. The phenomenology of motor tics is variable and can resemble that of other movement types such as dystonia or myoclonus.

Endocrine disorders

Thyroid disease

Hypothyroidism
Hypothyroidism and parkinsonism share several clinical signs in common, such as fatigue, constipation, depression, facial hypomimia, rigidity, slowed movements, and speech and gait abnormalities. Hypothyroidism can be differentiated from parkinsonian symptoms by measuring thyroid hormone levels and searching for other signs of thyroid deficiency such as coarse hair and temperature intolerance, and supportive laboratory features of endocrinologic abnormalities. The co-occurrence of hypothyroidism in patients with Parkinson's disease may be overlooked due to the similarity of the two disorders, and parkinsonism may improve after treatment of the underlying thyroid condition [9,10]. Chorea can occur with Hashimoto's thyroiditis, in association with Hashimoto's encephalopathy [11]. Of note, levodopa treatment may decrease TSH levels without affecting thyroid function [12].

Hyperthyroidism
Hyperthyroidism has been associated with a wide range of movement disorders, and may be due to enhanced catecholamine effects in the striatum, or alterations of dopaminergic pathways. Unusual and isolated cases of hyperthyroidism-associated syndromes of ballism, spasmodic truncal flexion, ataxia, platysmal and segmental myoclonus, Meige's syndrome with hemichorea, and stiff-person syndrome have also been reported [13]. Hyperthyroidism may mimic the hyperhydrosis or weight loss seen with Parkinson's disease. Hyperthyroidism may also exaggerate parkinsonian tremor, and improvement may occur with antithyroid treatments [14]. A case of reversible task-specific dystonia (writer's cramp) with hand tremor, as well as a case of acute chorea, have been reported as presenting signs of Graves' disease-related hyperthyroidism, which improved after treatment with carbimazole or propylthiouracil [15,16]. Chorea during the course of thyroid replacement therapy is uncommonly reported [17]. Hyperthyroid-related chorea will improve with normalization of thyroid hormone levels, although clinical improvement may lag behind hormone-level improvement by many weeks [18]. Propranolol or haloperidol may be effective as symptomatic treatments of hyperthyroid-related chorea and these drugs can be used for short-term control of the movement disorder while the thyroid function is being corrected [14,16].

Parathyroid disease

Hypoparathyroidism
Hypocalcemia from idiopathic hypoparathyroidism may cause paroxysmal dystonia and choreoathetosis, which rarely may be kinesigenic. It is associated with basal-ganglia calcification on neuroimaging [19]. Hypocalcemia-induced chorea, most frequently in the setting of hypoparathyroidism, improves when calcium is corrected [20,21]. Hypoparathyroidism can cause parkinsonism, either with or without the presence of basal-ganglia calcifications. Parkinsonism in these cases may occur as a late complication after thyroidectomy [22] and may be responsive to levodopa [23].

Hyperparathyroidism
Hyperparathyroidism related to parathyroid adenomas rarely causes parkinsonism, which can be reversible after removal of the tumor [24].

Pseudohypoparathyroidism
Pseudohypoparathyroidism (PHP), a condition that occurs when endogenous parathyroid hormone

(PTH) is adequate but is ineffective due to biological insensitivity to PTH, may be associated with parkinsonism in up to 4–12% of patients. Evidence of basal-ganglia calcifications may or may not be present [25]. Importantly, PTH-related parkinsonism may improve after normalizing serum calcium [26]. In one dramatic example, pseudohypoparathyroidism was discovered in one young girl presenting with paroxysmal, exercise-induced facial and upper extremity dystonic movements in association with hypocalcemia, which ceased with normalization of calcium levels [27].

Electrolyte and other metabolic disorders

Electrolyte disturbance

Extrapontine and central pontine myelinolysis may occur in multiple medical settings, including rapid correction of hyponatremia, liver disease, as a consequence of chronic alcohol abuse, or with malnutrition. Myelinolysis, particularly when extrapontine in location with basal-ganglia involvement, may be associated with subacute or delayed-onset parkinsonism, dystonia, or myoclonus, with accompanying neuropsychiatric symptoms [28]. Cases may respond to levodopa, but the majority have persistent symptoms [29]. Chorea may also result from this disorder [6].

Myoclonus is frequently seen in metabolic disturbances, and generally resolves with treatment of the underlying disease, including renal failure, hepatic failure, hyponatremia, hypoglycemia, nonketotic hyperglycemia, and metabolic alkalosis. It also results from intoxication from a great number of medications [30].

Disorders of calcium metabolism are often associated with parkinsonism. The term "Fahr's disease"—bilateral subcortical calcification involving the basal ganglia and cerebellum—is a label representing a heterogeneous collection of disorders, not necessarily associated with disorders of calcium metabolism. Affected patients most commonly have parkinsonism (55%), which occurs alongside other neurologic symptoms including ataxia, dementia, chorea, tremor, or dystonia [31].

Glucose metabolism

Nonketotic hyperglycemia-induced chorea occurs more often in women than men, in association with high blood-glucose levels (average 481 mg/dL) [32]. When treated promptly, nearly all patients recover fully by 6 months, although cases with prolonged symptoms may occur. Characteristic MRI findings include high signal in the striatum on T1-weighted imaging, which typically resolves on follow-up. The etiology is unclear, but most evidence suggests an ischemic process without calcification, and rare pathological reports show gliosis without hemorrhage. Hypoglycemia-induced chorea, myoclonus, and paroxysmal dyskinesias have also been reported [33].

Iron metabolism

Hereditary hemochromatosis (HH) is a genetic disorder in which excessive iron accumulates in systemic tissues due to an abnormality in iron handling, which can result in various clinical manifestations due to organ damage such as to the heart, pancreas, or liver. However, few cases of documented iron accumulation in the basal ganglia exist, typically with only the choroid plexus, pituitary gland, and periventricular/perivascular areas being affected [34]. Only rarely have movement disorders been reported, including eight cases of parkinsonism [35] and cases of dystonia, ataxia, and tremor. As pathological studies are conflicting and reports are rare, there is controversy as to the causality of HH in relation to movement disorders, with some experts arguing only a coincidental relationship [34].

Mitochondrial disease

Mitochondrial/respiratory chain disorders may cause all varieties of movement disorders, including parkinsonism, dystonia, chorea, tics, or myoclonus, and may occur as part of the well-recognized syndromes of mitochondrial encephalomyopathy, lactic acidosis, and stroke-like episodes (MELAS), Kearns–Sayre syndrome, or Leigh syndrome. Of special note, parkinsonism may be observed in up to 12% of adult patients with respiratory-chain disorders associated with mitochondrial dysfunction, including Leber hereditary optic neuropathy. Additional features of mitochondrial syndromes usually include myopathy, polyneuropathy, progressive external ophthalmoplegia, or premature menopause. Administration of levodopa may often improve parkinsonism in the context of mitochondrial dysfunction, and has resulted in drug-induced dyskinesias [36].

Other disorders

Conditions that increase catecholamine levels, such as mood disorders, pheochromocytoma, fever, and amphetamine use, commonly cause an enhanced physiological tremor. Tremor is a common feature of acute or subacute metabolic derangements including hypoglycemia, hyperthyroidism, and renal and hepatic dysfunction. Porphyria may cause paroxysmal tremulous episodes [5].

"Pseudodystonia" refers to conditions that may mimic dystonia, and often involve metabolic abnormalities. Examples include tetany-related carpopedal spasm due to alkalosis, hypocalcemia, or hypomagnesemia. Also included in this category is torticollis associated with retropharyngeal abscess or congenital injury; abnormal postures secondary to orthopedic or rheumatologic conditions; head tilt associated with hiatal hernia; or gastroesophageal reflux with Sandifer's syndrome [37].

Systemic autoimmune disorders

Systemic lupus erythematosus

Although neurologic symptoms occur in up to 60% of patients with systemic lupus erythematosus (SLE), movement disorders are uncommon. Chorea is most often described, followed by parkinsonism and myoclonus [38].

Case series and case reports identify at least 29 cases of SLE-associated parkinsonism [39], most being young women under the age of 30 years, with juvenile onset in one-third [40]. Hyperreflexia with an akinetic-rigid phenotype is more typical, with variably associated seizures, mutism, anorexia, encephalopathy, or psychiatric features, suggesting brain involvement outside the basal ganglia. Patients treated with immunomodulatory therapy and/or anti-parkinsonian medications generally improve, including one reported case with reversible subcortical enhancing fronto-striatal lesions [41]. The mechanisms of extrapyramidal symptoms in SLE are unclear; only a minority of patients have focal basal-ganglia lesions, and serum antidopaminergic antibodies have been detected [42]. Functional neuroimaging in one case

noted basal-ganglia hyperperfusion [43]. Patients with SLE may develop prominent basal-ganglia calcifications, and patients may also develop myoclonus, tremor, or ataxia [44].

Chorea occurs in 1–2% of patients with systemic lupus erythematosus, usually associated with the antiphospholipid antibody syndrome, and more commonly in women [45]. Antibody-related pathophysiology may underlie these conditions. Chorea may be the presenting symptom in a quarter of patients, may be present at the time of diagnosis in another quarter, and may manifest during flares of the disease. SLE-related chorea is rarely permanent [21].

Cases involving focal dystonia (blepharospasm and torticollis) have been uncommonly reported in association with systemic lupus erythematosus or myasthenia gravis. Dystonia in these cases was reported to respond to immunomodulatory therapies and correlated with autoimmune titers in the case of SLE [46].

Antiphospholipid antibody syndrome

Antiphospholipid antibody syndrome-related parkinsonism has a probable underlying main mechanism of a thrombo-occlusive vasculopathy, and is associated with cerebral infarctions, periventricular white-matter changes on neuroimaging, and poor response to levodopa [47]. A progressive supranuclear palsy phenotype may occur from cerebrovascular disease related to antiphospholipid antibody syndrome [48]. Other atypical movement disorders reported include tics, tremor, myoclonus, and a corticobasal degeneration-like syndrome, with resolution of involuntary movements after treatment with oral anticoagulation in a few cases, suggesting vasculopathy as an etiology [49].

Sydenham's chorea

Sydenham's chorea (SC) complicates about up to one-third of cases of rheumatic fever, usually occurring between 7 and 12 years of age (average age 9), with girls more commonly affected. Chorea develops weeks or months after infection with group A β-hemolytic streptococcus. Onset of chorea can occur up to 6 months after the initial infection, and may be accompanied by dysarthria (jerky and explosive speech), gait imbalance, facial grimacing, and ophthalmologic findings such as hypometric saccades [50] . Changes in

159

attention and behavior such as learning disabilities, obsessive compulsive disorder, anxiety, attention-deficit hyperactivity disorder, and tics may also be present [51]. Remission occurs in half the patients by 6 months, but mild chorea may persist for years [52].

The mechanism of action of chorea in Sydenham's chorea is thought to involve a cross-reaction between antibodies to group A β-hemolytic streptococcus and basal-ganglia structures, and anti-basal-ganglia anti-bodies have been identified in SC [53]. Pathologic studies show inflammation and neuronal loss in the basal ganglia [51]. Patients diagnosed with SC and rheumatic fever not only require treatment with anti-biotics (penicillin) for acute pharyngitis, but also chronic penicillin prophylaxis. Short courses of high-dose steroids can reduce chorea and improve remission time [54]. Disabling or persistent chorea can be treated with dopamine receptor blocking drugs (pimozide, haloperidol) although they should be employed with caution as patients with SC may be more susceptible to drug-induced parkinsonism [55]. Antiepileptic drugs (valproic acid, carbamazepine) may be effective as well.

Although controversial, other movement disorders have been reported and ascribed to autoimmune responses to streptococcal infections. In these disor-ders, proponents theorize that abnormal involuntary movements occur as a result of poststreptococcal autoimmunity in a manner similar to SC, with cross-reacting antibodies interfering with basal-ganglia function [56]. Under the general rubric of PANDAS (pediatric autoimmune neuropsychiatric disorders associated with streptococcal infections), several movement phenomenologies have been described, including paroxysmal dystonic choreoathe-tosis [57], a Tourette's-like syndrome, acute dissemi-nated encephalomyelitis, parkinsonism, or even isolated neuropsychiatric disorders such as obsessive-compulsive disorder or ADHD [58].

Sjögren syndrome

Sjögren syndrome, an autoimmune disorder associ-ated with exocrine gland dysfunction, may be associ-ated with a wide variety of central and peripheral neurological symptoms. Systemic symptoms classi-cally include dry eyes or dry mouth, with pathologic evidence of lymphocytic infiltration of the lacrimal and salivary glands. Several patients with Sjögren's

syndrome have been noted to have parkinsonism, some with associated white-matter lesions on neuro-imaging. Response to levodopa is generally poor, and there is variable improvement with immuno-suppressive therapy [59]. One case of Sjögren-related parkinsonism responded to corticosteroids despite lack of response to levodopa [60]. Rare cases of ataxia, either acute or chronic, have been noted with Sjögren disease [61].

Nonvasculitic autoimmune inflammatory meningoencephalitis

Nonvasculitic autoimmune inflammatory meningo-encephalitis (NAIM) is proposed as a rare auto-immune cause of acute or chronic encephalopathy that has multiple serologic autoimmune associations, including thyroid autoimmunity (Hashimoto ence-phalitis). This syndrome has presented with rapidly progressive parkinsonism accompanied by myoclo-nus and dementia, similar to the rapid progression of prion disease, including period sharp waves on elec-troencephalogram (EEG). However, unlike prion disease, this disease is exquisitely responsive to high-dose corticosteroids and may provide dramatic clinical recovery [62].

Celiac disease

Autoimmune diseases, including celiac disease, an immune-mediated gluten-sensitive enteropathy asso-ciated with malabsorption and development of auto-antibodies, may account for the etiology of many cases of idiopathic adult-onset sporadic ataxia [63]. Celiac disease may be associated with chronic neu-rological syndromes, including ataxia (also known as "gluten ataxia"), myoclonus, peripheral neuropathy, and dementia [64]. Ataxia may occur even in the absence of the typical gastrointestinal symptoms, in association with the characteristic antibodies that have been shown to be more prevalent in adult patients with sporadic ataxia of unknown etiology; however, some controversy surrounds this associa-tion [63]. Gluten ataxia patients may also present with a sensorimotor axonal neuropathy, or rarely chorea, palatal tremor, or opsoclonus-myoclonus. Unilateral dystonic limb posturing, in association with cortical tremor has been reported as the pre-senting neurological sign in a case of untreated celiac disease [65]. A gluten-free diet may improve symptoms [63].

Anti-GAD ataxia

Another uncommon immune-mediated ataxia is associated with anti-GAD-65 antibodies [66]. Clinically, women are more affected, and patients have a slowly progressive cerebellar syndrome that may show cerebellar atrophy on MRI imaging. The disease is often associated with insulin-dependent diabetes mellitus [8]. Anti-GAD ataxia may be linked to gluten sensitivity and has responded to immunomodulatory therapy [66,67]. Stiff-person syndrome, characterized by axial muscular rigidity and intermittent painful spasms, may be associated with anti-GAD antibodies, and may in some cases also be paraneoplastic, with the latter being more associated with amphiphysin antibodies [68].

Neuro-Behçet's disease

Behçet's disease is characterized by the triad of genital ulceration, uveitis, and apthous stomatitis. It may cause parkinsonism with myoclonus due to brain involvement, with MRI showing abnormalities in the brainstem and the basal ganglia [69]. One case of Neuro-Behçet's disease presented as a jaw-opening dystonia in association with chorea as part of generalized cerebral, meningeal, and brainstem involvement, with good response to immunomodulatory treatment [70]. Another young patient developed paroxysmal focal dystonia of the arm with an ipsilateral thalamic lesion seen on MRI [71].

Other autoimmune associations

A small number of reports illustrate the possible interaction of dystonia and autoimmune disease. In a series of 100 patients with Meige syndrome, a specific autoimmune disease was diagnosed in 7% and a high antinuclear antibody (ANA) titer (>1:80) was found in 26% [72]. Anti-basal-ganglia antibodies were found in 65% of a series of 65 patients with atypical tics and dystonia (adult onset generalized dystonia or fixed limb dystonia), suggesting an underlying autoimmune pathophysiology in more clinically unusual presentations [73]. Three patients with dystonia and positive anti-basal-ganglia

antibodies responded favorably to immunomodulatory therapy, suggesting that an autoimmune mechanism may underlie a certain number of patients with dystonia [74].

Myoclonus and/or ataxia may occur in conjunction with opsoclonus as an autoimmune or paraneoplastic phenomenon, and has been termed the opsoclonus-myoclonus ataxia syndrome [75]. Other causes of chorea with a presumed autoimmune etiology have occurred in the course of rheumatoid arthritis, Behçet's syndrome, Henoch Schönlein syndrome, periarteritis nodosa, and Churg–Strauss syndrome [76].

Organ dysfunction and failure

Liver failure

Wilson's disease

Wilson's disease is a rare autosomal recessive disorder caused by a mutation in the ATP7B gene. Expression of the abnormal protein results in progressive accumulation of copper in multiple organs including the liver, brain, and eyes. Patients are symptomatic by the second or third decade of life, and can present with a wide variety of neurological, psychiatric, or hepatic phenotypes. In general, older patients present more commonly with neurologic symptoms [77]. Up to 50% of patients may present with neurological signs, with tremor being most frequent; however, patients may also have an akinetic-rigid syndrome similar to Parkinson's disease, ataxia, dystonia, or myoclonus [78]. Comorbid behavioral and cognitive changes are common, including psychosis, depression, or anxiety. More specific signs may include the characteristic "wing-beating" tremor or dystonic "sardonic smile" [37]. Other systemic findings include cardiac, renal, pancreatic, hematologic, and endocrinologic signs. Patients with younger age of onset for any movement disorder, especially with comorbid liver disease, should be worked up for Wilson's disease, which may reveal low serum ceruloplasmin, elevated 24-h urine copper, and a slit-lamp examination showing Kaiser–Fleischer rings. Brain MRI shows decreased T1/increased T2 signal in the basal ganglia, cerebellum, and/or brainstem. Treatment modalities include copper chelation to promote copper excretion, zinc to reduce copper absorption, a reduced copper diet, or possibly liver transplantation [77]. However, new-onset neurologic signs may occur in some cases after transplantation, possibly due to immunosuppressive medication, myelinolysis, or mobilization of liver copper stores with higher brain deposition [79]. Although the disease is rare, it represents a treatable disorder; therefore, any patient with young-onset movement disorders of any phenomenology should be screened with the full workup.

Non-Wilsonian hepatocerebral degeneration

Acquired hepatocerebral degeneration (non-Wilsonian) describes a syndrome of cognitive, psychiatric, and motor abnormalities associated with chronic liver failure of any cause. These symptoms are distinct from the acute and transient symptoms associated with hepatic encephalopathy (i.e., tremor, myoclonus, acute parkinsonism, ataxia) [80]. Basal-ganglia involvement is suggested by a wide variety of involuntary movements including choreoathetosis, tremor, dystonia, myoclonus, and other signs. Neuropathological features are similar to Wilson's disease [81]. Common clinical phenotypes have been described, and can be grouped into three major categories: parkinsonism (most common); cognitive impairment with psychiatric symptoms; and gait ataxia with other neurologic findings (tremor, dystonia, cognitive impairment) [82]. Magnetic resonance imaging (MRI) demonstrates T1 basal-ganglia hyperintensities, which are believed to correlate with brain manganese deposition [82]. A prospective evaluation of 51 liver-transplant candidates documented 11 patients with rapidly progressive parkinsonism characterized by postural (not rest) tremor, early gait and postural impairment, focal dystonia (in 50%), frontal lobe impairment, and symmetric bradykinesia and rigidity. These patients had T1 hyperintensities in the substantia nigra, globus pallidus, ventral midbrain, and hypothalamus, elevated serum and cerebrospinal fluid manganese levels, and response to levodopa therapy in several cases [81]. Optimal treatment of the movement disorder in this context is unclear, but there are reports of parkinsonism, cognition, and MRI findings improving after liver transplantation [82,83].

Renal failure

Several movement disorders have been reported in patients with uremia due to end-stage renal disease, particularly in patients with concomitant diabetes and diabetic nephropathy [84]. Most typical is cortical involvement causing myoclonus (asterixis, multifocal myoclonus), encephalopathy, and seizures; however, involvement of the basal-ganglia structures is an increasingly recognized syndrome [85]. Features of basal-ganglia dysfunction include acute or subacute onset of parkinsonian symptoms sometimes associated with added ataxia, dysarthria, encephalopathy, myoclonus, and metabolic acidosis. Brain-imaging findings in these patients are striking and show evidence of symmetric, bilateral, and reversible enhancing basal-ganglia lesions with associated vasogenic edema and mass effect [86]. Pathophysiology is unclear, and clinical improvement lags the improvements in neuro-imaging, with diverse long-term outcomes.

Uremia has also been associated with the sudden onset of chorea, mainly in elderly Asian patients. Patients with diabetes and end-stage renal disease who develop chorea have MRI changes in basal ganglia consistent with vasogenic edema [87]. Treatment with more frequent dialysis leads to resolution of the chorea [88], although the chorea has been described as occurring suddenly during the course of dialysis [89].

Cardiopulmonary arrest

Various movement disorders can occur in survivors of cardiac arrest. While post-hypoxic myoclonus is the most commonly described syndrome, patients may also develop akinetic-rigid parkinsonism, choreoathetosis, tremor, tics, or dystonia, due to injury to the basal ganglia, cerebellum, or thalamus [90]. Acute posthypoxic myoclonus consists of severe generalized myoclonic jerks in comatose patients, with poor outcomes despite attempts at treatment of the movement disorder due to the severity of underlying brain injury [91]. Chronic posthypoxic myoclonus, also known as Lance–Adams syndrome, emerges within days to weeks after the hypoxic injury, with prominent action myoclonus, which prohibits most voluntary coordinated actions [92]. Negative myoclonus may also cause frequent falls due to loss of muscle tone in the legs. Treatment is difficult, but myoclonus may improve spontaneously or with benzodiazepines, antiepileptic drugs, or serotonergic drugs (5-hydroxytryptophan) [90].

Hypoxic brain injury may cause many patterns of dystonia, and is typically generalized. Dystonia occurs in ~1% of survivors of perinatal asphyxia, and may have clinical onset up to 32 years after the initial event [93]. In a review of 12 patients recovering from hypoxic injury due to various causes, putamenal damage was frequently noted on neuroimaging, and progressive dystonia developed postinjury between 1 week and 36 months. Older age at time of insult and more prominent involvement of the globus pallidum were associated with an akinetic-rigid motor syndrome, which frequently later developed dystonic features [94].

Systemic cancer and paraneoplastic disorders

Neoplasm

Solid tumors may cause movement disorders due to the direct involvement of or mass effect on basal-ganglia structures, either from a primary tumor or metastases. They may also cause secondary involvement of the basal ganglia due to edema, metabolic or nutritional defects, coagulopathy and resultant secondary strokes, infections related to treatment or immune dysregulation, or toxic side effects of cancer treatment. CSF obstruction with hydrocephalus can cause a syndrome resembling parkinsonism, but with lower-body predominance and apraxic gait. Neuroimaging usually rules out movement disorders related to structural involvement.

Paraneoplastic

Paraneoplastic movement disorders are a heterogeneous group of rare disorders occurring independently from the direct effect of tumors, and are usually immune-mediated. Neurologic symptoms more often precede the diagnosis of the underlying tumor. The importance of recognizing these disorders is that prompt identification and treatment of the underlying tumor, often in conjunction with immunosuppression, may lead to improvement and sometimes complete neurological recovery of affected patients [95].

Parkinsonism
Reports of paraneoplastic parkinsonism are rare. Two cases were described in conjunction with breast cancer, one with a syndrome of parkinsonism and painful dystonia, with death 5 months after onset. Autopsy showed degeneration of the substantia nigra without Lewy bodies or inflammation [96]. Rapidly progressive parkinsonism with incontinence, impotence, and

levodopa-induced moaning was described in one patient with multiple myeloma. Pathology showed loss of pigmented neurons from the substantia nigra but no Lewy bodies [97]. Two reports of progressive supranuclear palsy-like presentations were described in association with B-cell lymphoma and bronchial carcinoma [98]. No immunological markers had been discovered for the above-mentioned cases.

More recent case series documenting the associated clinical features of paraneoplastic antibodies have identified more cases of paraneoplastic parkinsonism. Anti-Ma2-associated encephalitis, most often associated with testicular or lung cancer, has been more associated with atypical parkinsonian syndromes than other paraneoplastic neurological disorders. In a review of 38 Ma2 antibody positive patients, five had parkinsonism accompanied by dystonia, hypophonia, poor verbal output, hyperreflexia, and hypersomnolence [99]. Parkinsonism was reported in 11% of a series of 72 patients with voltage-gated potassium-channel autoimmunity, in addition to tremor (7%) and myoclonus (21%) or nonspecific gait disorders (5%), with these cases often mimicking prion disease but responding favorably to immunomodulatory therapy [100]. The collapsin response-mediator protein (CRMP)-5 antibody has been reported with a few cases of parkinsonism [101], and antineuronal nuclear antibody type 2/Anti-Ri has been reported with two cases of parkinsonism and breast cancer [102].

Ataxia
Paraneoplastic ataxia has a high association with tumors of the breast, ovary, lung (small cell lung cancer (SCLC)), and Hodgkin's lymphoma, but has been reported with many types of tumors. Paraneoplastic cerebellar degeneration has been reported with most paraneoplastic antibodies, including anti-Yo, anti-Tr, anti-Hu, anti-Ri, anti-CRMP-5, anti-PCA-2, anti-GluR1, anti-Ma, anti-amphiphysin, anti-voltage-gated potassium channel antibodies, and in Lambert–Eaton myasthenic syndrome. Other variable neurologic signs may accompany the ataxia, although anti-Yo and anti-Tr are more likely to present with pure cerebellar dysfunction. Pathology includes loss and degeneration of Purkinje cells or other cerebellar structures [103]. Ataxia may also be a frequent feature of paraneoplastic limbic encephalitis (18% in one review), and is rarely the presenting symptom of the

CHAPTER 9

disorder [95]. 13/38 of a series of patients with anti-Ma2 antibodies had varying levels of ataxia; 2 of the latter had stable cerebellar symptoms for years and cerebellar atrophy on brain imaging [99].

Dystonia

Paraneoplastic dystonia usually occurs in association with other movement disorders, and is rarely isolated. Two cases with prominent dystonia were reported with non-Hodgkin's lymphoma, including presentation with camptocormia (abnormal, severe forward flexion of the thoracolumbar spine, manifesting mainly with standing and walking) beginning 3 years before the development of the malignancy [104], and a patient who had cervical dystonia, dysphonia, blepharospasm, bradykinesia, and choreic/dystonic limb movements associated with the CRMP-5 antibody (101). Anti-Ri (ANNA-2) antibodies were found in four patients with laryngospasm and four patients with jaw-opening dystonia (two of the latter group had additional cervical dystonia and one had parkinsonism), in association with cervical, breast, and lung malignancies [102]. Anti-Ma2 antibodies were found in two patients with jaw-closing dystonia [99].

Chorea

Paraneoplastic chorea most often occurs in association with CRMP-5 antibodies. This antibody is most commonly noted in thymomas or small-cell lung cancer, although several malignancies have also been described [105]. Associated signs and symptoms include limbic encephalitis, neuropathy, ataxia, visual loss, and elevated white blood cells and protein in the cerebrospinal fluid. MRI of the brain may show T2 and FLAIR lesions in the basal ganglia. Chorea may improve with treatment of the underlying cancer and immunomodulatory therapy [106], but some cases can be refractory to medical treatment. Other antibodies have been associated with paraneoplastic chorea, including anti-Ri and voltage-gated potassium-channel antibodies [99,102,107].

Neuropathic tremor

Up to 90% of patients with benign IgM (particularly anti-MAG) demyelinating paraproteinemic neuropathy may have upper-limb tremor, which is typically action and postural predominant, although rest tremor has been noted. Distal tremor is irregular

and is slower and more prominent than proximal-arm regions. The tremor is postulated to occur from distortion of peripheral afferent sensory input, with resultant altered function of a central generator [108]. Other diseases causing polyneuropathy, such as chronic inflammatory demyelinating polyradiculoneuropathy (CIDP), recurrent Guillain–Barré syndrome (GBS), diabetes, uremia, and vasculitis have also been associated with tremor, although less commonly [109].

Polycythemia vera

Chorea occurs in up to 5% of patients with polycythemia vera, and while it is frequently attributed to a vascular cause, the pathophysiology is uncertain. Chorea may precede the characteristic hematologic findings and usually occurs acutely or subacutely [110]. Chorea manifests most commonly in elderly females with the disorder, although polycythemia vera is overall more common in men, suggesting a complex interaction of multiple factors in the genesis of the movement disorder. The chorea may improve with phlebotomy [111].

NMDA receptor antibody-related encephalitis

Anti-N-methyl-D-aspartate (NMDA) receptor encephalitis is characterized by seizures, psychosis, mental-status changes, and characteristic movements of the trunk and face, particularly involving jaw dystonia and opisthotonus. Anti-NMDA receptor encephalitis can affect all age groups and both sexes (though predominantly affecting young women). As a paraneoplastic syndrome, anti-NMDA receptor encephalitis is most commonly associated with ovarian teratoma. Removal of the tumor, if present, and immunomodulatory therapy may lead to dramatic recovery [112].

Systemic infectious diseases

Most types of movement disorders, including parkinsonism, dystonia, chorea, tremor, myoclonus, ataxia, or tics, may occur as a consequence of central nervous system infections, either as an acute or chronic manifestation, often displaying a combination of abnormal

164

movements. Infectious diseases with parkinsonism as their most frequent manifestation include Japanese encephalitis, encephalitis lethargica, influenza A encephalitis (as a long-term complication), and neurocysticercosis; the last disease is related to both focal basal-ganglia lesions and secondary hydrocephalus. Dystonia as a prominent symptom has been reported with viral encephalitis (Japanese encephalitis, influenza A, cytomegalovirus), tuberculous meningitis, cerebral malaria, and *M. pneumoniae* infection. Dystonia or chorea occurs in association with opportunistic infections related to HIV (particularly toxoplasmosis). Chorea is the most frequent movement disorder occurring with acute influenza A infection, herpes simplex virus, or mycobacterium tuberculosis-related intracranial involvement. Chorea may also be a complication of infection with HIV (associated with HIV encephalopathy—sometimes as an early, reversible presenting sign [113] or secondary to opportunistic infections such as toxoplasmosis), cysticercosis, diphtheria, neurosyphilis, scarlet fever, or viral encephalitis [6]. Myoclonus is a prominent feature of prion disease, often associated with ataxia and parkinsonism [114]. Ataxia may result from encephalitis (particularly with varicella virus in children), acute or chronic infection with HIV, Epstein–Barr Virus, Lyme borreliosis, syphilis, or prion disease (sporadic CJD) [8]. Tics developing later in life can rarely be secondary to postinfectious states, including Sydenham's chorea and levodopa-treated postencephalitic parkinsonism [115]. One adult patient developed a chronic throat-clearing vocal tic after an episode of severe pharyngitis [116].

HIV

Movement disorders may occur in the context of infection with HIV. Several mechanisms may account for the movements, including drug-induced disorders, secondary brain infections, or the primary pathological changes of HIV-associated dementia (HAD). Parkinsonism is commonly noted in HAD, with documented radiological and pathological findings in the basal ganglia and nigrostriatal dopaminergic system likely accounting for these symptoms [117–119], and may occur even with effective HIV treatments as a possible consequence of accelerated aging processes in chronically managed HIV patients [120]. Parkinsonism with focal hand dystonia has been

reported as a presenting syndrome of HIV infection, improving over several weeks with levodopa therapy (not required long-term) and highly active antiretroviral therapy (HAART) [121]. HIV-infected patients are more susceptible to the extrapyramidal side effects of dopamine receptor-blocking medications than HIV-negative patients due to underlying basal-ganglia dysfunction, and drug interactions between HIV medications and other classes of medications may predispose patients to parkinsonism [117]. Myoclonus, chorea-ballism, paroxysmal dyskinesias, tremor, and dystonia have all been described as secondary to HAD, HIV infection, or opportunistic infections.

Whipple's disease

Whipple's disease is caused by the bacillus *Tropheryma whippelii*, and classically presents with gastrointestinal symptoms including weight loss, abdominal pain, and diarrhea; fevers of unknown origin and arthralgias may occur. Central nervous system involvement of the infection has been recognized in many cases, and may be isolated to the CNS (<5%) or have no classic bowel involvement (15%) [122]. Neurological presentations include a progressive supranuclear palsy-like syndrome with vertical supranuclear ophthalmoplegia; memory loss or dementia; sleep disturbances; or other movement disorders including myoclonus of the limbs and facial muscles [123]. Several cases with prominent ataxia have been described. The classic sign of oculomasticulatory myorhythmia is only present in a minority of cases; therefore, its absence should not exclude a workup for Whipple's disease. While rare, Whipple's disease should be worked up in the appropriate clinical setting, as it is treatable with antibiotics such as intravenous ceftriaxone, which may result in significant clinical improvement [124].

Complications due to transplantation

Most movement disorders occurring after transplantation are secondary to immunosuppressive drugs, with tremor being the most common movement disorder seen. Cyclosporine is known to cause tremor in up to 40% of patients, sometimes in association with encephalopathy, leukoencephalopathy, or cerebellar dysfunction [125]; it may also cause reversible akinetic rigid parkinsonism. Other immunosupressants (such as FK-506 or azathioprine) may also cause tremor.

Neurologic disturbances occur in 60–70% of bone-marrow transplant cases, but movement disorders are uncommonly reported outside of tremor related to immunosuppressive medications. A case of an acute akinetic syndrome with prominent gait freezing, severe postural impairment, and bilateral hyperintense lesions on MRI in the basal ganglia has been reported to occur 6 months after bone marrow transplant, and was unresponsive to therapy [126].

Complications of critical medical illness

Stroke

Chorea is the most common movement disorder resulting from cerebrovascular disease, and stroke is the main cause of sporadic chorea. In a series of 1500 patients poststroke, 4% developed movement disorders, one-third of whom had chorea. Chorea caused by stroke is typically unilateral (called hemichorea), occurring contralateral to the side of the stroke, with thalamic lesions as the most common localization. Most of patients show partial or full recovery in 1 year [127].

Postpump chorea

Postpump chorea can occur in children after cardiac surgery. Most cases are mild and transient, but severe manifestations can be life-threatening; severe cases are associated with preoperative cyanosis and older age. Pathophysiology is unclear, and may result from a combination of effects from hypoxia or hypothermia [128].

Progressive supranuclear palsy-like syndrome after ascending aortic aneurysm surgery

There are a growing number of rare cases of patients with a progressive supranuclear palsy phenotype developing after ascending aorta surgery for aneurysm repair. Variable signs have included akinetic-rigid parkinsonism, dysphagia, ataxia, spasticity, seizures, various eye movement disorders including vertical supranuclear gaze palsy, dementia, or dystonia. Imaging is typically unremarkable without evidence of ischemia or stroke, and etiology is uncertain. The clinical course follows a biphasic development with an earlier, mild, improving phase followed by a more aggressive, progressive decline that may plateau [129].

Drugs, toxins, and vitamin and mineral deficiencies

Drugs

Many drugs used commonly for treatment of medical and psychiatric diseases can cause movement disorders. The prevalence of drug-induced movement disorders is high and likely under-recognized, and may account for up to 20% of cases of all movement disorders in elderly patients in a community setting [130].

Parkinsonism

Drug-induced parkinsonism can occur as a complication of treatment with dopamine receptor blocking agents including antipsychotics (e.g., haloperidol, risperidone, perphenazine), prokinetic agents (metoclopramide), or antiemetic agents (e.g., prochlorperazine, promethazine). The history of dopamine receptor-blocking medication use may not always be obvious, given their often transient or "as needed" use, requiring specific questioning and investigations of past drug treatments in suspect cases. Metoclopramide, frequently used for treatment of medical conditions including gastroparesis, nausea, vomiting, and esophagitis, may account for up to 29% of drug-induced parkinsonism in the elderly [131]. Drug-induced parkinsonism may be less prevalent in patients treated with atypical, newer-generation antipsychotics, but the risk is still clinically pertinent as most drugs have been implicated in several reports. Discontinuation of the offending agent usually leads to recovery in several weeks or months. In cases where parkinsonism persists, it is probable that the patient had early Parkinson's disease unmasked by the drug.

Reports of other drug classes causing parkinsonism include calcium channel blockers (diltiazem, nifedipine, verapamil), antiarrhythmic drugs (amiodarone), monoamine depleters (reserpine, tetrabenazine), lithium, buspirone, anticonvulsants (phenytoin, sodium valproate), immunosuppressants or chemotherapeutic agents (cyclosporine, vincristine, busulfan, cytosine arabinoside, doxorubicin), procaine, chloroquine, α-methyldopa, chloroquine, and high doses of diazepam [132].

Dystonia

Drug-induced dystonia is difficult to diagnose as it may otherwise appear clinically similar to primary dystonia, with isolated dystonic movements. Careful and specific questioning for a history of dystonia-causing medications is therefore crucial [37]. Many drugs that cause drug-induced parkinsonism also cause drug-induced dystonia, but, unlike parkinsonism, drugs that cause dystonia may be grouped by their tendency to cause acute or late (tardive) dystonic syndromes. Drugs that cause *acute* dystonia include neuroleptics, dopaminergic agents, antidepressants, anxiolytics, antihistamines, and antiepileptic drugs. Acute dystonic reactions typically localize in axial, craniocervical, or pharyngeal muscles. Treatment of acute dystonic reactions includes discontinuation of the causative agent and administration of intravenous diphenhydramine or anticholinergic medications [133]. *Tardive* dystonia is most often caused by dopamine receptor-blocking drugs including neuroleptics, antiemetics, and prokinetic gastrointestinal agents [134]. Of special note, next to haloperidol, metoclopramide is the second most common drug causing tardive dystonia and tardive dyskinesia, which has led to a specific United States Food and Drug Administration (FDA) "black box warning" to caution about the risks of tardive dyskinesia [135]. Patients with HIV-associated dementia may be particularly sensitive to dopamine receptor-blocking medications [117]. Dystonia occurs less commonly with antihistamine drugs, antidepressants (SSRIs, TCAs), or calcium-channel blockers.

Chorea

Tardive dyskinesia occurs with exposure to dopamine receptor antagonists [135], most characteristically presenting with oral–lingual–buccal movements. Chorea may affect other body regions as well, often being difficult to distinguish from other causes of chorea. A variety of other drugs have been reported to cause chorea, including anti-parkinsonian drugs, antiepileptic drugs (phenytoin, valproic acid, carbamazepine), psychostimulants (amphetamines, cocaine), anticholinergics, calcium-channel blockers, antihistamines, steroids, lithium, theophylline, digoxin, cyclosporine, or antidepressants (tricyclic antidepressants, SSRIs) [6]. Treatment with interferon for hepatitis C in HIV patients may result in a chorea syndrome, sometimes with akathisia or parkinsonism [136].

Chorea has also been associated with the use of oral contraceptives (OCPs), with evidence suggesting that estrogen enhances central dopaminergic sensitivity. However, many patients with chorea on OCPs had coexisting antiphospholipid antibody syndrome, lupus, or prior rheumatic fever, which suggests that OCPs alone are usually not sufficient to cause chorea [137]. Chorea gravidarum (chorea with onset during pregnancy) may share a similar mechanism of action to that of OCP-associated chorea. It usually begins in the first trimester of pregnancy and improves later in pregnancy or after delivery, and can occur in patients with a history of rheumatic fever or other infectious or autoimmune diseases [138,139].

Non-parkinsonian tremor

Drugs are a common cause of acquired tremor. Risk factors for drug-induced tremor include older age, impaired hepatic and renal function, or other underlying neurological and medical conditions. While the list of implicated medications is quite long, some frequently used medications for tremor deserve special note:

- Amiodarone causes dose-dependent postural and intention tremor in one third of treated patients, resembling essential tremor. Parkinsonism has also been described with this drug.
- Cyclosporin causes a postural tremor in as many as 40% of patients, which is usually mild [140].
- Tacrolimus causes more disabling tremors, with the most frequent reports in liver-transplant patients or patients with rheumatoid arthritis [5].
- Most antidepressants may cause tremor. Up to 20% of patients on selective serotonin reuptake inhibitors (SSRIs) may have tremor. Tricyclic antidepressants are also implicated. Tremor generally develops 1 to 2 months after starting antidepressant therapy and may take up to 1 month to resolve.
- Lithium frequently causes tremor, with at least 30% of lithium-treated patients developing tremor even at therapeutic levels. With toxic lithium levels, tremor is nearly universal. Concomitant treatment with SSRIs increases the risk of developing tremor.
- The most common antiepileptic drug to cause tremor is valproic acid, with tremor occurring in up to 25% of patients. Tremor severity does not always correlate with serum level, but dose reduction and longer-acting formulations may improve tremor [5].

167

• Other drugs that commonly cause tremor: antiviral agents (e.g., acyclovir, vidarabine) and chemotherapy drugs (e.g., thalidomide, cytarabine).

In general, the approach to treating drug-induced tremor is to taper the drug or substitute another drug with a lower risk of tremor. Drugs used to treat essential tremor such as propranolol can be added if tapering or changing the medicine is not feasible.

Tics
Tics are rarely secondary to drug use, although lamotrigine has been reported to cause tics in small case series [141].

Ataxia
Certain compounds can cause chronic cerebellar damage, with the most relevant being phenytoin, lithium, amiodarone, or antineoplastics including cytosine arabinoside or 5-fluorouracil [8].

Toxins

Parkinsonism
Exogenous environmental toxins may play a role in the development of parkinsonism, and, based on current models of the molecular pathogenesis of the disease, may be risk factors for the development of Parkinson's disease [142]. Organophosphates, cyanide, methanol, mercury, carbon disulphide, copper, mercury, aliphatic hydrocarbons, disulfiram, hydrocarbons, lacquer thinner, manganese, and addictive drugs (MPTP [1-methyl-4-phenyl-1,2,3,6-tetrahydropyridine]), heroin pyrolysate, amphetamine drugs, and inhaled solvents such as toluene, and ecstasy) have been implicated [132]. Biochemical assays, careful exposure history, and potential improvement after minimizing exposure from the putative toxic environmental source may help solidify the diagnosis.

Manganese-related parkinsonism Manganese is an essential trace element in the normal human diet, is absorbed through the bowel, and is excreted through the bile, and may be associated with parkinsonian syndromes. Manganism can develop in several contexts, and two are highlighted here. There have been concerns that low-dose chronic occupational exposure to manganese increases the risk of Parkinson's disease, but this issue has not been settled.

Ephedronic encephalopathy Case series and reports have described a new form of manganese toxicity causing a distinct syndrome of akinetic-rigid parkinsonism, severe hypophonia, and impaired postural reflexes in association with manganese-related hyperintense signal on T1-weighted MRI in the globus pallidus and substantia nigra. The syndrome is noted mainly in self-preparing methcathinone hydrochloride (Ephedrone) users in Eastern European countries and Russia, most with concomitant hepatitis C and/or HIV infection. Manganese intoxication stems from the use of potassium permanganate as an oxidant [143,144].

Total parenteral nutrition Patients on long-term total parenteral nutrition (TPN) may have T1 high-signal abnormalities in the basal ganglia, pituitary gland, and brainstem, but the relationship of these imaging abnormalities, presumably due to manganese deposition, to neurological symptoms is unclear, because they may occur in asymptomatic patients [145]. Symptomatic patients may have parkinsonism, psychiatric or cognitive changes, with clinical and radiologic improvement after discontinuation of trace-element infusion [146]. Symptoms and imaging findings are generally reversible but may be unremitting in rare cases [147].

Carbon monoxide poisoning Carbon monoxide poisoning results in postanoxic parkinsonism in up to 10% of affected patients, occurring up to 6 months after the initial insult; however, symptoms are usually apparent within the first month. Neuroimaging demonstrates symmetric changes in the globus pallidum. Clinical features include prominent gait disturbances, urinary incontinence, and impaired cognition, with occasional cerebellar signs [148]. Anti-parkinsonian drugs are generally not effective. Spontaneous recovery or improvement occurs in most patients after 6 months.

Dystonia
Many of the same toxins predisposing to parkinsonism may cause dystonia due to injury to the basal ganglia. Methanol, cyanide, carbon monoxide, manganese, mercury, carbon disulfide, and mycotoxin are potent examples [134]. As discussed above, treatment involves removal of the offending agent in addition to the use of dopaminergic drugs or anticholinergic agents in cases of residual dystonia.

Chorea

Choreic syndromes are noted to accompany poisoning with carbon monoxide, thallium, methanol, heroin, glue sniffing, cyanide, manganese, mercury, or organophosphates [6].

Ataxia

The most common known cause of toxic cerebellar degeneration is alcohol, which typically affects the lower limbs and gait more severely. Alcoholic cerebellar degeneration may occur subacutely in heavy drinkers and may progress with continued alcohol consumption. Pathology shows pathological loss of Purkinje cells in the vermis and anterior cerebellar hemispheres. Other drugs and toxins with low threshold for ataxic side effects include antiepileptic drugs (i.e., phenytoin, carbamazepine), lithium, several antineoplastics, metronidazole, heavy-metal toxicities, and solvent toxicity [149].

Vitamin deficiencies

Inadequate serum vitamin D levels may increase the risk of several chronic conditions, and has been linked to an increased risk of Parkinson's disease in several studies, although several confounders for this association may exist [150].

Two autosomal recessive diseases may cause ataxia in association with vitamin E deficiency, and are important to recognize as they may benefit from vitamin supplementation. Ataxia with vitamin E deficiency (AVED) is an autosomal recessive disorder that presents with progressive cerebellar and sensory ataxia, and may resemble the phenotype of Freidreich's ataxia. Abetalipoproteinemia, which causes a malabsorption syndrome, is associated with ataxic neuropathy and retinal pigmentary degeneration; acanthocystosis may be seen on blood smears as a diagnostic clue [149]. Vitamin E deficiency, with the above associated neurologic symptoms, can also occur as part of general malabsorption [8].

Other vitamin deficiencies that may cause ataxia include vitamin B1 (leading to Wernicke's encephalopathy, with accompanying mental confusion and ophthalmoplegia), or vitamin B12 (causing subacute combined degeneration of the spinal cord, associated with predominantly sensory ataxia). Nutritional deficiency of vitamin B1 may play a role in the pathophysiology of alcoholic cerebellar degeneration [151]. B12 deficiency less frequently causes cerebellar ataxia, chorea, parkinsonism, or focal dystonia, which may improve with vitamin replacement [152]

Acknowledgment

Salary for Dr. Barton and Dr. Goetz is supported by the Parkinson Disease Foundation.

Five things to remember about movement disorders due to systemic disease

1. Identification of a medical cause for a movement disorder may often offer the potential for treatment or stabilization of the neurologic symptoms after treatment of the underlying medical condition.
2. The phenomenology of a movement disorder alone is not necessarily specific to the underlying etiology, with a broad differential diagnosis to consider in each case.
3. A thorough medical history, physical examination, and careful review of medications is required for a patient presenting with either a new onset movement disorder or worsening of a pre-existing movement disorder.
4. Medical history and physical examination will guide the practitioner to order indicated ancillary studies, consultations, or investigations to correctly identify a movement disorder as primary, secondary to a medical illness, or both.
5. Regardless of rarity, certain medical conditions should be considered in patients presenting with a new onset of a movement disorder, as these conditions may be highly treatable; examples from the text include Wilson's disease, vitamin deficiencies, or Whipple's disease.

References

1 Tolosa E, Wenning G, Poewe W. The diagnosis of Parkinson's disease. *Lancet Neurol.* 2006;5(1):75–86.

2 Tarsy D, Simon DK. Dystonia. *N. Engl. J. Med.* 2006;355(8):818–829.

3 Breakefield XO, Blood AJ, Li Y, Hallett M, Hanson PI, Standaert DG. The pathophysiological basis of dystonias. *Nat. Rev. Neurosci.* 2008;9(3):222–234.

4 Németh AH. The genetics of primary dystonias and related disorders. *Brain* 2002;125(Pt 4):695–721. 9212397781.

5 Morgan JC, Sethi KD. Drug-induced tremors. *Lancet Neurol.* 2005;4(12):866–876.

6 Cardoso F, Seppi K, Mair KJ, Wenning GK, Poewe W. Seminar on choreas. *Lancet Neurol.* 2006;5(7):589–602.

7 Caviness JN. Myoclonus. *Parkinsonism Relat. Disord.* 2007;13:S375–S384.

8 Klockgether T. Sporadic ataxia with adult onset: classification and diagnostic criteria. *Lancet Neurol.* 2010;9 (1):94–104.

9 García-Moreno JM, Chacón-Peña J. Hypothyroidism and Parkinson's disease and the issue of diagnostic confusion. *Mov. Disord.* 2003;18(9):1058–1059.

10 Teive HA, Munhoz RP. Hypothyroidism and Parkinson's disease. *Mov. Disord.* 2004;19(9):1116–1117.

11 Taurin G, Golfier V, Pinel JF. et al. Choreic syndrome due to Hashimoto's encephalopathy. *Mov. Disord.* 2002;17(5):1091–1092.

12 Munhoz RP, Teive HAG, Troiano, et al. Parkinson's disease and thyroid dysfunction. *Parkinsonism Relat. Disord.* 2004;10:381–383.

13 Miao J, Liu R, Li J, Du Y, Zhang W, Li Z. Meige's syndrome and hemichorea associated with hypothyroidism. *J. Neurol. Sci.* 2010;288(1-2); 175–177.

14 Kim HT, Edwards MJ, Lakshmi Narsimhan R, Bhatia KP. Hyperthyroidism exaggerating parkinsonian tremor: a clinical lesson. *Parkinsonism Relat. Disord.* 2005;11(5):331–332.

15 Yu JH, Weng YM. Acute chorea as a presentation of Graves disease: case report and review. *Am. J. Emerg. Med.* 2009;27(3):369e1–369e3.

16 Tan EK, Chan LL. Movement disorders associated with hyperthyroidism: expanding the phenotype. *Mov. Disord.* 2006;21(7):1054–1057.

17 Hayashi R, Hashimoto T, Tako K. Efficacy of propranolol in hyperthyroid-induced chorea: a case report. *Mov. Disord.* 2003;18(9):1073–1076.

18 Isaacs JD, Rakshi J, Baker R, Brooks DJ, Warrens AN. Chorea associated with thyroxine replacement therapy. *Mov. Disord.* 2005;20(12):1656–1657.

19 Barabas G, Tucker SM. Idiopathic hypoparathyroidism and paroxysmal dystonic choreoathetosis. *Ann. Neurol.* 1988;24(4):585.

20 Topakian R, Stieglbauer K, Rotaru J, Haring HP, Aichner FT, Pichler R. Hypocalcemic choreoathetosis and tetany after bisphosphonate treatment. *Mov. Disord.* 2006;21(11):2026–2027.

21 Janavs JL, Aminoff MJ. Dystonia and chorea in acquired systemic disorders. *J. Neurol. Neurosurg. Psychiatry* 1998;65(4):436–445.

22 Tambyah PA, Ong BK, Lee KO. Reversible parkinsonism and asymptomatic hypocalcemia with basal ganglia calcification from hypoparathyroidism 26 years after thyroid surgery. *Am. J. Med.* 1993;94(4):444–445.

23 Vaamonde J, Legarda I, Jimenez-Jimenez J, Zubieta JL, Obeso JA. Levodopa-responsive parkinsonism associated with basal ganglia calcification and primary hypoparathyroidism. *Mov. Disord.* 1993;8(3):398–400.

24 Kovacs CS, Howse DC, Yendt ER. Reversible parkinsonism induced by hypercalcemia and primary hyperparathyroidism. *Arch. Intern. Med.* 1993;153(9):1134–1136.

25 Evans BK, Donley DK. Pseudohypoparathyroidism, parkinsonism syndrome, with no basal ganglia calcification. *J. Neurol. Neurosurg. Psychiatry* 1988;51(5):709–713.

26 Pearson DW, Durward WF, Fogelman I, Boyle IT, Beastall G. Pseudohypoparathyroidism presenting as severe Parkinsonism. *Postgrad. Med. J.* 1981;57 (669):445–447.

27 Siejka SJ, Knezevic WV, Pullan PT. Dystonia and intracerebral calcification: pseudohypoparathyroidism presenting in an eleven-year-old girl. *Aust. N. Z. J. Med.* 1988;18(4):607–609.

28 Maraganore DM, Folger WN, Swanson JW, Ahlskog JE. Movement disorders as sequelae of central pontine myelinolysis: report of three cases. *Mov. Disord.* 1992;7(2):142–148.

29 Prevett MC, Rossor MN. Central pontine and extrapontine myelinolysis presenting with parkinsonism in a patient with cystic fibrosis. *Mov. Disord.* 1999;14 (3):523–525.

30 Caviness JN, Brown P. Myoclonus: current concepts and recent advances. *Lancet Neurol.* 2004;3:598–607.

31 Manyam BV. What is and what is not 'Fahr's disease'. *Parkinsonism Relat. Disord.* 2005;11(2):73–80.

32 Oh SH, Lee KY, Im JH, Lee MS. Chorea associated with non-ketotic hyperglycemia and hyperintensity basal ganglia lesion on T1-weighted brain MRI study: a meta-analysis of 53 cases including four present cases. *J. Neurol. Sci.* 2002;200(1-2):57–62.

33 Lai SL, Tseng YL, Hsu MC, Chen SS. Magnetic resonance imaging and single-photon emission computed

tomography changes in hypoglycemia-induced chorea. *Mov. Disord.* 2004;19(4):475–478.

34 Russo N, Edwards M, Andrews T, O'Brien M, Bhatia KP. Hereditary haemochromatosis is unlikely to cause movement disorders: a critical review. *J. Neurol.* 2004;251(7):849–852.

35 Costello DJ, Walsh SL, Harrington HJ, Walsh CH. Concurrent hereditary haemochromatosis and idiopathic Parkinson's disease: a case report series. *J. Neurol. Neurosurg. Psychiatry* 2004;75(4):631–633.

36 Sedel F, Saudubray JM, Roze E, Agid Y, Vidailhet M. Movement disorders and inborn errors of metabolism in adults: a diagnostic approach. *J. Inherit. Metab. Dis.* 2008;31(3):308–318.

37 Geyer HL, Bressman SB. The diagnosis of dystonia. *Lancet Neurol.* 2006;5(9):780–790.

38 Joseph FG, Lammie GA, Scolding NJ. CNS lupus: a study of 41 patients. *Neurology* 2007;69(7):644–654.

39 García-Moreno JM, Chacón J. Juvenile parkinsonism as a manifestation of systemic lupus erythematosus: case report and review of the literature. *Mov. Disord.* 2002;17(6):1329–1335.

40 Khubchandani RP, Viswanathan V, Desai J. Unusual neurologic manifestations (I): Parkinsonism in juvenile SLE. *Lupus* 2007;16(8):572–575.

41 Tan EK, Chan LL, Auchus AP. Reversible parkinsonism in systemic lupus erythematosus. *J. Neurol. Sci.* 2001;193(1):53–57.

42 Kunas RC, McRae A, Kesselring J, Villiger PM. Antidopaminergic antibodies in a patient with a complex autoimmune disorder and rapidly progressing Parkinson's disease. *J. Allergy Clin. Immunol.* 1995;96(5 Pt 1): 688–690.

43 Lee PH, Joo US, Bang OY, Seo CH. Basal ganglia hyperperfusion in a patient with systemic lupus erythematosus-related parkinsonism. *Neurology* 2004;63(2):395–396.

44 Fady GJ, Lammie GA, Scolding NJ. CNS Lupus: a study of 41 patients. *Neurology* 2007;69(7):644–654.

45 Sanna G, Bertolaccini ML, Cuadrado MJ, et al. Neuropsychiatric manifestations in systemic lupus erythematosus: prevalence and association with antiphospholipid antibodies. *J. Rheumatol.* 2003;30(5):985–992.

46 Rajagopalan N, Humphrey PR, Bucknall RC. Torticollis and blepharospasm in systemic lupus erythematosus. *Mov. Disord.* 1989;4(4):345–348.

47 Huang YC, Lyu RK, Chen ST, Chu YC, Wu YR. Parkinsonism in a patient with antiphospholipid syndrome: case report and literature review. *J. Neurol. Sci.* 2008;267(1-2):166–169.

48 Reitblat T, Polishchuk I, Dorodnikov E, et al. Primary antiphospholipid antibody syndrome masquerading as progressive supranuclear palsy. *Lupus* 2003;12(1):67–69.

49 Martino D, Chew NK, Mir P, et al. Atypical movement disorders in antiphospholipid syndrome. *Mov. Disord.* 2006;21(7):944–949.

50 Gordon N. Sydenham's chorea, and its complications affecting the nervous system. *Brain Dev.* 2009;31(1):11–14.

51 Chorea, ballism, athetosis: phenomenology and etiology. In S Fahn, J Jankovic, editors, *Principles and Practice of Movement Disorders. 1st ed.* Philadelphia, PA: Elsevier 2007: 393–407.

52 Cardoso F, Vargas AP, Oliveira LD, Guerra AA, Amaral SV. Persistent Sydenham's chorea. *Mov. Disord.* 1999;14(5):805–807.

53 Church AJ, Cardoso F, Dale RC, Lees AJ, Thompson EJ, Giovannoni G. Anti-basal ganglia antibodies in acute and persistent Sydenham's chorea. *Neurology* 2002;59(2):227–231.

54 Paz JA, Silva CA, Marques-Dias MJ. Randomized double-blind study with prednisone in Sydenham's chorea. *Pediatr. Neurol.* 2006;34(4):264–269.

55 Teixeira AL, Cardoso F, Maia DP, Cunningham MC. Sydenham's chorea may be a risk factor for drug induced parkinsonism. *J. Neurol. Neurosurg. Psychiatry* 2003;74(9):1350–1351.

56 Snider LA, Swedo SE. PANDAS: current studies and direction for research. *Mol. Psychiatry* 2004;9(10):900–907.

57 Dale RC, Church AJ, Surtees RA, Thompson EJ, Giovannoni G, Neville BG. Post-streptococcal autoimmune neuropsychiatric disease presenting as paroxysmal dystonia choreoathetosis. *Mov. Disord.* 2002;17(4):817–820.

58 Martino D, Giovannoni G. Antibasal ganglia antibodies and their relevance to movement disorders. *Curr. Opin. Neurol.* 2004;17(4):425–432.

59 Walker RH, Spiera H, Brin MF, Olanow CW. Parkinsonism associated with Sjögren's syndrome: three cases and a review of the literature. *Mov. Disord.* 1999;14(2):262–268.

60 Nishimura H, Tachibana H, Makiura N, Okuda B, Sugita M. Corticosteroid-responsive parkinsonism associated with primary Sjogren's syndrome. *Clin. Neurol. Neurosurg.* 1994;96(4):327–331.

61 Wong S, Pollock AN, Burnham JM, Sherry DD, Dlugos DJ. Acute cerebellar ataxia due to Sjogren syndrome. *Neurology* 2004;62(12):2332–2333.

62 Hoffman Snyder C, Mishark KH, Caviness JN, Drazkowski JF, Caselli RJ. Nonvasculitic autoimmune inflammatory meningoencephalitis imitating Creutzfeldt–Jakob disease. *Arch. Neurol.* 2006;63(5):766–768.

63 Hadjivassiliou M, Sanders DS, Woodroofe N, Williamson C, Grünewalk RA. Gluten ataxia. *Cerebellum* 2008;7(3):494–498.

64 Bhatia KP, Brown P, Gregory R, et al. Progressive myoclonic ataxia associated with celiac disease: the myoclonus is of cortical origin, but the pathology is in the cerebellum. *Brain* 1995;118(Pt 5): 1087–1093.

65 Fung VS, Duggins A, Morris JG, Lorentz IT. Progressive myoclonic ataxia associated with celiac disease presenting as unilateral cortical tremor and dystonia. *Mov. Disord.* 2000;15(4):732–734.

66 Hadjivassiliou M, Boscolo S, Tongiorgi E, et al. Cerebellar ataxia as a possible organ-specific autoimmune disease. *Mov. Disord.* 2008;23(10):1370–1377.

67 Nociti V, Frisullo G, Tartaglione T, et al. Refractory generalized seizures and cerebellar ataxia associated with anti-GAD antibodies responsive to immunosuppressive treatment. *Eur. J. Neurol.* 2010;17(1):e5.

68 Grant R, Graus F. Paraneoplastic movement disorders. *Mov. Disord.* 2009;24(12):1715–1724.

69 Bogdanova D, Milanov I, Georgiev D. Parkinsonian syndrome as a neurological manifestation of Behçet's disease. *Can. J. Neurol. Sci.* 1998;25(1):82–85.

70 Revilla FJ, Racette BA, Perlmutter JS. Chorea and jaw-opening dystonia as a manifestation of NeuroBehcet's syndrome. *Mov. Disord.* 2000;15(4):741–744.

71 Guak TH, Kim YI, Park SM, Kim JS. Paroxysmal focal dystonia in neuro-Behcet by a small ipsilateral thalamic lesion. *Eur. Neurol.* 2002;47(3):183–184.

72 Jankovic J, Patten BM. Blepharospasm and autoimmune disease. *Mov. Disord.* 1987;2(3):159–163.

73 Edwards MJ, Dale RC, Church AJ, Giovannoni G, Bhatia KP. A dystonic syndrome associated with anti-basal ganglia antibodies. *J. Neurol. Neurosurg. Psychiatry* 2004;75(6):914–916.

74 Edwards MJ, Trikouli E, Martino D, et al. Anti-basal ganglia antibodies in patients with atypical dystonia and tics: a prospective study. *Neurology* 2004;63(1):156–158.

75 Barton BR. Opsoclonus-myoclonus syndrome. In K Kompoliti, ML Verhagen, editors. *Encyclopedia of Movement Disorders*, vol. 2Oxford: Academic Press, 2010, pp. 332–335.

76 Valldeoriola F. Movement disorders of autoimmune origin. *J. Neurol.* 1999;246(6):423–431.

77 Ala A, Walker AP, Ashkan K, Dooley JS, Schilsky ML. Wilson's disease. *Lancet* 2007;369(9559):397–408.

78 Pfeiffer RF. Wilson's disease. *Semin. Neurol.* 2007;27(2):123–132.

79 Litwin T, Gromadzka G, Czlonkowska A. Neurological presentation of Wilson's disease in a patient after liver transplantation. *Mov. Disord.* 2008;23(5):743–746.

80 Lewis M, Howdle PD. The neurology of liver failure. *QJM* 2003;96(9):623–633.

81 Burkhard PR, Delavelle J, Pasquier R, Spahr L. Chronic parkinsonism associated with cirrhosis: a distinct subset of acquired hepatocerebral degeneration. *Arch. Neurol.* 2003;60(4):521–528.

82 Klos KJ, Ahlskog JE, Josephs KA, Fealey RD, Cowl CT, Kumar N. Neurologic spectrum of chronic liver failure and basal ganglia T1 hyperintensity of magnetic resonance imaging: probable manganese toxicity. *Arch. Neurol.* 2005;62(9):1385–1390.

83 Shulman LM, Minagar A, Weiner WJ. Reversal of parkinsonism following liver transplantation. *Neurology* 2003;60(3):519.

84 Wang HC, Cheng SJ. The syndrome of acute bilateral basal ganglia lesions in diabetic uremic patients. *J. Neurol.* 2003;250:948–955.

85 Li JY, Yong TY, Sebben R, Khoo E, Disney AP. Bilateral basal ganglia lesions in patients with end-stage diabetic nephropathy. *Nephrology* 2008;13(1):68–72.

86 Lee PH, Shin DH, Kim JW, Song YS, Kim HS. Parkinsonism with basal ganglia lesions in a patient with uremia: evidence of vasogenic edema. *Parkinsonism Relat. Disord.* 2006;12(2):93–96.

87 Lee EJ, Park JH, Ihn Y, Kim YJ, Lee SK, Park CS. Acute bilateral basal ganglia lesions in diabetic uraemia: diffusion-weighted MRI. *Neuroradiology* 2007;49(12):1009–1013.

88 Park JH, Kim HJ, Kim SM. Acute chorea with bilateral basal ganglia lesions in diabetic uremia. *Can. J. Neurol. Sci.* 2007;34(2):248–250.

89 Yaltho TC, Schiess MC, Furr-Stimmung E. Acute bilateral basal ganglia lesions and chorea in a diabetic-uremic patient on dialysis. *Arch. Neurol.* 67(2):246–247.

90 Venkatesan A, Frucht S. Movement disorders after resuscitation from cardiac arrest. *Neurol. Clin.* 2006;24(1):123–132.

91 Hui ACF, Cheng C, Lam A, et al. Prognosis following postanoxic myoclonus status epilepticus. *Eur. Neurol.* 2005;54(1):10–13.

92 Werhahn KJ, Brown P, Thompson PD, et al. The clinical features and prognosis of chronic post-hypoxic myoclonus. *Mov. Disord.* 1997;12(2):216–220.

93 Cerovac-Cosić N, Petrović I, Klein C, Kostić V. Delayed-onset dystonia due to perinatal asphyxia: a prospective study. *Mov. Disord.* 2007;22(16):2426–2429.

94 Bhatt MH, Obeso JA, Marsden CD. Time course of postanoxic akinetic-rigid and dystonic syndromes. *Neurology* 1993;43(2):314–317.

95 Gultekin SH, Rosenfeld MR, Voltz R, Eichen J, Posner JB, Dalmau J. Paraneoplastic limbic encephalitis: neurological symptoms, immunological findings, and tumor

association in 50 patients. *Brain* 2000;123(Pt 7):1481–1494.

96 Golbe LI, Miller DC, Duvoisin RC. Paraneoplastic degeneration of the substantia nigra with dystonia and parkinsonism. *Mov. Disord.* 1989;4(2):147–152.

97 Fahn S, Brin MF, Dwork AJ, Weiner WJ, Goetz CG, Rajput AH. Case 1, 1996: rapidly progressive parkinsonism, incontinence, impotency, and levodopa-induced moaning in a patient with multiple myeloma. *Mov. Disord.* 1996;11(3):298–310.

98 Tan JH, Goh BC, Tambyah PA, Wilder-Smith E. Paraneoplastic progressive supranuclear palsy syndrome in a patient with B-cell lymphoma. *Parkinsonism Relat. Disord.* 2005;11(3):187–191.

99 Dalmau J, Graus F, Villarejo A. et al. Clinical analysis of anti-Ma2-associated encephalitis. *Brain* 2004;127(Pt 8):1831–1844.

100 Tan KM, Lennon VA, Klein CJ, Boeve BF, Pittock SJ. Clinical spectrum of voltage-gated potassium channel autoimmunity. *Neurology* 2008;70(20):1883–1890.

101 Yu Z, Kryzer TJ, Griesmann GE, Kim K, Benarroch EE, Lennon VA. CRMP-5 neuronal autoantibody: marker of lung cancer and thymoma-related autoimmunity. *Ann. Neurol.* 2001;49(2):146–154.

102 Pittock SJ, Lucchinetti CF, Lennon VA. Anti-neuronal nuclear autoantibody type 2: paraneoplastic accompaniments. *Ann. Neurol.* 2003;53(5):580–587.

103 Bataller L, Dalmau J. Paraneoplastic neurologic syndromes: approaches to diagnosis and treatment. *Semin. Neurol.* 2003;23(2);215–224.

104 Zwecker M, Iancu I, Zeilig G, Ohry A. Camptocormia: a case of possible paraneoplastic aetiology. *Clin. Rehabil.* 1998;12(2):157–160.

105 Samii A, Dahlen DD, Spence AM, et al. Paraneoplastic movement disorder in a patient with non-Hodgkin's lymphoma and CRMP-5 autoantibody. *Mov. Disord.* 2003;18(12):1556–1558.

106 Vernino S, Tuite P, Adler CH. et al. Paraneoplastic chorea associated with CRMP-5 neuronal antibody and lung carcinoma. *Ann. Neurol.* 2002;51(5):625–630.

107 Kujawa KA, Niemi VR, Tomasi MA, Mayer NW, Cochran E, Goetz CG. Ballistic-choreic movements as the presenting feature of renal cancer. *Arch. Neurol.* 2001;58(7):1133–1135.

108 Bain PG, Britton TC, Jenkins IH, et al. Tremor associated with benign IgM paraproteinaemic neuropathy. *Brain* 1996;119(Pt 3):789–799.

109 Said G, Bathien N, Cesaro P. Peripheral neuropathies and tremor. *Neurology* 1982;32(5):480–485.

110 Nazabal ER, Lopez JM, Perez PA, Del Corral PR. Chorea disclosing deterioration of polycythaemia vera. *Postgrad. Med. J.* 2000;76(900):658–659.

111 Midi I, Dib H, Köseoglu M, Afsar N, Gunal DI. Hemichorea associated with polycythaemia vera. *Neurol. Sci.* 2006;27(6):439–441.

112 Rosenfeld MR, Dalmau J. Anti-NMDA-receptor encephalitis and other synaptic autoimmune disorders. *Curr. Treat. Options Neurol.* 2011;13:324–332.

113 Passarin MG, Alessandrini F, Nicolini GG, Musso A, Gambina G, Moretto G. Reversible choreoathetosis as the early onset of HIV-encephalopathy. *Neurol. Sci.* 2005;26(1):55–56.

114 Alarcón F, Gimenéz-Roldán S. Systemic diseases that cause movement disorders. *Parkinsonism Relat. Disord.* 2005;11(1):1–18.

115 Eapen V, Lees AJ, Lakke JP, Trimble MR, Robertson MM. Adult-onset tic disorders. *Mov. Disord.* 2002;17(4):735–740.

116 Chouinard S, Ford B. Adult onset tic disorders. *J. Neurol. Neurosurg. Psychiatry* 2000;68(6):738–743.

117 Tse W, Cersosimo MG, Gracies JM, Morgello S, Olanow CW, Koller W. Movement disorders and AIDS: a review. *Parkinsonism Relat. Disord.* 2004;10(6):323–334.

118 Koutsilieri E, Sopper S, Scheller C, ter Meulen T, Riederer P. Parkinsonism in HIV dementia. *J. Neural Transm.* 2002;109(5-6):767–775.

119 Tanaka M, Endo K, Suzuki T, et al. Parkinsonism in HIV encephalopathy. *Mov. Disord.* 2000;15(5):1032–1033.

120 Tisch S, Brew B. Parkinsonism in HIV-infected patients on highly active antiretroviral therapy. *Neurology* 2009;73(5):401–403.

121 Hersh BP, Rajendran PR, Battinelli D. Parkinsonism as the presenting manifestation of HIV infection; improvement on HAART. *Neurology* 2001;56(2):278–279.

122 Gerard A, Sarrot-Reynauld F, Liozon E, et al. Neurologic presentation of Whipple disease: report of 12 cases and a review of the literature. *Med. (Balt.)* 2002;81(6):443–457.

123 Averbuch-Heller L, Paulson GW, Daroff RB, Leigh RJ. Whipple's disease mimicking progressive supranuclear palsy: the diagnostic value of eye movement recording. *J. Neurol. Neurosurg. Psychiatry* 1999;66(4):532–535.

124 Matthews BR, Jones LK, Saad DA, Aksamit AJ, Josephs KA. Cerebellar ataxia and central nervous system Whipple disease. *Arch. Neurol.* 2005;62(4):618–620.

125 Patchell RA. Neurological complications of organ transplantation. *Ann. Neurol.* 1994;36(5):688–703.

126 Pirker W, Baumgartner C, Brugger S, et al. Severe akinetic syndrome resulting from a bilateral basal ganglia lesion following bone marrow transplantation. *Mov. Disord.* 1999;14(3):525–528.

127 Alarcón F, Zijlmans JC, Dueñas G, Cevallos N. Post-stroke movement disorders: report of 56 patients.

J. Neurol. Neurosurg. Psychiatry 2004;75(11):1568–1574.

128 Du Plessis AJ, Bellinger DC, Gauvreau K. et al. Neurologic outcome of choreoathetoid encephalopathy after cardiac surgery. Pediatr. Neurol. 2002;27(1):9–17.

129 Mokri B, Ahlskog JE, Fulgham JR, Matsumoto JY. Syndrome resembling PSP after surgical repair of ascending aorta dissection or aneurysm. Neurology 2004;62:971–973.

130 Wenning GK, Kiechl S, Seppi K. et al. Prevalence of movement disorders in men and women aged 50-89 years (Bruneck Study cohort): a population-based study. Lancet Neurol. 2005;4(12):815–820.

131 Esper CD, Factor SA. Failure of recognition of drug-induced parkinsonism in the elderly. Mov. Disord. 2008;23(3):401–404.

132 Lees JA. Secondary Parkinson's syndromes. In: J Jankovic, E Tolosa, editors. Parkinson's Disease & Movement Disorders. 5th ed. Philadelphia, PA: Lippincott Williams & Wilkins, 2007, pp. 213–224.

133 Dressler D, Benecke R. Diagnosis and management of acute movement disorders. J. Neurol. 2005;252(11):1299–1306.

134 Yebenes JG, Cantarero S, Tabernero C, Vazquez AV. Symptomatic dystonias. In: R Watts, W Koller, editors. Movement Disorders: Neurologic Principles and Practice. New York, NY;McGraw-Hill, 2004, pp. 541–567.

135 Kenney C, Hunter C, Davidson A, Jankovic J. Metoclopramide, an increasingly recognized cause of tardive dyskinesia. J. Clin. Pharmacol. 2008;48(3):379–384.

136 Brito MO, Doyle T. Movement and extrapyramidal disorders associated with interferon use in HIV/hepatitis C coinfection. AIDS 2007;21(14):1987–1989.

137 Miranda M, Cardoso F, Giovannoni G, Church A. Oral contraceptive induced chorea: another condition associated with anti-basal ganglia antibodies. J. Neurol. Neurosurg. Psychiatry 2004;75(2):327–328.

138 Bordelon YM, Smith M. Movement disorders in pregnancy. Semin. Neurol. 2007;27(5):467–475.

139 Cardoso F. Chorea gravidarum. Arch. Neurol. 2002;59:868–870.

140 Gijtenbeek JM, van den Bent MJ, Vecht CJ. Cyclosporine neurotoxicity: a review. J. Neurol. 1999;246(5):339–346.

141 Seemuller F, Dehning S, Grunze H, Muller N. Tourette's symptoms provoked by lamotrigine in a bipolar patient. Am. J. Psychiatry 2006;163(1):159.

142 Thomas B, Beal MF. Parkinson's disease. Hum. Mol. Genet. 2007;16:R183–R194.

143 Stepens A, Logina I, Liguts V, et al. A parkinsonian syndrome in methcathinone users and the role of manganese. N. Engl. J. Med. 2008;358(10):1009–1017.

144 De Bie RMA, Gladstone RM, Strafella AP, Ko J, Lang AE. Manganese-induced parkinsonism associated with methcathinone (Ephedrone) abuse. Arch. Neurol. 2007;64(6):886–889.

145 Dietemann JL, Reimund JM, Diniz RLFC, et al. High signal in the adenohypophysis on T1-weighted images presumably due to manganese deposits in patients on long-term parenteral nutrition. Neuroradiology 1998;40(12):793–796.

146 Nagatomo S, Umehara F, Hanada K, et al. Manganese intoxication during total parenteral nutrition: report of two cases and review of the literature. J. Neurol. Sci. 1999;162(1):102–105.

147 Kamata N, Oshitani N, Oiso R, et al. Crohn's disease with parkinsonism due to long-term total parenteral nutrition. Digestive Dis. Sci. 2003;48(5):992–994.

148 Choi IS. Parkinsonism after carbon monoxide poisoning. Eur. Neurol. 2002;48(1):30–33.

149 Manto M, Marmolino D. Cerebellar ataxias. Curr. Opin. Neurol. 2009;22(4):1–11.

150 Knekt P, Kilkkinen A, Rissanen H, et al. Serum Vitamin D and the risk of Parkinson disease. Arch. Neurol. 2010;67(7):808–811.

151 Klockgether T. Ataxias. Parkinsonism Relat. Disord. 2007;13:S391–S394.

152 Shyambabu C, Sinha S, Taly AB, Vijayan J, Kovoor JM. Serum vitamin B12 deficiency and hyperhomocystinemia: a reversible cause of acute chorea, cerebellar ataxia in an adult with cerebral ischemia. J. Neurol. Sci. 2008;273(1-2):152–154.

10 Myelopathies due to systemic disease

Sital V. Patel & Steven L. Lewis
Rush University Medical Center, Chicago, IL, USA

Introduction

A number of systemic disorders can lead to spinal cord dysfunction (*myelopathy*). Similar to any cause of myelopathy, systemic diseases can cause myelopathy due to extrinsic spinal cord compression or due to intrinsic noncompressive spinal cord involvement. When intrinsic spinal cord dysfunction is felt to be related to an inflammatory process, the term *myelitis* is used.

This chapter reviews a variety of both common and rare systemic diseases that cause spinal cord dysfunction, focusing on the clinical presentation of the myelopathic complication, the pathophysiologic mechanism of injury if known, the diagnostic evaluation and MRI findings, and treatment options. Prompt recognition and treatment of a myelopathy—whether compressive or noncompressive—due to systemic disease is crucial to attempt to prevent irreversible and disabling spinal cord dysfunction.

Endocrine disorders

Adrenomyeloneuropathy

Though strictly not a complication of a systemic disease, but rather the co-occurrence of a myelopathy and endocrinopathy due to a genetic disorder, adrenomyeloneuropathy is included here, both because of its prominent medical features as well as the importance of considering this disorder in the differential diagnosis of a progressive myelopathy in an adult patient.

The first description of concurrent adrenal failure and spastic paraparesis was in 1910, though it was not until the 1970s that the term adrenomyeloneuropathy was coined to emphasize the prominent spinal cord and peripheral nerve disease in patients with this syndrome, considered a variant of X-linked adrenoleukodystrophy [1]. X-linked adrenoleukodystrophy is a peroxisomal disorder affecting the nervous system, adrenal cortex, and testes. The genetic defect is mapped to gene ABCD1 on chromosome Xq28 and this codes for the peroxisomal membrane protein, and hence in these patients there is an accumulation of very long-chain fatty acids in tissues [2]. Adrenomyeloneuropathy affects both the spinal cord and the peripheral nerves (*myeloneuropathy*); in the spinal cord, it particularly affects the dorsal columns and corticospinal tracts. Of the adult form of X-linked adrenoleukodystrophy, adrenomyeloneuropathy is the most common phenotype of the disease.

The typical adrenomyeloneuropathy patient presents in the second to fifth decade with stiffness and clumsiness of the lower extremities, which progresses over years to a severe spastic paraparesis. In addition to leg weakness and increased tone, patients may also have decreased vibration and position sense [3].

Neurological Disorders due to Systemic Disease, First Edition. Edited by Steven L. Lewis.
© 2013 Blackwell Publishing Ltd. Published 2013 by Blackwell Publishing Ltd.

Patients also exhibit signs of adrenal insufficiency such as thinned hair and skin changes and/or testicular insufficiency [1].

Approximately 40–50% of patients with adrenomyeloneuropathy will also have lesions in their cerebral white matter and these patients generally will have a poorer outcome compared to those without cerebral white-matter changes [1]. Patients with adrenomyeloneuropathy without cerebral involvement ("pure" adrenomyeloneuropathy) generally have a better prognosis although recent studies using MR spectroscopy have shown that these patients also have brain abnormalities [4] and these patients may also have mild cognitive deficits [1].

The diagnosis of adrenomyeloneuropathy is based on assessing serum levels of very long-chain fatty acids and by genetic testing. Neuroimaging can show spinal cord atrophy; diffusion tensor imaging has also been reported to show abnormalities in the dorsal columns and corticospinal tracts [2].

Treatment of adrenomyeloneuropathy predominantly involves correction of any hormonal deficit; there is currently no known specific treatment of the neurologic disorder. A clinical trial evaluating the efficacy of Lorenzo's oil, a mixture of the oils glyceryl trierucate and glyceryl trioleate, in adrenomyeloneuropathy is currently in progress [5].

Electrolyte and other metabolic disorders

Gout

Gout is an inflammatory arthropathy associated with hyperuricemia that occurs due to deposition of monosodium urate crystals in synovial fluid and other systemic tissues [6]. Although the appendicular (extremity) skeleton is typically symptomatically involved, gout can also affect the axial (spinal) skeleton. Spinal involvement by gout is typically asymptomatic or may cause back pain [7]. Rarely, however, gouty involvement of the spine can cause symptomatic spinal cord or cauda equina compression due to destruction and erosion of vertebral elements by the severe inflammatory process, requiring surgical decompression [7,8]. Spinal cord compression due to gout has even been described as the presenting manifestation of hyperuricemia in the absence of a known history of gout [8].

On MRI, axial gouty arthropathy causing spinal cord compression may show variable and heterogeneous gadolinium enhancement and the imaging findings can resemble other destructive processes such as metastatic disease and abscess. The diagnosis is typically made by finding monosodium urate crystals on pathologic analysis of the surgically removed compressive tissue [7,8].

Systemic autoimmune disorders

Atopic myelitis

Over recent years, the concept of the syndrome of atopic myelitis has emerged, proposed to be caused by an exaggerated IgE response to mite antigens with concomitant clinical symptoms of atopic disease in some patients [9]. Atopic myelitis was originally described by Kira et al. in Japan in 1997, who reported four patients with atopic dermatitis who had sensory myelopathies predominantly affecting the posterior columns [10]. Since that time, further studies have elaborated on the clinical, radiologic, and pathologic findings in these patients. Atopic myelitis is generally defined as myelitis in a patient with concomitant atopic disease such as atopic dermatitis, bronchial asthma, allergic rhinitis, or hyperIgEemia with specific IgE to mite antigens *Dermatotophagoides pteronyssinus* and *D. farina* [9]. Clinically, patients with atopic myelitis have prominent sensory disturbances rather then weakness and may have increased peripheral eosinophils. CSF studies are usually unrevealing. MRI shows cord swelling and enhancing lesions expanding two thirds the width of cord and often involve three to four vertebral levels, most often in the thoracic cord. These patients usually do not have brain lesions.

Patients with atopic myelitis typically have a poor response to intravenous corticosteroid treatment. The poor treatment response and the long duration of symptoms may be related to the findings of axonal loss on histopathology. In addition, histopathology has shown eosinophilic infiltration within these lesions which is unique to this entity and has not been described in other myelitides [11].

So far atopic myelitis has mostly been diagnosed in patients in Japan and Korea. This is felt to be related to the fact that Asian populations are most susceptible to atopic disorders in comparison to Western populations [11]. However, atopic myelitis should be considered in all patients with atopic diseases and concomitant idiopathic myelitis.

Neurosarcoidosis

The prevalence of sarcoidosis is approximately 40 per 100,000 people, with a typical age of onset of symptoms between 20 to 30 years. Pathologically, the hallmark of sarcoidosis is noncaseating granulomas that are composed of epithelioid macrophages, lymphocytes, monocytes, and fibroblasts [12]. Neurosarcoidosis is estimated to occur in 5–15% of sarcoidosis cases and is most commonly associated with granulomatous infiltrates involving the meninges, hypothalamus, pituitary gland, and cranial nerves. Cranial nerve palsies are the most common manifestation. Other presentations of neurosarcoidosis include aseptic meningitis, hydrocephalus, parenchymal disease and mass lesions, seizures, peripheral neuropathy, and myopathy [12]. Less than 1% of patients have spinal or spinal cord involvement due to neurosarcoidosis and these patients can present with intramedullary, extramedullary (intradural or extradural) lesions, cauda equina syndrome, or arachnoiditis, due to inflammatory granulomatous infiltration of the leptomeninges or the cord itself [12,13].

Spinal cord MRI in intramedullary neurosarcoidosis may show increased T2 signal and contrast enhancement; intramedullary lesions can be multiple, diffuse, or nodular, usually involving one or two spinal cord levels in length [13], although very extensive longitudinal myelitis has also been reported [14]. CSF may show low glucose, high protein, and a lymphocytic predominant pleocytosis. There is no defined role for CSF angiotensin-converting enzyme levels in the diagnosis of neurosarcoidosis. The finding of biopsy-proven systemic sarcoidosis provides circumstantial evidence to support the possibility of neurosarcoidosis as the cause of the myelopathic process, though other etiologies should be considered and excluded as clinically appropriate.

Treatment of myelopathy due to neurosarcoidosis is empiric and typically involves first-line intravenous corticosteroid therapy followed by a slow oral taper. For refractory cases, immunosuppressive medication and immunomodulating drugs can be used. Tumor necrosis factor (TNF)-alpha antagonist drugs, such as infliximab, have been used in some steroid-refractory neurosarcoidosis cases [12–14].

Systemic lupus erythematosis and Sjögren syndrome

Systemic lupus erythematosis (SLE) and Sjögren syndrome can both be associated with a severe acute or subacute myelopathy [15–18]. When myelopathies occur in either of these autoimmune conditions, the MRI may show longitudinally extensive lesions (defined as greater than three vertebral segments in length) similar to lesions seen in neuromyelitis optica (NMO). In addition, when myelitis or optic neuritis occurs in the setting of SLE and Sjögren syndrome, aquaporin-4 antibodies may also be found [19].

Based on these observations and findings, there is growing consensus that myelitis occurring in the setting of SLE or Sjögren syndrome likely usually represents an NMO spectrum disorder rather than a specific (e.g., vasculitic) complication of the systemic autoimmune disorder [19,20]. Treatment of acute severe myelitis typically involves intravenous methylprednisolone (or plasmapheresis for refractory or very severe attacks). Prophylaxis of an NMO-spectrum disorder typically involves chronic immunosuppression, often with azathioprine, although other agents such as rituximab, mycophenolate mofetil, or cyclophosphamide are therapeutic options; however, there is limited evidence base to specifically guide the choice of prophylactic immunosuppressive agent [20,21].

Behçet's disease

Behçet's disease is an inflammatory multisystem disease of unknown cause characterized by recurrent oral aphthous ulcers, genital ulcers, uveitis, and skin lesions [22]. Behçet's disease is most commonly seen in the Middle East, Mediterranean basin, and the Far East [23]. Neurologic involvement has been estimated to occur in approximately 10–20% of patients with Behçet's disease and is more common in males [22]. There are two major manifestations of neuro-Behçet's disease: a more common *parenchymal* immune-mediated meningoencephalitis characterized pathologically by an inflammatory perivasculitis, and a less-common *non-parenchymal* complication involving thrombosis of the large cerebral veins [23].

Parenchymal meningoencephalitis typically affects the upper brainstem, thalamus, and basal ganglia; however, the spinal cord can also rarely be involved, causing a symptomatic myelopathy, and in some cases the spinal cord may be the only site of neurologic parenchymal disease [23]. Spinal cord involvement by

Behçet's may be longitudinally extensive and multifocal, and show contrast enhancement in the acute phase [24]. Fukae et al. described a case of longitudinally extensive myelitis due to Behçet's extending from the medulla down through the entire spinal cord [25]. Similar to other manifestations of Behçet's disease, treatment of myelopathy due to Behçet's usually involves corticosteroids and possibly other immunosuppressants; currently TNF antagonists are also a therapeutic option for aggressive or poorly responsive disease [23]. Though spinal cord involvement by Behçet's disease is classically associated with a poor response to therapy, recent cases have been reported showing good clinical and MRI improvement with corticosteroid therapy of the acute myelitis [24,25].

Rheumatoid arthritis

Rheumatoid arthritis is a systemic autoimmune disease characterized by synovial inflammation (synovitis) which may lead to damage and erosion of adjacent cartilage and bone. The cervical spine is commonly involved in rheumatoid arthritis due to the presence of synovial joints in the cervical spine; there are no synovial joints in the thoracic or lumbar spine so these regions are spared in this condition [18].

Cervical spine involvement by rheumatoid arthritis is a well-described cause of compressive cervical myelopathy, which can occur in any of three ways. Rheumatoid involvement of the atlantoaxial synovial joint can lead to atlantoaxial subluxation, resulting in compression of the upper cervical cord with symptomatic quadriparesis and sensory loss. Rheumatoid involvement of the lateral masses of C2 can lead to descent of the skull into the cervical spine (basilar invagination) resulting in compression of the lower brainstem and upper cervical spine, and symptomatic brainstem and cranial nerve dysfunction and myelopathy. Finally, rheumatoid involvement of the cervical spine below C1/C2 (subaxial subluxation) can result in symptomatic compression of the cervical spinal cord, particularly at C2–C3 and C3–C4 [18,26]. In each of these scenarios, inflammatory synovial tissue (called pannus) results in destruction of adjacent cartilage, ligaments, and bone. Asymptomatic cervical spine involvement by rheumatoid arthritis is common; indications for decompressive surgery include symptomatic myelopathy, spinal instability, or brainstem dysfunction [26].

Rheumatoid arthritis can also rarely be associated with inflammation of the dura mater (*pachymeningitis*), which typically, though not invariably, occurs in the setting of long-standing seropositive disease with rheumatoid nodules. This unusual complication of rheumatoid arthritis has primarily been described in relation to its involvement of the meninges around the brain, with symptoms of headaches, seizures, cranial neuropathies, and various focal neurologic symptoms [18]. However, rheumatoid pachymeningitis may also be a very rare cause of a symptomatic progressive compressive myelopathy [27]. Pachymeningitis occurring outside of the setting of rheumatoid arthritis or other rheumatologic disease is described in the next section.

"Idiopathic" hypertrophic spinal pachymeningitis and IgG-4-related sclerosing disease

The term *idiopathic hypertrophic pachymeningitis* refers to localized or diffuse dural thickening, pathologically typically associated with chronic inflammation, and in which alternative specific systemic or infectious etiologies (such as rheumatoid arthritis, Wegener's granulomatosis, neoplasm, or tuberculosis) have been excluded [28]. Idiopathic hypertrophic pachymeningitis can involve the meninges of the brain or of the spinal cord. In the brain, this uncommon disorder is typically associated with headache and optic or other cranial-nerve dysfunction.

Patients with spinal dural involvement by hypertrophic pachymeningitis typically present with a progressive compressive cervical or thoracic myelopathy. MRI in these patients shows dural thickening and enhancement, most commonly involving multiple contiguous levels of the cervical and/or thoracic spine, which may be compressing the spinal cord [29].

Treatment of idiopathic hypertrophic spinal pachymeningitis typically involves surgical decompression. Pathologic analysis of the abnormal dura shows thickened, dense fibrous tissue with associated chronic lymphoplasmacytic inflammation. In addition to surgical decompression, treatment of this condition typically includes steroids or other immunosuppressants, which have been associated anecdotally with clinical and imaging improvement; relapses, however, are sometimes seen [29].

Recently, IgG4-related sclerosing disease has been reported as a potential etiology for at least some cases of previously "idiopathic" hypertrophic (cerebral or spinal) pachymeningitis. IgG4-related sclerosing disease is a systemic disorder characterized histopathologically by IgG4-positive plasma-cell infiltrates involving various organs, most frequently the pancreas, the salivary glands, or lacrimal glands [30,31]. In 2009, Chan et al. reported a 37-year-old man who presented with a progressive myelopathy due to a thoracic hypertrophic pachymeningitis with spinal cord compression, and who also had evidence of a chronic sialadenitis [30]. After surgical decompression, pathologic analysis of the involved dura showed a dense infiltrate of plasma cells and lymphocytes within the fibrotic stroma, with immunohistochemical staining confirming a high percentage of IgG4-positive plasma cells in addition to CD3-positive T-lymphocytes. The authors suggested that some proportion of cases of idiopathic hypertrophic pachymeningitis may actually represent cases of IgG4-related sclerosing disease [30]. Subsequently, Choi et al. reported a 46-year-old woman with a progressive and recurrent myelopathy due to T9–T12 hypertrophic pachymeningitis who was found on pathologic analysis of her previously excised surgical specimen to have IgG4-bearing plasma cells within the lymphocytoplasmic infiltrate, consistent with IgG4-related sclerosing disease [31]. In another recent case of (cranial) hypertrophic pachymeningitis that was found to be related to IgG4-related disease, the authors noted that the diagnosis can be suggested by the following laboratory and clinical features: high serum IgG and IgG4 levels; infiltration of IgG4-positive plasma cells in the dural lesion; involvement of other organs typically associated with IgG4-related disease; exclusion of other diseases associated with high serum IgG4 levels (including atopic dermatitis, parasitic infections, and pemphigus); exclusion of other diseases that can cause pachymeningitis; and good response to steroids [32].

Organ dysfunction and failure

Liver failure

The relationship between hepatic dysfunction and neurologic dysfunction has been known for many years, with the most common neurologic manifestation being hepatic encephalopathy. However, spinal cord dysfunction can also occur in chronic liver disease, and is referred to as hepatic myelopathy or portosystemic myelopathy. Although hepatic myelopathy is a rare complication of liver disease, its impact on morbidity in these patients is significant. Clinical features of hepatic myelopathy include gait disturbance with spastic paraparesis. Examination findings include bilateral lower extremity weakness, hyperreflexia, extensor plantar reflexes, and increased tone; sensory examination may be normal [33]. Symptoms of hepatic myelopathy occur and worsen after repeated bouts of hepatic encephalopathy with hyperammonemia [33]. Workup is usually unrevealing, with normal spinal cord imaging, normal findings for other causes of myelopathy (e.g., B12 level), and acellular CSF. Nardone et al. evaluated 13 patients with liver cirrhosis and surgical or spontaneous portosystemic shunts using motor-evoked potentials and found that six of the patients had clinical symptoms of hepatic myelopathy, often with severe neurophysiological abnormalities [34]. Hepatic myelopathy has a male predominance and usually occurs in patients with cirrhosis and associated portosystemic shunts (either surgically or spontaneously formed).

The pathophysiology behind the syndrome is unclear [35]. Some authors suggest that the spinal cord insult is due to nitrogenous toxins such as ammonia that are bypassed by the diseased liver. However, treatments directed at decreasing such exposure has not shown to help with the symptoms or progression of the disease. Pathologically, these patients have greater corticospinal tract demyelination in caudal than cervical spinal segments and often have greater number of Alzheimer type II cells in cerebral cortex than other liver-disease patients [33]. More progressive cases of hepatic myelopathy have shown pathological changes including axonal loss within the spinal cord [34].

Unlike hepatic encephalopathy, conservative medical treatments for hepatic myelopathy are usually considered insufficient. Liver transplantation has shown varying outcomes for hepatic myelopathy patients [36]. Nardone et al. found that patients with milder neurophysiological abnormalities and milder neurologic symptoms had improvement with transplantation versus the more severely affected patients [34]. This clinical observation corroborates previous pathologic descriptions of early demyelination loss within corticospinal tracts and later progression with axonal loss and cord degeneration. Qu et al. describe two cases where orthotopic liver transplantation was performed 2–3 months after onset of clinical symptoms of hepatic myelopathy [36]. Both patients had significant improvement of their spastic paraparesis after liver transplantation. These observations suggest that, given there is no significant improvement with medical treatments and there is significant clinical progression and morbidity associated with hepatic myelopathy, early aggressive treatment with liver transplantation should be considered in hepatic myelopathy patients with the hope of reversing neurologic dysfunction.

Extramedullary hematopoiesis

Extramedullary hematopoiesis is a complication of chronic anemic states such as beta-thalassemia, sickle cell anemia, myelofibrosis, and polycythemia vera. Frequent sites for extramedullary hematopoiesis include the spleen, liver, kidney, and less commonly the adrenal gland, heart, lymph nodes, or thymus [37].

On rare occasions, the site of this hematopoiesis is within the epidural space, and this can lead to compressive myelopathy. Early symptoms may include focal back pain and paresthesias, and may progress to sensory loss, spastic weakness, hyperreflexia, and bowel or bladder dysfunction, typically progressing over months [37]. There are two main hypotheses in regards to the source of the epidural hematopoietic tissue: (1) blood-forming elements in the vertebral marrow may extrude through weakened trabecular bone into the epidural space; or (2) primitive hematopoietic stem cells located in the epidural space become proliferative under stress [37].

The first reported case of spinal cord compression due to extramedullary hematopoiesis was in 1954, and subsequently a number of additional cases have been reported, although the incidence of extramedullary hematopoiesis causing spinal cord compression appears to be very low. There appears to be an increased preponderance of men over women with a ratio of 5:1. MRI is the most sensitive test for spinal cord pathology, however, the signal intensities are variable in each case depending on the contents (fat, iron, etc.) within the extramedullary hematopoiesis [38]. The most common area for extramedullary hematopoiesis causing spinal cord compression is the lower thoracic levels. Lack of gadolinium enhancement of extramedullary hematopoiesis helps to differentiate it from other epidural masses such as abscesses or metastases that typically show enhancement [39].

However it may still be necessary to biopsy the lesion if the diagnosis is unclear based on MRI. Biopsies reveal friable fleshy masses which on pathological analysis show hematopoietic cells consistent with medullary hematopoiesis [40].

Treatment options are controversial and there this no clear standard. Options include hypertransfusion that is believed to decrease erythropoietin production although it is felt that this alone is insufficient treatment. Radiation therapy can be effective since hematopoietic tissue is radiosensitive; however, this can cause the patient to become more hematologically compromised. Also, if the spinal cord is already damaged by the extramedullary hematopoiesis, radiation may cause further damage. Decompressive surgery is effective to relieve pressure on the spinal cord, but given the nature of the masses, bleeding is a significant risk for such surgery [41]. The general consensus is to diagnose early and treat with a combination of hypertransfusions to improve symptoms, with decompressive surgery and/or radiation if necessary. Other agents that are cytostatic such as hydroxyurea may also be helpful as adjunctive therapies [39].

Systemic cancer and paraneoplastic disorders

Spinal cord compression due to metastatic cancer

Spinal cord compression due to metastatic disease is a common and potentially devastating complication of systemic cancer or lymphoproliferative disorders, and in some cases may be the presenting manifestation of the illness [42,43]. Cancers of the breast, prostate, and lung are the most common primary malignancies associated with cord compression. Patients with metastatic spinal cord compression commonly, but not invariably, present with back pain and a progressive myelopathy. The diagnosis should be considered and excluded as early as possible, since the ambulatory status at diagnosis is a strong predictive factor of ultimate ambulatory status and survival [42].

Although a detailed discussion of spinal cord compression due to metastatic cancer is beyond the scope of this chapter, it is important to underscore that spinal cord compression should be considered as a potential emergent etiology in any patient (with or without cancer) who presents with a myelopathy, and especially immediately excluded by spinal cord MRI in any patient with a known cancer who presents with a possible myelopathy, even in the absence of pain.

The finding of spinal cord compression due to metastasis warrants immediate high-dose steroids and emergent neurosurgical decompression or radiation [42,44,45]. Taylor and Schiff recently outlined an algorithm for the evaluation and treatment of metastatic spinal cord compression [42].

Paraneoplastic myelopathy

Myelopathies can rarely occur as a paraneoplastic syndrome, and these syndromes have been associated with a variety of paraneoplastic antibody markers, most frequently antiamphiphysin, antinuclear autoantibody type 2 (ANNA-2 or anti-Ri), ANNA-3, collapsin response-mediator protein 5, and ANNA-1 (anti-Hu), in addition to others [43,46].

Flanagan et al. recently reported the clinical, imaging, and laboratory findings of 31 patients who presented with isolated myelopathy with coexisting cancer [46]. All of their patients presented with a progressive myelopathy that was either insidious or subacute, and a neural autoantibody was found in 25 of their 31 patients; none of their patients had the aquaporin-4 antibody. A characteristic MRI finding in these patients was the presence of symmetric longitudinally extensive T2 signal abnormalities, often showing enhancement, involving lateral or dorsal white-matter tracts or gray matter [46]. Unfortunately, the patients with this syndrome typically progressed quickly to significant disability despite treatment of the underlying cancer and immunotherapy.

Paraneoplastic necrotizing myelopathy

Some patients with cancer have been reported to have an even more aggressive disorder with rapid ascending paraplegia and death from respiratory dysfunction, described as a *paraneoplastic necrotizing myelopathy* [47]. Histologically, this disorder is characterized by necrosis of both white and gray matter of the spinal cord, usually without inflammation [48]. Paraneoplastic necrotizing myelopathy has been reported in association with several carcinomas and lymphoproliferative disorders. Patients usually initially present with thoracic cord symptoms including ascending sensory deficits, sphincter dysfunction, and paraplegia and often also complain of back pain [48]. There is rapid progression over days to weeks to respiratory

failure and duration of symptoms prior to death has been reported to range from 5 days to 16 months [47]. CSF studies show elevated protein without pleocytosis and MRI imaging often shows a longitudinal lesion on T2 imaging without inflammation and without enhancement [47,48]. Evaluation for serum and CSF onconeural antibodies has also often been negative in these cases. Accurate diagnosis of paraneoplastic necrotizing myelopathy can only be made postmortem by spinal cord pathologic examination. This usually reveals frank necrosis of the central cord involving gray and white matter, and histological findings of necrosis of white and gray matter and accumulation of foamy macrophages. There is usually no evidence of inflammation [49].

There is little information on successful treatments or interventions for patients with this devastating and aggressive disorder. Urai et al. described a case involving a woman who presented with bilateral lower extremity numbness, weakness, and difficulty voiding. During the workup, their patient was diagnosed with Stage 4 esophageal carcinoma and MRI images and CSF elevated protein supported the diagnosis of a paraneoplastic necrotizing myelopathy. She was then treated with high-dose intravenous steroids and had some improvement with strength of bilateral lower extremities. She died 1 year later from complications of her primary cancer [48].

Of note, Pittock and Lennon reported the association of cancer with the aquaporin 4 antibody in some patients, suggesting that this antibody may occasionally occur in a paraneoplastic context [50]. Whether some of the previously reported cases of paraneoplastic necrotizing myelopathy, such as those described above, may have represented myelopathy from neuromyelitis optica spectrum disorders is unclear.

Myelopathy due to treatment of systemic cancer

Spinal cord dysfunction can occur as a result of cancer treatment, mainly due to complications from radiation and intrathecal chemotherapy.

Radiation myelopathy

Radiation myelopathy can occur as an "early-delayed" complication (1–6 months after radiation exposure) or as a "late-delayed" complication (beyond 6 months). The median time to the development of symptoms of radiation myelopathy is 3 months [45]. Early-delayed phase myelopathy usually resolves spontaneously without treatment; Lhermitte's sign can occur with cervical spine involvement. Late-delayed phase radiation myelopathy, however, is often persistent or progressive, with varying response to corticosteroids, and is postulated to occur due to radiation-induced vascular damage and injury to oligodendrocytes [45]. The dose limit for radiation to the spinal cord is felt to be generally between 45 and 50 Gy although radiation myelopathy can occur below this limit [45,51]. Patients with hypertension and diabetes mellitus appear to be at higher risk of developing radiation myelopathy [52]. MRI findings are typically nonspecific and may be normal, though can include T2 hyperintensity and contrast enhancement which may progress to spinal cord atrophy [51].

Myelopathy due to chemotherapy
Intrathecal chemotherapeutic agents such as ara-C and methotrexate, as well as systemic high doses of these agents, can rarely cause myelopathy. In the past, myelopathy due to intrathecal methotrexate was believed to occur due to additives such as benzyl alcohol that were then used to dilute the formulation of the intrathecal agent [53]. Watterson et al. reviewed 23 cases of myelopathy that occurred in association with intensive central nervous system (CNS)-directed therapy, both from their own experience and the literature. These patients had received intrathecal and/or systemic ara-C, methotrexate, or thiotepa without such preservatives. Some of these patients had also received radiation therapy. These patients developed myelopathy with varying clinical presentations, and outcome ranging from recovery to death. The authors concluded that high doses and long-term cumulative dosing of CNS-penetrating chemotherapeutic agents lead to a higher risk of developing a myelopathy. In addition, concomitant intrathecal ara-C and systemic high-dose ara-C may be particularly toxic [53].

Systemic infectious diseases

Many types of infectious organisms can lead to myelopathy, including viruses, bacteria, fungi, and parasitic organisms. Spinal cord dysfunction can occur due to direct infection by the agent, compression by an infectious mass (abscess), or by a postinfectious immune response. A detailed discussion of each of the pathogens that might directly or indirectly lead to spinal cord dysfunction is beyond the scope of this review and the reader is referred to detailed reviews on these topics [54,55]. This section discusses several specific and classic myelopathic syndromes that mainly occur as a consequence of chronic systemic infection.

HIV vacuolar myelopathy

Vacuolar myelopathy has been described as a common pathological finding at post mortem examination of HIV-positive patients, but only approximately 10% of these patients will have clinical symptoms. These symptoms include progressive painless spastic paraparesis, sensory loss with sensory ataxia, and sphincter dysfunction [56,57]. Some of the patients are also simultaneously suffering from AIDS dementia and peripheral neuropathies and may have these complaints as well. There is usually no complaint of back pain, and on examination a sensory level is rarely found.

Vacuolar myelopathy is a diagnosis of exclusion and therefore other causes of myelopathy including metabolic, infectious (e.g., CMV, VZV, HSV, HTLV), and neoplastic disorders should be ruled out [57]. In HIV myelopathy, MRI imaging will often (reported up to 80% of the time) show either atrophy of the spinal cord or T2 hyperintensities in the posterior columns, especially in the thoracic cord over multiple levels [56].

Definitive diagnosis is made based on pathologic examination. Petito et al. examined the spinal cords of 89 HIV-positive patients who had progressive spastic paraparesis and described pathological findings of vacuoles within myelin lamella and between myelin and axons in the dorsolateral white-matter tracts. There was little destruction of the axons themselves in his series [56]. There were also lipid-laden macrophages and microglia expressing IL-1 and TNF alpha.

Clinically, radiologically, and histologically, HIV vacuolar myelopathy is very similar to subacute combined degeneration of the spinal cord due to vitamin B12 deficiency. It is therefore very important to also check vitamin B12 and, if necessary, methylmalonic acid levels to rule out vitamin B12 deficiency as the etiology of patients' symptoms [57]. Also due to this striking similarity, one of the main hypotheses behind the pathophysiology of vacuolar myelopathy is impaired repair mechanisms in the vitamin B12-dependent transmethylation pathways [58]. Other theories include direct HIV infection into the cells of the spinal cord, or an unknown infectious agent causing the syndrome given that vacuolar myelopathy can also be seen in other immunosuppressed states [56,58]. Serum copper levels should also be performed in these patients due to the clinical similarity of B12 deficiency to copper deficiency.

Treatment is supportive with some reports of improvement with initiation of HAART [57].

HTLV-1

It is thought that approximately 15–20 million people worldwide are infected with HTLV-1, a double-stranded RNA oncogenic retrovirus that is endemic in Japan, sub-Saharan Africa, Americas, Seychelles, and the Middle East [59]. Initially the disorder was called "Jamaican neuropathy" as it was initially described in the Jamaican population in 1956. It was later described in the Japanese population and found to have atypical "flower" shaped lymphocytes in the CSF. It was then also found to be associated with antibodies to HTLV-1 and therefore the term HTLV-1 associated myelopathy has been used [60]. The three major routes of transmission include through breast milk, sexual contacts, and transmission of infected blood [61]. With increasing migration, this infection has become more prevalent throughout the world, and its transmission (including sexual intercourse and sharing IV needles) puts even more people at risk. HTLV-1 is associated with several clinical conditions including uveitis, adult T-cell leukemia/lymphoma and HTLV-1-associated myelopathy (HAM), which is also known as tropical spastic paraparesis (TSP) (the neurologic syndrome is sometimes referred to as HAM/TSP). The lifetime risk of a patient with HTLV-1 developing HTLV-1-associated myelopathy has been reported to be 0.25–3% [59]. An elevated HTLV-1 proviral load is the single best marker of symptomatic neurologic disease in individuals with HTLV-1 [61].

There are three main theories about how HTLV-1 causes myelopathy. The first theory is the direct toxicity theory, where HTLV-1-infected glial cells are lysed by specific CD8+ cytotoxic T lymphocytes. The second theory involves molecular mimicry causing normal glial cells being mistaken for infected glial

cells. The third, and most popular, theory is known as the "bystander theory" where HTLV-infected CD4+ cells are recognized by specific cytotoxic T CD8 lymphocytes that induce microglia to secrete cytokines such as TNF alpha that are myelinotoxic [60].

HTLV-1-associated myelopathy is a meningomyelitis of the white and gray matter that is followed by axonal degeneration, and usually affects the lower thoracic cord. Histopathologically, there is perivascular and parenchymal infiltration of T cells, and later on in the disease there is loss of cellularity, and atrophy develops. Degeneration is usually seen in the lateral columns, and to varying degrees in the anterior and posterior columns, of the spinal cord [59,61,62].

Clinically, patients present with a slowly progressive spastic paraparesis as well as bladder dysfunction, and often complain of low back pain. The weakness often beings unilaterally and then later becomes symmetric. An important feature is that the motor weakness and spasticity is much more significant in comparison to mild sensory disturbances such as tingling of the hands or feet. On examination, these patients often have a spastic gait, bilateral lower extremity weakness, hyperreflexia, extensor plantar response, and usually no sensory level. Symptoms can become worse over several years. The diagnosis is often delayed due to the slow development of symptoms, but when tested these patients will have positive serum antibodies to HTLV-1 and usually will have higher levels of antibodies to HTLV-1 in the CSF than in the serum. CSF studies will also typically show mild pleocytosis and increase in protein [59]. Usually neuroimaging of the spinal cord in HTLV-1-associated myelopathy patients reveals cord atrophy, especially involving the thoracic cord, and this is likely due to the fact that imaging is typically done after the patient has had disease for several years. There have been cases, however, where the disease course has been more subacute, and in these cases MRI has shown some cord edema and contrast-enhancing lesions [63].

Effective treatment to alter long-term disability for patients with HTLV-1-associated myelopathy is still not established. Corticosteroids, plasmapheresis, and intravenous immunoglobulin have been used, but long-term benefits have not been proven, although transient benefits have been reported anecdotally. Interferon alpha is a mainstay of treatment in Japan where one study did show clinical benefit but long-term therapy has not been well established [61]. Treatment with the antiretroviral agents zidovudine and lamivudine also have been studied with no clear clinical benefit. Valproate was found to substantially decrease the proviral load of HTLV-1 in one study but did not have clinical benefits [59]. Therefore, to date, the mainstay of treatment is symptomatic treatment with antispasticity agents, analgesics, medications for neurogenic bladder, laxatives, and neurorehabilitation [60].

It is important to note the high coincidence of HIV and HTLV-1, so if a patient with HIV and normal CD4 count presents with a similar clinical picture as described above, testing for HTLV-1 myelopathy should be considered [60].

Tuberculosis

Tuberculosis of the spine was first described by Sir Percival Pott in 1782 and hence spinal tuberculosis is often referred to as Pott's disease. This occurs in about 1–2% of all tuberculosis patients. Tuberculosis can affect patients in endemic countries as well as in developed countries, especially in those who are immunocompromised [64]. In the 1980s, there was a rise in the incidence of tuberculosis in the United States, and this was speculated to be due to increased number of people living in an immunocompromised state due to HIV infection [65]. The initial route of *M. tuberculosis* is through the respiratory tract, which is then followed by hematologic dissemination. Tuberculosis is believed to spread to the spine via the Batson venous plexus [64].

Presenting symptoms of spinal tuberculosis include pain (usually at the overlying site), fever, kyphosis, weight loss, and night sweats [66]. A progressive myelopathy can develop in these patients due to either marked bone collapse with spinal canal compromise, or due to granulomatous epidural or subdural abscess causing spinal compression. Very rarely, patients can develop intramedullary tuberculomas that can also lead to neurologic dysfunction.

MRI is very useful in diagnosis [65]. Spinal tuberculosis can be seen on MRI images with vertebral bodies showing low signal on T1 and high signal on T2 consistent with osteomyelitis. Other abnormalities that can be seen include pyogenic disciitis, extradural abscess, bone fragments, or rarely intramedullary tubercular granuloma. The spinal cord itself may be edematous with abnormal signal, or atrophy [67]. The diagnosis can be aided by positive culture from the abscess or from blood, as well as specific serological testing. Often, serum cultures may not be positive [64,67]. Delay in diagnosing and treating spinal involvement of tuberculosis can lead to devastating outcomes. Depending on the degree of spinal cord injury and the exact location of the infection, treatment may consist of only antituberculous medications versus additional surgical intervention [65].

Schistosomiasis

Schistosomiasis is an infection that affects over 200 million people worldwide and is caused by parasites belonging to the *Schistosoma* genus [68]. Larvae are released by fresh-water snails and upon contact with human skin will penetrate into body tissues or travel through the blood stream to different organs. Symptoms often include fever, chills, pruritis at penetration site, as well as splenomegaly, hepatic dysfunction, diarrhea, and urinary dysfunction. Specific species of the *Schistosoma* genus can infect the spinal cord leading to neurologic dysfunction. The prevalence of schistosomal myeloradiculopathy is unknown and likely underestimated. Clinically patients present with varying degrees of neurologic deficits and symptoms can occur anywhere from days to years after initial infection. Patients present with conus medullaris involvement, acute transverse myelitis, spastic paraplegia, painful radiculopathy, or cauda equina syndrome. Initial symptoms often include a triad of lumbar/lower extremity pain, paraparesis and/or sensory changes in the lower limbs and urinary dysfunction [68–70].

In a patient with these clinical symptoms who are in, or recently visited, an endemic country such as Brazil or African countries, the diagnosis is supported by CSF studies, serologic testing and neuroimaging. CSF shows normal glucose, elevated protein and lymphocytic predominant pleocytosis with presence of eosinophils in CSF in 41–90% of cases. Anti-schistosoma antibodies can be detected in blood and CSF by ELISA. Eggs can also be found in fecal, urine, or tissue biopsy. There is however cross-reactivity between other helminths and therefore the finding of positive anti-schistosoma antibodies is not very specific. Neuroimaging shows enlargement of the spinal cord on T1-weighted images with hyperintensity on T2-weighted images, and heterogeneous diffuse granular enhancement with postcontrast imaging.

Usually, the conus or lower spinal cord from T12 to L1 levels are affected [69,70].

Pathophysiologically, *Schistosoma japonicum* is known to affect the cerebrum and *Schistosoma mansoni* to cause myeloradicular damage [70]. Often, the spinal involvement of *Schistosoma* precedes other systemic manifestations. It is believed that there is in-situ deposition of ova within the spinal cord forming necrotic exudative granulomas. Another hypothesis includes embolic travel of eggs via retrograde venous flow throughout valveless Batson's vertebral venous plexus. These granulomas enlarge to intramedullary masses that are seen on MRI as a widened spinal cord with heterogeneous enhancement [69].

Treatment is important as the patient will often have ameliorations of these neurologic symptoms with treatment with steroids and praziquantel. There is no clear evidence to guide the duration of treatment [70].

Neurocysticercosis

Neurocysticercosis, the most common helminthic infection of the central nervous system worldwide, occurs due to the presence of the larval stage of the pork tapeworm *Taenia solium* within nervous system tissues, or within the subarachnoid space [71,72]. Cysticercal involvement of the spinal cord, causing a progressive clinical myelopathy, is a rare but well-described manifestation of this condition.

Spinal cord dysfunction from neurocysticercosis can occur due to cord compression by single or multiple extramedullary cysts in the subarachnoid space, or due to direct cord involvement from an intramedullary cyst [71–73]. The MRI findings of intramedullary or subarachnoid cysticercosis vary depending on the viability of the cyst and the nature of the patient's immune response to the cyst; that is, viable early cysts may show an obvious scolex, lack of contrast enhancement of the cyst wall, and no perilesional edema, while degenerating cysts may show contrast enhancement of a thickened cyst capsule and perilesional edema [73]. Cysticercosis should be considered as a diagnostic possibility in any patient with a cystic lesion within, or compressing, the spinal cord, and should be especially strongly considered in a patient from (or with previous travel to) a highly endemic country.

The optimal treatment of symptomatic spinal subarachnoid or intramedullary neurocysticercosis is unclear, but surgical therapy is most typically employed, often followed by cysticidal therapy with albendazole [72,73].

Drugs, toxins, and vitamin and mineral deficiencies

Vitamin B12 deficiency

Vitamin B12 deficiency leads to hematologic disorders, in particular megaloblastic anemia, as well as gastrointestinal and psychiatric disorders. It also causes neurologic impairment with myelopathy, neuropathy, neuropsychiatric disease, and optic atrophy; these neurologic symptoms can occur in the absence of the hematologic manifestations of vitamin B12 deficiency. The myelopathy of vitamin B12 deficiency is also known as subacute combined degeneration of the spinal cord, due to the typical time course of symptom development and the "combined" posterior column and corticospinal tract involvement. These patients present with sensory ataxia and paraparesis and it is important to diagnose and treat patients promptly and aggressively to prevent further progression of the disease [74]. Vitamin B12 deficiency can occur due to decreased oral intake (such as in strict vegans or severe alcoholics), inadequate absorption (such as can occur from pernicious anemia, gastrectomy, bariatric surgery intestinal infection, tropical sprue, or other malabsorptive states) or due to inactivation of the active form of cobalamin (nitrous oxide exposure).

Vitamin B12 deficiency causes decreased activity in the cobalamin-dependent methylcobalamin esterase enzyme. This subsequently causes increased levels of methylmalonic acid that is toxic to myelin. The deficient state causes dysfunction of the posterior columns and lateral corticospinal tracts. Neuropathologically, these patients have reversible swelling of myelin sheaths on posterior and lateral columns but later on in the disease, axonal degeneration will occur if treatment is not initiated. Usually the cervical cord and thoracic cord are involved, and MRI imaging may show longitudinal hyperintensity on T2-weighted images in the dorsal columns. Usually there is no change in signal in the lateral corticospinal tracts, likely due to MRI imaging not being sensitive enough to date to detect these changes [75].

185

The clinical symptoms of vitamin B12 deficiency include progressive, ascending parasthesias in the hands and feet, disturbance of deep sensation in the legs more than the arms and sensory ataxia—all of which reflect the involvement of the posterior columns. Additional symptoms of spastic paraparesis, increased deep tendon reflexes, and extensor plantar responses represent dysfunction of the lateral corticospinal tracts that are affected in the disease. With aggressive and prompt cobalamin treatment, most patients will have no further progression of disease and often clinically improve. Repeat MRI after treatment may show resolution of previously seen abnormalities in the dorsal columns [75].

More recently the incidence of subacute combined degeneration from vitamin B12 deficiency has been increasing likely due to two different factors. First, more patients have been receiving bariatric surgeries and therefore are at higher risk for vitamin deficiencies. Also, there has been an increase in the recreational use of nitrous oxide which causes subacute combined degeneration due to dysfunction of the active form of vitamin B12 in the body (see section on "Nitrous Oxide" below).

Copper deficiency

Copper deficiency leading to ataxia is a well-known disorder in ruminant animals known as swayback disease [76]. Copper deficiency in humans was first described in 2001 by Schleper and Stuerenburg [77]. They described a patient with a history of gastrectomy and partial colonic resection who presented with severe tetraparesis and painful parasthesias and who was found on imaging to have dorsomedial cervical cord T2 hyperintensity. Upon further analysis, it was found that the patient had decreased levels of serum ceruloplasmin, serum copper, and CSF copper. The patient was treated with parenteral copper and although the paresis did not improve, the patient's parasthesias did resolve. Since this discovery, there has been heightened awareness of copper-deficiency myelopathy and its treatment, and this disorder has been studied and reviewed extensively by Kumar [76,78].

Copper is an essential trace element that has a critical role in the structure and function of the central nervous system and is ubiquitous in normal diet foods [78]. Acquired copper deficiency can occur due to insufficiently supplemented parental feeds, malabsorptive states (especially with gastric bypass, as described in numerous cases), and with excessive zinc intake [78].

Excessive zinc intake is now a well-described cause of copper-deficiency myelopathy [79,80]. Increased zinc intake causes copper deficiency by inducing higher concentrations of metallothionein in enterocytes that then bind copper. These enterocytes are then sloughed off in the gastrointestinal tract and copper is lost [80]. Recently, ingestion of denture cream containing zinc has been found to be an important environmental cause of excess zinc intake leading to copper deficiency and copper-deficiency myelopathy [81].

Patients with copper-deficiency myelopathy present with prominent gait difficulty due to sensory ataxia from dorsal column dysfunction with loss of vibratory sensation and proprioception, as well as lower limb spasticity. Copper-deficiency myelopathy clinically mimics subacute combined degeneration of the spinal cord due to vitamin B12 deficiency (and B12 deficiency can sometimes coexist with copper deficiency). Patients with copper deficiency myelopathy may have evidence of peripheral neuropathy as well, causing a myeloneuropathy syndrome [78].

Diagnostically these patients have decreased serum copper, low serum ceruloplasmin levels, and may have decreased CSF copper if tested [77]. There is commonly evidence of axonal neuropathy on EMG, and MRI studies may show increased signal on T2-weighted imaging involving the dorsal columns (similar to vitamin B12 deficiency), particularly involving the cervical cord [76].

Patients with copper-deficiency myelopathy may or may not also demonstrate other systemic effects of copper deficiency such as anemia or leukopenia at the time of their presentation with neurologic changes [80]. Treatment with intravenous or oral copper supplementation has been associated with variable degrees of neurologic improvement, but should prevent further deterioration; it is therefore important to make the diagnosis and initiate treatment as promptly as possible [78].

Due to its potential irreversibility if not diagnosed and treated promptly, copper deficiency (whether due to nutritional deficiency or excessive zinc intake), similar to vitamin B12 deficiency, should be included in the differential diagnosis, and excluded, in any progressive noncompressive myelopathy [80].

Nitrous oxide

The association of nitrous-oxide exposure and the development of a myeloneuropathy, clinically identical to subacute combined degeneration of the spinal cord from vitamin B12 deficiency, was first described in 1978 [82]. Multiple cases have subsequently been reported due to recreational abuse of nitrous oxide or exposure to nitrous oxide during surgical or dental procedures [83].

Nitrous oxide irreversibly oxidizes the cobalt core of cobalamin, therefore inactivating methylcobalamin. Patients who have subtle or minor B12 deficiency are particularly at risk of developing subacute combined degeneration due to exposure to nitrous oxide, but the neurologic syndrome can occur despite normal vitamin B12 levels. Treatment of myelopathy due to nitrous exposure consists of discontinuation of nitrous oxide exposure and prompt and aggressive repletion of vitamin B12. Some authors suggest that exogenous methionine supplementation may also be of benefit [83].

Clioquinol

Clioquinol is a copper–zinc chelating antibiotic that caused an epidemic of subacute myelo-optico-neuropathy in Japan in the 1970s that affected nearly 10,000 patients before its use as an antibiotic was banned (though this agent remains of current investigational interest for other conditions). Several authors have recently suggested that this devastating neurologic disorder may have been due to copper-deficiency myelopathy (and optico-myelopathy) induced by hypocupremia from this agent [80,84,85]. Recently, Kimura and colleagues performed cervical MRIs in a group of patients who developed subacute myelo-optico-neuropathy from clioquinol in the 1960s and found faint T2 hyperintensities in the dorsal columns suggestive of the findings seen in copper-deficiency myelopathy [86].

Heroin myelopathy

The first reports of myelopathy in heroin users was in 1968 and since that time there have been many cases reported in the medical literature. It is still unclear as to how heroin use causes myelopathy [87]. Clinically, patients present with weakness and sensory deficits, often with urinary retention, after the use of heroin, particularly after a period of abstinence from the drug. Most cases occur following use of intravenous delivery of heroin, although there are reports of similar myelopathic presentations after insufflation or inhalation of heroin vapors. On exam, patients will have evidence of myelopathy including weakness, sensory level, hyperreflexia, and extensor plantar reflexes [88–91]. Neuroradiologically, the injury appears to be a transverse myelopathy and one popular theory is that this syndrome occurs due to a hypersensitivity reaction causing an autoimmune-mediated attack on spinal cord tissue [87]. This is further supported by the fact that many of these reported cases of heroin myelopathy have occurred in patients who have abstained from use for some time prior to relapse. Other hypotheses include a direct toxic effect on spinal cord tissue, or injury due to hypotension (a hypothesis that is deemed less likely since the affected areas are not typical watershed regions) [87,88]. For the same reason, heroin-induced vasculitis is felt to be less likely as the territories affected are not particularly highly vascular. Other cases have also been reported where the whole width of the cord is not affected but rather just the posterior columns or corticospinal tracts are involved [90]. Most authors do recommend an empiric trial of high-dose steroids as a treatment option given that the most popular theory of injury is an autoimmune hypersensitivity reaction. Patients have varying degrees of recovery, with some patients recovering without intervention over time, and others with poor recovery despite steroid or plasma-exchange therapies [87,89].

Neurolathyrism

Neurolathyrism occurs in famined countries in Africa and Asia where people are dependent on certain diets for prolonged periods of time. The chickling pea from the *Lathyrus sativus* plant, when consumed for prolonged periods (200–400 g per day for 2–3 months), can cause neurologic dysfunction. Neurolathyrism is predominantly a motor neuron disease causing spastic paraparesis. These symptoms include increased muscle tone, patellar and ankle clonus, extensor plantar responses, and spastic gait. If consumption is

187

ceased early enough, symptoms may improve, otherwise if exposure has been for too long, patients may not improve [92]. It is believed that the non-protein L-beta-oxalyl aminoalanine (L-BOAA) in the chickling pea is the neurotoxic agent and specifically targets the anterior horn cell and Betz cells but that also other areas of the nervous symptom are affected, as patients can also have myoclonus, parasthesias, urinary incontinence, increased nocturnal dreaming, and short-term memory loss in initial stages. Histopathologically, these patients have degeneration of the anterior horn cells and loss of axons in the pyramidal tracts [93]. These neurotoxic effects of L-BOAA have been reproduced in animal models. Treatment is early recognition and discontinuation of neurotoxin.

Konzo

Konzo is a less-well-defined neurotoxin-related disease in people who have prolonged consumption of the protein-poor root cassava *Manihot esculenta*, which is grown in Africa. This cassava contains linamarin and lotaustralin which are both cyanogenic glycosides and are felt to be the specific neurotoxic agents in this disease. These patients present with visual and speech disturbances as well as spastic paraparesis similar to neurolathyrism. Consumption should be stopped immediately to prevent progression of symptoms. The reversibility of these symptoms is unclear [92].

Conclusion

Many systemic diseases can be associated with the development of a symptomatic myelopathy, whether due to compression, inflammation, infection, or metabolic or toxic dysfunction. Compressive, inflammatory, or infectious causes are more likely to cause a "level" of spinal cord dysfunction, whereas metabolic or toxic disorders are less likely to be associated with a discrete motor or sensory level. However, these clinical distinctions are not invariable, and in each patient with myelopathy the clinician should take care to immediately consider and exclude—typically with MRI—compressive causes which would likely require emergent decompression. MRI will also suggest the presence of inflammatory or infectious causes requiring immunosuppressive or more specific therapy. Finally, patients with clinical syndromes resembling subacute combined degeneration of the spinal cord should be urgently assessed for both vitamin B12 and copper deficiency, and if found should be treated promptly and aggressively to decrease the likelihood of irreversible spinal cord dysfunction.

 Five things to remember about myelopathies due to systemic disease

1. Systemic disease can cause myelopathy due to compression of the spinal cord or by direct (structural or functional) involvement of the spinal cord itself.
2. Spinal cord compression from systemic disease can occur due to commonly considered causes such as malignancy, abscess, and cervical spine involvement from rheumatoid arthritis, but can also occur from unusual causes such as extramedullary hematopoiesis and gout.
3. Paraneoplastic myelopathy typically causes an insidious or subacute myelopathy with characteristic longitudinally extensive high signal in the white-matter tracts or gray matter.
4. Myelopathies from both vitamin B12 deficiency and copper deficiency are clinically very similar, may be associated with similar MRI findings, may occur with or without hematologic abnormalities, and may lead to irreversible posterior column and corticospinal tract dysfunction if not recognized and treated urgently.
5. Schistosomal myelopathy should be considered in a patient with a subacute myelopathy involving the lower spinal cord or conus medullaris, who has traveled to an endemic area.

References

1 Powers JM, DeCiero DS, Ito M, Moser AB, Moser HW. Adrenomyeloneuropathy: a neuropathologic review featuring its non-inflammatory myelopathy. *J. Neuropathol. Exp. Neurol.* 2000;59:89–102.

2 Zackowski KM, Dubey P, Raymond GV, et al. Sensorimotor function and axonal integrity in adrenomyeloneuropathy. *Arch. Neurol.* 2006;63:74–80.

3 Dubey P, Fatemi A, Huang H, Nagae-Poetscher L, Wakana S, et al. Diffusion tensor-based imaging reveals occult abnormalities in adrenomyeloneuropathy. *Ann. Neurol.* 2005;58:758–766.

4 Marino S, DeLuca M, Dotti MT, Stromillo ML, Formichi P, et al. Prominent brain axonal damage and functional reorganization in 'pure' adrenomyeloneuropathy. *Neurology* 2007;69:1261–1269.

5 U.S. National Institutes of Health: ClinicalTrials.gov. A phase III trial of Lorenzo's oil in adrenomyeloneuropathy http://clinicaltrials.gov/ct2/show/NCT00545597. Accessed February 4, 2012.

6 . Neogi T. Gout. *N. Engl. J. Med.* 364;443–452.

7 Ibrahim GM, Ebinu JO, Rubin LA, Noel de Tilly L, Spears J. Gouty arthropathy of the axial skeleton causing cord compression and myelopathy. *Can. J. Neurol. Sci.* 2011;38:918–920.

8 Dharmadhikari R, Dildey P, Hide IG. A rare cause of spinal cord compression: imaging appearances of gout of the cervical spine. *Skeletal Radiol.* 2006;35:942–945.

9 Yoon JH, Joo IS, Li WY, Sohn SY. Clinical and laboratory characteristics of atopic myelitis: Korean experience. *J. Neurol. Sci.* 2009;285:154–158.

10 Kira J, Yamasaki K, Kawano Y, Kobayashi T. Acute myelitis associated with hyperIgEemia and atopic dermatitis. *J. Neurol. Sci.* 1997;148:199–203.

11 Kikuchi H, Osoegawa M, Ochi H, et al. Spinal cord lesions of myelitis with hyperIgEemia and mite antigen specific IgE (atopic myelitis) manifest eosinophilic inflammation. *J. Neurol. Sci.* 2001;183:73–78.

12 Stern BJ. Neurological complications of sarcoidosis. *Curr. Opin. Neurol.* 2004;17:311–316.

13 Hashmi M, Kyritsis AP. Diagnosis and treatment of intramedullary spinal cord sarcoidosis. *J. Neurol.* 1998;245:178–180.

14 Dolhun R, Sriram S. Neurosarcoidosis presenting as longitudinally extensive transverse myelitis. *J. Clin. Neurosci.* 2009;16:595–597.

15 Kovacs B, Lafferty TL, Brent LH, DeHoratius RJ. Transverse myelopathy in systemic lupus erythematosus; an analysis of 14 cases and review of the literature. *Ann. Rheum. Dis.* 2000;59:120–124.

16 Theodoridou A, Settas L. Demyelination in rheumatic diseases. *Postgrad. Med. J.* 2008;84:127–132.

17 Birnbaum J, Petri M, Thompson R, et al. Distinct subtypes of myelitis in systemic lupus erythematosus. *Arthritis Rheum.* 2009;60:3378–3387.

18 Lewis SL. Neurologic complications of Sjögren syndrome and rheumatoid arthritis. *Continuum Lifelong Learning Neurol.* 2008;14:120–144.

19 Pittock SJ, Lennon VA, de Seze J. Neuromyelitis optica and non-organ specific immunity. *Arch. Neurol.* 2008;65:78–83.

20 Flanagan EP, Lennon VA, Pittock SJ. Autoimmune myelopathies. *Continuum Lifelong Learning Neurol.* 2011;17:776–799.

21 Scott TF, Frohman EM, DeSeze J, et al. Evidence-based guideline: clinical evaluation and treatment of transverse myelitis. *Neurology* 2011;77:2128–2134.

22 Sakane T, Takeno M, Suzuki N, Inaba G. Behçet's disease. *N. Engl. J. Med.* 1999;341:1284–1291.

23 Al-Araji A, Kidd DP. Neuro-Behçet's disease: epidemiology, clinical characteristics, and management. *Lancet Neurol.* 2009;8:192–204.

24 Moskau S, Urbach H, Hartmann A, et al. Multifocal myelitis in Behçet's disease. *Neurology* 2003;60:517.

25 Fukae J, Kazuyuki N, Fujishima K, et al. Subacute longitudinal myelitis associated with Behçet's disease. *Inter. Med.* 2010;49:343–347.

26 Kim DH, Hilibrand AS. Rheumatoid arthritis in the cervical spine. *J. Am. Acad. Orthop. Surg.* 2005;13:463–474.

27 Gutmann L, Hable K. Rheumatoid pachymeningitis. *Neurology* 1963;13:901–905.

28 Kupersmith MJ, Martin V, Heller G, et al. Idiopathic hypertrophic pachymeningitis. *Neurology* 2004;62:686–694.

29 Ranasinghe MG, Zalatimo O, Rizk E, et al. Idiopathic hypertrophic spinal pachymeningitis: report of 3 cases. *J. Neurosurg. Spine* 2011;15:195–201.

30 Chan S-K, Cheuk W, Chan K-T, Chan JKC. IgG-4 related sclerosing pachymeningitis: a previously unrecognized form of central nervous system involvement in IgG-4 related sclerosing disease. *Am. J. Surg. Pathol.* 2009;33:1249–1252.

31 Choi SH, Lee SH, Khang SK, et al. IgG4-related sclerosing pachymeningitis causing spinal cord compression. *Neurology* 2010;75:1388–1390.

32 Kosakai A, Ito D, Yamada S, et al. A case of definite IgG4-related pachymeningitis. *Neurology* 2010;75:1390–1392.

33 Campellone JV, Lacomis D, Giuliani MJ, Kroboth FJ. Hepatic myelopathy. Case report with review of the literature. *Clin. Neurol. Neurosurg.* 1996;98:242–246.

34 Nardone R, Buratti T, Oliviero A, Lochmann A, Tezzon F. Corticospinal involvement in patients with a portosystemic shunt due to liver cirrhosis: a MEP study. *J. Neurol.* 2006;253:81–85.

35 Lewis M, Howdle PD. The neurology of liver failure. *Q. J. Med.* 2003;96:623–633.

36 Qu B, Liu C, Guo L, et al. The role of liver transplantation in the treatment of hepatic myelopathy: case report with review of the literature. *Transplant Proc.* 2009;41:1987–1989.

37 Dibbern DA, Loevner LA, Lieberman AP, et al. MR of thoracic cord compression caused by epidural extramedullary hematopoiesis in myelodysplastic syndrome. *Am. J. Neuroradiol.* 1997;18:363–366.

38 Moncef B, Hafedh J. Management of spinal cord compression caused by extramedullary hematopoiesis in beta-thalassemia. *Intern. Med.* 2008;47:1125–1128.

39 Michel L, Auffray-Calvier E, Raoul S, Derkinderen P. Spinal cord compression secondary to extra medullary hematopoiesis. *Clin. Neurol. Neurosurg.* 2008;11.

40 Dewan U, Kumari N, Jaiswal A, Behari S, Jain M. Extramedullary hemopoiesis with undiagnosed, early myelofibrosis causing spastic compressive myelopathy: case report and review. *Indian J. Orthop.* 2010;44:98–103.

41 Salehi SA, Koski T, Ondra SL. Spinal cord compression in beta-thalassemia: case report and review of the literature. *Spinal Cord.* 2004;42:117–123.

42 Taylor JW, Schiff D. Metastatic epidural spinal cord compression. *Semin. Neurol.* 2010;30:245–253.

43 Graber JJ, Nolan CP. Myelopathies in patients with cancer. *Arch. Neurol.* 2010;76:298–304.

44 Patchell RA, Tibbs PA, Regine W, et al. Direct decompressive surgical resection in the treatment of spinal cord compression caused by metastatic cancer: a randomized trial. *Lancet* 2005;366:643–648.

45 Giglio P, Gilbert MR. Neurologic complications of cancer and its treatment. *Curr. Oncol. Rep.* 2010;12:50–59.

46 Flanagan EP, McKeon A, Lennon VA. Paraneoplastic isolated myelopathy: clinical course and neuroimaging clues. *Neurology* 2011;76:2089–2095.

47 Misumi H, Ishibashi H, Kanayama K, et al. Necrotizing myelopathy associated with hepatocellular carcinoma. *Jpn. J. Med.* 1988;27:333–336.

48 Urai Y, Matsumoto K, Shimamura M, et al. Paraneoplastic necrotizing myelopathy in a patient with advanced esophageal cancer: an autopsied case report. *J. Neurol. Sci.* 2009;280:113–117.

49 Lins H, Kanakis D, Dietzmann K, et al. Paraneoplastic necrotizing myelopathy with hypertrophy of the cauda equina. *J. Neurol.* 2003;250:1388–1389.

50 Pittock SJ, Lennon VA. Aquaporin-4 autoantibodies in a paraneoplastic context. *Arch. Neurol.* 2008;65:629–632.

51 Counsel P, Khangure M. Myelopathy due to intrathecal chemotherapy: magnetic resonance imaging findings. *Clin. Radiol.* 2007;62:172–176.

52 Uchida K, Nakajima H, Takamura T, et al. Neurologic improvement associated with resolution of irradiation-induced myelopathy: serial magnetic resonance imaging and positron emission tomography findings. *J. Neuroimaging* 2009;19:274–276.

53 Watterson J, Toogood I, Nieder M, et al. Excessive spinal cord toxicity from intensive central nervous-system directed therapies. *Cancer* 1994;74:3034–3041.

54 Kincaid O, Lipton HL. Viral myelitis: an update. *Curr. Neurol. Neurosci. Rep.* 2006;6:469–474.

55 Berger Jr., Infectious myelopathies. *Continuum Lifelong Learn. Neurol.* 2011;17:761–775.

56 Sartoretti-Schefer S, Blattler T, Wichmann W. Spinal MRI in vacuolar myelopathy, and correlation with histopathological findings. *Neuroradiology* 1997;39:865–869.

57 Bizaare M, Dawood H, Moodley A. Vacuolar myelopathy: a case report of functional, clinical, and radiological improvement after highly active antiretroviral therapy. *Int. J. Infect. Dis.* 2008;12:442–444.

58 Stacpoole SR, Phadke R, Jacques TS, et al. Vacuolar myelopathy associated with optic neuropathy in an HI-negative, immunosuppressed liver transplant recipient. *J. Neurol. Neurosurg. Psychiatry* 2009;80:581–583.

59 Cooper SA, van der Loeff MS, Taylor GP. The neurology of HTLV-1 infection. *Pract. Neurol.* 2009;9:16–26.

60 Araujo AQ, Silva MT. The HTLV-1 neurological complex. *Lancet Neurol.* 2006;5:1068–1076.

61 Oh U, Jacobson S. Treatment of HTLV-1-associated myelopathy/tropical spastic paraparesis: toward rational targeted therapy. *Neurol. Clin.* 2008;26:781–797.

62 Saito M. Immunogenetics and the pathological mechanisms of human T-cell leukemia virus type 1-(HTLV-1-) associated myelopathy/tropical spastic paraparesis (HAM/TSP). *Interdiscip. Perspect. Infect. Dis.* 2010;2010:478461. Published online.

63 Silva MT, Araujo A. Spinal cord swelling in human T-lymphotropic virus 1-associated myelopathy/tropical spastic paraparesis: magnetic resonance indication for early anti-inflammatory treatment? *Arch. Neurol.* 2004;61:1134–1135.

64 Dass B, Puet TA, Watanakunakorn C. Tuberculosis of the spine (Pott's disease) presenting as 'compression fractures'. *Spinal Cord* 2002;40:604–608.

65 Nussbaum ES, Rockswold GL, Bergman TA, et al. Spinal tuberculosis: a diagnostic and management challenge. *J. Neurosurg.* 1995;83:243–247.

66 Turgut M. Spinal tuberculosis (Pott's disease): its clinical presentation, surgical management, and outcome: a survey study on 694 patients. *Neurosurg. Rev.* 2001;24:8–13.

67 Jain AK. Tuberculosis of the spine: a fresh look at an old disease. *J. Bone Joint Surg. Br.* 2010;92:905–913.

68 Makinson A, Morales RJ, Basset D, et al. Diagnostic approaches to imported schistosomal myeloradiculopathy in travelers. *Neurology* 2008;71:66–67.

69 Carod Artal FJ, Vargas AP, Horan TA, et al. *Schistosoma mansoni* myelopathy: clinical and pathologic findings. *Neurology* 2004;63:388–391.

70 Lambertucci JR, Silva LC, do Amaral RS. Guidelines for the diagnosis and treatment of schistosomal myeloradiculopathy. *Rev. Soc. Bras. Med. Trop.* 2007;40:574–581.

71 Del Brutto OH, Roman GC, Sotel J. Chapter 6, Clinical manifestations. In: *Neurocysticercosis, A Clinical Handbook*, Lisse: Swets & Zeitlinger, 1998, pp. 57–72.

72 Sinha S, Sharma BS. Neurocysticercosis: a review of current status and management. *J. Clin. Neurosci.* 2009;16:867–876.

73 Qi B, Ge P, Yang H, et al. Spinal intramedullary cysticercosis: a case report and literature review. *Int. J. Med. Sci.* 2011;8:42–423.

74 Hemmer B, Glocker FX, Schumacher M, et al. Subacute combined degeneration: clinical, electrophysiological, and magnetic resonance imaging findings. *J. Neurol. Neurosurg. Psychiatry* 1998;65:822–827.

75 Srikanth SG, Jayakumar PN, Vasudev MK, et al. MRI in subacute combined degeneration of spinal cord: a case report and review of literature. *Neurol. India* 2002;50:310–312.

76 Kumar N. Copper deficiency myelopathy (human swayback). *Mayo Clin. Proc.* 2006;81:1371–184.

77 Schleper B, Stuerenburg HJ. Copper deficiency-associated myelopathy in a 46-year-old woman. *J. Neurol.* 2001;248:705–706.

78 Kumar N, Gross JB, Ahlskog JE. Copper deficiency myelopathy produces a clinical picture like subacute combined degeneration. *Neurology* 2004;63:33–39.

79 Kumar, N. Myelopathy due to copper deficiency. *Neurology* 2003;61:273–274.

80 Rowin J, Lewis SL. Copper deficiency myeloneuropathy and pancytopenia secondary to overuse of zinc supplementation. *J. Neurol. Neurosurg. Psychiatry* 2005;76:750–751.

81 Nations SP, Boyer PJ, Love LA, et al. Denture cream: an unusual source of excess zinc, leading to hypocupremia and neurologic disease. *Neurology* 2008;71:639–643.

82 Layzer RB. Myeloneuropathy after prolonged exposure to nitrous oxide. *Lancet* 1978;2:1227–1230.

83 Renard D, Dutray A, Remy A, et al. Subacute combined degeneration of the spinal cord caused by nitrous oxide anaesthesia. *Neurol. Sci.* 2009;30:75–76.

84 Kumar N, Knopman DS. SMON, clioquinol, and copper. *Postgrad. Med. J.* 2005;81:227.

85 Schaumburg H, Herskovitz S. Copper deficiency myeloneuropathy: a clue to clioquinol-induced myelo-optic neuropathy? *Neurology* 2008;71:622–623.

86 Kimura E, Hirano T, Yamashita S, et al. Cervical MRI of subacute myelo-optico-neuropathy. *Spinal Cord* 2011;49:182–185.

87 McGuire JL, Beslow LA, Finkel RS, et al. A teenager with focal weakness. *Pediatr. Emerg. Care* 2008;24:875–879.

88 McCreary M, Emerman C, Hanna J, Simon J. Acute myelopathy following intranasal insufflation of heroin: a case report. *Neurology* 2000;55:316–317.

89 Riva N, Morana P, Cerri F, et al. Acute myelopathy selectively involving lumbar anterior horns following intranasal insufflations of ecstasy and heroin. *J. Neurol. Neurosurg. Psychiatry* 2007;78:908–909.

90 Nyffeler T, Stabba A, Sturzenegger M. Progressive myelopathy with selective involvement of the lateral and posterior columns after inhalation of heroin vapour. *J. Neurol.* 2003;250:496–498.

91 Ell JJ, Uttley D, Silver Jr., Acute myelopathy in association with heroin addiction. *J. Neurol. Neurosurg. Psychiatry* 1981;44:448–450.

92 Ludolph AC, Spencer PS. Toxic models of upper motor neuron disease. *J. Neurol. Sci.* 1996;139:53–59.

93 Ravindranath V. Neurolathyrism: mitochondrial dysfunction in excitotoxicity mediated by L-beta-oxalyl aminoalanine. *Neurochem. Int.* 2002;40:505–509.

11 Peripheral nerve disorders in systemic disease

Michelle L. Mauermann[1] and Ted M. Burns[2]
[1]Mayo Clinic, Rochester, MN, USA
[2]University of Virginia, Charlottesville, VA, USA

Endocrine disorders

Diabetes mellitus

Peripheral neuropathy is common in diabetic patients, affecting 66% of type 1 diabetics and 59% of type 2 diabetics [1]. It is the most common cause of neuropathy in developed Western countries [2]. The most common type of neuropathy affecting diabetic patients is diabetic distal polyneuropathy. Other less common types of neuropathy include diabetic radiculoplexus neuropathies, diabetic autonomic neuropathy, diabetic cachexia, insulin neuritis, hypoglycemic neuropathy, polyneuropathy after ketoacidosis, diabetic cranial neuropathy, and diabetic mononeuropathies (Table 11.1) [3].

Diabetic polyneuropathy
The frequency of diabetic polyneuropathy (DPN) increases with the duration of diabetes and hyperglycemia [2]. The severity of DPN correlates with the microvascular complications of DPN such as retinopathy and nephropathy [4] and alternative diagnoses should be considered in their absence. The development of 24-h microalbuminuria is a significant risk factor for worsening of nerve function due to diabetes [5].

Clinical symptoms of DPN are often predated by silent dysfunction of the nerves that can be demonstrated by progressive subclinical abnormalities seen on nerve conduction studies [5]. With progression there is a gradual onset of predominantly positive neuropathic symptoms (pain, tingling, or burning). In more severe cases, motor fibers are involved and can produce distal lower limb weakness. The neuropathy is length-dependent, slowly progressive, and symmetrical, almost exclusively involving the distal lower limbs (Figure 11.1). Symptoms and signs of autonomic dysfunction may be present. The most common electrodiagnostic test (EDX) abnormality is reduced lower extremity sensory nerve action potential amplitudes. However, in some instances, a purely small fiber neuropathy can be seen with normal nerve conduction studies and electromyography [6,7].

Diabetic radiculoplexus neuropathy
Diabetes mellitus appears to be a risk factor for the development of lumbosacral radiculoplexus neuropathy. Diabetic lumbosacral radiculoplexus neuropathy (DLRPN) occurs in approximately 1% of diabetic patients [1] and is more frequent in type 2 diabetics. In general, these patients have better glycemic control compared to diabetic distal polyneuropathy patients [8] and have a lower rate of coexistent end-organ damage related to diabetes mellitus [9].

DLRPN presents with acute to subacute onset of severe pain in the lower extremity that can be in the leg or thigh but ultimately spreads to the entire limb. The pain is described as sharp or lancinating, deep aching, burning, or contact allodynia. Weakness follows and is the cause of morbidity in these

Neurological Disorders due to Systemic Disease, First Edition. Edited by Steven L. Lewis.
© 2013 Blackwell Publishing Ltd. Published 2013 by Blackwell Publishing Ltd.

Table 11.1 Neuropathies associated with diabetes mellitus

Symmetric
    Diabetic polyneuropathy
    Diabetic autonomic neuropathy
    Diabetic cachexia
    Insulin neuritis
    Hypoglycemic neuropathy
    Neuropathy after ketoacidosis
    Diabetic cranial neuropathy
    CIDP
    Neuropathy associated with impaired glucose intolerance
Focal or asymmetric
    Diabetic mononeuropathy
    Diabetic thoracic radiculopathy
    Diabetic lumbosacral radiculoplexus neuropathy
    Diabetic cervical radiculoplexus neuropathy

CIDP, chronic inflammatory demyelinating polyradiculoneuropathy.

patients. In general the process begins unilaterally but often becomes bilateral within 3 months [8]. When the neuropathic process affects both lower extremities it is almost always asymmetric [8].

Many patients require narcotic pain medication. Patients almost always have coincident weight loss (more than 10 pounds), which can sometimes be an important diagnostic clue [9]. The course is typically self-limited with initial progression lasting weeks to months with incomplete recovery. Concurrent cervical radiculoplexus neuropathies can occur in 10–15% of patients [8,10]. Cerebrospinal fluid (CSF) examination typically demonstrates a mildly elevated protein concentration with normal cell count [11]. EDX confirms asymmetrical involvement usually with more widespread abnormalities than suspected based on clinical evaluation. There is evidence of an axonal process involving the roots, plexus, and peripheral nerves [11]. Nerve biopsy, when performed, demonstrates ischemic injury with multifocal fiber loss, axonal degeneration, focal perineurial degeneration, neovascularization, and injury neuroma due to microscopic vasculitis (epineurial vascular and perivascular inflammation, vessel wall necrosis, and previous bleeding) [11]. Preliminary data from a controlled clinical trial demonstrated improvement in symptoms but failed to show significant improvement in neurologic deficits with immunotherapy [12].

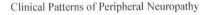

Clinical Patterns of Peripheral Neuropathy

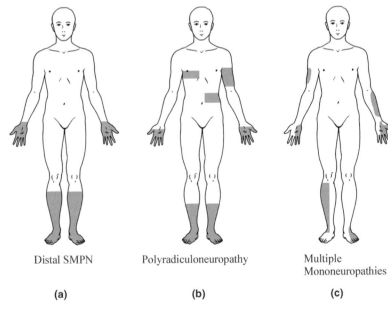

Distal SMPN

Polyradiculoneuropathy

Multiple Mononeuropathies

(a)

(b)

(c)

Fig 11.1 Typical peripheral neuropathy patterns: (a) length-dependent peripheral neuropathy, (b) polyradiculoneuropathy, and (c) multiple mononeuropathies.

193

Impaired glucose metabolism and neuropathy

The American Diabetes Association defines impaired fasting glucose as a plasma glucose level greater than 100 and less than 126 mg/dL, and impaired glucose tolerance as a 2 h glucose level between 140 and 199 mg/dL after a 75-g oral glucose load. Impaired glucose metabolism is suggested as a cause of chronic idiopathic axonal polyneuropathy (CIAP) [13–17]. The neuropathy is reported to most commonly affect small nerve fibers, although involvement of both large and small nerve fibers is also reported. Published studies on this subject have conflicting results, suggesting further research is needed before concluding an association.

Hypothyroidism

Hypothyroidism is a common disorder, often affecting women. The diagnosis should be considered in patients with symptoms such as fatigue, weakness, weight gain, cold intolerance, coarse dry hair and skin, constipation, depression, and abnormal menstrual cycles. Symptoms suggesting neuropathy are common; one study of newly diagnosed patients reported 42% had clinical symptoms and signs of distal, symmetrical, sensory-predominant neuropathy with decreased ankle reflexes, however, only 17% were confirmed by EDX [18]. The symptoms often include paresthesias, numbness, and pain. Patients often complain of weakness but do not often have abnormalities on examination.

Acromegaly

Peripheral neuropathy occurs in the majority of patients with acromegaly by clinical and/or electrophysiological studies [19]. Median mononeuropathy at the wrist, consistent with carpal tunnel syndrome, is also common. Symptoms of peripheral neuropathy include paresthesias in the hands and feet, depressed or absent ankle reflexes, and distal muscle wasting and sensory loss. In some cases, the peripheral neuropathy is thought to be related to diabetes mellitus, a frequent comorbidity in these patients. EDX demonstrates reduction in motor conduction velocities and in sensory nerve action potentials [19]. Nerve biopsy demonstrates a reduction in the number of myelinated fibers and an increase in endoneurial tissue. In addition there are features of remyelination following segmental demyelination [19].

Systemic autoimmune disorders

Vasculitis

The various forms of vasculitis make up a heterogeneous group of disorders that can affect different organ systems and different blood vessel calibers [20]. Several forms of vasculitis can affect the peripheral nervous system. Vasculitis can be roughly classified as primary vasculitis, with no known cause, and secondary vasculitis, which are those associated with a drug, virus, or connective tissue disease (Table 11.2). Vasculitis can also be classified by the kind and size of blood vessel that is involved, organ involvement, disease associations, underlying mechanisms, and sometimes autoantibody profiles [20–22]. The histopathology of peripheral nerve vessel involvement also allows some separation of the different types of vasculitis into two groups, nerve large arteriole vasculitis and nerve microvasculitis [20,23]. Large arteriole vasculitis of nerve has involvement of small arteries, large arterioles, and a varying degree of smaller vessels (vessels 75–200 microns) [23] and is usually associated with rheumatoid arthritis, polyarteritis nodosa, Churg–Strauss syndrome, or Wegener's granulomatosis. Nerve microvasculitis involves small arterioles, microvessels, and venules (usually vessels smaller that 40 μm). Nerve microvasculitis occurs in microscopic polyangiitis, nonsystemic vasculitis, immune sensorimotor polyneuropathies sometimes associated with sicca (i.e., Sjögren's

Table 11.2 Vasculitides associated with peripheral nerve involvement

Primary systemic vasculitides
  Polyarteritis nodosa
  Wegener's granulomatosis
  Churg–Strauss syndrome
  Microscopic polyangiitis
Secondary causes of systemic vasculitides
  Rheumatoid arthritis
  Systemic lupus erythematosis
  Sjögren's syndrome
  Mixed cryoglobulinemia
Nonsystemic vasculitic neuropathy

syndrome), paraneoplastic neuropathies, virus-associated neuropathies (HIV, CMV, and hepatitis C), diabetic and nondiabetic radiculoplexus neuropathies and immune and inherited brachial plexus neuropathies.

The most common presentation of vasculitic neuropathy is mononeuritis multiplex (Figure 11.1). Mononeuritis multiplex presents with acute to subacute onset of painful sensory or sensorimotor deficits. It can present in the upper or lower limbs, typically at watershed zones, especially the sciatic nerve in the mid-thigh region [24]. Often the progression of mononeuropathies is so rapid that on presentation the deficits appear confluent [20]. Taking a detailed history about the sequence of neuropathic events is of paramount importance. Less often, these present with a painful asymmetrical or distal, symmetrical sensorimotor peripheral neuropathy [20,22]. Systemic vasculitis almost always occurs in the setting of constitutional symptoms such as weight loss, respiratory symptoms, hematuria, abdominal pain, rash, myalgias, arthralgias, fever. and night sweats [22].

Evaluation of suspected vasculitic neuropathy should include a detailed laboratory investigation checking CBC, electrolytes, creatinine, BUN, sedimentation rate, C-reactive protein (CRP), antinuclear antibody (ANA), angiotensin converting enzyme (ACE), myeloperoxidase/p-antineutrophil cytoplasmic antibody (MPO/p-ANCA), proteinase3 (PR3/c-ANCA), extractable nuclear antigen (ENA), SSA and SSB, anti-cyclic citrullinated peptide (CCP), hepatitis B and C panels, cryoglobulins, serum monoclonal protein studies, and human immunodeficiency virus (HIV). A urinalysis and chest x-ray should also be performed. CSF analysis is usually not helpful except in the exclusion of mimickers including Lyme disease and other inflammatory etiologies including carcinomatous root involvement [20]. Nerve conduction studies can establish multiple individual nerve involvement or an asymmetric peripheral neuropathy. Needle electromyography typically shows subacute axonal injury in a patchy multifocal pattern.

Tissue biopsy is recommended for diagnosis given the likely need for long-term treatment with potentially toxic medications. A sensory nerve biopsy (sural or superficial peroneal) is recommended to confirm the diagnosis before embarking on potentially toxic treatments. In general, the sensitivity of a nerve or nerve and muscle biopsy is believed to be approximately 60% for vasculitis, if inflammation and vessel wall destruction are mandatory criteria [25,26]. Sensitivity of nerve biopsy increases, but specificity decreases, if other features, such as ischemic injury (multifocal fiber loss) with inflammation but without vessel wall destruction, are considered sufficient for diagnosis (Figure 11.2) [25–27].

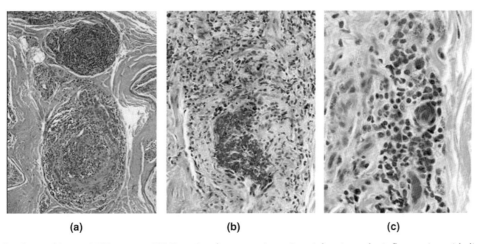

| (a) | (b) | (c) |

Fig 11.2 Sural nerve biopsy. (a) Transverse H&E section demonstrating epineurial perivascular inflammation with disruption of the vessel wall. (b) Longitudinal Masson-Trichrome section demonstrating fibrinoid necrosis. (c) Longitudinal Masson-Trichome preparation demonstrating hemosiderin-laden macrophages. Findings are diagnostic for necrotizing vasculitis. (See also Plate 11.2.).

Primary systemic vasculitides
Primary systemic vasculitides have no known cause. The most common primary systemic vasculitides are polyarteritis nodosa, Wegener's granulomatosis, Churg–Strauss syndrome, and microscopic polyangiitis. In patients with biopsy proven nerve vasculitis, microscopic polyangiitis is perhaps the one that most commonly causes vasculitic neuropathy [28].

Polyarteritis nodosa Polyarteritis nodosa (PAN) affects larger blood vessels (small and medium muscular arteries) than those in the other vasculitides that affect nerve; PAN typically does not involve arterioles, capillaries and venules [29,30]. There is often renal and gastrointestinal involvement [31]. Vasculitic neuropathy occurs in up to 75% of patients with PAN [32,33]. PAN is commonly associated with hepatitis B in one-third to one-half of patients [34,35].

Wegener's granulomatosis Wegener's granulomatosis affects the upper and lower airways and kidneys, and involves capillaries, arterioles, and venules. Peripheral nerve involvement is reported in 14 to 40% of cases [36,37]. The majority of patients are c-ANCA positive [38].

Churg–strauss syndrome Churg–Strauss syndrome usually presents with asthma, pulmonary infiltrates, fever, and eosinophilia, and affects the small to medium-sized vessels. Neuropathy occurs in 65–80% of patients [27,39–41]. P-ANCA is positive in more than half of patients [40].

Microscopic polyangiitis Microscopic polyangiitis often presents with systemic, renal, or cutaneous manifestations of vasculitis. More than half of the patients develop a neuropathy [33]. P-ANCA is positive in 58–76% of patients [33,42].

Secondary causes of systemic vasculitides
Secondary systemic vasculitides are those in which a virus, drug, or connective tissue disease is responsible for vessel wall inflammation. The common causes include rheumatoid arthritis, systemic lupus erythematosus, Sjögren's syndrome, and mixed type II or type III cryoglobulinemic vasculitis associated with HCV infection.

Rheumatoid arthritis Vasculitis associated with rheumatoid arthritis (RA) typically occurs as a late manifestation of severe seropositive disease. Rheumatoid vasculitis affects 5–10% of rheumatoid arthritis patients; half of these vasculitis patients will develop neuropathy secondary to vasculitis [43]. With modern therapies, the incidence of rheumatoid vasculitis appears to be declining. The vasculitis typically affects small to medium-sized arteries. In addition to, or instead of, vasculitic neuropathy, many patients with RA develop an insidious, mild, symmetric, distal sensory or sensorimotor neuropathy that is not caused by vasculitis [44]. Evaluation for vasculitis in patients with rheumatoid arthritis should include CCP antibodies, which in early disease have a sensitivity of 57% and specificity of 96% [45].

Systemic lupus erythematosus Systemic lupus erythematous (SLE) is a multisystem disorder that can present with variable combinations of fever, rash, alopecia, arthritis, pleuritis, pericarditis, nephritis, anemia, leukopenia, thrombocytopenia, and nervous system disease. Neuropathy is reported in 5–27% of patients with SLE [46]. In less than 5% of SLE patients the pattern is of multiple mononeuropathies, likely secondary to vasculitis [47]. Other types of neuropathy include a mild, modestly progressive, length-dependent, sensory or sensorimotor neuropathy. Patients have positive (prickling, tingling, pain) and negative (dead-type numbness) sensory symptoms. Less commonly, patients have a pure small-fiber neuropathy [48]. Laboratory testing for autoimmune markers includes ANA (sensitivity is 99% and specificity is 80%), anti-dsDNA (sensitivity of 70% and specificity of 95%) and anti-Smith (sensitivity of 25% and a specificity of 99%) [49].

Sjögren's syndrome Sjögren's Syndrome (SS) is a systemic autoimmune disease that primarily affects middle-aged women [50]. The criteria for diagnosis include sicca symptoms (dry eyes, dry mouth), objective evidence of keratoconjunctivitis, evidence of chronic lymphocytic sialoadenitis, and the presence of either anti-SS-A or anti-SS-B antibodies [51,52]. Rash, arthralgias, and Raynaud's phenomenon are also common [53,54]. However, there is considerable confusion and disagreement on the classification of SS-associated immune-mediated neuropathies, in part because different case series use different clinical criteria for study inclusion. Furthermore, presence of sicca complex does not always imply glandular inflammation as sometimes these may be a manifestation of concurrent autonomic ganglionopathy or a side effect of a medication. Some have proposed that these neuropathies be instead classified as immune-sensory and autonomic neuropathies with or without sicca [55].

Peripheral neuropathy is reported to occur in 10–30% of patients with SS [56,57]. The neuropathy of SS is secondary to vasculitis in some cases and secondary to mononuclear cell infiltration without vasculitis (e. g., ganglionitis) in some other cases. There are also other mechanisms of neuropathy in these patients. For example, the etiology of the small-fiber neuropathy seen in some cases of SS may be different. Several patterns of neuropathy are seen in association with SS: sensory ataxic neuropathy, painful sensory neuropathy without ataxia, multiple mononeuropathies, multiple cranial neuropathies, trigeminal sensory neuropathy, autonomic neuropathy with anhidrosis, and radiculoneuropathy (Table 11.3) [54,58]. Abnormal pupils and orthostatic hypotension are common accompaniments to many of these neuropathies. Sensory ataxic neuropathy typically presents with asymmetric paresthesias and ataxia and gradually becomes more widespread [50,59]. Painful sensory neuropathy without ataxia may present insidiously with asymmetric, painful neuropathic symptoms that gradually progresses in a length-dependent manner [54,60].

The ANA titer is elevated (>1:160) in one-third to one-half of patients in some series [53]. Anti-SS-A or anti-SS-B antibodies have also been reported to be present in approximately one-third to one-half of SS patients with neuropathy [50]. Evidence of salivary gland dysfunction can be obtained by measuring salivary flow rates or by imaging salivary glands with radiographic contrast agents or technetium scanning.

Table 11.3 Neuropathies associated with Sjögren's syndrome

Sensory ataxic neuropathy
Painful sensory neuropathy without ataxia
Multiple mononeuropathies
Multiple cranial neuropathies
Trigeminal sensory neuropathy
Autonomic neuropathy with anhidrosis
Radiculoneuropathy

Biopsy of the minor salivary glands provides a means of assessing the extent and nature of infiltration by lymphocytes and plasma cells and glandular destruction [50]. The Schirmer test can assess for lacrimal gland dysfunction.

Hepatitis C associated cryoglobulinemia See "Systemic infectious diseases" section.

Nonsystemic vasculitic neuropathy

Vasculitis can also be confined to the nerve and muscle without systemic involvement, which is termed nonsystemic vasculitic neuropathy (NSVN). Untreated NSVN is usually not fatal in contrast to the primary systemic vasculitides. Importantly, it is estimated that approximately 10% of cases that initially appear to be nonsystemic ultimately become systemic vasculitis, so it may be difficult to differentiate early, and continued follow-up is recommended [25,61].

Sarcoidosis

Sarcoidosis is an inflammatory multisystem disorder characterized by the development of noncaseating epithelioid-cell granulomas. Sarcoidosis most commonly affects the lungs, in up to 90% of patients [62]. Cases affecting the spinal roots or peripheral nerves are rare, representing only about 1% of total sarcoidosis cases [63–66].

The onset of the neuropathy is typically abrupt with a definite date of onset [66,67]. The pattern is asymmetric, non-length-dependent (often involving proximal roots), and affects sensory and motor nerve fibers. There are often positive neuropathic sensory symptoms (P-NSS) including pain, which is usually prominent and can require narcotic medications [67]. The most common patterns are a polyradiculoneuropathy followed by polyneuropathy [67]. Less common patterns are multiple mononeuropathies, polyradiculopathy, and radiculoplexus neuropathy. A small-fiber neuropathy has also been reported to occur in sarcoidosis [68]. Accompanying cranial neuropathies and/or thoracic radiculopathies are seen in about one-third of patients [67]. The neuropathy often occurs in the setting of fatigue, malaise, fever, and unexplained weight loss in many patients [67]. At the time of the diagnosis of neuropathy, arthralgias, skin, and eye involvement are also commonly encountered [67].

197

MRI in sarcoid

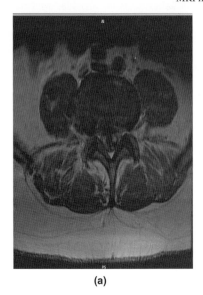
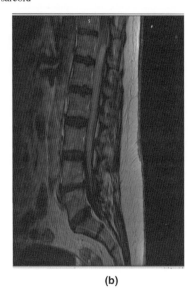

(a)　　　　　　　　　　　　　　　　　**(b)**

Fig 11.3 Lumbosacral MRI of a patient with a polyradiculopathy due to sarcoidosis. (a) Axial T1-weighted fat suppressed echo (FSE) image after gadolinium administration demonstrating abnormally thickened and enhancing cauda equina nerve roots. (b) Sagittal T1-weighted FSE after gadolinium demonstrates intradural extramedullary enhancement around the conus medullaris.

Abnormalities on chest imaging (chest radiograph or computed tomography), such as hilar adenopathy, are found in the majority of cases [67]. Serum ACE is elevated in about one-fourth of patients with peripheral nerve sarcoidosis [67]. CSF protein is usually elevated, and one-third of patients demonstrate CSF pleocytosis [62,67]. MR imaging can also sometimes be helpful by demonstrating nerve enlargement or enhancement of affected nerves (Figure 11.3) [67]. EDX usually reveals an asymmetric, multifocal axonal process [62,67].

Celiac disease

Celiac disease is a T-cell mediated chronic immune-mediated inflammatory disorder in response to gluten and related proteins in wheat, rye, and barley, that leads to inflammation, villous atrophy, and crypt hyperplasia in the proximal part of the intestine [69]. It is more common in people who are HLA DQ2 and DQ8 positive [70]. Current diagnostic standards require positive antibodies (IgA endomysial antibody or IgA tissue transglutaminase) and/or positive histopathology from small bowel biopsy (increased epithelial lymphocytes, enlarged crypts, and villous atrophy). Some of the neurological complications due to celiac disease are thought to be due to malabsorption. An example of this would be malabsorption leading to vitamin B12

deficiency, which can cause a peripheral neuropathy and/or myelopathy.

Peripheral neuropathy associated with celiac disease remains controversial, in part due to lack of diagnostic standards. All reports are case reports or small case series [71–75]. Common symptoms include burning, tingling, and numbness in the hands and feet with distal sensory loss [71]. EDX is often normal or only mildly abnormal in these cases. Less often, motor or multifocal neuropathies have been reported. There has been conflicting evidence regarding improvement in symptoms with a gluten-free diet.

Organ dysfunction and failure

Uremia

Peripheral neuropathy due to uremia occurs in 10–83% of patients with chronic renal failure who are on dialysis, but has become less frequent due to renal transplantation [76–79]. The neuropathy in uremia is similar to other neuropathies from a metabolic cause. The neuropathy is often distal, symmetric, sensory predominant, and slowly progressive. Patients often have symptoms of numbness and imbalance as well as paresthesias and burning indicating involvement of both large and small fibers [78,79]. Other common symptoms include restless legs, cramps, and weakness. The diagnosis should be considered especially in patients with end-stage renal disease with a creatinine of 5 mg/dL or higher, or creatinine clearance less than 12 mL/min.

Systemic cancer and paraneoplastic disorders

Monoclonal gammopathy of undetermined significance

Monoclonal gammopathy of underdetermined significance (MGUS) occurs in 3.2% of persons over age 50 and more than 5% of persons over age 70 [80]. The criteria for MGUS have been defined previously [81,82]. Monoclonal proteins are not necessarily benign, in that there is a risk of conversion to multiple myeloma and related serious B-cell disorders of approximately 1% per year [83]. The rate of malignant disease progression in one large series was 17% at 10 years, 34% at 20 years, and 39% at 25 years [84]. The monoclonal (M) protein can be of IgM, IgG, or IgA heavy chain. High-risk factors for conversion to serious B-cell disorders include non-IgG MGUS, serum M-protein levels ≥1.5 g/dL and an abnormal serum free light chain ratio (<0.26 or >1.65) [85].

IgG is the most common class of paraprotein associated with MGUS in the general population, however, IgM with a kappa light chain is most frequent in patients with neuropathy [86,87]. A monoclonal protein is found in the serum of about 10% of patients with a peripheral neuropathy [88]. Evaluation of patients with a neuropathy associated with a paraprotein can be challenging and should focus on whether there is an association or whether the presence is just due to chance.

Neuropathies associated with paraproteinemias include distal acquired demyelinating symmetric (DADS-M) neuropathy (also known as a CIDP variant), primary systemic amyloidosis, POEMS syndrome (polyneuropathy, organomegaly, endocrinopathy, M protein, and skin changes), Waldenström's macroglobulinemia, multiple myeloma, and Castleman's syndrome (Table 11.4). The history and EDX testing are particularly helpful in sorting this out: accompanying systemic symptoms raise concern for primary systemic amyloidosis, POEMS or malignancy; autonomic symptoms and signs are common in primary systemic amyloidosis; EDX features of primary demyelination are commonly seen in neuropathies of DADS-M, POEMS, and Castleman's syndrome, whereas the neuropathy is usually axonal when associated with primary systemic amyloidosis

Table 11.4 Monoclonal gammopathies associated with neuropathy

IgM neuropathy—DADS (associated with anti-MAG antibodies)
Primary systemic amyloidosis
Waldenström's macroglobulinemia
Multiple myeloma
Osteosclerotic myeloma (POEMS syndrome)
Castleman's syndrome

DADS, distal acquired demyelinating symmetric neuropathy; MAG, myelin associated glycoprotein; POEMS, polyneuropathy, organomegaly, endocrinopathy, monoclonal gammopathy and skin changes.

and Waldenström's macroglobulinemia [89]. Neuropathies that are not primarily demyelinating and lack systemic symptoms and concurrent autonomic nervous system involvement are often coincidental.

Primary systemic amyloidosis

Primary systemic amyloidosis is a disorder characterized by deposition of insoluble monoclonal immunoglobulin light-chain fragments in various tissues [90]. 90% of cases have an M protein in either the serum or the urine, and 75% have lambda light chain [91]. Primary systemic amyloidosis presents more commonly in men after age 40 years [91]. Patients usually present with prominent systemic symptoms such as fatigue, weight loss, and edema [92]. Diagnostic periorbital or facial purpura, or macroglossia, are present in only 10–15% of patients [91]. Often there is multiorgan involvement, with the heart, liver, and kidney being most commonly affected [90].

The frequency of neuropathy is between 15% and 20% [90]. It most often presents as a symmetric, lower limb predominant, small-fiber neuropathy with pain (sharp, stabbing, burning, and aching) and autonomic dysfunction (postural hypotension, diarrhea, constipation, and impotence) [90,93]. The neuropathy is diffuse and progressive, and over time both motor and sensory (large and small fibers) become involved. There are rare cases presenting with multiple mononeuropathies [94,95], focal nerve involvement due to localized deposition of amyloid (amyloidoma) [96,97], or cranial neuropathies [93,94,98].

Evaluation for a monoclonal protein should include serum and urine protein electrophoresis (SPEP, UPEP) and immunofixation (SIFE, UIFE) [99,100]. In those

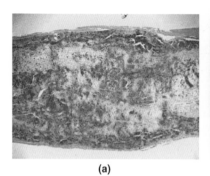
(a)

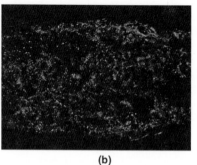
(b)

Fig 11.4 Targeted fascicular sciatic nerve biopsy. (a) Transverse paraffin section demonstrating amorphous congophilic material throughout the endoneurium and (b) apple-green birefringence with polarized light, diagnostic of amyloid. (See also Plate 11.4.)

without detectable monoclonal proteins, bone-marrow examination usually detects a clonal population of plasma cells [91]. There is mild anemia in approximately 50% of patients [90]. EDX examination usually demonstrates a symmetric, axonal sensorimotor neuropathy. Diagnosis depends on the demonstration of amyloid deposits in bone-marrow aspirate (positive in 50% of patients), abdominal fat aspirate (70%), rectal biopsy (80%), or nerve biopsy (80%) [101]. Nerve biopsy may demonstrate a marked decrease in myelinated fiber density with axonal degeneration, and endoneurial/epineurial perivascular amyloid deposition (Figure 11.4) [90].

Multiple myeloma

Multiple myeloma is a clonal plasma-cell disorder characterized by the presence of a monoclonal protein in the serum or urine, osteolytic lesions, increased plasma cells in the bone marrow, anemia, and hypercalcemia [102]. Peripheral neuropathy has been reported to occur in as few as 1–10% [88,103,104]. The major differential diagnosis is radicular or myelopathic symptoms due to compressive disease, toxic neuropathy due to chemotherapies for multiple myeloma such as bortezomib and thalidomide [105], or primary systemic amyloidosis [88]. Peripheral neuropathy can be the presenting feature of multiple myeloma, or occur during the course of the disease [88]. The neuropathy can be sensory or motor predominant, or sensory and motor. Often the neuropathy is mild, with distal numbness or tingling, and mild large and small-fiber sensory loss, and distal weakness on examination. Pain and autonomic symptoms are not prominent [88].

Poems syndrome

POEMS syndrome is a rare paraneoplastic syndrome secondary to a plasma-cell dyscrasia. The diagnostic criteria require the presence of peripheral neuropathy and a monoclonal plasma-cell-proliferative disorder, as well as one other major criterion, such as: sclerotic bone lesions, Castleman disease, or elevation of vascular endothelial growth factor (VEGF). Patients must have one other minor criterion which include: organomegaly, endocrinopathy, skin changes, thrombocytosis, extravascular volume overload, or papilledema [106].

The neuropathy associated with POEMS syndrome is often the dominant feature of the syndrome. Initial symptoms are typically sensory and include paresthesias and coldness that begin at the feet. Weakness follows, beginning distally and spreading proximally. Often the weakness predominates and causes significant functional impairment [107]. Reflexes are reduced or absent. Cranial nerves are often spared except for possible papilledema. Autonomic symptoms are rare except for erectile dysfunction which often relates to hypotestosternism. The clinical phenotype is very similar to chronic inflammatory demyelinating polyradiculoneuropathy (CIDP) and therefore POEMS is often initially diagnosed as CIDP. However systemic symptoms and signs, and a monoclonal protein—almost always IgG or IgA lambda—help in distinguishing these two entities [108].

Cerebrospinal fluid demonstrates albuminocytological dissociation, sometimes with very high protein levels [107,108] Nerve conduction studies demonstrate features of segmental demyelination as well as axonal loss, typically without features of temporal dispersion or conduction block, [108] which can also aid in distinguishing from CIDP.

Lymphoma

Neurolymphomatosis (NL) is the least common neurological manifestation of lymphoma. NL is the infiltration

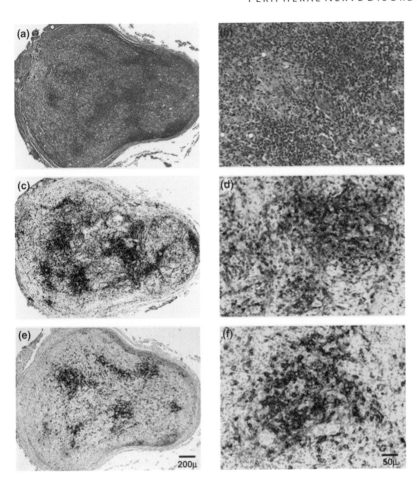

Fig 11.5 Targeted fascicular sciatic nerve biopsy. Transverse paraffin sections demonstrating immature mononuclear cells extensively infiltrating the endoneurium of a nerve fascicle (a, b) with reactivity for CD45 (lymphocytes) (c, d) and CD20 (B-cells) (e, f) diagnostic of B-cell neurolymphomatosis (See also Plate 11.5.).

of the cranial and peripheral nerves and roots. There are four recognized clinical presentations: (1) painful involvement of nerves and roots; (2) cranial neuropathy with or without pain; (3) painless involvement of peripheral nerves; and (4) painful or painless involvement of a single peripheral nerve [109]. Suggestive clinical symptoms include severe pain, asymmetric distribution, and rapid resolution. NL is almost always due to B-cell non-Hodgkins lymphoma [109]. CSF examination can be helpful in demonstrating lymphocytic pleocytosis and malignant lymphocytes on cytology. Nerve biopsy demonstrates an increased rate of segmental demyelination and axonal degeneration, and sheets of lymphoma cells predominantly involving the endoneurium (Figure 11.5) [110]. Rarely, intravascular lymphoma can cause a mononeuritis multiplex syndrome associated with stroke due to embolic phenomenon.

Paraneoplastic syndromes

Paraneoplastic syndromes are rare complications of malignancy. More than half of patients with a paraneoplastic syndrome present with neurologic symptoms that precede tumor detection [111–114]. Paraneoplastic syndromes are found more commonly in women in the 6th decade but can occur at any age [115]. History of tobacco use is common in these syndromes. The cancer is most commonly a small cell lung cancer (SCLC) but other cancers have been described. As many of these patients are found to have limited disease burden, they often do not have systemic evidence of malignancy. Neuropathy may be the most common presentation, especially in those with autoantibodies directed against antineuronal nuclear antibody ANNA-1 (anti-Hu) or collapsin response mediating protein 5 (CRMP-5/anti-CV2) [114,116]. Other presentations include a cerebellar syndrome, limbic encephalitis, brainstem dysfunction, and dysautonomia, and often there is multifocal nervous system involvement [111,114,117].

The neuropathy may present as a sensory ganglionopathy or sensory predominant neuropathy. Subacute onset with rapid progression is typical [111,114]. Sensory symptoms, including paresthesias, dysesthesias and pain predominate, whereas motor involvement is typically mild and may only be found on EDX evaluation [112,113]. There may be prominent upper extremity involvement and pseudoathetosis [111,112]. Autonomic involvement, most commonly orthostatic hypotension and gastroparesis, is found in up to one-fourth of patients [111,112,118]. Most patients develop severe disease with significant disability [117].

Paraneoplastic antibody evaluation is helpful in identifying these disorders. These antibodies usually do not predict the neurological syndrome but rather predict the malignancy [119]. EDX often shows axonal sensory or sensorimotor neuropathy or sensory ganglionopathy [112]. Once an antibody is identified, investigation for a malignancy should follow [111,112,114,117]. This should begin with a chest radiograph and proceed to a CT, MRI, or PET if necessary [114,115,120,121].

Systemic infectious diseases

Hepatitis C virus

Hepatitis C virus (HCV) is the most common chronic bloodborne viral infection in the United States. Patients with HCV may be asymptomatic or can have systemic symptoms such as fatigue, loss of appetite, nausea, weight loss, fever, weakness, and arthralgias [122,123]. Neuropathy associated with HCV may affect approximately 10% of patients [122,124]. There is a higher prevalence (up to 30%) in those positive for type II or type III cryoglobulins [125]. Different pathophysiological mechanisms have been suggested included virus-triggered nerve microvasculitis, and intravascular deposits of cryoglobulins leading to interference of the vasa nervorum microcirculation [122,125]. The peripheral neuropathy may present as a distal, asymmetric sensory or sensorimotor polyneuropathy, or as multiple mononeuropathies (Table 11.5) [122,125]. Patients often have prominent symptoms of pricking, burning, or pain [126]. Palpable purpura, for example on the ankles, is common and should be looked for during the examination [127].

Screening for HCV infection is accomplished by an enzyme immunoassay that is able to detect antibodies within 4–10 weeks after infection, missing only 0.5–1% of cases. Recombinant immunoblot assays are used to confirm the serologic assay. HCV RNA tests are used to confirm viremia [128]. Cryoglobulins are tested for in the serum and assessed at 24 h and 7 days for precipitate [129]. EDX will demonstrate an axonal sensorimotor neuropathy that is often asymmetric [122] or involves multiple nerves as a mononeuritis multiplex. Pathological findings include multifocal fiber loss with perivascular epineurial inflammation, sometimes suggestive of nerve microvasculitis [122].

Leprosy

Leprosy remains an important cause of treatable neuropathy worldwide. It is most prevalent in Southeast Asia, India, Africa, and Central and South America. Leprosy is caused by *Mycobacterium leprae*, an obligate intracellular acid-fast bacillus, which is transmitted by nasal droplets and then hematogenously spreads to skin and nerves. The average incubation period is approximately 7 years [130].

Leprosy neuropathies have three key features: anesthetic skin lesions, enlarged peripheral nerves, and acid-fast bacilli in skin smears/biopsy or nerve biopsy. There are two main types: tuberculoid and lepromatous. Tuberculoid leprosy presents with an asymmetric sensory polyneuropathy, with injury confined to nerves adjacent to hypopigmented skin lesions (Table 11.5). Lepromatous leprosy presents as a symmetric distal neuropathy due to more widespread involvement of the skin and nerves. Weakness ultimately develops due to motor involvement, often involving the ulnar nerve [130]. A third intermediate type, borderline leprosy, can also occur. Approximately 10% of patients may present without skin lesions, often presenting as a mononeuritis multiplex [130]. The initial symptoms are decreased thermal sense, followed by loss of pain and pressure sensations [131]. As the bacilli favor the cooler areas of the body, the sensory examination should focus on the chin, malar areas of the face, earlobes, buttocks, knees, and distal extremities, so sensory testing should be performed on these regions in suspected cases. In contrast to most other infectious neuropathies, the neuropathy is painless. Sensory involvement precedes motor involvement [130].

The most widely used serologic test is an antibody to phenolic glycolipid-1 (PGL-1), but it has a low

Table 11.5 Neuropathy patterns seen in systemic infectious diseases

Distal sensory-predominant neuropathy
   Lepromatous leprosy
   AIDS neuropathy
   HIV with DILS
   Lyme disease
Asymmetric or multiple mononeuropathies
   Hepatitis C (with or without cryoglobulins)
   Tuberculoid leprosy
   Advanced HIV with CMV co-infection
Polyradiculoneuropathy
   HIV at seroconversion (AIDP), CIDP, or associated with
      CMV infection
   Diphtheria
   Lyme disease

HIV, human immunodeficiency virus; DILS, diffuse infiltrative lymphocytosis syndrome; CMV, cytomegalovirus; AIDP, acute inflammatory demyelinating polyradiculoneuropathy; CIDP, chronic inflammatory demyelinating polyradiculoneuropathy.

sensitivity [130]. EDX testing demonstrates axonal loss and demyelination [132]. Definitive diagnosis is made by nerve biopsy, with strikingly different findings in the two forms. Tuberculoid leprosy shows significant destruction of nerve architecture with granulomas extending from the perineurium into the endoneurium. Bacilli are usually not abundant [130]. Lepromatous leprosy shows splitting of the perineurium by edema and foamy cells, infiltration of the endoneurium and perineurium by foamy cells, and bacilli in macrophages and Schwann cells with Fite preparation [130].

HIV

Symptomatic neuropathies occur in approximately 10–15% of HIV-1-infected patients, and the incidence increases as the CD4 count declines and the immunodeficiency worsens [133]. Rapid HIV testing has a sensitivity of 99–100% and specificity of 99–100% depending on the test [134].

Distal symmetric sensory polyneuropathy (DSPN) is the most common HIV neuropathy presentation, present in 35–44% of patients with AIDS (e.g., CD4 counts <200) (Table 11.5) [133]. DSPN presents with distal pain, paresthesias, and numbness in a symmetric length-dependent manner. It involves sensory or sensorimotor

nerve fibers and is gradually progressive. The neuropathy is very similar to that associated with nucleoside-analog reverse-transcriptase inhibitors (NRTIs—ddI, ddC, d4T), used in the treatment of HIV [135]. Helpful aspects in establishing a relationship between the neuropathy and the NRTIs are: (1) there is a temporal association with the onset of neuropathy and the initiation of NRTIs; (2) there is an improvement in symptoms and signs with reduction or cessation of NRTIs; (3) the patient might experience "coasting", that is, 2–4 weeks of worsening symptoms after discontinuation of NRTIs with subsequent improvement [135].

Polyradiculopathy is a much less common presentation for neuropathy in an HIV-infected patient. Acute inflammatory demyelinating polyradiculopathy (AIDP) can rarely occur at the time of seroconversion (CD4 counts ≥500). Polyradiculopathy can also be seen in moderately advanced HIV (CD4 counts 200–500) as a CIDP. In both cases, CSF examination typically demonstrates lymphocytosis of 10–50 cells/mm^3 [136]. Co-infection with other viruses, such as hepatitis C virus, CMV, and HTLV1, may occur [133,136].

Mononeuritis multiplex is an infrequent complication of HIV (0.1–3% of patients). Mononeuritis multiplex can occur at seroconversion or late stages [133,137]. At seroconversion, the neuropathy is self-limited and either immune or vasculitic in nature [133]. In advanced HIV (CD4 counts <50), coinfection with CMV can cause painful mononeuritis multiplex, polyradiculoneuropathy, or polyradiculopathy [133,136,138]. CSF demonstrates polymorphonuclear pleocytosis in only 15%, but CMV PCR in CSF is positive in 90% of cases [136].

Diffuse infiltrative lymphocytosis syndrome (DILS) (CD4 counts <260) is a rare cause of neuropathy in HIV. DILS is characterized by persistent peripheral blood polyclonal CD8 lymphocytosis and by visceral CD8 T-cell infiltration, including salivary glands, lungs, kidneys, gastrointestinal tract, and peripheral nerves [139]. It presents as an acute or subacute, painful, symmetric, length-dependent, axonal neuropathy which mainly involves the distal lower limbs [140]. EDX demonstrates axonal features with reduction in motor and sensory amplitudes and neurogenic abnormalities on electromyography. CSF usually shows lymphocytosis with elevated protein. Nerve biopsy reveals dense perivascular epineurial and endoneurial mononuclear infiltration which demonstrate predominantly CD8 reactivity [140].

Diphtheria

Diphtheria has seen resurgence in eastern European countries due to a lack of vaccination in adults who no longer had sufficient immunity to protect against the infection. Respiratory diphtheria presents with a low-grade fever, sore throat, neck swelling, and an adherent membrane of the tonsils, pharynx, or nose [141].

Diphtheric neuropathy occurs in up to 68% of infected patients, and the incidence is directly proportional to the severity of the infection [141]. It usually occurs within 2 months after infection. Initial symptoms may include numbness of the gingivae, tongue and face, distal paresthesias, dysphonia, and dysphagia [141]. These symptoms are followed by bilateral multiple cranial neuropathies and quadriparesis or quadriplegia requiring artificial ventilation in over half of patients (Table 11.5) [141,142]. Many patients have a sensory ataxia and autonomic involvement [141]. EDX findings are of demyelination with axonal degeneration in severe cases. Diagnosis can be made by bacterial culture from pharyngeal swab or from elevated serum titers of diphtheria antibodies.

Lyme

Lyme disease is caused by *Borellia burgdorferi* infection transmitted by the *Ixodes* tick. Lyme disease has a predilection for certain seasons and geographic locations. In approximately 80% of infected individuals, Lyme disease manifests first with erythema migrans, a painless and nonpruritic skin lesion that evolves over days to weeks [143]. Patients typically have flu-like symptoms and may have infection of large joints, heart, meninges, or peripheral nerve.

Approximately 15% of patients develop neurological complications days to weeks following untreated infection [143]. The most typical neurological manifestations are one or more elements of the triad of polyradiculoneuritis, lymphocytic meningitis, accompanied by cranial neuritis [144]. The polyradiculopathy or polyradiculoneuropathy is typically sensorimotor, painful, asymmetric and non-length-dependent due to involvement of nerve roots (Table 11.5). Rarely patients present with what looks like mononeuritis multiplex [145]. EDX confirms a polyradiculopathy or polyradiculoneuropathy and reveals primarily axonal damage [146]. Approximately 5% of untreated patients develop a chronic axonal neuropathy, occurring a median of 16 months after the initial

infection [143,147], with symptoms of relatively symmetric, distal paresthesias. The chronic axonal neuropathy may occur in the setting of encephalopathy or encephalomyelitis [147]. The pathology is not well described, although perineurial thickening associated with a lymphocytic infiltrate has been reported in acute infection [148].

Serum IgM for *B. burgdorferi* infection has a sensitivity of 32% in acute disease, and the IgG has a sensitivity of 83% in established disease [149]. Serologies may be negative early in the course and should be repeated if the clinical suspicion is high. Positive serologies should be confirmed by Western Blot. CSF in acute disease typically shows modest lymphocytic pleocytosis and mild increase in protein [149]. In chronic infection the IgG synthesis rate should be increased, and oligoclonal bands may be present [144]. CSF Lyme PCR has 40–50% sensitivity and 97% specificity [147].

Complications due to transplantation

Bone-marrow transplantation

Several autoimmune diseases are reported post transplantation. These are more commonly seen after allogeneic bone-marrow transplantation for hematologic disease versus solid organ transplantation. These complications often occur after the development of graft-versus-host disease (GVHD) following transplantation. Examples of autoimmunity include CIDP and AIDP [150–154]. The phenotype is typical for these acquired demyelinating diseases, with evidence of proximal and distal weakness, distal sensory loss, and reduced or absent reflexes. Nerve conduction studies demonstrate demyelinating features (slowed conduction velocities, prolonged distal latencies) with distal denervation [151]. CSF protein is elevated without pleocytosis. The neuropathy improves with resolution of the underlying transplantation rejection and with associated immunosuppressive therapy.

Complications of critical medical illness

Critical illness polyneuropathy

Peripheral neuropathy occurs in the setting of critical illness in 50–70% of patients with systemic inflammatory response syndrome (SIRS) and is referred to as critical illness polyneuropathy (CIP) [155,156]. SIRS includes two or more of the following clinical manifestations: (1) a body temperature of $>38\,°C$ or $<36\,°C$; (2) heart rate of >90 beats/min; (3) tachypnea, as manifested by a respiratory rate of >20 breaths/min or hyperventilation, as indicated by a $PaCO_2$ of <32 torr; and (4) an alteration of the white blood cell count of $>12,000$ cells/mm^3, $<40,000$ cells/mm^3, or the presence of $>10\%$ immature neutrophils (bands) [157]. SIRS occurs in 20–50% of patients in major Intensive Care Units (ICUs) [158]. The pathophysiology is uncertain but presumed to relate to the same defect that affects all organ systems in critical illness [156]. Number of days in the intensive care unit, increasing blood glucose, and decreasing serum albumin, correlate with decreasing peripheral nerve function [156]. Recent studies of CIP have demonstrated that the peripheral nerves are depolarized and that the membrane depolarization may relate to endoneurial hyperkalemia and/or hypoxia [159].

CIP is often preceded by a septic encephalopathy, which is an early neurological complication of sepsis [160]. It is usually first recognized as difficulty in weaning from the ventilator as the septic encephalopathy improves. It can be difficult to recognize the neuropathy because of technical issues in performing a sensory examination in a patient with an altered level of consciousness [161].

EDX is important in the evaluation of CIP. Often there is a reduction in compound muscle action potential (CMAP) and sensory nerve action potential (SNAP) amplitudes, usually without significant slowing of conduction velocities or prolongation of distal latencies [162]. The interpretation of the motor and sensory responses can be technically challenging in the ICU patient due to lower extremity edema and cold body temperatures. The polyneuropathy may be not identified in up to 50% of patients, in part because the patient infrequently complains of neuropathic symptoms and EDX testing in the ICU is technically challenging [156].

The improvement in neuropathy is first noted by improvement in limb strength, although reappearance of reflexes is the most objective sign. Improvement occurs first in the upper limbs and proximal lower limbs, followed by the respiratory system, and later the distal lower limbs [162]. EDX often normalize

6 months to 1 year after diagnosis [162]. Nerve biopsy demonstrates loss of fibers and active degeneration without inflammation [162].

CIP may coexist with critical illness myopathy (CIM). On EDX in CIM, the CMAP's often demonstrate increased duration with low amplitude. The needle examination may show abnormal spontaneous activity and short duration motor unit potentials with rapid recruitment. If the patient is not able to voluntarily activate the muscle, direct muscle stimulation may help in differentiating between CIP and CIM (CIM demonstrates no activation with direct muscle stimulation) [163].

Drugs, toxins, and vitamin and mineral deficiencies

Many drugs in clinical practice are known to be associated with the development of neuropathy (Table 11.6) and will not be specifically discussed here. Most of these drugs cause dose-related axonal dysfunction.

Alcohol

The prevalence of neuropathy in alcohol use is uncertain, however, one study prospectively identified neuropathy in 58% of alcoholics, and the incidence

Table 11.6 Some medications that may be associated with neuropathy

Amiodarone
Bortezomib
Chloroquine
Cisplatinum
Colchicine
Dapsone
Disulfiram
Hydralazine
Isoniazid
Metronidazole
Nucleoside-analog reverse-transcriptase inhibitors
Perhexiline
Phenytoin
Propafenone
Pyridoxine
Taxanes—paclitaxel and docetaxel
Thalidomide
Vincristine

correlated with age of the patient and the duration of alcohol use [164]. The pathophysiology is uncertain but the direct toxic effect of alcohol on peripheral nerves seems to be the most important etiology [164].

Alcoholic neuropathy has a similar phenotype to other metabolic neuropathies. The neuropathy is often distal, symmetrical, pure sensory or sensory predominant, and slowly progressive. There are often positive neuropathic sensory symptoms such as tingling, pain and/or burning, as well as loss of nociceptive sensation.

There is no specific laboratory test to make the diagnosis of alcoholic neuropathy. One study demonstrated 47% of alcohol-dependent patients with neuropathy had macrocytosis compared with 7% of alcohol-dependent patients without neuropathy [164]. A higher incidence of liver dysfunction and elevated blood sugars occurred in those with neuropathy [164]. Patients should be evaluated for other vitamin deficiencies or causes of malnutrition, as alcohol neuropathy often coexists with neuropathy due to thiamine deficiency [165].

Cobalamin (vitamin B12)

Cobalamin deficiency is a common problem, especially in people older than 60 years where the prevalence is up to 15% [166]. The most common cause of cobalamin deficiency is pernicious anemia. Other causes include dietary avoidance (vegetarians), gastric bypass surgery, gastrectomy, and nitrous oxide abuse. In a cohort of patients undergoing evaluation for neuropathy, cobalamin deficiency was found in 8% [167].

The neuropathy associated with cobalamin deficiency can be very similar to other metabolic neuropathies, with an insidious onset of distal symmetric numbness and paresthesias. However, a large percentage of patients actually present with sudden onset, painless, non-length-dependent symptoms [167]. This may be due to the concurrent development of a myelopathy. The development of sensory symptoms solely in the hands, or in the hands and feet at the same time, is not uncommon in cobalamin-deficiency neuropathy with or without myelopathy.

The evaluation of cobalamin deficiency should include a serum B12 level. In those with a low-normal level, for example, less than 300 pg/mL, further testing with homocysteine and methylmalonic acid should be carried out, as 5–10% will demonstrate characteristic elevations suggestive of cobalamin deficiency. Treatment of cobalamin deficiency consists of prompt parenteral administration of vitamin B12.

Thiamine (vitamin B1)

Thiamine (vitamin B1) deficiency most commonly occurs in chronic alcohol abuse, chronic gastrointestinal problems (including recurrent vomiting and other malnourished states, such as in patients receiving total parenteral nutrition, cancer patients and the elderly), and following weight-reduction surgery (i.e., bariatric surgery) [168]. Severe deficiency causes congestive heart failure (wet beriberi), peripheral neuropathy (dry beriberi), Wernicke's encephalopathy, and Korsakoff's syndrome.

Neuropathy associated with thiamine deficiency may present with acute onset or insidiously, with distal, symmetric, sensory or sensorimotor neuropathy with positive neuropathic sensory symptoms (i.e., prickling, tingling, pain, allodynia) [169]. Thiamine deficient patients have more large fiber involvement including weakness, numbness, and loss of balance, rather than small fiber impairment, in contrast to alcoholic neuropathy [165]. Patients with thiamine deficiency may also complain of fatigue, irritability. and muscle cramps that develop within days to weeks of nutritional deficiency [168].

Neuropathy due to thiamine deficiency should be especially considered in patients following bariatric surgery. Patients most likely to develop neuropathy following gastric bypass surgery are those with risk factors for malnutrition, including extreme weight loss, rapid weight loss, postoperative nausea and vomiting, and lack of nutrition counseling [169]. In a large series of patients who underwent weight-reduction surgery, approximately 6% developed neuropathy, and in some of these cases it appeared that nutritional deficiency, including thiamine deficiency, was pathogenic [169].

High-performance liquid chromatography (HPLC) analysis of whole blood thiamine is the most sensitive, specific, and precise method for determining the nutritional status of thiamine and is a reliable indicator of total body stores [170]. As discussed in Chapter 3, however, treatment for possible thiamine deficiency should not await results of laboratory testing and should include emergent parenteral administration of thiamine.

Five things to remember about peripheral nerve disorders in systemic disease

1. Diabetes is the most common cause of peripheral neuropathy. Abnormalities on electrodiagnostic testing precede symptoms of neuropathy. This presents with a progressive, distal, and symmetric sensorimotor neuropathy.

2. Systemic vasculitides are an important cause of peripheral neuropathy and can be associated with morbidity and mortality. The most common presentation is mononeuritis multiplex with associated systemic symptoms. Tissue biopsy is recommended for diagnosis.

3. Monoclonal gammopathies may be associated with peripheral neuropathy, the most frequent of which are IgM kappa. The neuropathy associated with IgM kappa has been described as DADS-M and is often associated with anti-MAG antibodies.

4. HIV is responsible for many different presentations of neuropathy. A distal neuropathy can occur from the disease or the treatment. A polyradiculoneuropathy can occur with seroconversion or coinfection (CMV).

5. A careful review of a patient's medications is necessary as there are many drugs associated with peripheral neuropathy, the most common of which are antineoplastic medications.

References

1 Dyck PJ, Kratz KM, Karnes JL, Litchy WJ, Klein R, Pach JM, et al. The prevalence by staged severity of various types of diabetic neuropathy, retinopathy, and nephropathy in a population-based cohort: the Rochester Diabetic Neuropathy Study. *Neurology* 1993;43(4): 817–824.

2 Pirart J. [Diabetes mellitus and its degenerative complications: a prospective study of 4,400 patients observed between 1947 and 1973 (3rd and last part) (author's transl)]. *Diab. Metab.* 1977;3(4):245–256.

3 Tracy JA, Dyck PJB. The spectrum of diabetic neuropathies. *Phys. Med. Rehab. Clin. N. Am.* 2008;19(1):1–26, v.

4 Dyck PJ, Davies JL, Wilson DM, Service FJ, Melton LJ, 3rd, O'Brien PC. Risk factors for severity of diabetic polyneuropathy: intensive longitudinal assessment of the Rochester Diabetic Neuropathy Study cohort. *Diab. Care.* 1999;22(9):1479–1486.

5 Dyck PJ, O'Brien PC, Litchy WJ, Harper CM, Klein CJ, Dyck PJB. Monotonicity of nerve tests in diabetes: subclinical nerve dysfunction precedes diagnosis of polyneuropathy. *Diab. Care.* 2005;28(9):2192–2200.

6 Casey EB, Le Quesne PM. Digital nerve action potentials in healthy subjects, and in carpal tunnel and diabetic patients. *J. Neurol. Neurosurg. Psychiatr.* 1972;35(5): 612–623.

7 Gilliatt RW, Willison RG. Peripheral nerve conduction in diabetic neuropathy. *J. Neurol. Neurosurg. Psychiatr.* 1962;25:11–18.

8 Dyck PJB, Windebank AJ. Diabetic and nondiabetic lumbosacral radiculoplexus neuropathies: new insights into pathophysiology and treatment. *Muscle Nerve* 2002;25(4):477–491.

9 Dyck PJB, Norell JE, Dyck PJ. Non-diabetic lumbosacral radiculoplexus neuropathy: natural history, outcome and comparison with the diabetic variety. *Brain* 2001;124(Pt 6):1197–1207.

10 Simmons Z, Feldman EL. Update on diabetic neuropathy. *Curr. Opin. Neurol.* 2002;15(5):595–603.

11 Dyck PJB, Norell JE, Dyck PJ. Microvasculitis and ischemia in diabetic lumbosacral radiculoplexus neuropathy. *Neurology* 1999;53(9):2113–2121.

12 Thaisetthawatkul P, Dyck PJB. Treatment of diabetic and nondiabetic lumbosacral radiculoplexus neuropathy. *Curr. Treat. Options Neurol.* 2010;12(2):95–99.

13 Novella SP, Inzucchi SE, Goldstein JM. The frequency of undiagnosed diabetes and impaired glucose tolerance in patients with idiopathic sensory neuropathy. *Muscle Nerve* 2001;24(9):1229–31.

14 Singleton JR, Smith AG, Bromberg MB. Painful sensory polyneuropathy associated with impaired glucose tolerance. *Muscle Nerve* 2001;24(9):1225–1228.

15 Sumner CJ, Sheth S, Griffin JW, Cornblath DR, Polydefkis M. The spectrum of neuropathy in diabetes and impaired glucose tolerance. *Neurology* 2003;60(1):108–111.

16 Hoffman-Snyder C, Smith BE, Ross MA, Hernandez J, Bosch EP. Value of the oral glucose tolerance test in the evaluation of chronic idiopathic axonal polyneuropathy. *Arch. Neurol.* 2006;63(8):1075–1079.

17 Hughes RA, Umapathi T, Gray IA, Gregson NA, Noori M, Pannala AS, et al. A controlled investigation of the cause of chronic idiopathic axonal polyneuropathy. *Brain* 2004;127(Pt 8):1723–1730.

18 Duyff RF, Van den Bosch J, Laman DM, van Loon BJ, Linssen WH. Neuromuscular findings in thyroid dysfunction: a prospective clinical and electrodiagnostic study. *J. Neurol. Neurosurg. Psychiatr.* 2000;68(6): 750–755.

19 Low PA, McLeod JG, Turtle JR, Donnelly P, Wright RG. Peripheral neuropathy in acromegaly. *Brain* 1974;97(1):139–152.

20 Burns TM, Schaublin GA, Dyck PJB. Vasculitic neuropathies. *Neurol. Clin.* 2007;25(1):89–113.

21 Saleh A, Stone JH. Classification and diagnostic criteria in systemic vasculitis. *Best Practice Res.* 2005;19(2): 209–221.

22 Schaublin GA, Michet CJ, Jr., Dyck PJB, Burns TM. An update on the classification and treatment of vasculitic neuropathy. *Lancet Neurol.* 2005;4(12): 853–865.

23 Dyck PJB, Engelsatd J, Dyck PJ. In PJ Dyck and PK Thomas, editors, *Microvasculitis*, 4th ed., 2005.

24 Dyck PJ, Conn DL, Okazaki H. Necrotizing angiopathic neuropathy. Three-dimensional morphology of fiber degeneration related to sites of occluded vessels. *Mayo Clin. Proc.* 1972;47(7):461–475.

25 Collins MP, Periquet MI. Non-systemic vasculitic neuropathy. *Curr. Opin. Neurol.* 2004;17(5):587–98.

26 Said G, Lacroix-Ciaudo C, Fujimura H, Blas C, Faux N. The peripheral neuropathy of necrotizing arteritis: a clinicopathological study. *Ann. Neurol.* 1988;23(5): 461–465.

27 Hattori N, Ichimura M, Nagamatsu M, Li M, Yamamoto K, Kumazawa K, et al. Clinicopathological features of Churg–Strauss syndrome-associated neuropathy. *Brain* 1999;122(Pt 3):427–439.

28 Vital C, Vital A, Canron MH, Jaffre A, Viallard JF, Ragnaud JM, et al. Combined nerve and muscle biopsy in the diagnosis of vasculitic neuropathy. A 16-year retrospective study of 202 cases. *J. Peripher. Nerv. Syst.* 2006;11(1):20–29.

29 Younger DS. Vasculitis of the nervous system. *Curr. Opin. Neurol.* 2004;17(3):317–336.

30 Stone JH. Polyarteritis nodosa. *JAMA* 2002;288 (13):1632–1639.

31 Moore PM, Richardson B. Neurology of the vasculitides and connective tissue diseases. *J. Neurol. Neurosurg. Psychiatr.* 1998;65(1):10–22.

32 Guillevin L, Le Thi Huong D, Godeau P, Jais P, Wechsler B. Clinical findings and prognosis of polyarteritis nodosa and Churg–Strauss angiitis: a study in 165 patients. *Br. J. Rheumatol.* 1988;27(4):258–264.

33 Agard C, Mouthon L, Mahr A, Guillevin L. Microscopic polyangiitis and polyarteritis nodosa: how and when do they start? *Arthritis Rheumatism* 2003;15;49(5): 709–715.

34 Guillevin L, Lhote F, Cohen P, Jarrousse B, Lortholary O, Genereau T, et al. Corticosteroids plus pulse cyclophosphamide and plasma exchanges versus corticosteroids plus pulse cyclophosphamide alone in the treatment of polyarteritis nodosa and Churg–Strauss syndrome patients with factors predicting poor prognosis. A prospective, randomized trial in sixty-two patients. *Arthritis Rheumatism* 1995;38(11): 1638–1645.

35 Guillevin L, Lhote F, Cohen P, Sauvaget F, Jarrousse B, Lortholary O, et al. Polyarteritis nodosa related to hepatitis B virus. A prospective study with long-term observation of 41 patients. *Medicine* 1995;74(5):238–253.

36 Hoffman GS, Kerr GS, Leavitt RY, Hallahan CW, Lebovics RS, Travis WD, et al. Wegener granulomatosis: an analysis of 158 patients. *Ann. Inter. Med.* 1992;116 (6):488–98.

37 Reinhold-Keller E, Beuge N, Latza U, de Groot K, Rudert H, Nolle B, et al. An interdisciplinary approach to the care of patients with Wegener's granulomatosis: long-term outcome in 155 patients. *Arthritis Rheumatism* 2000;43(5):1021–1032.

38 de Groot K, Schmidt DK, Arlt AC, Gross WL, Reinhold-Keller E. Standardized neurologic evaluations of 128 patients with Wegener granulomatosis. *Arch. Neurol.* 2001;58(8):1215–21.

39 Lane SE, Watts RA, Shepstone L, Scott DG. Primary systemic vasculitis: clinical features and mortality. *QJM* 2005;98(2):97–111.

40 Noth I, Strek ME, Leff AR. Churg–Strauss syndrome. *Lancet* 2003;361(9357):587–594.

41 Sehgal M, Swanson JW, DeRemee RA, Colby TV. Neurologic manifestations of Churg–Strauss syndrome. *Mayo Clin. Proc.* 1995;70(4):337–341.

42 Sugiura M, Koike H, Iijima M, Mori K, Hattori N, Katsuno M, et al. Clinicopathologic features of non-systemic vasculitic neuropathy and microscopic polyangiitis-associated neuropathy: a comparative study. *J. Neurol. Sci.* 2006;241(1–2):31–37.

43 Vollertsen RS, Conn DL, Ballard DJ, Ilstrup DM, Kazmar RE, Silverfield JC. Rheumatoid vasculitis: survival and associated risk factors. *Medicine* 1986;65(6): 365–375.

44 Good AE, Christopher RP, Koepke GH, Bender LF, Tarter ME. Peripheral neuropathy associated with rheumatoid arthritis. A clinical and electrodiagnostic study of 70 consecutive rheumatoid arthritis patients. *Ann. Inter. Med.* 1965;63:87–99.

45 Whiting PF, Smidt N, Sterne JA, Harbord R, Burton A, Burke M, et al. Systematic review: accuracy of anticitrullinated peptide antibodies for diagnosing rheumatoid arthritis. *Ann. Inter. Med.* 2010;152(7):456–464; W155–W166.

46 Omdal R, Loseth S, Torbergsen T, Koldingsnes W, Husby G, Mellgren SI. Peripheral neuropathy in systemic lupus erythematosus—a longitudinal study. *Acta Neurol. Scand.* 2001;103(6):386–391.

47 D'Cruz D. Vasculitis in systemic lupus erythematosus. *Lupus* 1998;7(4):270–274.

48 Goransson LG, Tjensvoll AB, Herigstad A, Mellgren SI, Omdal R. Small-diameter nerve fiber neuropathy in systemic lupus erythematosus. *Arch. Neurol.* 2006; 63(3):401–404.

49 Crow MK. In L Goldman and D Auseillo, editors, *Systemic Lupus Erythematosus*, 23rd ed. Philadelphia, WB: Saunders Company, 2007.

50 Kaplan JG, Rosenberg R, Reinitz E, Buchbinder S, Schaumburg HH. Invited review: peripheral neuropathy in Sjogren's syndrome. *Muscle Nerve* 1990;13(7): 570–579.

51 Fujibayashi T, Sugai S, Miyasaka N, Toujou T, Miyawaki S, Ichikawa Y. Revised Japanese diagnostic criteria for Sjogren's syndrome. Annual Report of Research Committee for Immune Disease. Tokyo 1999.

52 Vitali C, Bombardieri S, Jonsson R, Moutsopoulos HM, Alexander EL, Carsons SE, et al. Classification criteria for Sjogren's syndrome: a revised version of the European criteria proposed by the American-European Consensus Group. *Ann. Rheum. Dis.* 2002;61(6): 554–558.

53 Gorson KC, Ropper AH. Positive salivary gland biopsy, Sjogren syndrome, and neuropathy: clinical implications. *Muscle Nerve.* 2003;28(5):553–560.

54 Mori K, Iijima M, Koike H, Hattori N, Tanaka F, Watanabe H, et al. The wide spectrum of clinical manifestations in Sjogren's syndrome-associated neuropathy. *Brain* 2005;128(Pt 11):2518–2534.

55 Dyck PJ. The clinical heterogeneity of immune sensory and autonomic neuropathies with (or without) sicca. *Brain* 2005;128(Pt 11):2480–2482.

56 Mochizuki H, Kamakura K, Masaki T, Hirata A, Nakamura R, Motoyoshi K. Motor dominant neuropathy in Sjogren's syndrome: report of two cases. *Int. Med. (Tokyo, Japan).* 2002;41(2):142–146.

57 Gemignani F, Marbini A, Pavesi G, Di Vittorio S, Manganelli P, Cenacchi G, et al. Peripheral neuropathy associated with primary Sjogren's syndrome. *J. Neurol. Neurosurg. Psychiatry* 1994;57(8):983–986.

58 Gono T, Kawaguchi Y, Katsumata Y, Takagi K, Tochimoto A, Baba S, et al. Clinical manifestations of neurological involvement in primary Sjogren's syndrome. *Clin. Rheumatol* 2011;30(4):485–490.

59 Takahashi Y, Takata T, Hoshino M, Sakurai M, Kanazawa I. Benefit of IVIG for long-standing ataxic sensory neuronopathy with Sjogren's syndrome. IV immunoglobulin. *Neurology* 2003;60(3):503–505.

60 Mellgren SI, Conn DL, Stevens JC, Dyck PJ. Peripheral neuropathy in primary Sjogren's syndrome. *Neurology* 1989;39(3):390–394.

61 Said G, Lacroix C. Primary and secondary vasculitic neuropathy. *J. Neurol.* 2005;252(6):633–641.

62 Hoitsma E, Faber CG, Drent M, Sharma OP. Neurosarcoidosis: a clinical dilemma. *Lancet Neurol.* 2004; 3(7):397–407.

63 Stern BJ, Krumholz A, Johns C, Scott P, Nissim J. Sarcoidosis and its neurological manifestations. *Arch. Neurol.* 1985;42(9):909–917.

64 Colover J. Sarcoidosis with involvement of the nervous system. *Brain* 1948;71:451–475.

65 Oksanen V. Neurosarcoidosis: clinical presentations and course in 50 patients. *Acta Neurol. Scand.* 1986;73(3):283–290.

66 Said G, Lacroix C, Plante-Bordeneuve V, Le Page L, Pico F, Presles O, et al. Nerve granulomas and vasculitis in sarcoid peripheral neuropathy: a clinicopathological study of 11 patients. *Brain* 2002;125(Pt 2):264–275.

67 Burns TM, Dyck PJB, Aksamit AJ, Dyck PJ. The natural history and long-term outcome of 57 limb sarcoidosis neuropathy cases. *J. Neurol. Sci.* 2006;244(1–2):77–87.

68 Hoitsma E, Drent M, Verstraete E, Faber CG, Troost J, Spaans F, et al. Abnormal warm and cold sensation thresholds suggestive of small-fibre neuropathy in sarcoidosis. *Clin. Neurophysiol.* 2003;114(12): 2326–2333.

69 Grossman G. Neurological complications of coeliac disease: what is the evidence? *Practical Neurol.* 2008;8(2):77–89.

70 Branski D, Fasano A, Troncone R. Latest developments in the pathogenesis and treatment of celiac disease. *J. Pediatr.* 2006;149(3):295–300.

71 Chin RL, Sander HW, Brannagan TH, Green PH, Hays AP, Alaedini A, et al. Celiac neuropathy. *Neurology* 2003;60(10):1581–1585.

72 Briani C, Zara G, Alaedini A, Grassivaro F, Ruggero S, Toffanin E, et al. Neurological complications of celiac disease and autoimmune mechanisms: a prospective study. *J. Neuroimmunol.* 2008;195(1–2):171–175.

73 Hadjivassiliou M, Chattopadhyay AK, Davies-Jones GA, Gibson A, Grunewald RA, Lobo AJ. Neuromuscular disorder as a presenting feature of coeliac disease. *J. Neurol. Neurosurg. Psychiatr.* 1997; 63(6):770–775.

74 Rigamonti A, Magi S, Venturini E, Morandi L, Ciano C, Lauria G. Celiac disease presenting with motor neuropathy: effect of gluten free-diet. *Muscle Nerve* 2007;35 (5):675–677.

75 Chin RL, Tseng VG, Green PH, Sander HW, Brannagan TH, 3rd, Latov N. Multifocal axonal polyneuropathy in celiac disease. *Neurology* 2006;66(12):1923–1925.

76 Said G, Boudier L, Selva J, Zingraff J, Drueke T. Different patterns of uremic polyneuropathy: clinicopathologic study. *Neurology* 1983;33(5):567–574.

77 Laaksonen S, Metsarinne K, Voipio-Pulkki LM, Falck B. Neurophysiologic parameters and symptoms in chronic renal failure. *Muscle Nerve* 2002;25(6):884–890.

78 Krishnan AV, Kiernan MC. Uremic neuropathy: clinical features and new pathophysiological insights. *Muscle Nerve* 2007;35(3):273–290.

79 Zochodne DW. In PJ Dyck, PK Thomas, editors, *Neuropathies Associated with Renal Failure, Hepatic Disorders, Chronic Respiratory, and Crtical Illness*, 4th ed. Philadelphia: Elsevier Saunders, 2005.

80 Kyle RA, Therneau TM, Rajkumar SV, Larson DR, Plevak MF, Offord JR, et al. Prevalence of monoclonal gammopathy of undetermined significance. *N. Engl. J. Med.* 2006;354(13):1362–1369.

81 Criteria for the classification of monoclonal gammopathies, multiple myeloma and related disorders: a report of the International Myeloma Working Group. *Br. J. Haematol.* 2003;121(5):749–757.

82 Eurelings M, Lokhorst HM, Kalmijn S, Wokke JH, Notermans NC. Malignant transformation in polyneuropathy associated with monoclonal gammopathy. *Neurology* 2005;64(12):2079–2084.

83 Kyle RA, Therneau TM, Rajkumar SV, Offord JR, Larson DR, Plevak MF, et al. A long-term study of prognosis in monoclonal gammopathy of undetermined significance. *N. Engl. J. Med.* 2002;346(8):564–569.

84 Kyle RA, Therneau TM, Rajkumar SV, Larson DR, Plevak MF, Melton LJ, 3rd. Long-term follow-up of 241 patients with monoclonal gammopathy of undetermined significance: the original Mayo Clinic series 25 years later. *Mayo Clin. Proc.* 2004;79(7):859–866.

85 Rajkumar SV, Kyle RA, Therneau TM, Melton LJ, 3rd, Bradwell AR, Clark RJ, et al. Serum free light chain ratio is an independent risk factor for progression in monoclonal gammopathy of undetermined significance. *Blood* 2005;106(3):812–817.

86 Ropper AH, Gorson KC. Neuropathies associated with paraproteinemia. *N. Engl. J. Med.* 1998;338(22):1601–1607.

87 Latov N. Pathogenesis and therapy of neuropathies associated with monoclonal gammopathies. *Ann. Neurol.* 1995;37(Suppl 1):S32–S42.

88 Kelly JJ, Jr., Kyle RA, Miles JM, O'Brien PC, Dyck PJ. The spectrum of peripheral neuropathy in myeloma. *Neurology* 1981;31(1):24–31.

89 Mauermann ML, Burns TM. The evaluation of chronic axonal polyneuropathies. *Semin. Neurol.* 2008;28(2):133–151.

90 Rajkumar SV, Gertz MA, Kyle RA. Prognosis of patients with primary systemic amyloidosis who present with dominant neuropathy. *Am. J. Med.* 1998;104(3):232–237.

91 Gertz MA, Rajkumar SV. Primary systemic amyloidosis. *Curr. Treat. Options Oncol.* 2002;3(3):261–271.

92 Gertz MA, Merlini G, Treon SP. Amyloidosis and Waldenstrom's macroglobulinemia. *Hematology (Am. Soc. Hematol. Educ. Program)* 2004:257–282.

93 Kelly JJ, Jr., Kyle RA, O'Brien PC, Dyck PJ. The natural history of peripheral neuropathy in primary systemic amyloidosis. *Ann. Neurol.* 1979;6(1):1–7.

94 Sadek I, Mauermann ML, Hayman SR, Spinner RJ, Gertz MA. Primary systemic amyloidosis presenting with asymmetric multiple mononeuropathies. *J. Clin. Oncol.* 2010;28(25):e429–32.

95 Tracy JA, Dyck PJB, Dyck PJ. Primary amyloidosis presenting as upper limb multiple mononeuropathies. *Muscle Nerve* 2010; 41(5):710–715.

96 Ladha SS, Dyck PJB, Spinner RJ, Perez DG, Zeldenrust SR, Amrami KK, et al. Isolated amyloidosis presenting with lumbosacral radiculoplexopathy: description of two cases and pathogenic review. *J. Peripher. Nerv. Syst.* 2006;11(4):346–352.

97 Antoine JC, Baril A, Guettier C, Barral FG, Bady B, Convers P, et al. Unusual amyloid polyneuropathy with predominant lumbosacral nerve roots and plexus involvement. *Neurology* 1991;41(2 (Pt 1)):206–208.

98 Traynor AE, Gertz MA, Kyle RA. Cranial neuropathy associated with primary amyloidosis. *Ann. Neurol.* 1991;29(4):451–454.

99 Kyle RA. Sequence of testing for monoclonal gammopathies. *Arch. Pathol. Lab. Med.* 1999;123(2):114–118.

100 Kyle RA. Monoclonal gammopathy of undetermined significance (MGUS): a review. *Clin. Haematol.* 1982;11(1):123–150.

101 Kissel JT, Mendell JR, Neuropathies associated with monoclonal gammopathies. *Neuromuscul. Disord.* 1996;6(1):3–18.

102 Bataille R, Harousseau JL. Multiple myeloma. *N. Engl. J. Med.* 1997;336(23):1657–1664.

103 Chaudhry V, Cornblath DR, Polydefkis M, Ferguson A, Borrello I. Characteristics of bortezomib- and thalidomide-induced peripheral neuropathy. *J. Peripher. Nerv Syst.* 2008;13(4):275–282.

104 Plasmati R, Pastorelli F, Cavo M, Petracci E, Zamagni E, Tosi P, et al. Neuropathy in multiple myeloma treated with thalidomide: a prospective study. *Neurology* 2007;69(6):573–581.

105 Mohty B, El-Cheikh J, Yakoub-Agha I, Moreau P, Harousseau JL, Mohty M. Peripheral neuropathy and new treatments for multiple myeloma: background and practical recommendations. *Haematologica* 2010; 95(2):311–319.

106 Dispenzieri A. POEMS syndrome. *Blood Rev.* 2007;21(6):285–299.

107 Kelly JJ, Jr., Kyle RA, Miles JM, Dyck PJ. Osteosclerotic myeloma and peripheral neuropathy. *Neurology* 1983;33(2):202–210.

108 Mauermann ML, Sorenson EJ, Dispenzieri A, Mandrekar J, Suarez GA, Dyck PJ, Dyck PJB. Uniform demyelination and more severe axonal loss distinguish POEMS syndrome from CIDP. *J. Neurol. Neurosurg. Psychiatr.* 2012;83(5):480–6.

109 Baehring JM, Damek D, Martin EC, Betensky RA, Hochberg FH. Neurolymphomatosis. *Neuro-oncol.* 2003;5(2):104–115.

110 Taghavi V, Dyck PJB, Spinner RJ, Amrami KK, Kurtin PJ, Engelsatd J, et al. Clinical and neuropathological characteristics of peripheral nerve lymphoma. *J. Peripher. Nerv. Syst.* 2007;12(Supp):85.

111 Dalmau J, Graus F, Rosenblum MK, Posner JB. Anti-Hu-associated paraneoplastic encephalomyelitis/sensory neuronopathy. A clinical study of 71 patients. *Med. (Balt.)* 1992;71(2):59–72.

112 Camdessanche JP, Antoine JC, Honnorat J, Vial C, Petiot P, Convers P, et al. Paraneoplastic peripheral neuropathy associated with anti-Hu antibodies. A clinical and electrophysiological study of 20 patients. *Brain* 2002;125(Pt 1):166–175.

113 Oh SJ, Gurtekin Y, Dropcho EJ, King P, Claussen GC. Anti-Hu antibody neuropathy: a clinical, electrophysiological, and pathological study. *Clin. Neurophysiol.* 2005;116(1):28–34.

114 Lucchinetti CF, Kimmel DW, Lennon VA. Paraneoplastic and oncologic profiles of patients seropositive for type 1 antineuronal nuclear autoantibodies. *Neurology* 1998;50(3):652–657.

115 Amato AA, Collins MP. Neuropathies associated with malignancy. *Semin. Neurol.* 1998;18(1):125–144.

116 Yu Z, Kryzer TJ, Griesmann GE, Kim K, Benarroch EE, Lennon VA. CRMP-5 neuronal autoantibody: marker of lung cancer and thymoma-related autoimmunity. *Ann. Neurol.* 2001;49(2):146–154.

117 Graus F, Keime-Guibert F, Rene R, Benyahia B, Ribalta T, Ascaso C, et al. Anti-Hu-associated paraneoplastic encephalomyelitis: analysis of 200 patients. *Brain* 2001;124(Pt 6):1138–1148.

118 Molinuevo JL, Graus F, Serrano C, Rene R, Guerrero A, Illa I. Utility of anti-Hu antibodies in the diagnosis of paraneoplastic sensory neuropathy. *Ann. Neurol.* 1998;44(6):976–980.

119 Pittock SJ, Kryzer TJ, Lennon VA. Paraneoplastic antibodies coexist and predict cancer, not neurological syndrome. *Ann. Neurol.* 2004;56(5):715–719.

120 Antoine JC, Cinotti L, Tilikete C, Bouhour F, Camdessanche JP, Confavreux C, et al. [18F]fluorodeoxyglucose positron emission tomography in the diagnosis of cancer in patients with paraneoplastic neurological

syndrome and anti-Hu antibodies. *Ann. Neurol.* 2000;48(1):105–108.

121 Rees JH, Hain SF, Johnson MR, Hughes RA, Costa DC, Ell PJ, et al. The role of [18F]fluoro-2-deoxyglucose-PET scanning in the diagnosis of paraneoplastic neurological disorders. *Brain* 2001;124(Pt 11):2223–2231.

122 Authier FJ, Bassez G, Payan C, Guillevin L, Pawlotsky JM, Degos JD, et al. Detection of genomic viral RNA in nerve and muscle of patients with HCV neuropathy. *Neurology* 2003;60(5):808–812.

123 Ferri C, La Civita L, Cirafisi C, Siciliano G, Longombardo G, Bombardieri S, et al. Peripheral neuropathy in mixed cryoglobulinemia: clinical and electrophysiologic investigations. *J. Rheumatol.* 1992;19(6):889–895.

124 Santoro L, Manganelli F, Briani C, Giannini F, Benedetti L, Vitelli E, et al. Prevalence and characteristics of peripheral neuropathy in hepatitis C virus population. *J. Neurol. Neurosurg. Psychiatr.* 2006;77(5):626–629.

125 Nemni R, Sanvito L, Quattrini A, Santuccio G, Camerlingo M, Canal N. Peripheral neuropathy in hepatitis C virus infection with and without cryoglobulinaemia. *J. Neurol. Neurosurg. Psychiatr.* 2003;74(9):1267–1271.

126 Apartis E, Leger JM, Musset L, Gugenheim M, Cacoub P, Lyon-Caen O, et al. Peripheral neuropathy associated with essential mixed cryoglobulinaemia: a role for hepatitis C virus infection? *J. Neurol. Neurosurg. Psychiatr.* 1996;60(6):661–666.

127 Zaltron S, Puoti M, Liberini P, Antonini L, Quinzanini M, Manni M, et al. High prevalence of peripheral neuropathy in hepatitis C virus infected patients with symptomatic and asymptomatic cryoglobulinaemia. *Ital. J. Gastroenterol. Hepatol.* 1998;30(4):391–395.

128 Lauer GM, Walker BD. Hepatitis C virus infection. *N. Engl. J. Med.* 2001;345(1):41–52.

129 Kallemuchikkal U, Gorevic PD. Evaluation of cryoglobulins. *Arch. Pathol. Lab. Med.* 1999;123(2):119–125.

130 Ooi WW, Srinivasan J. Leprosy and the peripheral nervous system: basic and clinical aspects. *Muscle Nerve* 2004;30(4):393–409.

131 Thomas PK. Tropical neuropathies. *J. Neurol.* 1997;244 (8):475–482.

132 Chad DA, Hedley-Whyte ET. Case records of the Massachusetts General Hospital. Weekly clinico-pathological exercises. Case 1-2004. A 49-year-old woman with asymmetric painful neuropathy. *N. Engl. J. Med.* 2004;350(2):166–176.

133 Verma A. Epidemiology and clinical features of HIV-1 associated neuropathies. *J. Peripher. Nerv. Syst.* 2001;6 (1):8–13.

134 Greenwald JL, Burstein GR, Pincus J, Branson B. A rapid review of rapid HIV antibody tests. *Curr. Infect. Dis. Rep.* 2006;8(2):125–131.

135 Dalakas MC. Peripheral neuropathy and antiretroviral drugs. *J. Peripher. Nerv. Syst.* 2001;6(1):14–20.

136 Brew BJ. The peripheral nerve complications of human immunodeficiency virus (HIV) infection. *Muscle Nerve* 2003;28(5):542–552.

137 Brannagan TH, III, McAlarney T, Latov N. In N Latov, JH Wokke, JJ Kelly, Jr., editors, *Peripheral Neuropathy in HIV-1 Infection*, Cambridge, UK: Cambridge University Press, 1998.

138 Roullet E, Assuerus V, Gozlan J, Ropert A, Said G, Baudrimont M, et al. Cytomegalovirus multifocal neuropathy in AIDS: analysis of 15 consecutive cases. *Neurology* 1994;44(11):2174–2182.

139 Ferrari S, Vento S, Monaco S, Cavallaro T, Cainelli F, Rizzuto N, et al. Human immunodeficiency virus-associated peripheral neuropathies. *Mayo Clin. Proc.* 2006;81(2):213–219.

140 Chahin N, Temesgen Z, Kurtin PJ, Spinner RJ, Dyck PJB. HIV lumbosacral radiculoplexus neuropathy mimicking lymphoma: diffuse infiltrative lymphocytosis syndrome (DILS) restricted to nerve? *Muscle Nerve* 2010; 41(2):276–282.

141 Piradov MA, Pirogov VN, Popova LM, Avdunina IA. Diphtheritic polyneuropathy: clinical analysis of severe forms. *Arch. Neurol.* 2001;58(9):1438–1442.

142 Logina I, Donaghy M. Diphtheritic polyneuropathy: a clinical study and comparison with Guillain–Barre syndrome. *J. Neurol. Neurosurg. Psychiatr.* 1999;67(4): 433–438.

143 Steere AC. Lyme disease. *N. Engl. J. Med.* 2001;345 (2):115–125.

144 Halperin JJ. Nervous system Lyme disease. *Infect. Dis. Clin. N. Am.* 2008;22(2):261–274, vi.

145 Pachner AR, Steere AC. The triad of neurologic manifestations of Lyme disease: meningitis, cranial neuritis, and radiculoneuritis. *Neurology* 1985;35(1):47–53.

146 Halperin J, Luft BJ, Volkman DJ, Dattwyler RJ. Lyme neuroborreliosis. Peripheral nervous system manifestations. *Brain* 1990;113(Pt 4):1207–1221.

147 Thaisetthawatkul P, Logigian EL. Peripheral nervous system manifestations of lyme borreliosis. *J. Clin. Neuromusc. Dis.* 2002;3(4):165–171.

148 Elamin M, Alderazi Y, Mullins G, Farrell MA, O'Connell S, Counihan TJ. Perineuritis in acute lyme neuroborreliosis. *Muscle Nerve* 2009;39(6):851–854.

149 Halperin JJ. Lyme disease and the peripheral nervous system. *Muscle Nerve* 2003;28(2):133–143.

150 Adams C, August CS, Maguire H, Sladky JT. Neuromuscular complications of bone marrow transplantation. *Pediatr. Neurol.* 1995;12(1):58–61.

151 Amato AA, Barohn RJ, Sahenk Z, Tutschka PJ, Mendell JR, Polyneuropathy complicating bone marrow and solid organ transplantation. *Neurology* 1993;43(8): 1513–1518.

152 Wen PY, Alyea EP, Simon D, Herbst RS, Soiffer RJ, Antin JH. Guillain–Barre syndrome following allogeneic bone marrow transplantation. *Neurology* 1997;49 (6):1711–1714.

153 Rodriguez V, Kuehnle I, Heslop HE, Khan S, Krance RA. Guillain–Barre syndrome after allogeneic hematopoietic stem cell transplantation. *Bone Marrow Transpl.* 2002;29(6):515–517.

154 El-Sabrout RA, Radovancevic B, Ankoma-Sey V, Van Buren CT. Guillain–Barre syndrome after solid organ transplantation. *Transplantation* 2001;71(9):1311–1316.

155 Leijten FS, De Weerd AW, Poortvliet DC, De Ridder VA, Ulrich C, Harink-De Weerd JE. Critical illness polyneuropathy in multiple organ dysfunction syndrome and weaning from the ventilator. *Intensive Care Med.* 1996;22(9):856–861.

156 Witt NJ, Zochodne DW, Bolton CF, Grand'Maison F, Wells G, Young GB, et al. Peripheral nerve function in sepsis and multiple organ failure. *Chest* 1991; 99(1):176–184.

157 American College of Chest Physicians/Society of Critical Care Medicine Consensus Conference: definitions for sepsis and organ failure and guidelines for the use of innovative therapies in sepsis. *Crit. Care Med.* 1992; 20(6):864–874.

158 Tran DD, Groeneveld AB, van der Meulen J, Nauta JJ, Strack van Schijndel RJ, Thijs LG. Age, chronic disease, sepsis, organ system failure, and mortality in a medical intensive care unit. *Crit. Care Med.* 1990;18(5): 474–479.

159 Z'Graggen WJ, Lin CS, Howard RS, Beale RJ, Bostock H. Nerve excitability changes in critical illness polyneuropathy. *Brain* 2006;129(Pt 9):2461–2470.

160 Bolton CF, Young GB, Zochodne DW. The neurological complications of sepsis. *Ann. Neurol.* 1993;33(1):94–100.

161 Bolton CF. Neuromuscular manifestations of critical illness. *Muscle Nerve* 2005;32(2):140–163.

162 Zochodne DW, Bolton CF, Wells GA, Gilbert JJ, Hahn AF, Brown JD, et al. Critical illness polyneuropathy. A complication of sepsis and multiple organ failure. *Brain* 1987;110(Pt 4):819–841.

163 Rich MM, Bird SJ, Raps EC, McCluskey LF, Teener JW. Direct muscle stimulation in acute quadriplegic myopathy. *Muscle Nerve* 1997;20(6):665–673.

164 Zambelis T, Karandreas N, Tzavellas E, Kokotis P, Liappas J. Large and small fiber neuropathy in chronic alcohol-dependent subjects. *J. Peripher. Nerv. Syst.* 2005;10(4):375–381.

165 Koike H, Iijima M, Sugiura M, Mori K, Hattori N, Ito H, et al. Alcoholic neuropathy is clinicopathologically

distinct from thiamine-deficiency neuropathy. *Ann. Neurol.* 2003;54(1):19–29.

166 Lindenbaum J, Rosenberg IH, Wilson PW, Stabler SP, Allen RH. Prevalence of cobalamin deficiency in the Framingham elderly population. *Am. J. Clin. Nutr.* 1994;60(1):2–11.

167 Saperstein DS, Wolfe GI, Gronseth GS, Nations SP, Herbelin LL, Bryan WW, et al. Challenges in the identification of cobalamin-deficiency polyneuropathy. *Arch. Neurol.* 2003;60(9):1296–1301.

168 Saperstein DS, Barohn RJ. In PJ Dyck, PK Thomas, editors, *Polyneuropathy Caused by Nutritional and Vitamin Deficiency*, 4th ed. Philadelphia: Elsevier Saunders, 2005.

169 Thaisetthawatkul P, Collazo-Clavell ML, Sarr MG, Norell JE, Dyck PJB. A controlled study of peripheral neuropathy after bariatric surgery. *Neurology* 2004; 63(8):1462–1470.

170 Herve C, Beyne P, Letteron P, Delacoux E. *Comparison of erythrocyte transketolase activity with thiamine and thiamine phosphate ester levels in chronic alcoholic patients.* Clin. Chim. Acta; Int. J. Clin. Chem. 1995;234(1–2):91–100.

12 Neuromuscular junction disorders due to systemic disease

Jaffar Khan
Emory University School of Medicine, Atlanta, GA, USA

Introduction

The neuromuscular junction plays an important role in coupling electrical and chemical communication for the purpose of, among many functions, producing muscle contraction and volitional movement. In order to understand the pathophysiology underlying defective neuromuscular transmission, one must fully comprehend the normal function of the NMJ. The NMJ consists of a presynaptic nerve terminal of the motor neuron and a postsynaptic muscle membrane that are separated by a very small space, the synaptic cleft. Initiation of the NMJ process begins with the arrival of an action potential at the nerve terminal that depolarizes and opens transmembrane voltage-gated calcium channels, allowing the influx of calcium ions into the cytosol of the presynaptic nerve terminal. As intracytosolic calcium concentration rises, vesicles of immediately available Ach fuse in specialized regions of the presynaptic membrane, called active zones, and exocytose their contents into the synaptic cleft. Once in the synaptic cleft, Ach is able to freely bind to Ach-receptors on the postsynaptic muscle membrane and result in depolarizing end-plate potentials (EPPS). If enough EPPs are generated, and the postsynaptic membrane reaches threshold, an action potential is generated. At this point, communication across the NMJ is complete and successful muscle contraction ensues.

This chapter begins with a discussion of myasthenia gravis, the prototypical and most common disorder of the NMJ, to provide an underpinning to the discussion that follows on the association of systemic diseases with NMJ disorders.

Myasthenia gravis

Myasthenia gravis (MG) is the most common disease of the NMJ; the prevalence of MG is 20 cases per 100,000 people, with an overall female to male ratio of 2:1 [1]. However, this ratio approaches 1:1 at ages greater than 60, and in the very elderly the prevalence is slightly higher among men as compared with age-matched women. Review of epidemiologic studies of myasthenia gravis suggests that the incidence is increasing in patients over the age of 50 and that the increase cannot be explained by improved recognition of disease or improved diagnostic testing alone [2,3]. Additional factors include improved treatment resulting in patients living longer with the MG, as well as the longer life span of the general population, resulting in an increase in the pool of patients susceptible to developing myasthenia gravis [4].

The antigenic target of myasthenia gravis is the Ach receptor on the postsynaptic membrane. Due to a breakdown in the process of T-cell immunotolerance, a process that should protect against the development of autoantibodies, antibodies against Ach-receptors

Neurological Disorders due to Systemic Disease, First Edition. Edited by Steven L. Lewis.
© 2013 Blackwell Publishing Ltd. Published 2013 by Blackwell Publishing Ltd.

expressed on myogenic cells in the thymus are produced [5]. Induction of autoantibodies from exposure to virus, such as cytomegalovirus and poliovirus, has also been suggested as a mechanism for the production of self-reactive T-cells [6,7].

Ach-receptor antibodies bind to acetylcholine receptors on the postsynaptic membrane of the NMJ and induce a complement-mediated attack against the receptors. This process results in a reduction of the total number of receptors available to bind Ach once released from the presynaptic nerve terminal, thereby reducing the ability of the postsynaptic membrane to reach the electrical threshold required for action-potential generation. Additionally, the architecture of the postsynaptic membrane undergoes a morphologic change. Instead of the complex infolding of the postsynaptic membrane, thought to allow for a greater surface area for the Ach-receptors to cluster in the normal state, the membrane folds are simplified and provide less surface area to which Ach can interact with the receptors. The net effect of these changes in the postsynaptic membrane is failure of the muscle fiber to contract, which results in the clinical manifestation of weakness [8].

The presenting complaint of a patient with MG is muscle weakness, and the clinical hallmark of MG is neuromuscular fatigue, with weakness occurring upon repetitive use of a muscle or group of muscles. The weakness resolves upon resting symptomatic muscles. In the generalized form of MG, symptoms and signs of weakness are more common in proximal greater than distal muscles. Patients may report difficulty in performing tasks mediated by proximal muscle groups, such as washing hair, reaching for objects above the head, climbing stairs, or rising from chairs. Additionally slurred speech, as well as difficulty chewing and swallowing may occur. Weakness of extraocular muscles is common, and patients often report fluctuating eyelid droop and intermittent diplopia. On examination, ptosis, ophthalmoparesis, and weakness of facial expression are often present in symptomatic patients. Patients may exhibit weakness of the shoulders and hips with sparing of the intrinsic muscles of the hands and feet. Muscle-stretch reflexes are usually spared and the sensory examination is normal. In contrast to botulism, the pupils are spared in MG.

Many patients are asymptomatic at the time of evaluation and have a normal neurologic examination.

In these patients, the induction of weakness with sustained muscle contraction should be attempted. This can be accomplished by assessing for ptosis and ophthalmoparesis after having the patient sustain eye gaze superiorly for 1–2 min, as well as checking muscle strength before and after having the patient hold the arms in an abducted position for several minutes.

A life-threatening consequence of MG occurs when weakness of the diaphragm and accessory respiratory muscles result in respiratory failure (myasthenic crisis). In contrast to generalized MG, ocular MG results in isolated weakness of the eyelids and ocular motility. At the onset of symptoms, patients with ocular MG are indistinguishable from those with generalized MG. However if after 2 years, signs and symptoms of MG remain isolated to the ocular musculature, generalized MG is unlikely to develop [9].

Do to relative ease and patient comfort, a reasonable first step in confirming a clinical diagnosis of MG is to assess for autoantibodies in the serum. Autoantibodies are detected in up to 90% of patients with MG. The majority, approximately 80%, of all patients with MG have antibodies to the Ach-receptor on the postsynaptic membrane of the NMJ [10]. In most cases, the detection of Ach-receptor antibodies in serum is enough to confirm the diagnosis of MG. Approximately 40% of patients without detectable Ach-receptor antibodies (sero-negative MG) will have antibodies against muscle-specific tyrosine kinase (MuSK), a protein responsible for grouping Ach-receptors together on the postsynaptic membrane [11].

Neurophysiologic testing offers another relatively easily attained method for immediate confirmation of the diagnosis [12]. Standard motor and sensory nerve conduction responses and electromyography are commonly unrevealing; however, repetitive nerve stimulation (RNS) can be helpful. In MG, supramaximal nerve stimulation at slow, 2–3 Hz, rates may result in the electrical hallmark of a gradual decrement in the amplitude of the compound muscle action potential. This decrement correlates with a progressive drop in the number of muscle fibers contracting with subsequent stimulations. A 10% decrement in amplitude of the fourth or fifth motor response compared with the first is suggestive of MG. The median, ulnar, spinal accessory, and facial nerve are commonly selected for testing. However, proximal muscle testing has a higher sensitivity for displaying the classic decremental response as compared with distal muscles. Unfortunately, proximal nerve stimulation of the face and neck are poorly tolerated, and prone to movement artifact which may limit the interpretation of the results. Lastly, single fiber electromyography (SFEMG) is a neurophysiologic technique that compares the latency difference of action-potential generation between two muscle fibers in the same motor unit [13]. This difference, referred to as "jitter," is present to a small degree in normal muscles, but when jitter is abnormally increased, an underlying defect in neuromuscular transmission is suggested. In extreme cases, one of the muscles fibers in the pair may fail to fire, a process referred to as "blocking." Similar to jitter, blocking correlates highly with the presence of defective neuromuscular transmission.

A gratifying feature of MG is that most patients respond very well to treatment, which includes both symptomatic treatment of the weakness and suppression of the immune-mediated attack of Ach-receptors. Acetylcholinesterase inhibitors, of which pyridostigmine is the most commonly used, are used for symptomatic improvement of weakness. This class of medication inactivates acetylcholinesterase, thereby allowing Ach to act at the postsynaptic membrane for a longer period of time. Its rapid onset of action (10–15 min), easy titration, and availability of both short and long-acting formulations, make pyridostigmine an ideal drug for symptomatic management. Several immunomodulatory drugs have been used to suppress the immune-mediated destruction of Ach-receptors and architecture of the post-synaptic membrane. These include prednisone, azathioprine, cyclosporine, and mycophenolate mofetil. Each drug has a distinct profile for onset of clinical response, tolerability, laboratory monitoring, risk of long-term development of cancer, and other adverse effects. As a result, the selection of these drugs should be tailored to the individual patient, and discussed in detail with the patient, before initiating therapy [14].

Plasmapheresis and intravenous immune globulin (IVIg) are excellent treatment options for patients with acute exacerbations of weakness or when initiating other immunomodulatory therapies that have a delayed onset of action. These modalities offer the advantage of having a clinical response in days to weeks; however, the effect is short-lived, ending after several weeks. Overall, plasmapheresis and IVIg are felt to be equivalent in their efficacy, and the clinician should evaluate the risk versus benefits of each therapy, and the clinical characteristics of the patient, when selecting one over the other. Although typically reserved for patients in a myasthenic crisis or those awaiting surgery, intermittent therapy may be provided at weekly or monthly intervals over a defined period of time while observing for a clinical response. The role of thymectomy in patients with MG (with or without thymoma) is discussed below in the section on Systemic Cancer and Paraneoplastic Disorders.

Endocrine disorders

Several reports in the medical literature have cited an association of MG with hyperthyroidism or hypothyroidism [15,16]. Although the exact etiology is not known, it is hypothesized that thyroid hormone may have a direct effect on the function of the neuromuscular junction, or that a common etiology underlies both diseases. The diagnosis of weakness due to MG in the setting of thyroid dysfunction can be difficult due to the concomitant thyrotoxic myopathy. However, the results of neurophysiologic testing (e.g., showing the decremental response seen with MG) can support the diagnosis of defective NMJ transmission. Resolution of the myasthenic symptoms upon normalization of thyroid function serves as additional evidence of an association between the two diseases. As a result, clinical signs and symptoms of thyroid dysfunction, as well as laboratory assessment of thyroid function, should be assessed in all patients with MG.

The association of MG with autoimmune thyroid disease is discussed in the next section.

Systemic autoimmune disorders

Several systemic autoimmune disorders are reported to be associated with MG. These include pernicious anemia, systemic lupus erythematosis, rheumatoid arthritis, and autoimmune thyroid disease. With the exception of autoimmune thyroid disease, a clear-cut increase in the incidence of these diseases in patients with MG has not been found [17]. However, the frequency of autoimmune thyroid disease in patients with MG is approximately 10% and has been reported with both Graves disease and Hashimoto's thyroiditis [18]. Lambert–Eaton Myasthenic syndrome (LEMS) has been reported to occur with systemic autoimmune-mediated diseases including hypothyroidism, pernicious anemia, celiac disease, and juvenile onset diabetes; however, its strongest association is with systemic cancer as described below.

Systemic cancer and paraneoplastic disorders

Thymoma and myasthenia gravis

Thymoma is a rare tumor with a prevalence of 0.15 new cases per 100,000 in the United States [19]. Patients with detectable Ach-receptor antibodies have a high incidence of thymic tissue pathology; however, only the minority (approximately 10%) of patients have thymoma, and the remainder typically have thymic hyperplasia [20]. The incidence of thymoma in patients with MG is equal in males and females with a peak onset of occurrence at the age of 50 [21]. Antibodies to striated muscle highly correlate with the presence of thymoma in both patients with and without MG, however antistriated muscle antibodies are present in up to 50% of patients without thymoma who are over the age of 60 at the onset of disease. As a result, testing for this antibody is better suited to identify thymoma in MG patients with an onset younger than age 60. Patients newly diagnosed with MG should have a CT of the chest to assess for thymoma. The presence of thymoma is an absolute indication for thymectomy due to the tumor's malignant natural history and risk of local invasion into nearby surrounding structures in the thoracic cavity.

In the absence of an associated cancer, thymectomy remains a controversial but widely practiced treatment option for patients with MG. This invasive surgery is usually reserved for select populations of patients. Overall there is enough evidence to recommend thymectomy in noncancer associated MG; however, exactly who should undergo this surgical intervention is not well agreed upon [22]. Factors such as age, sex, and response to conventional therapies are considered with the understanding that, although desired,

remission my not be seen for several years and in many cases may not be achieved at all.

Lambert–Eaton myasthenic syndrome

The LEMS best exemplifies the impact of systemic disease on the neuromuscular junction. LEMS is an autoimmune disorder affecting older men more than women. This syndrome is associated with carcinoma in approximately half of the patients diagnosed [23]. LEMS is most strongly associated with small cell lung cancer (SCLC), although it has also been reported to occur with thymoma, some subtypes of lymphoma, leukemia, and sarcoma, as well as systemic autoimmune-mediated diseases including hypothyroidism, pernicious anemia, celiac disease, and juvenile onset diabetes [24–27].

The underlying pathophysiology in LEMS results from the inability to adequately release Ach from the presynaptic terminal. This process, which is dependent upon an influx of calcium into the presynaptic cytosol, is mediated by opening voltage-gated calcium channels (VGCC) during axon depolarization. The presence of circulating IgG antibodies to the P/Q subunit of the VGCC prevents normal function by binding to the channels and blocking entry of calcium ions into the cytosol at the presynaptic nerve terminal [28,29]. This effectively reduces fusion of Ach vesicles with "active zones" in the presynaptic membrane, thereby reducing exocytosis of Ach into the synaptic cleft. The reduced amount of Ach available to bind to postsynaptic Ach receptors results in reduced number of EPP depolarizations of the postsynaptic membrane, which lessens the likelihood of muscle contraction and volitional strength generation. In addition to this, there is evidence of a second mechanism contributing to the reduction in exocytosis of Ach. The same IgG antibody that blocks calcium entry into the nerve cell is also thought to bind to membrane proteins in the "active zones" of the presynaptic membrane and reduce the number of active zones available for binding of Ach vesicles [30,31]. Subsequently, in LEMS, not only is there a reduction in the entry of calcium ions into the presynaptic nerve terminal, but there is also a reduced number of regions for the Ach vesicles to attach and release their contents into the synaptic cleft. These two mechanisms work together to reduce the total amount of Ach entering the synaptic cleft and available to depolarize the postsynaptic muscle membrane, resulting in the clinical manifestation of weakness. Similar to the VGCC found on the presynaptic membrane of the neuromuscular junction, muscarinic Ach-receptors also contain a P/Q subunit. This explains the signs and symptoms of autonomic dysfunction common to patients with LEMS [32,33].

As with MG, the presenting complaint of LEMS is the insidious development of weakness and muscle fatigue. In conjunction with these difficulties, patients may experience autonomic symptoms of dry mouth, light-headedness, constipation, and impotence [34]. The typical clinical presentation is that of gait dysfunction with reduced or absent muscle stretch reflexes. The examination reveals weakness of the proximal lower extremities more than upper extremities, producing a waddling gait. Extraocular movements, bulbar muscles, and facial strength are commonly unaffected. Respiratory distress is also uncommon. The clinical hallmark of this syndrome is the improvement of strength with continued volitional activity. This is classically demonstrated by Lambert's sign, in which hand strength improves after several seconds of sustained or repetitive gripping [32]. The improvement in strength noted after a very brief period of volitional muscle contraction is directly attributable to the accumulation of calcium within the presynaptic nerve terminal, which augments Ach release into the synaptic cleft, increasing the likelihood of muscle membrane depolarization and subsequent muscle contraction [34]. The same phenomenon underlies the clinical finding of a return or enhancement of muscle stretch reflexes after a brief period of volitional contraction [35]. Due to involvement of the autonomic nervous system, poorly reactive pupils may be seen on examination [24].

Once the diagnosis of LEMS is considered, the presence of anti-VGCC antibodies provides laboratory support for diagnosis and may eliminate the need for additional testing [36]. This IgG antibody is detected in approximately 70–90% of patients with cancer-associated LEMS and is felt to develop from calcium channels expressed on tumor cells [37]. Additional support of the diagnosis can be found with neurophysiologic testing. Routine motor nerve conduction testing reveals normal conduction velocities and distal latencies, however, reduced response amplitudes can be suggestive of the diagnosis, especially when amplitudes increase immediately after

brief volitional exercise of the muscle tested. Additional support is found with repetitive nerve conduction studies. Although LEMS behaves electrophysiologically similar to myasthenia gravis, with a decrement in the motor response amplitude with low-frequency repetitive nerve stimulation, the electrical hallmark of LEMS is the finding of an incremental response of the motor amplitude with fast, 20–50 Hz, repetitive nerve stimulation. The increment is typically greater than 200% and in some cases may be greater than eight times the amplitude of the initial response [24]. With continued stimulation the response may sustain itself for 30 s. This electrical response represents an electrophysiologic correlate to the physical finding of increased strength and enhancement of muscle stretch reflexes after maximal volitional muscle activation. Additional testing includes checking a serum creatine kinase level to exclude the possibility of an inflammatory myopathy.

Once a diagnosis of LEMS is established, a vigilant search for an underlying cancer should occur. When detected, treatment is directed at the etiology of the pathophysiology by removing or medically treating the associated cancer. Since LEMS can occur up to 2 years prior to the detection of cancer, all initial evaluations that do not detect cancer in high-risk patients with a new diagnosis of LEMS should be repeated at frequent intervals, especially in high-risk individuals such as those with a significant smoking history, and the elderly. In patients with cancer-associated LEMS, overall prognosis is dictated by the response to cancer treatment [38].

Symptomatic treatment of LEMS is provided with 3,4-diaminopyridine, a potassium channel blocker, that prolongs action potentials by delaying repolarization [39,40]. This allows for a greater time for calcium to enter the cytosol at the nerve terminus, and augments Ach release. Pyridostigmine can be helpful when used in conjunction with 3,4-diaminopyridine. By reducing the breakdown of Ach in the synaptic cleft, pyridostigmine allows Ach more time to act at the postsynaptic membrane and initiate an action potential. Immunosuppression with prednisone, cyclosporine, azathioprine, methotrexate, or myocophenolate mofetil has been used. However, these agents have resulted in limited success when compared to their use with other immune-mediated diseases. Other possible treatment considerations include plasma exchange and intravenous immunoglobulin. Similar to the other immuno-suppressive therapies, these treatments have limited benefit and are commonly reserved for acute exacerbations. In general, immunosuppressive therapies are now largely reserved for patients who do not respond to symptomatic treatment [41].

Systemic infectious diseases

Botulism

The clinical botulism syndrome is associated with the anaerobic gram-positive bacteria *Clostridium botulinum*. Seven strains of *C. botulinum* exist, serotype A through E, but almost all human cases of botulism are caused by one of three serotypes (A, B, or E) [42]. Botulism may result from either intoxication due to the ingestion of preformed toxin proteins made by the bacteria, or infection due to the ingestion of *C. botulinum spores* or seeding of soft tissue wounds. Five clinical syndromes have been described. These are the classic, infantile, wound, hidden, and inadvertent. The classic form of botulism results from the ingestion of toxin produced by bacteria in contaminated food products. Home-canning, fermenting, inadequate cooking, and food left unrefrigerated for extended periods of time are common sources. While cooking usually denatures preformed toxin, botulinum spores are very heat-resistant and may survive inadequate boiling. The infantile form, the most common of the five, results from the ingestion of spores in contaminated food. This form typically occurs in infants less than 6 months old and is thought to result from an intestine that has not developed the normal flora and pH found in the adult [43]. Both factors create an environment conducive for the growth of *C. botulinum* spores and the production of toxin. Classically, honey has been implicated in the infection of infants [44]. As a result, it is recommended to avoid feeding honey to infants less than 1 year old. In the modern era, wound botulism had been fairly rare; however, a resurgence of cases associated with illicit drug use among heroin and cocaine users has been noted over the last few decades. Abscesses from needle injection or seeding the sinuses from inhalation of cocaine are implicated in the development of wound botulism [45]. Hidden botulism is diagnosed when the evaluation for a typical clinical picture does not reveal evidence of the toxin, spore, or contaminated food product. In contrast to the usual intoxication that occurs in adults, many reports point to this form resulting from the ingestion of spores as in infantile botulism. Inadvertent botulism may occur as an undesired complication of injecting muscles with botulinum toxin to treat neurologic and non-neurologic disease. Diffusion of the toxin away from the target muscle may result in weakness of surrounding muscles. Weakness of oropharyngeal muscles and autonomic dysfunction become unintended consequences of the medical use of botulinum toxin.

The pathophysiologic basis of botulism is that of a presynaptic NMJ disorder. Botulinum toxin enters the presynaptic nerve terminal and prevents the exocytosis of Ach into the synaptic cleft [42]. Similar to the pathophysiology of LEMS, the postsynaptic membrane does not reach its depolarization threshold and fails to initiate an action potential resulting in muscle weakness. The toxin also prevents the release of Ach in the autonomic nervous system and results in prominent autonomic dysfunction.

In classical botulism, symptoms and signs commonly develop within 24 h after ingesting contaminated food. Symptoms begin with diplopia, dysarthria, and dysphagia, followed soon by weakness of the arms and then legs. This pattern of descending weakness is in contrast to the development of weakness with the Guillain–Barre syndrome which is typically described as beginning in the legs and ascending to the arms and craniobulbar region. The neurologic examination reveals oculomotor dysfunction, facial weakness, tongue weakness, and dilatation of the pupils. Flaccid weakness or paralysis of the arms and legs may be prominent, and in severe cases, botulism may result in respiratory compromise. Muscle stretch reflexes may be diminished but are usually retained and augmented by brief volitional exercise of the associated weak muscle. Autonomic symptoms are prominent and result in symptoms of dry mouth, light-headedness, nausea, vomiting, constipation or diarrhea, and accompany clinical signs of pupillary dilatation, tachycardia, and hypotension. The clinical picture of the wound, hidden, and inadvertent forms of botulism are typically indistinguishable from the classic, food-borne form. However, in the infantile form of the disease, constipation, weak cry, and poor suck are early findings; these signs are followed by generalized hypotonia from progressive weakness of the neck, arms, and legs.

219

Confirmation of botulism is obtained through the identification of botulinum spores in stool cultures, or toxin in stool, wound, serum or contaminated food products. When laboratory tests are unrevealing, electrophysiology can be used to demonstrate presynaptic dysfunction of neuromuscular transmission [46]. As in LEMS, classic electrophysiology reveals the augmentation of low motor amplitudes with a single stimulation after brief volitional exercise of a weak muscle, and an incremental response of motor amplitudes with fast rates of repetitive nerve stimulation. In contrast to LEMS, the incremental response may be maintained for several minutes with continued stimulation, and the actual increase in amplitude is not as large. Slow, less than 2–3 Hz, repetitive nerve stimulation results in a similar decremental response noted with MG and LEMS. Sensory nerve responses are normal.

Although several therapies have been proposed, first-line therapy of botulism is largely supportive [47]. These patients should be observed closely, preferably in a critical-care environment with cardiac and respiratory monitoring and appropriate nursing care. Intubation and mechanical ventilation should be provided promptly in the event of impending respiratory failure. With appropriate supportive care, recovery over several weeks is expected. When found, wounds suspected of harboring the bacteria should be surgically drained, debrided, and treated with antibiotics. In a recent Cochrane review examining the medical therapies of all forms of botulism, the literature only provided good evidence to support the use of human-derived immune globulin for the infantile form [48]. There was no evidence to support or refute other therapies for botulism, including equine serum trivalent botulism antitoxin, human-derived botulinum immune globulin, plasma exchange, 3,4-diaminopyridine, and guanidine. Until further investigation is completed, these therapies should be viewed as experimental. Lastly, any case of botulism suspected to result from exposure at a restaurant or other public event should be reported to the local health department in order to prevent the development of a possible epidemic.

Drugs and toxins

Medications

Many drugs are associated with the development of neuromuscular fatigue. This occurs by multiple mechanisms. Drugs may induce the development of Ach-receptor antibodies, augment defective neuromuscular transmission in patients with MG, or unmask MG in clinically asymptomatic MG. Most of these drugs are known to interfere with neuromuscular transmission and worsen symptoms in patients with preexisting symptomatic or unrecognized asymptomatic MG, while the minority induce the production of Ach-receptor antibodies and result in clinical myasthenia gravis.

The best-recognized drug that induces production of antibodies to the Ach-receptor is D-penicillamine [49]. Although less frequently used now, D-penicillamine has been used in the treatment of rheumatoid arthritis, systemic lupus erythematosis, scleroderma, cystinuria, Wilson's disease, and primary biliary sclerosis. The development of drug-induced MG is thought to be very rare and to occur in only a very small minority of patients treated with D-penicillamine for these conditions. In fact, these patients may or may not develop clinical evidence of fluctuating weakness despite the presence of Ach-receptor antibodies in their serum. When neuromuscular fatigue is clinically evident, it is identical to patients with MG, and when recognized, discontinuation of the offending drug is recommended. While symptomatic treatment with acetylcholinesterase inhibitors may improve weakness, this symptom resolves in most patients upon stopping the drug, or several months later, and long-term treatment is usually not necessary.

In addition to obvious drugs that interfere with neuromuscular junction transmission, such as neuromuscular blocking agents used in critical illness and during surgery, the medical literature contains hundreds of reports citing the association of various drugs with clinical worsening of MG [50]. A complete description of all of the drugs reported to result in clinical worsening of MG, and their mechanism of interfering with the NMJ, is beyond the scope of this chapter. However two facts are worth noting. First, the association is stronger with some drugs more than others and the clinician should be familiar with more commonly prescribed drugs reported to interfere with neuromuscular transmission (Table 12.1). Second, the literature should be searched before prescribing any drug to a patient with myasthenia gravis. If a drug is proposed to worsen weakness in a patient with MG, alternative treatments

Table 12.1 Commonly prescribed drugs associated with worsening neuromuscular transmission

Definite association	Probable association	Possible association
Nondepolarizing neuromuscular blocking agents	Aminoglycosides	Ampicillin
	Ciprofloxacin	Anticholinergic drugs
	Lithium	Erythromycin
Anesthetic agents	Phenytoin	Radiocontrast agents
	Procainamide	Verapamil
	Quinidine sulfate	Chloroquine
	Beta-adrenergic receptor blocking agents (including eye drops)	Combination of imipenem and cilastatin
		Levonorgestrel
		Methocarbamol
		Phenothiazines
		Propafenone
		Pyrantel
		Transdermal nicotine

should be sought. If alternatives are not available and the treatment is deemed essential, the patient should be closely observed for worsening weakness. Otherwise, weakness may be incorrectly attributed to the natural history of MG resulting in unnecessary adjustments to their current therapeutic regimen, exposure to higher risk of adverse events from the medications, and at the extreme, may induce a myasthenia crisis.

Toxins

Envenomation from a poisonous snake may produce profound weakness or paralysis of the bulbar, ocular, and limb muscles. In severe cases, paralysis of respiratory muscles develops and death may occur if medical attention is not immediately sought. Snake venom contains a mixture of toxins and enzymes that may cause systemic injury to the snake's prey. Systemic targets of snake venom included the kidney, cardiovascular system, muscle, skin, and the coagulation cascade [51]. Neurotoxins are among the most lethal components of snake venom and are well-known to act at the NMJ. Although there are hundreds of species of venomous snakes, each with their

own specific makeup of venom, the neurotoxins can be broadly divided into two categories, beta-neurotoxin and alpha-neurotoxin [52,53]. Beta-neurotoxins act as phospholipases at the presynaptic nerve terminal and typically block release of Ach; however, some beta-neurotoxins act to enhance its release. In contrast, alpha-neurotoxins are active at the postsynaptic membrane, where they reversibly bind the Ach-receptor and prevent depolarization. The net effect of these mechanisms is to produce progressive weakness.

Prior treatment interventions of incising the area of the bite, applying suction to remove the venom, and placing a tourniquet on the symptomatic limb to limit systemic spread of the venom, are no longer recommended. Current recommendations include maintaining the patient's airway, breathing, and circulation, as well as immediate transport to the nearest medical facility for clinical observation, supportive care, and assessing for signs of envenomation. Treatment with antivenom is determined on case-by-case based upon the likelihood of envenomation, severity of the bite wound, progression of local edema and erythema, presence of muscle weakness, and development of coagulopathy [54].

221

Five things to remember about neuromuscular junction disorders due to systemic disease

1. Disorders of neuromuscular transmission can be associated with other non-nervous system immune-mediated disorders.
2. All patients with a new diagnosis of myasthenia gravis should be screened for thyroid dysfunction and thymoma.
3. All patients with a new diagnosis of LEMS should be screened for systemic cancer. Since LEMS may precede the detection of cancer by up to 2 years, patients with a negative initial evaluation (especially those at high risk for cancer) should undergo repeat cancer screening.
4. Before prescribing a medication to a patient with a disease of the NMJ, the clinician should perform a detailed review of a medication's impact on neuromuscular transmission. Likewise, the evaluation of progressive weakness in a patient with known dysfunction of neuromuscular transmission should include a detailed review of all previously and newly prescribed medications to avoid incorrectly ascribing the weakness to progression of disease.
5. Due to the risk of respiratory failure, patients with possible botulism, or MG patients in possible crisis, should be monitored closely in an intensive care unit setting.

REFERENCES

1 Isbister CM, Makenzie PJ, Anderson D, et al. Co-occurrence of multiple sclerosis and myasthenia gravis in British Columbia: a population-based study. *Neurology* 2002;58:A185–A186.

2 Carr AS, Cardwell CR, McCarron PO, et al. A systematic review of population based epidemiological studies in myasthenia gravis. *BMC Neurol.* 2010;10:46.

3 Vincent A, Clover L, Buckley C, et al. Evidence of under-diagnosis of myasthenia gravis in older people. *J. Neurol. Neurosurg. Psychiatry* 2003;74:1105–1108.

4 Phillips LH. The epidemiology of myasthenia gravis. *Semin. Neurol.* 2004;24:17–20.

5 Giraud M, Taubert R, Vandiedonck C, et al. An IRF8-binding promoter variant and AIRE control CHRNA1 promiscuous expression in thymus. *Nature* 2007;448:934–937.

6 Tackenberg B, Schlegel K, Happel M, et al. Expanded TCR Vbeta subsets of CD8(þ) T-cells in late-onset myasthenia gravis: novel parallels with thymoma patients. *J. Neuroimmunol.* 2009;216:85–91.

7 Cavalcante P, Barberis M, Cannone M, et al. Detection of poliovirus-infected macrophages in thymus of patients with myasthenia gravis. *Neurology* 2010;74:1118–1126.

8 Hughes BW, Moro de Casillas ML, Kaminski HJ. Pathophysiology of myasthenia gravis. *Semin. Neurol.* 2004;24:21–30.

9 Penn AS, Rowland LP. Myasthenia gravis. In: LP Rowland, editor. *Merritt's Neurology.* Philadelphia: Lippincott Williams and Wilkins, 2005, pp. 877–88415.

10 Lindstrom JM, Seybold ME, Lennon VA, et al. Antibody to acetylcholine receptor in myasthenia gravis: prevalence, clinical correlates, and diagnostic value. *Neurology* 1976;26:1054–1059.

11 Hoch W, McConville J, Helms S, et al. Auto-antibodies to the receptor tyrosine kinase MuSK in patients with myasthenia gravis without acetylcholine receptor antibodies. *Nat. Med.* 2001;7:365–368.

12 Howard JF, Sanders DB, Massey JM. The Electrodiagnosis of myasthenia gravis and Lambert–Eaton myasthenic syndrome. *Neurol. Clin.* 1994;12:305–329.

13 Sanders DB, Stlberg E. AAEM minimonograph #25: single-fiber electromyography. *Muscle Nerve* 1996;19:1069–1083.

14 Kumar K, Kaminski HJ. Treatment of myasthenia gravis. *Curr. Neurol. Neurosci. Rep.* 2011;11:89–96.

15 Puvanendran K, Cheah JS, Naganathan N, et al. Neuromuscular transmission in thyrotoxicosis. *J. Neurol. Sci.* 1979;43:47–57.

16 Norris F. Neuromuscular transmission in thyroid disease. *Ann. Intern. Med.* 1966;64:81–86.

17 Christensen PB, Jenson TS, Tsiropoulos I, et al. Associated autoimmune diseases in myasthenia gravis. A population-based study. *Acta Neurol. Scand.* 1995; 192–195

18 Weetman AP. Non-thyroid autoantibiodies in autoimmune thyroid disease. *Best Practice Res. Clin. Endocrinol. Meta.* 2005;19:27–32.

19 Engels EA, Pfeiffer RM. Malignant thymoma in the United States: demographic patterns in incidence and

associations with subsequent malignancies. *Int. J. Cancer* 2003;105:546e51.

20 Hohlfeld R, Wekerle H. The thymus in myasthenia gravis. *Neurol. Clin.* 1994;12:331–342.

21 Romi F. Thymoma in myasthenia gravis: from diagnosis to treatment. *Autoimmune Dis.* 2011;474512:1–5.

22 Gronseth G, Barohn R. Practice parameter: Thymectomy for autoimmune myasthenia gravis (an evidence-based review): report of the Quality Standards Subcommittee of the American Academy of Neurology. *Neurology* 2000;55:7–15.

23 Gutmann L, Phillips L, Gutmann L. Trends in the association of Lambert–Eaton myasthenic syndrome with carcinoma. *Neurology* 1992;42:848–850.

24 O'neil JH, Murray NM, Newsom-Davis J. The Lambert–Eaton myasthenic syndrome. *Brain* 1988;111:577–596.

25 Argov Z, Shapira Y, Averbuch-Heller L, et al. Lambert Eaton myasthenic syndrome (LEMS) in lymphoproliferative disorders (LPD). *Muscle Nerve* 1994;18:715–719.

26 Gutmann L, Crosby T, Takamori M, et al. The Eaton–Lambert syndrome and autoimmune disorders. *Am. J. Medi.* 1972;53:354–356.

27 Lennon VA, Lambert EH, Whittington S, et al. Autoimmunity in the Lambert–Eaton myasthenic syndrome. *Muscle Nerve* 1982;5:S21–S25.

28 Lang B, Newsom-Davis J, Peers C, et al. The effect of myasthenic syndrome antibody on presynaptic calcium channels in the mouse. *J. Physiol.* 1987;390:257–270.

29 Lennon VA, Kryzer T, Griesmann G, et al. Calcium-channel antibodies in the Lambert–Eaton syndrome and other paraneoplastic syndromes. *N. Engl. J. Med.* 1995;332:1467–1474.

30 Fukunaga H, Engel AG, Osame M, Lambert EH. Paucity and disorganization of presynaptic membrane active zones in the Lambert–Eaton myasthenic syndrome. *Muscle Nerve* 1982;5:686–697.

31 Engel AG. Review of evidence for loss of motor nerve terminal calcium channels in Lambert–Eaton myasthenic syndrome. *Ann. N. Y. Acad. Sci.* 1991;635:246–258.

32 Pascuzzi R. Myasthenia and Lambert–Eaton syndrome. *Therapeutics Apheresis* 2002;6:57–68.

33 O'Suilleabhain P, Low PA, Lennon VA. Autonomic dysfunction in the Lambert–Eaton myasthenic syndrome: serologic and clinical correlates. *Neurology* 1998;50:88–93.

34 Oh SJ, Kurokawa K, Claussen GC, et al. Electro-physiological diagnostic criteria of Lambert–Eaton syndrome. *Muscle Nerve* 2005;32:515–520.

35 Nilsson O, Rosén I. The stretch reflex in the Eaton Lambert syndrome, myasthenia gravis and myotonic dystrophy. *Acta Neurol. Scand.* 1978;58:350–357.

36 Lennon VA, Lambert EH. Autoantibodies bind solubilized calcium channel-omega-conotoxin complexes from small cell lung carcinoma: a diagnostic aid for Lambert–Eaton myasthenic syndrome. *Mayo Clin. Proc.* 1989;64:1498–1504.

37 Johnston I, Lang B, Lyes K, et al. Heterogeneity of calcium channel autoantibodies detected using a small-cell lung cancer line derived from a Lambert–Eaton myasthenic syndrome patient. *Neurology* 1994;44:334–338.

38 Chalk CH, Murray NM, Newsom-Davis J, et al. Response of the Lambert–Eaton myasthenic syndrome to treatment of associated small-cell lung carcinoma. *Neurology* 1990;40:1552–1556.

39 Linquist S, Stangel M. Update on treatment options for Lambert–Eaton myasthenic syndrome: focus on use of amifampridine. *Neuropsychiatr. Dis. Treat.* 2011;7:341–349.

40 Keogh M, Sedehizadeh S, Maddison P. Treatment for Lambert–Eaton myasthenic syndrome. *Cochrane Database Syst. Rev.* 2011;2:CD003279.

41 Skeie GO, Apostolski S, Evoli A, et al. Guidelines for treatment of autoimmune neuromuscular transmission disorders. *Eur. J. Neurol.* 2010;17:893–902.

42 Cherington M. Clinical spectrum of botulism. *Muscle Nerve* 1998;21:701–710.

43 Brook I. Infant botulism. *J. Perinatol.* 2007;27:175–180.

44 Tanzi MG, Gabay MP. Association between honey consumption and infant botulism. *Pharmacotherapy* 2002;22:1479–1483.

45 Yuan J, Inami G, Mohle-Boetani J, et al. Recurrent wound botulism among injection drug users in California. *Clin. Infect. Dis.* 2011;52:862–866.

46 Cherington M. Clinical spectrum of botulism. *Muscle Nerve* 1998;21:701–710.

47 Zhang JC, Sun L, Nie QH. Botulism, where are we now? *Clin. Toxicol.* 2010;48:876–879.

48 Chalk C, Benstead TJ, Keezer M. Medical treatment for botulism. *Cochrane Database Syst. Rev.* 2011; (3).

49 Penn AS, Low BW, Jaffe IA, et al. Drug-induced autoimmune myasthenia gravis. *Ann. N. Y. Acad. Sci.* 1998;841:433–449.

50 Wittbrodt ET. Drugs and myasthenia gravis: an update. *Arch. Intern. Med.* 1997;157:399–408.

51 Harris JB. Snake venoms in science and clinical medicine 3. Neuropharmacologic aspects of the activity of snake venoms. *Trans. R. Soc. Trop. Med. Hyg.* 1989;83:745–747.

52 Hodgson WC, Wickramaratna JC. In vitro neuromuscular activity of snake venoms. *Clin. Exp. Pharmacol. Physiol.* 2002;29:807–814.

53 Warrell DA. Snakebite. *Lancet* 2010;375:77–88.

54 Lavonas EJ, Ruha AM, Banner W. Unified treatment algorithm for the management of crotaline snakebite in the United States: results of an evidence-informed consensus workshop. *BMC Emerg. Med.* 2011;11:1–15.

13 Myopathies due to systemic disease

Hannah R. Briemberg
University of British Columbia, Vancouver BC, Canada

Endocrine disorders

Although most endocrine disorders have an associated myopathy, it is often overlooked as it is usually mild and rarely the presenting complaint. Most endocrine myopathies are reversible with correction of the underlying hormonal imbalance.

Thyroid disease

Both hypo- and hyperthyroid states are associated with the development of clinical myopathy. Virtually all patients with hypothyroidism demonstrate some elevation in creatine phosphokinase (CK). Myalgias and limb girdle pattern of weakness may also be seen. Although not often the chief complaint, up to one third of patients presenting with hypothyroidism have detectable weakness on manual muscle testing [1]. The degree of CK elevation does not correlate with this weakness. Classical signs of hypothyroidism that can be seen in some, but not all, patients are delayed relaxation of muscle stretch reflexes and painless mounding of muscle tissue when percussed (myoedema).

Electromyography (EMG) may be normal or show myopathic motor units. Diagnosis is based on abnormalities in thyroid stimulating hormone (TSH) in association with decreased free T3 and T4 levels. Serum CK normalizes rapidly with thyroid-replacement therapy. However, the weakness can take longer to recover and does not always recover completely.

Approximately 60% of hyperthyroid patients develop some degree of muscle weakness [1]. In contrast to hypothyroidism, the severity of the weakness seems to correlate with the degree of hyperthyroidism. Hyperthyroid myopathy primarily localizes to the hip flexors and quadriceps, although weakness of virtually all muscle groups has been described, including involvement of bulbar and respiratory muscles. However, because of the association between myasthenia gravis and autoimmune thyroid disease, it is important to consider myasthenia in hyperthyroid patients presenting with generalized or atypical patterns of weakness. Reflexes are usually preserved, if not slightly brisk. Weakness improves rapidly with correction of the hyperthyroid state. Propranolol also results in some improvement in the weakness [2].

Thyrotoxic periodic paralysis is a recognized complication of thyrotoxicosis associated with hypokalemia. This complication is more common in the Asian population and more common in men than in women. It is seen in approximately 2% of thyrotoxic patients in China and Japan compared with 0.1–0.2% of thyrotoxic patients in North America [3]. The male to female ratio is at least 17:1 and may be higher [3]. When it occurs, it is usually the presenting symptom of hyperthyroidism and, in fact, other signs and symptoms of hyperthyroidism may be absent or relatively subtle. Hypokalemia and the subsequent paralysis results from a sudden intracellular shift of potassium and is not due to potassium deficiency.

Thyrotoxic periodic paralysis usually presents in patients between 20 and 40 years of age. This differs from familial hypokalemic periodic paralysis where the age of presentation is generally in the first and second decades. Patients present with a history of recurrent episodes of limb weakness. The legs are affected first

Neurological Disorders due to Systemic Disease, First Edition. Edited by Steven L. Lewis
© 2013 Blackwell Publishing Ltd. Published 2013 by Blackwell Publishing Ltd.

and then the arms. The degree of weakness corresponds with the degree of hypokalemia. Proximal muscles are more affected than distal. Deep tendon reflexes are usually, but not always, depressed or absent. Respiratory, bulbar, and cranial musculature are generally spared although paralysis of these muscles may occur in a severe attack [4]. In approximately half of cases, only the lower extremities are affected [5].

Weakness may last anywhere from a few hours to several days. Attacks usually occur on awakening the morning after eating a carbohydrate-laden meal. They can also occur with rest following exercise or with alcohol. As a rule, they do not come on during exercise itself. This is likely because exercise results in movement of potassium out of muscle cells and into the circulation.

Diagnosis is based on the clinical presentation supported by laboratory evidence of hyperthyroidism and hypokalemia. Interestingly, however, serum thyroid levels are often only mildly elevated. Potassium levels are generally less than 3.0 mmol/L. Phosphate and magnesium levels are also commonly low, but return to normal with correction of the hypokalemia, indicating that the hypomagnesemia and hypophosphatemia are also likely secondary to intracellular ion flux rather than depletion of body stores. Potassium may be normal if the patient is already in the recovery phase. Serum CK is elevated in two thirds of patients and occasional patients with severe weakness develop rhabdomyolysis [6].

Treatment of the acute episode entails immediate potassium supplementation to prevent the potential cardiac complications of hypokalemia. However, because the low potassium does not represent total body depletion, one must take care not to overshoot. Weakness resolves with correction of the hypokalemia. Nonselective beta-adrenergic blockers (i.e., propranolol) can ameliorate and prevent recurrence of the paralytic attacks. Potassium supplementation in between attacks will not prevent further attacks. However, the episodic paralysis will remit with definitive control of the hyperthyroidism.

Increased sodium–potassium ATPase pump activity and enhanced insulin response in hyperthyroid patients is postulated to contribute to the hypokalemia. This response is more marked in patients with thyrotoxic periodic paralysis than in hyperthyroid patients without this complication. The enhanced insulin response may explain the association with carbohydrate-rich meals. The enhanced β-adrenergic response in thyrotoxicosis further increases Na/K-ATPase activity and may explain why nonselective β-adrenergic blockers can abort or prevent paralytic attacks.

Diabetes

Diabetic muscle infarction is a rare myopathic complication of diabetes. Patients present with the acute onset of focal muscle swelling and pain. The most frequently involved muscles are those in the anterior/medial thigh followed by the calf muscles. Two percent of patients have involvement of both thigh and calf muscles, and 8% have bilateral involvement [7]. The most common laboratory abnormalities are an elevated erythrocyte sedimentation rate (ESR) and/or a mildly elevated CK (up to 700 IU/L). However, both of these measures may be normal. In a minority of patients fever and/or leukocytosis are present [7]. Understandably, the clinical presentation of diabetic muscle infarction can be confused with multiple more common entities, such as muscle abscess, diabetic amyotrophy, deep vein thrombosis, cellulitis, and even focal myositis [8].

The precise etiology is unknown. Mean duration of diabetes prior to the development of diabetic muscle infarction is approximately 14 years. Most patients have diabetic microvascular complications (i.e., retinopathy, nephropathy, and neuropathy) at the time of presentation with diabetic muscle infarction. It is also more common in patients whose diabetes is complicated by end-stage renal disease [7]. In diabetic patients on dialysis, it has an estimated incidence of one per 233 patient-years [9]. In larger series, women are affected more frequently than men by a 3:2 ratio. Recurrence of diabetic muscle infarction was found in 48% of published cases [7]. Although most patients recover uneventfully, it has been associated with a mortality rate of around 10%, with most deaths occurring 6–12 months from diagnosis [8].

Electrophysiological studies may be normal or, more commonly, demonstrate the typical length-dependent polyneuropathy seen in the later stages of diabetes. Electromyography commonly demonstrates muscle membrane irritability (fibrillation potentials and positive sharp waves) in affected muscles. Motor units may be small and polyphasic (myopathic) or normal in appearance. Some insertional points can be electrically silent even with active contraction, indicating areas of fibrosis.

Although not specific, the abnormalities seen on MRI can be diagnostic in the appropriate clinical

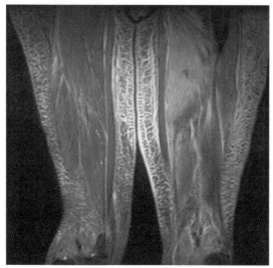

Fig 13.1 Diabetic muscle infarction: Coronal MRI of thighs demonstrating swelling of the left adductor magnus and partial loss of normal intermuscular septa with hyperintense signal on T2 FSEIR sequences.

setting. The characteristic findings are increased signal from the affected muscle and surrounding perimysial tissue on T2 and fast spin echo inversion recovery (FSEIR) sequences (Figures 13.1, 13.2) [10]. T1 sequence usually shows isointense or hypointense signal in the affected region, secondary to increased water content from edema and inflammation accompanying the infarction. Gadolinium enhancement on T1 sequences suggests an area of necrosis within the inflamed muscle. The affected muscle is usually diffusely enlarged with ill-defined borders due to loss of fatty intramuscular septa. Tiny foci of hemorrhage

can also be present and are seen as increased signal on T1 sequences.

Findings on muscle biopsy are nonspecific and depend on the time line between symptom onset and biopsy. Gross specimens show nonhemorrhagic, pale, whitish muscle [9,11]. On light microscopy, large areas of muscle necrosis, and phagocytosis of necrotic muscle fibers are early findings. Late in the disease course, one sees replacement of necrotic muscle fibers by fibrous tissue, myofiber regeneration, and mononuclear cellular infiltration. In general, however, muscle biopsy is discouraged due to a possible increased risk of hemorrhage and/or localized recurrence of symptoms at the biopsy site in this population of patients [12].

Patients with diabetic muscle infarction are generally treated with supportive measures only, primarily bed rest and analgesia to control their pain. It is not clear whether glycemic control influences the natural history of the attack. Some clinicians have advocated treatment with antiplatelet therapy or anticoagulation [8,13,14]. Others have advocated treatment with corticosteroids [8,14]. However, it is not clear that either of these interventions influences the natural history [8]. Given the absence of any evidence of benefit from these specific treatment modalities, treatment should remain supportive, directed at pain control and physical therapy to prevent joint contractures.

Diagnosis can be made based on the clinical presentation and characteristic magnetic resonance imaging findings, avoiding the need for muscle biopsy in most cases. Although the pain can be extremely debilitating, most patients appear to recover with time, so the key is to make an accurate diagnosis and avoid iatrogenic complications.

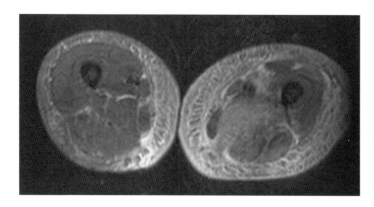

Fig 13.2 Diabetic muscle infarction: Axial images of thighs (same patient as in Fig 13.1) again demonstrating swelling of the left adductor magnus with hyperintense signal on T2 sequences.

Cushing's syndrome

Proximal muscle weakness develops in patients with Cushing's syndrome. This myopathy is identical to the myopathy induced by exogenous steroids discussed later in this chapter.

Electrolyte and other metabolic disorders

A number of electrolyte abnormalities can be associated with the development of muscle weakness. This includes hypo- and hypercalcemia, hypo- and hyperkalemia, hypo- and hyperphosphatemia, and hypermagnesemia. In general, patients present with symmetric, proximal, or generalized weakness. CK is sometimes, but not always, elevated. EMG may show muscle membrane irritability and myopathic-appearing motor units, or may be normal. Hypocalcemia, usually secondary to hypoparathyroidism, has been associated with a spectrum of myopathic features, including elevation in CK, myalgias, easy fatiguability, and mild limb girdle weakness. Regardless of the etiology, the weakness virtually always resolves rapidly with correction of the underlying electrolyte abnormality.

Systemic autoimmune disorders

Rheumatological disease and myositis

Approximately 20% of patients with dermatomyositis and polymyositis have a concurrent connective-tissue disorder [15]. The most common association is with mixed connective tissue disease (MCTD), also known as "overlap syndrome." This is an undifferentiated connective tissue disease that has features of scleroderma, systemic lupus erythematosus (SLE), rheumatoid arthritis, and myositis. Dermatomyositis and polymyositis also occur in association with isolated SLE, rheumatoid arthritis, Sjogren's syndrome, and scleroderma. Most commonly, the myositis and the systemic symptoms of the associated connective tissue disease present within a year of one another.

Dermatomyositis has a bimodal age distribution with peaks at 5–24 years and 45–64 years of age [16]. Polymyositis is generally not seen in childhood. Both present with the subacute onset of symmetric proximal weakness progressing over weeks to months. Pain is a feature in approximately 30% of patients and

is thought to be related to involvement of muscle fascia. Although weakness is maximal proximally, patients can also exhibit milder distal weakness. Mild, asymptomatic facial weakness is sometimes found, but as a rule, extraocular muscles are spared. Some patients develop dysphagia, manifested by difficulties swallowing solids. They complain that food gets stuck in their throat and that they have to wash it down. This is in contrast to dysphagia secondary to neuropathic or neuromuscular junction disorders where the most difficult consistency to swallow is typically liquid.

The skin manifestations of dermatomyositis are characteristic. Patients typically exhibit a macular erythematous and pruritic rash over their face, scalp, anterior chest, and/or posterior neck and upper back (Figures 13.3, 13.4). Other potential skin changes include a periorbital heliotrope rash, Gottron's papules over extensor tendon surfaces, and periungual capillary telangiectasias. The heliotrope rash is a lilac discoloration of the upper eyelids, frequently associated with periorbital edema. Gottron's papules are raised erythematous lesions over extensor tendon surfaces. There is often associated scaling of the skin overlying these erythematous plaques. They are most frequently found on the metacarpophalangeal

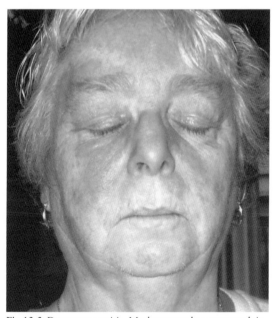

Fig 13.3 Dermatomyositis. Moderate erythematous rash is appreciated over the forehead, around the eyes, and across the malar region of the face. (See also Plate 13.3.)

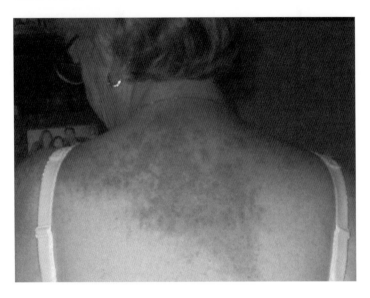

Fig 13.4 Dermatomyositis. Maculopapular erythematous rash across the upper back and posterior neck (shawl sign). (See also Plate 13.4.)

and interphalangeal joints of the hands but may also be seen over the extensor surface of the elbows and knees or over the malleoli. The rash may precede the development of the muscle weakness or may occur simultaneously with the weakness.

Although occasionally serum CK can be normal, particularly early in dermatomyositis, most often it is elevated and may be as high as 50 times the upper limit of normal (10,000 IU/L). Other muscle-related enzymes (AST, ALT, LDH, aldolase) may also be elevated. Antinuclear antibodies are present in 24–60% of patients, but not all of these patients will manifest evidence of concurrent connective tissue disease [17,18]. ESR is frequently elevated when concurrent connective tissue disease is active but ESR, itself, has no relationship to myositis disease activity. EMG demonstrates muscle membrane irritability, in the form of fibrillation potentials, positive sharp waves, and/or complex repetitive discharges [19,20]. These abnormalities are usually most pronounced proximally, particularly in the paraspinal muscles.

The gold standard for diagnosis of autoimmune myositis is muscle biopsy. Because inflammation is patchy, the yield for a positive diagnosis is increased if the muscle chosen for biopsy is moderately weak (Grade 4 to 4−) and if it demonstrates clear myopathic abnormality on EMG or evidence of inflammation on MRI. To avoid EMG artifact, it is suggested that the muscle chosen for biopsy be on the opposite side to that where the EMG was done (i.e., if the right biceps is

moderately weak and demonstrates fibrillation potentials, the biopsy should be taken from the left biceps). If at all possible, it is best to do the biopsy before immunosuppressive treatment is started.

Although inflammation is the hallmark histopathological finding in both polymyositis and dermatomyositis, the distribution and predominant type of inflammatory cell differ, reflecting their different underlying pathophysiologies. Dermatomyositis is a humorally-mediated vasculopathy and the most specific histopathologic abnormalities are associated with endomysial capillaries. The earliest histological abnormality is the deposition of membrane attack complex (MAC) on capillaries and arterioles, which can be shown by immunohistochemistry stains. The subsequent necrosis of vessels results in a reduction in the capillary density [21–23]. Electron microscopy (EM) demonstrates endothelial hyperplasia with tubuloreticular inclusions. Inflammatory cells are typically seen in the perimysium, especially around blood vessels, but are less common within fascicles. The inflammatory infiltrate is composed primarily of B-cells, CD4+ cells, and macrophages [24]. Perifascicular atrophy occurs in only about one-third of patients and may be even less common in adults [22,25].

Blood-vessel changes and perifascicular atrophy are not seen in polymyositis, which is characterized by endomysial inflammation and the invasion of nonnecrotic muscle fibers by inflammatory cells. Polymyositis is a T-cell mediated disease and, as such, the invading inflammatory cells consist primarily of activated CD8+ (cytotoxic) T-cells and macrophages [24]. It is important to be aware that not all endomysial inflammation is indicative of a primary inflammatory myopathy, as it is not uncommon to see reactive inflammation in the muscular dystrophies. However, in the dystrophies, the inflammatory cells are always surrounding and invading necrotic or degenerating muscle fibers (reactive inflammation). Invasion of healthy muscle fibers by inflammatory infiltrate is specific for the primary inflammatory myopathies.

Autoimmune necrotizing myositis is an increasingly recognized entity that may also be associated with an underlying mixed connective-tissue disease. The clinical presentation is identical to that of polymyositis. Serum CPK is usually markedly elevated (8000–10,000 IU/L) and EMG demonstrates muscle membrane irritability. However, in contrast to polymyositis, muscle biopsy demonstrates widespread muscle fiber necrosis and degenerating and regenerating muscle fibers without inflammation. Despite the absence of inflammation, these patients also respond to treatment with immunomodulating therapies, although they often seem to require higher doses of steroids for longer periods of time than most patients with polymyositis [26].

The most frequent systemic complication of the immune-mediated myopathies is interstitial lung disease; therefore, it is recommended that all patients have a baseline high-resolution computed tomography (CT) scan to assess for this. Less frequent complications include pericarditis or myocarditis. Inflammation of the skeletal and smooth muscle of the gastrointestinal tract can also occur, leading to dysphagia and delayed gastric emptying.

Although no prospective, randomized, controlled clinical trials have studied the efficacy of corticosteroids in the treatment of autoimmune myositis, there is no doubt, based on clinical experience, that their use results in moderate to significant improvement in most patients. Other immunomodulating agents, including azathioprine, methotrexate, cyclophosphamide, cyclosporine, mycophenolate mofetil, or intravenous immunoglobulin may add additional benefit as well as provide a steroid-sparing effect in patients who do not respond adequately to steroids alone. There is still little experience with biologics in these diseases so it is difficult to make recommendations in this regard.

Currently, most authorities recommend high-dose prednisone as the first-line treatment of the immune-mediated myopathies (dermatomyositis, polymyositis, and autoimmune necrotizing myositis) and most patients demonstrate clinical improvement within 3–6 months of starting therapy. Methotrexate or azathioprine are the most commonly used prednisone-sparing agents. Intravenous immunoglobulin (IVIg) is recommended for patients with severe involvement or those who do not respond adequately to the combination of prednisone and methotrexate or azathioprine. Third-line agents include mycophenolate, cyclosporine, or cyclophosphamide. One of these is generally added in patients who do not respond adequately to the preceding regimen. Of note, both mycophenolate and IVIg appear to be particularly helpful for severe skin manifestations in dermatomyositis. Plasmapheresis has been shown *not* to be effective in these disorders.

Sarcoidosis

Symptomatic myopathy associated with systemic sarcoidosis is relatively rare, with an incidence of approximately 2% while asymptomatic muscle involvement can be seen in 50–80% of cases [27,28]. Because of its rarity, little is known about this disorder. The literature is limited to case reports and small case series, the largest including eight patients with systemic sarcoidosis and symptomatic myopathy [28]. It appears that, in most patients, the diagnosis of systemic sarcoidosis is already established at the time of presentation of the myopathy. However, in occasional myopathy patients the finding of noncaseating granulomata in muscle tissue leads to further investigation with the simultaneous diagnosis of systemic sarcoid.

Most commonly, sarcoid myopathy presents with the insidious onset of proximal, primarily hip girdle, weakness. Occasionally, a subacute onset occurs, mimicking polymyositis [27–29]. In the subacute form, serum CK can be markedly elevated. In the insidious, chronic form, CK may be normal to moderately elevated (usually less than 2000 IU/L). EMG almost always shows fibrillation potentials and positive sharp waves in affected muscles along with myopathic-appearing motor units.

One series suggested that dysphagia is a prominent symptom in granulomatous myopathy associated with systemic sarcoidosis and that these patients respond well to treatment with prednisone [30]. However, other series have not found dysphagia to be prominent and have reported a variable response to prednisone and other immunosuppressive agents [28]. In the author's personal experience, dysphagia has not been a significant feature of symptomatic myopathy in sarcoidosis. Two of this author's patients, with the chronic form, refused immunosuppressive treatment and their weakness has remained relatively stable over several years. One additional patient has had a moderate, although incomplete response to long-term treatment with prednisone. It is the general consensus that the subacute form, mimicking polymyositis, is more responsive to immunosuppressive treatment than is the chronic form.

Organ dysfunction and failure

No significant muscle disease has been directly associated with specific organ failure. However, a number of myopathies are related to systemic diseases that also cause organ failure. These myopathies are discussed in the relevant sections in this chapter.

Systemic cancer and paraneoplastic disorders

Dermatomyositis and autoimmune necrotizing myositis can also occur in the setting of underlying malignancy. Their clinical presentation is essentially identical to that outlined earlier in this chapter. However, there is the general impression that paraneoplastic myositis is more resistant to treatment than idiopathic myositis or that associated with connective-tissue disease. Although polymyositis is not generally thought to be associated with underlying malignancy, because it may be challenging to differentiate it from either dermatomyositis or autoimmune necrotizing myositis (i.e., a mild skin rash may be missed; reactive inflammation in a necrotizing myopathy may lead to the misdiagnosis of polymyositis) many practitioners also screen patients with presumed polymyositis for malignancy [31,32].

There is no common malignancy associated with these autoimmune myopathies. Thus, a widespread malignancy screen is recommended in all patients presenting with these disorders. Unfortunately, there

is also no consensus on what this malignancy screen should entail. In general, it is recommended that all patients undergo CT scan of the chest and either CT or ultrasound of the abdomen and pelvis. Patients over 50 years of age should have a colonoscopy to screen for the presence of colorectal cancers. Women should undergo mammography and men should have a testicular and prostate examination. Reports suggest that nasopharyngeal cancer is the most common cancer associated with dermatomyositis in Hong Kong and Singapore [33,34]. Gastric cancer is commonly associated with dermatomyositis in Japan [31]. This likely reflects the increased incidence of these cancers in these specific populations. Thus, in our increasingly global society, it is important to remain cognizant of the epidemiology of various malignancies and screen at-risk patients accordingly. It is recommended that malignancy screening be repeated annually in myositis patients for at least 3 years [32].

Amyloidosis

Amyloid myopathy is a rare complication of primary amyloidosis. This is the form of amyloidosis associated with the proliferation of free light chains. It is rarely seen in familial amyloidosis and does not occur in secondary amyloidosis. The latter is associated with inflammatory or infectious disease [35,36]. The majority of patients present with progressive proximal weakness. Macroglossia and muscle pseudohypertrophy are frequently reported; however, muscle atrophy may also be seen. Occasional patients have been reported to present with respiratory failure [37]. Only a minority of patients have an associated peripheral neuropathy or carpal tunnel syndrome [36]. Although there are occasional reports of very high CK levels in association with amyloid myopathy, in general CK is normal or only mildly elevated (<1200 IU/L). EMG demonstrates myopathic motor units with or without evidence of muscle membrane irritability (fibrillation potentials and positive sharp waves). Muscle biopsy is required for definitive diagnosis. Usually, the amyloid is found surrounding intramuscular blood vessels and is identified on Congo red staining. It may also be found in the perimysial or endomysial connective tissue and occasionally surrounding muscle fibers. Immunohistochemistry confirms that the amyloid deposits consist of lambda or kappa light chains.

Amyloid myopathy may be an underdiagnosed entity. The diagnosis may be missed if muscle biopsy specimens are not routinely stained with Congo red [35,36]. All patients with unexplained myopathy should also undergo serum and urine protein electrophoresis and immunofixation. The sensitivity of serum protein electrophoresis alone is approximately 66%. The addition of serum and urine electrophoresis increases sensitivity for detecting primary amyloidosis to approximately 94% [38].

Unfortunately, the prognosis in amyloid myopathy is poor with a mean survival of 21 months, although occasional long-term survival does occur [36]. Treatment is targeted at decreasing or eliminating the serum free light chains. Treatment with high-dose intravenous melphalan followed by autologous stem-cell transplantation seems to be most effective in inducing hematological remission. There is little data on its effect on the myopathy; however, at least one case report and personal experience suggests that stabilization of the myopathy can occur with successful hematological treatment.

Systemic infectious diseases

Human immunodeficiency virus

The most common myopathic complications of human immunodeficiency virus (HIV) include zidovudine (AZT) toxicity and polymyositis. In addition, HIV-infected individuals are more susceptible to developing focal pyomyositis. Infectious myopathies associated with systemic opportunistic infections (i.e., microsporidiosis, cryptococcus neoformans, and toxoplasmosis) have also been reported [39].

Patients infected with HIV can develop polymyositis as a direct complication of the HIV, itself. This appears to be a relatively rare complication. One study in Texas found a prevalence of 0.2% among HIV-infected individuals [39]. However, there is a suggestion that the incidence has declined since the advent of highly active antiretroviral therapy (HAART) [39,40]. As with other HIV-associated autoimmune disorders, HIV-associated polymyositis can occur at any stage of the infection. The clinical presentation is identical to that of idiopathic polymyositis with the subacute onset of symmetric, proximal greater than distal, weakness [41]. Although serum CK can be normal, it is most often elevated. EMG demonstrates muscle membrane irritability (fibrillation

potentials, positive sharp waves, and/or complex repetitive discharges) in weak muscles. Muscle biopsy is identical to that in idiopathic polymyositis, demonstrating perimysial and endomysial inflammatory infiltrates, consisting primarily of CD8+ cytotoxic T cells and macrophages [42]. Perivascular inflammation may also be seen. Occasionally ragged red fibers and rimmed vacuoles are seen, suggestive of inclusion body myositis (IBM). In this situation, the typically younger age at onset, the pattern of weakness, and the associated HIV infection should tip the clinician off to the fact that the correct diagnosis is likely HIV-related polymyositis rather than IBM.

HIV antigen has been found in interstitial mononuclear cells but not in myocytes. Therefore, it is assumed that the HIV-associated polymyositis is due to HIV-related immune dysregulation rather than to direct viral infection of the muscle fibers [42]. The optimal treatment for HIV-associated polymyositis is unclear. It appears to respond well to treatment with prednisone, but obviously immunosuppressive therapies need to be used with caution in patients who are already immunocompromised [39,41]. IVIg is not generally felt to be that effective in HIV-associated polymyositis [39]. There are isolated reports of improvement with institution of antiretroviral therapies alone but at this point their role in the treatment of HIV-associated polymyositis is unclear [41].

Nemaline rods have also been reported with apparently increased frequency in muscle biopsies of HIV-infected individuals. Whether this represents sporadic late-onset nemaline myopathy or is an epiphenomenon of another underlying disease process is unclear. Some of these patients have been reported to respond to treatment with IVIg [43].

Zidovudine myopathy is a reversible toxic myopathy that occurs in patients who have received high cumulative doses of this anti-retroviral medication (also known as azidothymidine, or AZT) [44,45]. Clinically, it mimics HIV-associated polymyositis; however, the histopathological findings differentiate zidovudine myopathy from polymyositis. Muscle biopsies are characterized by the presence of multiple atrophic ragged red fibers with scant if any inflammation. Typically, multiple cytochrome c oxidase (COX) negative fibers are also present. EM demonstrates loss of thick myofilaments [45]. Symptoms resolve with withdrawal of zidovudine. In patients whose weakness does not improve, or worsens, after stopping

231

zidovudine, consideration should be given to an alternate diagnosis, most commonly HIV-associated polymyositis.

Rhabdomyolysis has been reported in all stages of HIV infection. Again, whether this is directly related to the underlying HIV and/or associated antiretrovirals is unclear. Antiretrovirals that have been implicated in rhabdomyolysis in HIV patients include didanosine, lamivudine, ritonavir, and indinavir [40]. Of note, protease inhibitors may increase statin concentrations in patients receiving treatment for HAART-associated hyperlipidemia. This may increase the risk of rhabdomyolysis in these patients.

Human T-cell leukemia virus type 1

Human T-cell leukemia virus, type 1 (HTLV-1) can also be associated with myositis. The clinical presentation is similar to that of HIV-associated polymyositis. Many, but not all, patients also demonstrate the tropical spastic paraparesis that is more commonly associated with this virus. Clues to a concurrent myositis include the presence of neck and upper-extremity weakness in addition to a spastic paraparesis. Serum CK is typically elevated. EMG may show muscle membrane irritability and myopathic motor units. Muscle biopsy is similar to that seen in polymyositis. As with HIV-polymyositis, the pathophysiology is thought to relate to immune dysregulation rather than to direct muscle infection by the virus [46]. Case reports suggest possible improvement with immunosuppression but the response does not appear to be as robust or as prolonged as with idiopathic or HIV-associated polymyositis [47,48].

Influenza viruses

Benign acute myositis occurs in the pediatric population in association with various strains of influenza. It is characterized by the acute onset of symmetrical calf muscle pain and tenderness, weakness of the lower extremities, and an inability or refusal to walk. CK levels are invariably elevated. The symptom onset is usually about 48 h after onset of influenza symptoms but these symptoms can also begin as the child is recovering from the influenza. Most affected children are 2–10 years of age. Boys may be affected more frequently than girls [49]. Symptoms are self-limiting

and generally resolve within 3 to 7 days. Although most commonly seen in association with influenza, benign acute myositis has also been reported with parainfluenza, coxsackie virus, adenovirus, and *Mycoplasma pneumoniae* [50].

Rhabdomyolysis can also be seen in association with seasonal influenza and can occur in any age group. It can be associated with myoglobinuria and acute renal failure. The incidence is unknown. A number of cases were reported in association with the Influenza A (H1N1) pandemic in 2009; whether this represents reporting bias due to increased vigilance or a true increased association with the H1N1 strain is unknown. Treatment is supportive with bed rest and hydration to avoid renal failure from myoglobinuria.

Complications due to transplantation

Myopathy of graft versus host disease

Chronic graft versus host disease (GVHD) occurs in 30–70% of allogeneic hematopoietic stem-cell recipients [51]. It is the result of an immunological reaction against recipient antigens by the immunocompetent donor graft. The main target organs of chronic GVHD are skin, eyes, mouth, liver, esophagus, bowel, lung, and serosa. The syndrome has features resembling autoimmune disorders such as scleroderma, Sjögren's syndrome, primary biliary cirrhosis, and bronchiolitis obliterans [51]. Muscle-related complications of GVHD include myositis, fasciitis, and steroid myopathy.

GVHD-associated myositis resembles idiopathic polymyositis. Patients present with subacute-onset, symmetrical, proximal greater than distal weakness. CK is typically elevated. EMG demonstrates muscle-membrane irritability and myopathic motor units. Muscle biopsy demonstrates endomysial greater than perimysial inflammation with a predominance of CD8+ T-cells, similar to idiopathic polymyositis. Degenerating and regenerating fibers, along with endomysial fibrosis have also been reported [51].

GVHD-associated fasciitis can sometimes be mistaken for polymyositis. This begins rather abruptly with sudden painful skin swelling that does not respond to immunosuppression but that appears to resolve spontaneously over 2–6 months. Following resolution of the edema, patients develop sclerodermatous skin changes (peau d'orange) and restriction of joint mobility. As with polymyositis, these changes are symmetric and the restriction of joint mobility can be accompanied by apparent weakness, although usually strength is relatively preserved within the patient's active range of motion. Interestingly, CK is often elevated in these patients, although muscle biopsies appear relatively normal [52].

MRI can be useful in differentiating GVHD-associated myositis from fasciitis as the MRI images of patients with fasciitis show high intensity along the fascia in short T1 inversion recovery (STIR) sequences whereas in polymyositis one sees high signal intensity in the muscle itself. Fascial biopsy shows fascial thickening and fibrosis with lymphocytic infiltration within the fibrotic fascia. As with polymyositis, the lymphocytes are primarily CD8+ T-cells.

Time to onset of GVHD-associated myositis and/or fasciitis can be anywhere from 3 to 55 months posttransplant [51,52]. The exact incidence is unknown but the prevalence of myositis in two studies of chronic GVHD patients appears to be approximately 0.6% [51,53]. Virtually all patients have manifestations of chronic GVHD concurrent with, or preceding, the development of the polymyositis. The polymyositis responds well to increasing or restarting immunosuppressive medications. The fasciitis is also managed with immunosuppression; unfortunately, the response does not appear as robust as in polymyositis [51,52].

Complications of critical medical illness

Critical illness myopathy

Critically ill patients who receive a combination of intravenous corticosteroids and neuromuscular blocking agents are at risk of developing critical illness myopathy. However, occasional cases of critical illness myopathy have also been reported in patients who have received intravenous corticosteroids alone or who have not received either intravenous corticosteroids or neuromuscular blocking agents [54]. The clinical presentation is identical to that of critical illness polyneuropathy with flaccid quadriparesis and difficulty weaning from the ventilator. Although CK may be elevated initially, it is typically normal at the time the myopathy is identified.

Electrophysiological testing demonstrates low-amplitude compound muscle action potentials

(CMAPs) with relatively preserved sensory responses. Severe critical illness myopathy is characterized by an inability to elicit muscle contraction even with direct electrical stimulation using an EMG needle electrode. This is in contrast to critical-care polyneuropathy, where the muscle remains easily excitable with direct muscle stimulation even if CMAPs are absent on stimulation of the nerve. This test is not useful in differentiating the two in less severe cases, where the muscle remains partially excitable, as normative data for this response has not been established. EMG may show fibrillation potentials, positive sharp waves, and small polyphasic motor units. Early recruitment may be seen. However, in some severe cases, no motor units can be elicited.

Aside from the inability to elicit muscle contraction with direct needle stimulation, the other specific test for differentiating critical illness myopathy from polyneuropathy is the muscle biopsy. This demonstrates widespread loss of myosin, a finding that is felt to be pathognomic for critical illness myopathy [54].

If the critical illness can be treated successfully, muscle strength usually recovers over a prolonged period of weeks to months. Interestingly, the rate of recovery is virtually identical to that of critical care polyneuropathy [55].

Drugs, toxins (including alcohol), and vitamin and mineral deficiencies

Many drugs used in the treatment of systemic disease have been associated with the risk of developing myopathy as a side effect. However, the incidence of medication-induced myopathy remains relatively low. Probably the most frequently encountered toxic myopathies, because of the prevalence of their use, are myopathies associated with statins and with glucocorticoids. Vitamin and mineral deficiencies are not a significant cause of myopathy.

Statin-induced myopathy

Myalgias with or without elevation in CK are the most common side effect of statin therapy with an incidence of 10–15% [56]. More serious myopathic complications, such as weakness or rhabdomyolysis, are less common [57,58]. It should be noted that fibrates, nitrates, and ezetimibe have also been associated with a similar myopathy, although again the exact incidence is unknown [59]. The risk of developing a statin myopathy correlates with statin dose, patient age, female gender, smaller body build, concurrent systemic disease (i.e., diabetes, renal, or liver disease), family history of statin myopathy and the use of multiple medications, primarily including fibrates, nitrates and/or other cytochrome p450 metabolized drugs [60]. Symptoms typically start within one month of starting statin therapy although onset 4 years after starting a statin agent has been reported.

The weakness, when it occurs, is symmetric with proximal greater than distal involvement. The hip girdle muscles are usually the most severely affected. Weakness is virtually always associated with an elevation in CK. In patients with muscle weakness, EMG typically shows irritability (positive sharp waves, fibrillation potentials, and myotonic discharges). Motor units may be normal or myopathic in appearance. Treatment involves withdrawing the statin. The time to symptom resolution is not well documented but generally is less than 4 months.

Interestingly, there have been several case series of patients developing immune-mediated myopathies (polymyositis, dermatomyositis, necrotizing myositis) during treatment with a statin or within 12–18 months of discontinuing a statin medication [61]. Therefore, this needs to be considered in the differential of patients who do not improve, or who relapse, following statin discontinuation Although patients who develop myalgias with minimal elevation in CK (<10 times upper limit of normal) can be rechallenged with another statin once symptoms resolve, the National Lipid Association (NLA) guidelines recommend that further statin use be avoided in patients who develop rhabdomyolysis, muscle weakness, or a CK greater than ten times normal during treatment [59].

In vitro studies suggest that coenzyme Q10 depletion may play a role in the development of statin-induced myopathy, as serum coenzyme Q10 levels are known to decrease in statin-treated patients. However, although several uncontrolled trials suggested Coenzyme Q10 may be of benefit in preventing statin-induced myopathy, the one randomized placebo-controlled trial that has been published did not demonstrate any benefit of Coenzyme Q10 over placebo [62]. Thus, at this point, the NLA guidelines recommend against using Coenzyme Q10 prophylactically in statin-treated patients.

Steroid (glucocorticoid) myopathy

Steroid myopathy, when it occurs, is typically associated with doses of prednisone of at least 30 mg daily, or its equivalent [63]. Symptom onset is usually after several weeks of high-dose steroid or several weeks after a sudden increase in steroid dose. It is unusual to present in a patient who does not have other signs of steroid toxicity (i.e., a Cushingoid appearance). The myopathy itself manifests as proximal weakness affecting the hip girdle more than shoulder girdle. Neck flexors are generally spared. Serum CK is normal. EMG is usually normal. Occasionally, small, polyphasic (myopathic) motor units are noted. Muscle biopsy shows atrophy of type IIb fibers. However, muscle biopsy is rarely required to make the diagnosis.

Myopathy is more common with fluorinated steroids (i.e., dexamethasone) than nonfluorinated ones (i.e., prednisone). One study found clinically significant myopathy in 10% of brain tumor patients after receiving at least 2 weeks of daily dexamethasone [64]. It is recommended that these patients be switched to nonfluorinated steroids if they are unable to be weaned. Steroid myopathy is unusual in patients treated with prednisone 10 mg daily or less.

In most cases, the diagnosis of steroid myopathy is fairly straightforward. Treatment is to decrease the steroid dose. Improvement is usually seen within 3–4 weeks. If the patient can be completely weaned off the steroids, complete recovery is the rule.

One challenge can be differentiating relapse of an inflammatory myopathy from a steroid-induced myopathy. If CK is normal and the EMG does not demonstrate abnormal spontaneous activity, it is likely steroid-induced weakness. If the CK is increased and/or there is abnormal spontaneous activity on EMG, it is likely a relapse of the underlying inflammatory myopathy, in which case an increase in steroid dose would be recommended.

Chloroquine and hydroxychloroquine myopathy

Chloroquine and hydroxychloroquine are quinolones used primarily in the treatment of malaria, SLE, and other connective-tissue diseases. Occasional patients treated with these medications develop an associated myopathy characterized by the insidious onset of proximal greater than distal weakness. Usually it is the hip girdle muscles that are maximally affected. Although most cases are relatively mild, there are reports in the literature of severe myopathies with neuromuscular respiratory failure related to chloroquine/hydroxychloroquine toxicity [65,66]. The myopathy improves after discontinuation of the offending medication. Hydroxychloroquine is said to be less myotoxic than chloroquine.

EMG is similar to that seen in inflammatory myopathies. Specifically, there is muscle membrane irritability in the form of fibrillation potentials, positive sharp waves, and/or complex repetitive discharges in weak muscles. Motor units are myopathic in appearance. CK is usually elevated.

Muscle biopsy demonstrates autophagic vacuoles, primarily in type 1 myofibers. These vacuoles stain positive for acid phosphatase. Electron microscopy shows them to contain concentric lamellar myeloid debris and curvilinear structures [67]. It is believed that the chloroquine forms a complex with intracellular lipids that is resistant to lysosomal digestion, resulting in the formation of these autophagic vacuoles [68]. Interestingly, chloroquine and hydroxychloroquine cardiomyotoxicity have also been reported with similar pathological changes to that seen in skeletal muscle biopsies [69].

Colchicine

Colchicine is another commonly used medication that exhibits potential myotoxicity. Risk factors include chronic renal failure and concurrent administration of a statin medication or of cyclosporine [70,71]. Colchicine is hepatically metabolized and 80% of the drug is excreted through the biliary system. However, 20% is renally excreted, likely explaining the increased risk of colchicine toxicity with renal failure. Colchicine is not removed by dialysis [70].

Patients present with new-onset proximal weakness, often with associated myalgias. The onset of symptoms is usually quite abrupt and typically begins within days to weeks of starting colchicine or with a change in underlying disease state (i.e., addition of a statin, new-onset renal failure) [70]. CK is almost always elevated and EMG shows muscle membrane irritability and myopathic motor units. Clinical and electromyographic myotonia has been observed [72,73]. Muscle biopsy demonstrates vacuolar changes without prominent necrosis or inflammation. The pathological changes are believed to be due to colchicine-mediated disruption of cytoskeletal microtubules. In the majority of cases, weakness resolves within weeks of discontinuing the colchicine.

Amiodarone

Amiodarone is also reported to cause a vacuolar myopathy; however, the evidence for this is primarily based on case reports [74,75]. Many patients with amiodarone-associated myopathy are also identified to be hypothyroid, a well-recognized complication of long-term amiodarone therapy. As peripheral neuropathy is another well-recognized complication of long-term therapy, it is likely that, in many cases, weakness from the neuropathy and/or hypothyroidism is misinterpreted as being secondary to concurrent amiodarone-induced myopathy. Nevertheless, there are case reports of patients presenting with proximal greater than distal weakness, elevated CK and EMG studies demonstrating myopathic changes (fibrillation potentials, positive sharp waves and short duration, polyphasic motor units) with vacuolar changes on muscle biopsy. As with other toxic myopathies, strength generally improves with discontinuation of the amiodarone.

Alcohol

Alcohol abuse has been associated both with acute episodes of rhabdomyolysis and also with the development of a chronic alcoholic myopathy. The pathogenesis of both of these entities remains obscure. The rhabdomyolysis is characterized by muscle pain, swelling, cramping, and generalized weakness associated with marked elevation in CK. It generally occurs during, or soon after, an intense drinking binge. Severe cases are associated with myoglobinuria and acute renal failure. Treatment is supportive with intravenous hydration, close monitoring of renal function and dialysis, if significant renal failure develops.

Chronic alcoholic myopathy is characterized by the insidious onset of proximal weakness after years of alcohol abuse. Muscle biopsy may demonstrate scattered muscle fiber atrophy with necrosis and regeneration [76]. Whether this represents true myotoxicity from alcohol or is a secondary effect from poor nutrition and/or disuse atrophy is unclear. Because of the ambiguity surrounding this disorder, it should be a diagnosis of exclusion, as patients presenting with limb girdle weakness and a history of alcoholism are not immune from other causes of muscle weakness.

> ### Five things to remember about myopathies due to systemic disease
>
> **1.** Myopathies due to drug toxicity are important to identify as they virtually all resolve with removal of the offending agent, potentially saving the patient from invasive investigations and/or trials of potentially toxic immunosuppressive treatment.
> **2.** Steroid myopathy is more common with fluorinated steroids (i.e. dexamethasone);it rarely occurs at doses of less than prednisone 30 mg daily (or its equivalent).
> **3.** Inflammatory myopathies can generally be differentiated from toxic myopathies by the pattern of weakness: in most toxic myopathies, the weakness primarily affects the hip girdle muscles; whereas in inflammatory myopathies, the degree of weakness in the hip and shoulder girdle tends to be similar.
> **4.** Polymyositis is associated with a number of systemic diseases in addition to the connective tissue diseases, including HIV infection, HTLV-1 infection, and graft versus host disease.
> **5.** The diagnosis of an inflammatory or autoimmune necrotizing myopathy necessitates a thorough malignancy screen, which should be repeated annually for at least 3 years following diagnosis.

References

1 Duyff RF, Van den Bosch J, Laman DM, et al. Neuromuscular findings in thyroid dysfunction: a prospective clinical and electrodiagnostic study. *J. Neurol. Neurosurg. Psychiatry* 2000;68:750–755.

2 Olson BR, Klein I, Benner R, et al. Hyperthyroid myopathy and the response to treatment. *Thyroid* 1991;1:137–141.

3 Kung AW. Clinical review: thyrotoxic periodic paralysis: a diagnostic challenge. *J. Clin. Endocrinol. Metab.* 2006;91:2490–2495.

4 Liu YC, Tsai WS, Chau T, Lin SH. Acute hypercapnic respiratory failure due to thyrotoxic periodic paralysis. *Am. J. Med. Sci.* 2004;327:264–267.

5 Li J, Yang XB, Zhao Y. Thyrotoxic periodic paralysis in the Chinese population: clinical features in 45 cases. *Exp. Clin. Endocrinol. Diabetes* 2010;118:22–26.

6 Manoukian MA, Foote JA, Crapo LM. Clinical and metabolic features of thyrotoxic periodic paralysis in 24 episodes. *Arch. Intern. Med.* 1999;159:601–606.

7 Trujillo-Santos AJ. Diabetic muscle infarction: an underdiagnosed complication of long-standing diabetes. *Diabetes Care* 2003 Jan; 26:211–215.

8 Kapur S, McKendry RJ. Treatment and outcomes of diabetic muscle infarction. *J. Clin. Rheumatol.* 2005;11:8–12.

9 Lentine K, Guest S. Diabetic muscle infarction in end-stage renal disease. *Nephrol. Dial. Transplant* 2004;19:664–669.

10 Jelinek JS, Murphey MD, Aboulafia AJ, et al. Muscle infarction in patients with diabetes mellitus: MR imaging findings. *Radiology* 1999;211:241–247.

11 Sahin I, Taskapan C, Taskapan H, et al. Diabetic muscle infarction: an unusual cause of muscle pain in a diabetic patient on hemodialysis. *Int. Urol. Nephrol.* 2005;37:629–632.

12 Chester CS, Banker BQ. Focal infarction of muscle in diabetics. *Diabetes Care* 1986;9(6):623–630.

13 Bjornskov EK, Carry MR, Katz FH, et al. Diabetic muscle infarction: a new perspective on pathogenesis and management. *Neuromuscul. Disord.* 1995;5:39–45.

14 Palmer GW, Greco TP. Diabetic thigh muscle infarction in association with antiphospholipid antibodies. *Semin. Arthritis Rheum.* 2001;30:272–280.

15 Amato AA, Dumitru D. Acquired myopathies. In D Dumitru, AA Amato, MJ Zwarts, editors, *Electrodiagnostic Medicine*, 2nd ed. Philadelphia: Hanley & Belfus, Inc, 2002, pp. 1371–1432.

16 Dalakas MC. Polymyositis, dermatomyositis, and inclusion body myositis. *N. Engl. J. Med.* 1991;325:1487–1498.

17 Hochberg MC, Feldman D, Stevens MB. Adult-onset polymyositis/dermatomyositis: analysis of clinical and laboratory features and survival in 76 cases with a review of the literature. *Semin. Arthritis Rheum.* 1986;15:168–178.

18 Targoff IN. Immune manifestations of inflammatory disease. *Rheum. Dis. Clin. N. Am.* 1994;20:857–880.

19 Streib EW, Wilbourn AJ, Mitsumoto H. Spontaneous electrical muscle fiber activity in polymyositis and dermatomyositis. *Muscle Nerve* 1979;2:14–18.

20 Mitz M, Chang GJ, Albers JW, Sulaiman AR. Electromyographic and histologic paraspinal abnormalities in polymyositis/dermatomyositis. *Arch. Phys. Med. Rehabil.* 1981;62:118–121.

21 Kissel JT, Mendell JR, Rammohan KW. Microvascular deposition of complement membrane attack complex in dermatomyositis. *N. Engl. J. Med.* 1986;314:331–334.

22 Kissel JT, Halterman RK, Rammohan KW, Mendell JR, The relationship of complement-mediated microvasculopathy to the histologic features and clinical duration of disease in dermatomyositis. *Arch. Neurol.* 1991;48:26–30.

23 De Visser M, Emslie-Smith AM, Engel AG. Early ultrastructural alterations in adult dermatomyositis: capillary abnormalities precede other structural changes in muscle. *J. Neurol. Sci.* 1989;94:181–192.

24 Arahata K, Engel AG. Monoclonal antibody analysis of mononuclear cells in myopathies. I: Quantitation of subsets according to diagnosis and sites of accumulation and demonstration and counts of muscle fibers invaded by T cells. *Ann. Neurol.* 1984;16:193–208.

25 Carpenter S, Karpati G. *Pathology of Skeletal Muscle*, 2nd ed. New York: Oxford University Press, 2001.

26 Bronner IM, Hoogendijk JE, Wintzen AR, et al. Necrotizing myopathy, an unusual presentation of a steroid-responsive myopathy. *J. Neurol.* 2003;250:480–485.

27 Douglas AC, Macleod JG, Matthews JD. Symptomatic sarcoidosis of skeletal muscle. *J. Neurol. Neurosurg. Psychiatry* 1973;36:1034–1040.

28 Le Roux K, Streichenberger N, Vial C, et al. Granulomatous myositis: a clinical study of 13 cases. *Muscle Nerve* 2007;35:171–177.

29 Wolfe SM, Pinals RS, Aelion JA, et al. Myopathy in sarcoidosis: clinical and pathologic study of four cases and review of the literature. *Semin. Arthritis Rheum.* 1987;16:300–306.

30 Mozaffar T, Lopate G, Pestronk A. Clinical correlates of granulomas in muscle. *J. Neurol.* 1998;245:519–524.

31 Azuma K, Yamada H, Ohkubo M, et al. Incidence and predictive factors for malignancies in 136 Japanese patients with dermatomyositis, polymyositis and clinically amyopathic dermatomyositis. *Mod. Rhematol.* 2010 Oct 5 [Epub ahead of print].

32 Dalakas MC. An update on inflammatory and autoimmune myopathies. *Neuropathol. Appl. Neurobiol.*, "Accepted Article"; doi: 10.1111/j.1365-2990.2010.01153.x.

33 Yamauchi K, Kogashiwa Y, Nagafuji H, et al. Head and neck cancer with dermatomyositis: a report of two clinical cases. *Int. J. Otolaryngol.*, [Epub 2010 May 31].

34 Teh Cl, Wong JS, Soo HH. Polymyositis and dermatomyositis in Sarawak: a profile of patients treated in the Sarawak general hospital. *Rheumatol. Int.* 2011 [Epub ahead of print] DOI 10.1007/s00296-010-1745-2.

35 Spuler S, Emslie-Smith A, Engel AG. Amyloid myopathy: an underdiagnosed entity. *Ann. Neurol.* 1998;43:719–728.

36 Chapin JE, Kornfeld M, Harris A. Amyloid myopathy: characteristic features of a still underdiagnosed disease. *Muscle Nerve* 2005;31:266–272.

37 Ashe J, Borel CO, Hart G, et al. Amyloid myopathy presenting with respiratory failure. *J. Neurol. Neurosurg. Psychiatry* 1992;55:162–165.

38 Katzmann JA, Kyle RA, Benson J, et al. Screening panels for detection of monoclonal gammopathies. *Clin. Chem.* 2009;55:1517–1522.

39 Johnson RW, Williams FM, Kazi S, et al. Human immunodeficiency virus-associated polymyositis: a longitudinal study of outcome. *Arthritis Rheum.* 2003;49:172–178.

40 Authier FJ, Chariot P, Gherardi RK. Skeletal muscle involvement in human immunodeficiency virus (HIV)-infected patients in the era of highly active antiretroviral therapy (HAART). *Muscle Nerve.* 2005;32:247–260.

41 Heckmann JM, Pillay K, Hearn AP, Kenyon C. Polymyositis in African HIV-infected subjects. *Neuromusular Disorders* 2010;20:735–739.

42 Illa I, Nath A, Dalakas M. Immunocytochemical and virological characteristics of HIV associated inflammatory myopathies: similarities with seronegative polymyositis. *Ann. Neurol.* 1991;29:474–481.

43 de Sanctis JT, Cumbo-Nacheli G, Dobbie D, et al. HIV-associated nemaline rod myopathy: role of intravenous immunoglobulin therapy in two persons with HIV/AIDS. *AIDS Read.* 2008;18:90–94.

44 Dalakas MC, Illa I, Pezeschkpour GH, et al. Mitochondrial myopathy caused by long-term zidovudine therapy. *N. Engl. J. Med.* 1990;322:1098–1105.

45 Mhiri C, Baudrimont M, Bonne G, et al. Zidovudine myopathy: a distinctive disorder associated with mitochondrial dysfunction. *Ann. Neurol.* 1991;29:606–614.

46 Saito M, Higuchi I, Saito A, et al. Molecular analysis of T cell clonotypes in muscle-infiltrating lymphocytes from patients with human T lymphotropic virus type 1 polymyositis. *J. Infect. Dis.* 2002;186:1231–1241.

47 Gilbert DT, Morgan O, Smikle MF, et al. HTLV-1 associated polymyositis in Jamaica. *Acta Neurol. Scand.* 2001;104:101–104.

48 Inose M, Higuchi I, Yoshimine K, et al. A study of clinical symptoms, muscle pathology, therapeutic response, and prognosis of myositis in patients with HTLV-1 associated myelopathy (HAM). *Rinsho Shinkeigaku* 1999;39:807–811.

49 Agyeman P, Duppenthaler A, Heininger U, et al. Influenza-associated myositis in children. *Infection* 2004;32:199–203.

50 Meier PW, Bianchetti MG. An 8-year-old boy with a 4-day history of fever, cough and malaise, and a 2-day history of painful calves and difficulty walking. *Eur. J. Pediatr.* 2003;162:731–732.

51 Oda K, Nakaseko C, Ozawa S, et al. Fasciitis and myositis: an analysis of muscle-related complications caused by chronic GVHD after allo-SCT. *Bone Marrow Transplant* 2009;43:159–167.

52 Janin A, Socie G, Devergie A, et al. Fasciitis in chronic graft-versus-host disease. A clinicopathologic study of 14 cases. *Ann. Intern. Med.* 1994;120:993–998.

53 Stevens AM, Sullivan KM, Nelson JL. Polymyositis as a manifestation of chronic graft versus-host disease. *Rheumatol. (Oxf.)* 2003;42:34–39.

54 Lacomis D, Zochodne DW, Bird SJ. Critical illness myopathy. *Muscle Nerve* 2000;23:1785–1788.

55 Lacomis D, Petrella JT, Giuliani MJ. Causes of neuromuscular weakness in the intensive care unit: a study of ninety-two patients. *Muscle Nerve* 1998;21:610–617.

56 Bruckert E, Hayem G, Dejager S, et al. Mild to moderate muscular symptoms with high-dosage statin therapy in hyperlipidemic patients—The PRIMO Study. *Cardiovasc. Drugs Ther.* 2005;19:403–414.

57 Gaist D, Rodriguez G, Huerta C, et al. Lipid-lowering drugs and risk of myopathy—a population-based follow-up study. *Epidemiology* 2001;12:565–569.

58 Shanahan RL, Kerzee JA, Sandhoff BG, et al. Clinical Pharmacy Cardiac Risk Service (CPCRS) Study Group. Low myopathy rates associated with statins as monotherapy or combination therapy with interacting drugs in a group model health maintenance organization. *Pharmacotherapy* 2005;25:345–351.

59 Harper CR, Jacobson TA. The broad spectrum of statin myopathy: from myalgia to rhabdomyolysis. *Curr. Opin. Lipidol.* 2007;18:401–408.

60 Sewright KA, Clarkson PM, Thompson PD. Statin myopathy: incidence, risk factors, and pathophysiology. *Curr. Atheroscler. Rep.* 2007;9:389–396.

61 Grable-Esposito P, Katzberg HD, Greenberg SA, et al. Immune-mediated necrotizing myopathy associated with statins. *Muscle Nerve* 2010;41:185–190.

62 Young JM, Florkowski CM, Molyneux S.L. et al. Effect of coenzyme Q(10) supplementation on simvastatin-induced myalgia. *Am. J. Cardiol.* 2007;100:1400–1403.

63 Bowyer SL, LaMothe MP, Hollister JR., Steroid myopathy: incidence and detection in a population with asthma. *J. Allergy Clin. Immunol.* 1985;76:234–242.

64 Dropcho EJ, Soong SJ. Steroid-induced weakness in patients with primary brain tumors. *Neurology* 1991;41:1235–1239.

65 Siddiqui AK, Huberfeld SI, Weidenheim KM, et al. Hydroxychloroquine-induced toxic myopathy causing respiratory failure. *Chest* 2007;131:588–590.

66 Abdel-Hamid H, Oddis CV, Lacomis D. Severe hydroxychloroquine myopathy. *Muscle Nerve* 2008;38:1206–1210.

67 Casado E, Gratacos J, Tolosa C, et al. Antimalarial myopathy: an underdiagnosed complication? Prospective longitudinal study of 119 patients. *Ann. Rheum. Dis.* 2006;65:385–390.

68 Suzuki T, Nakagawa M, Yoshikawa A, et al. The first molecular evidence that autophagy relates rimmed vacuole formation in chloroquine myopathy. *J. Biochem.* 2002;131:647–651.

69 Nord JE, Shah PK, Rinaldi RZ, et al. Hydroxychloroquine cardiotoxicity in systemic lupus erythematosus: a report of 2 cases and review of the literature. *Semin. Arthritis Rheum.* 2004;33:336–351.

70 Wilbur K, Makowsky M. Colchicine myotoxicity: case reports and literature review. *Pharmacotherapy* 2004;24:1784–1792.

71 Sahin G, Korkmaz C, Yalcin AU. Which statin should be used together with colchicine? Clinical experience in three patients with nephritic syndrome due to AA type amyloidosis. *Rheumatol. Int.* 2008;28:289–291.

72 Rutkove SB, De Girolami U, Preston DC, et al. Myotonia in colchicine myoneuropathy. *Muscle Nerve.* 1996;19:870–875.

73 Caglar K, Odabasi Z, Safali M, et al. Colchicine-induced myopathy with myotonia in a patient with chronic renal failure. *Clin. Neurol. Neurosurg.* 2003;105:274–276.

74 Carella F, Riva E, Morandi L, et al. Myopathy during amiodarone treatment: a case report. *Ital. J. Neurol. Sci.* 1987;8:605–608.

75 Pulipaka U, Lacomis D, Omalu B. Amiodarone-induced neuromyopathy: three cases and a review of the literature. *J. Clin. Neuromuscul. Dis.* 2002;3:97–105.

76 Amato AA, Russell JA. *Neuromuscular Disorders*, China: The McGraw-Hill Companies, Inc., 2008.

14 Autonomic manifestations of systemic disease

Brent P. Goodman[1] and Eduardo E. Benarroch[2]
[1]Mayo Clinic, Scottsdale, AZ, USA
[2]Mayo Clinic, Rochester, MN, USA

Introduction

The autonomic nervous system is diffuse, with pathways that pervade every organ system. As a result, autonomic nervous system dysfunction can accompany systemic disease affecting virtually any organ system. Signs and symptoms of autonomic nervous system impairment can occur in conjunction with other neurological disorders, such as sensorimotor peripheral neuropathy in a patient with amyloidosis, or can occur without any other apparent neurological dysfunction. Recognition of autonomic nervous system impairment may play a vital role in establishing a diagnosis of a particular systemic disease, and treatment of autonomic symptoms (in addition to treatment of the underlying systemic condition when possible) may be necessary.

The evaluation of a patient with suspected impairment of the autonomic nervous system involves a thorough history and examination, and when possible, autonomic testing. The general categories of autonomic nervous system disease that should be queried during the history include cardiovascular adrenergic, skin vasomotor, sudomotor, secretomotor, gastrointestinal, and genitourinary function (see Table 14.1). Postural lightheadedness and syncope suggest cardiovascular adrenergic impairment, and demonstration of orthostatic hypotension on examination can provide objective evidence of adrenergic failure. Symptoms such as flushing or coldness of the extremities may indicate the presence of skin vasomotor impairment. Sudomotor dysfunction may manifest as excessive sweating (hyperhidrosis), which may be generalized, segmental, or focal, and diminished or absent sweating (hypohidrosis or anhidrosis), which typically manifests as heat intolerance. Dry eyes and mouth may indicate secretomotor dysfunction. Symptoms such as early satiety, nausea, vomiting, and weight loss may be a clue to gastroparesis. Constipation, and occasionally constipation alternating with diarrhea, may indicate intestinal autonomic impairment. Typical symptoms of genitourinary impairment include urinary dysfunction with incomplete emptying or urinary retention, and erectile dysfunction.

An important aspect of the clinical evaluation is a complete medication review. Medications used to treat systemic disease can result in autonomic nervous system impairment, and depending upon symptom severity and the underlying condition the medication is being used to treat, it may be necessary to discontinue a medication to determine whether or not medication side effect is the cause. For example, alpha-1-receptor antagonists used to treat benign prostatic hypertrophy in the elderly may cause postural lightheadedness due to orthostatic hypotension. Medications with anticholinergic properties may cause dry eyes and dry mouth, constipation, or decreased sweating.

Supine and standing heart rate and blood pressure should be checked. An initial standing blood pressure at 1 min, and then later at 5 or even 10 min can be performed to assess fluctuations in blood pressure and heart rate, or orthostatic hypotension that may

Neurological Disorders due to Systemic Disease, First Edition. Edited by Steven L. Lewis.
© 2013 Blackwell Publishing Ltd. Published 2013 by Blackwell Publishing Ltd.

Table 14.1 Clinical assessment of the autonomic nervous system

Autonomic system	Symptoms
Cardiovascular adrenergic	Postural lightheadedness
	Syncope
	Head, neck pain w/standing
Vasomotor	Flushing
	Cold extremities
Sudomotor	Hyperhidrosis
	Anhidrosis
	Hypohidrosis
	Heat intolerance
Secretomotor	Dry eyes, mouth
Gastrointestinal	Early satiety
	Nausea, vomiting
	Weight loss
	Constipation
	Diarrhea
	Abdominal pain
	Bloating
Genitourinary	Urinary retention
	Erectile dysfunction
	Retrograde ejaculation

become more prominent with prolonged standing. Orthostatic hypotension in the absence of a compensatory tachycardia provides objective evidence of adrenergic and cardiovagal failure. Pupillary responses to light and accommodation test the integrity of sympathetic and parasympathetic pupillary pathways. Examination of the skin for abnormal color, temperature, or sweating changes can suggest vasomotor or sudomotor impairment.

Autonomic testing

Autonomic nervous system testing provides additional objective and quantifiable information regarding the integrity of the autonomic nervous system. Such testing can identify the distribution and severity of autonomic nervous system dysfunction. Analysis of beat-to-beat blood pressure and heart responses during tilt-table testing appraises cardiovascular

adrenergic function. Patients with adrenergic failure demonstrate a progressive decrease in blood pressure (>20 mmHg decrease in systolic blood pressure; >10 mmHg decrease in diastolic blood pressure) and reduction in pulse pressure during head-up tilt. Other abnormalities that can be seen during tilt-table testing in those with disorders of orthostatic intolerance include syncope, fluctuations in blood pressure, and excessive increase in heart rate during head-up tilt (see Table 14.2). Beat-to-beat blood pressure response during the Valsalva maneuver provides additional analysis of cardiovascular adrenergic function.

Cardiovagal function can be assessed through a number of different means including heart-rate variation during deep breathing, the Valsalva ratio, and

Table 14.2 Autonomic testing

Modality tested	Tests	Findings in autonomic disorders
Cardiovascular adrenergic	Tilt-Table	Orthostatic hypotension
		Syncope
		Excessive heart rate increment
		BP fluctuations
	BP Valsalva	Impairment late phase II
		Impairment phase IV
		Excessive early phase II
Cardiovagal	HR Variation DB	Reduction heart rate variation
	Valsalva Ratio	
	Spectral Analysis HR	
Sudomotor	QSART	Hyperhidrosis
	TST	Hypohidrosis, anhidrosis
	PASP	
	Silastic imprint	

BP, blood pressure; HR, heart rate; DB, deep breathing; QSART, quantitative sudomotor axon reflex testing; TST, thermoregulatory sweat test; PASP, peripheral autonomic surface potential.

spectral analysis of heart-rate variation. Disorders of the autonomic nervous system can result in a reduction in heart-rate variation on such tests, indicating cardiovagal dysfunction. Sudomotor function can be formally assessed through quantitative sudomotor axon reflex testing (QSART), thermoregulatory sweat testing, silastic imprinting, or skin potential recording. These tests provide an assessment of sympathetic sudomotor pathways, and can demonstrate excessive sudomotor output in patients with hyperhidrosis, or deficient sudomotor output in patients with hypohidrosis or anhidrosis with various autonomic disorders.

Gastrointestinal motility studies are essential in establishing the presence, distribution, and severity of gastrointestinal dysmotility. Gastric emptying studies can provide evidence of gastroparesis in individuals with symptoms of early satiety, and small and large bowel transit studies can demonstrate delayed transit times in patients with constipation resulting from intestinal dysmotility. Urodynamic studies provide a quantitative assessment of urologic function in patients with urinary symptoms.

Anatomy of the autonomic nervous system

The autonomic nervous system (ANS) refers to the visceral internal-regulation system responsible for the control of automatic functions necessary for health and survival. The ANS can be generally characterized as consisting of a system of efferent and afferent pathways. The visceral efferent pathways innervate blood vessels, heart, viscera, glands, and smooth muscles, and afferent visceral pathways transmit impulses from these structures to the central nervous via autonomic and peripheral somatic nerves. The visceral afferent nerves are thinly myelinated or unmyelinated and terminate in the spinal cord and brain stem.

The ANS consists of three divisions, including the craniosacral or parasympathetic division, the thoracolumbar or sympathetic division, and the enteric nervous system located in the wall of the gastrointestinal system. The preganglionic parasympathetic nerves originate in the brainstem and the second, third, and fourth segments of the sacral spinal cord, and synapse on ganglia close to the structures they innervate. In the brainstem, the dorsal nucleus of the vagus is the origin of the preganglionic, parasympathetic efferent pathway, which travels via the vagus nerve to cardiac, pulmonary, and gastrointestinal ganglia where they synapse with short, postganglionic neurons that innervate these organs. The sacral parasympathetic visceral efferent pathways leave the spinal cord, forming the pelvic splanchnic nerves, and then synapse in the ganglia of the pelvic plexus, bladder, and large bowel. Preganglionic sympathetic nerves originate in the interomediolateral gray matter in the thoracolumbar spinal cord (T1–L2) and synapse in one of several paravertebral and prevertebral ganglia. Gray communicating rami connect the paravertebral ganglia with the spinal nerves, which carry the postganglionic sympathetic nerves to the body.

Acetylcholine is the primary neurotransmitter between the preganglionic and postganglionic neurons in the sympathetic and parasympathetic nervous system, is present at the parasympathetic postganglionic nerve terminals, and is the neurotransmitter involved in postganglionic sympathetic nerve fibers innervation of the sweat glands. The primary neurotransmitter involved in all other postganglionic sympathetic nervous system function is norepinephrine.

A variety of systemic conditions can be associated with peripheral autonomic neuropathies. The presence of neuropathic signs and symptoms such as extremity paresthesias, and sensorimotor impairment on neurological examination, is a potential clue to the presence of a peripheral autonomic neuropathy in a patient with symptoms of autonomic nervous system impairment. Conditions associated with autonomic neuropathies can be broadly categorized as being due to various metabolic, infectious, immunologic, and hematologic disorders. Because symptoms of an autonomic neuropathy can be the initial, and in some cases, sole harbinger of these systemic conditions, establishing an accurate diagnosis requires knowledge of these conditions and an appropriate diagnostic evaluation. Furthermore, the severity of autonomic symptom involvement in these conditions can range from mild, requiring no treatment, to severe, necessitating treatment.

Diabetic autonomic neuropathy

Diabetes mellitus affects 220 million people worldwide [1]. Neuropathy, including autonomic neuropathy, is a frequent complication of both type I and type II diabetes mellitus, and is the cause of significant morbidity and mortality. Reported incidence and prevalence rates of autonomic neuropathy in diabetics vary, but many of these studies have been hampered by methodological issues, and there remain a paucity of population-based studies. Based upon a population-based study of diabetic patients in Rochester, Minnesota, the prevalence of autonomic impairment was 54% in type I and 73% in patients with type II diabetes [2]. It is notable that these prevalence rates are similar to the reported prevalence rates of peripheral neuropathy in the earlier population-based Rochester diabetic neuropathy study [3].

Most patients with diabetic autonomic neuropathy have mild autonomic impairment, however, 14% of diabetic patients in the Rochester study had generalized autonomic failure, including up to 8.4% of patients with orthostatic hypotension [2]. Autonomic symptoms generally increase over time, and generally correlate with the duration of diabetes, severity of peripheral neuropathy, and advancing age [4]. Other commonly encountered autonomic symptoms in diabetic patients include constipation, urinary symptoms, impotence, and diarrhea [2,5]. Diabetic patients with significant orthostatic hypotension may experience syncope.

There has been considerable interest in the concept of cardiac autonomic neuropathy (CAN) [6,7]. Cardiac rate and performance is primarily controlled through autonomic pathways, and an early manifestation of autonomic dysfunction in patients with diabetes mellitus is cardiovagal (parasympathetic) impairment [8,9]. This results in a reduction in heart-rate variability, and can be established through the tests of cardiovagal function discussed earlier in this chapter. In conjunction with this reduction of cardiovagal or parasympathetic modulation of heart rate, there is evidence of early enhancement of sympathetic tone [10,11]. It has been suggested that this pattern of autonomic dysregulation underlies the increased risk of cardiac dysrhythmia and sudden death in diabetic patients. Longitudinal studies of subjects with type I and II diabetes who have autonomic neuropathy have shown 5 year mortality rates

of 16–50% [12–14]. Furthermore, meta-analysis of 12 studies comparing diabetic patients with and without CAN, demonstrated that those with CAN had double the risk of having experienced silent myocardial ischemia than those without [15].

The pathogenesis of diabetic autonomic neuropathy has not been established, though a number of different theories have been proposed. Chronic hyperglycemia is an important factor, and it has long been assumed that maintenance of normoglycemia is important in reducing the risk of developing or worsening an autonomic neuropathy. Indeed, data from the Diabetes Control and Complications Trial (DCCT) showed that intensive insulin therapy in type I diabetics resulted in a 53% reduction in the incidence of CAN compared with conventional treatment [16]. In a more recent report of this same DCCT cohort, the prevalence of CAN remained significantly lower in the group given intensive insulin therapy 14 years after termination of the DCCT trial despite no difference in insulin treatment or glycemic levels between the groups [17].

Symptomatic treatment of autonomic failure may be necessary in individuals with significant autonomic symptoms. Because patients with autonomic failure may also have a significant concomitant neuropathy, patient education to prevent complications (such as trauma to joints and skin) related to reduced sensation should be emphasized. Pharmacologic treatment of neuropathic pain may also be necessary in some patients. Treatment of orthostatic hypotension through pharmacologic and nonpharmacologic measures may be necessary in a minority of patients (see Table 14.3). Important nonpharmacologic interventions for orthostatic hypotension include compression stockings, abdominal binder, exercise regimen to strengthen lower limb and abdominal muscles, and plasma expansion through liberalization of salt and fluid intake. Midodrine, an α_1-receptor agonist, is often used in the first-line pharmacologic treatment of orthostatic hypotension. It is currently the only medication approved by the United States Food and Drug Administration for the treatment of orthostatic hypotension. Fludrocortisone may be beneficial in the treatment of orthostatic hypotension through plasma expansion. Pyridostigmine has more recently been reported to be of potential benefit in patients with orthostatic hypotension by increasing vascular adrenergic tone, and appears to not worsen supine

Table 14.3 Treatment of orthostatic hypotension

Nonpharmacologic treatment	Pharmacologic treatment
Compression stockings	Midodrine
Abdominal binder	Fludrocortisone acetate
Leg and abdominal strengthening exercises	Pyridostigmine
Increase salt intake	Erythropoietin
Increase fluid intake	Desmopressin

hypertension, which is a potential side effect of both midodrine and fludrocortisone [18]. Erythropoietin may be considered in refractory patients or in those with a normochromic normocytic anemia.

Amyloidosis

Amyloidosis results from the deposition of insoluble amyloid proteins in various organs and tissues. The deposition of these protein fibrils in a beta-pleated sheet configuration disrupts organ structure and function, with a particular propensity to impair cardiac, renal, and hepatic function. Amyloid is selectively stained with Congo red stain, and exhibits a green birefringence when viewed under a polarizing microscope. Peripheral nerve impairment, including peripheral autonomic neuropathy, is common in some but not all forms of amyloidosis.

Amyloidosis may be generally considered as acquired or hereditary. The acquired amyloidoses are further classified as primary, in which the fibrils consist primarily of light chains (AL), or secondary, with fibrils consisting of protein A (AA) [19]. The AA amyloid protein is produced in the liver in response to proinflammatory cytokines in various infectious and inflammatory conditions [20]. Significant peripheral nerve impairment does not typically occur in AA amyloidosis [21]. Peripheral nervous system involvement, including autonomic neuropathy, is frequent in AL amyloidosis and in certain forms of hereditary amyloidosis.

Primary systemic amyloidosis

AL amyloidosis is an uncommon disorder with an estimated incidence of 0.89 per 100,000 [22], but is

thought be the most common form of amyloidosis in the developed world. AL amyloidosis is a systemic disorder that can affect virtually any organ system including the peripheral autonomic nerves. The median age at diagnosis is 65, and in a large series of 229 patients, 99% were older than 40 years of age [19]. Systemic symptoms, such as weakness, fatigue, or weight loss, are the most common initial symptom in AL amyloidosis, and orthostatic hypotension was present prior to or at the time of diagnosis in 14% of patients [19]. Postural lightheadedness, "dizziness," and syncope suggest the possibility of orthostatic hypotension in these patients.

Familial amyloidosis due to transthyretin mutation

There are many different forms of hereditary amyloidosis, which are characterized by the type of protein contained in the amyloid deposits. Transthyretin, apolipoprotein AI, and gelsolin are the only hereditary forms known to affect the peripheral nervous system. Of these, transthyretin (TTR-A) amyloidosis is the most common, and results from mutation in the TTR molecule. TTR-A is an autosomal dominant disorder, and there are now approximately 100 different known mutations in the transthyretin gene [23]. The median age at diagnosis is 64 and a male-to-female ratio of 3.7:1 has been reported [24]. Autonomic neuropathy ultimately developed in 70% of this cohort, with orthostatic hypotension being the most common manifestation, followed by symptoms of gastrointestinal dysmotility. A more recent report of 36 patients with TTR-A who underwent autonomic testing suggested that autonomic symptoms were the initial symptom in 11% of patients, and were present in 91% of patients at the time of evaluation [25]. Rarely, recurrent syncope may be an isolated, persistent feature of TTR-A [26].

Familial amyloidosis due to gelsolin and apolipoprotein A-1 mutations

Familial amyloid polyneuropathy resulting from a mutation in gelsolin is a rare, autosomal dominant disorder that has been reported in Finland, several European countries, the United States, and Japan [27]. The primary clinical manifestations of this form of familial amyloidosis include progressive cranial neuropathy, corneal lattice dystrophy, a typically mild polyneuropathy, and carpal tunnel syndrome [28]. Autonomic nervous system impairment can occur in this form of familial amyloidosis, but is typically milder than that seen with AL amyloidosis and familial amyloidosis due to transthyretin mutation [29].

Multiple mutations in the apolipoprotein A-1 (ApoA1) gene have been identified, with some resulting in systemic amyloid deposition. However, only one of these mutations has been associated with peripheral neuropathy, as originally described by Van Allen and colleagues in an Iowa cohort [46]. The peripheral neuropathy and autonomic involvement is similar to that seen with transthyretin amyloidosis, and renal failure secondary to amyloid deposition is frequently encountered.

Manifestations of autonomic neuropathy in amyloidosis

In a review of 65 patients with primary systemic and familial amyloidosis referred to the Mayo Clinic Autonomic laboratory, the most common symptom of autonomic dysfunction was orthostatic intolerance (see Figure 14.1) in 74% of patients, followed by gastrointestinal symptoms in 71%, 35% of patients with secretomotor (dry eyes and dry mouth) failure, and 25% with genitourinary symptoms [30]. Within this cohort, signs and symptoms of generalized autonomic failure in conjunction with a painful peripheral neuropathy was present in most (62%) patients, though 11% of patients in this series had autonomic failure without signs or symptoms or EMG evidence of neuropathy.

Gastrointestinal involvement by amyloidosis is common and varied. Diarrhea is the most common gastrointestinal symptom associated with AL amyloidosis and likely results from a number of different mechanisms, including gastrointestinal dysmotility [31]. Disordered motility can affect the esophagus, stomach, small intestine, and large intestine. Impairment in esophageal motility may result in dysphagia, and gastric dysmotility may result in early satiety, abdominal pain, nausea, and vomiting. Diarrhea is a typical manifestation of small intestinal motility, and impairment in large intestinal function may result in constipation or even pseudo-obstruction [31].

Impairment of the genitourinary system is an indicator of autonomic neuropathy in patients with amyloidosis. Symptoms suggesting genitourinary dysfunction include erectile dysfunction, incomplete bladder emptying, urinary retention, and urinary overflow incontinence [22]. Disturbances in sweating are frequently observed on autonomic studies of patients with primary systemic and transthyretin amyloidosis [30]. Sweating impairment may be subclinical, or may result in symptoms of heat intolerance. Light and electron microscopic studies of patients with transthyretin familial amyloidosis have demonstrated loss of nerve terminals and unmyelinated axons in the region of eccrine sweat glands, indicating that sweat gland denervation is the likely cause of anhidrosis in amyloid patients [32]. Rarely, anhidrosis may be particularly severe in gelsolin amyloidosis [33].

Diagnosis

The diagnosis of amyloidosis requires the pathological demonstration of amyloid tissue deposition. Amyloid deposits demonstrate apple-green birefringence under polarizing light with Congo red staining.

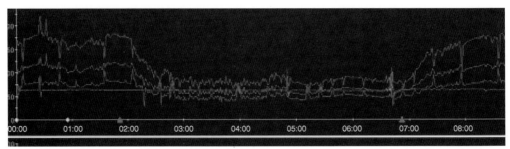

Fig 14.1 Tilt-table testing in familial amyloidosis. This figure demonstrates orthostatic hypotension on head-up tilt-table testing in a patient with transthyretin (Phe64Leu) amyloidosis, due to severe autonomic neuropathy. (See also Plate 14.1.)

Distinguishing primary systemic from familial amyloidosis can prove challenging but is critical given differences in prognosis and treatment. A family history of amyloidosis is absent in over half of patients with familial amyloidosis [34]. Therefore, a negative family history does not exclude hereditary amyloidosis. Furthermore, it is well established that a monoclonal gammopathy is not uncommon in patients with hereditary amyloidosis [35,36]. In a study from the United Kingdom, a monoclonal gammopathy was discovered in 24% of patients with hereditary amyloidosis [35]. A later study reported that 6% of patients screened had both a monoclonal gammopathy and hereditary amyloidosis [36]. These authors have suggested that genetic screening should be performed in all patients with amyloidosis, including those with a monoclonal gammopathy. There may also be a role for mass spectrometry on clinical biopsy specimens in classifying amyloidosis [34,37].

Treatment

Treatment options for primary systemic amyloidosis include high-dose chemotherapy and stem-cell transplantation. Melphalan, often used in conjunction with corticosteroids, has been the standard chemotherapeutic agent used in the treatment of AL amyloidosis [38], but clinical response rates are only 20% with this standard regimen [39]. Peripheral blood stem-cell transplantation has also been utilized in AL amyloidosis, with some suggestion of improved survival in select patients who underwent this treatment regimen [40]. Mortality rates with peripheral blood stem-cell transplantation remain between 15% and 25% [41–43]. Recent research suggests that survival in AL amyloidosis has improved over time [44], but a recent systematic review comparing chemotherapy with stem-cell transplantation has failed to show any definitive survival advantage of one treatment approach over the other [45].

Transthyretin amyloidosis results from mutations in tranthyretin, which is a plasma transport protein for thyroid hormone and retinol-binding protein/vitamin A [46]. The transthyretin gene is localized on chromosome 18 and is synthesized in the liver. This is the basis for liver transplantation, which was first performed in Sweden in 1990 [47], and has become the treatment of choice for this condition [48]. Liver transplantation does reduce circulating

levels of mutant transthyretin, and may stop neurological progression if performed in patients with mild neurological deficits [49]. Impact of liver transplantation on autonomic dysfunction is variable. Improvement in anhidrosis has been reported following liver transplantation [50]. Orthostatic hypotension improved in some patients [50,51], but was reported to be unchanged in some patients following transplantation [49]. In one series, orthostatic hypotension developed following liver transplantation [49]. Gastrointestinal symptoms may improve following liver transplantation [49–51].

Rheumatologic disorders

Sjögren syndrome

Sjögren syndrome (SS) is an autoimmune disorder that is characterized by a lymphocytic infiltration of salivary and lacrimal glands, resulting in xerostomia and xerophthalmia. Systemic, extraglandular manifestations occur in at least 1/3 of patients, and may include neurological, pulmonary, rheumatologic, or gastrointestinal signs and symptoms [52]. SS can occur in isolation (termed primary Sjögren syndrome) or may occur in conjunction with other connective tissue disorders (secondary Sjögren syndrome).

Autonomic symptoms may occur in up to 50% of patients with SS [53]. Signs and symptoms of generalized autonomic failure have been reported [54,55] but are uncommon. Rarely, autonomic symptoms can be the initial manifestation of SS [54,56]. Autonomic symptoms may accompany any of the different forms of peripheral nerve disease associated with SS [55,57]. In a large cohort study of over 1000 SS patients, 11% had peripheral neuropathy [58]. A number of different types of neuropathy have been described in SS including a small fiber sensory neuropathy, sensorimotor peripheral neuropathy, sensory ataxic neuropathy, multiple mononeuropathies, cranial neuropathy, and autonomic neuropathy [53,57]. Sensory neuropathy or neuronopathy are the most common forms of peripheral neuropathy [55,60–61], and in one series of patients with sensory neuronopathy, orthostatic hypotension was noted in 40%, and 70% had abnormal sweating [55,62]. Other signs and symptoms of autonomic nervous system impairment reported in SS patients include abnormal pupillary responses, diarrhea, constipation, vomiting, and urinary dysfunction [55]. Rarely, patients with SS may develop profound autonomic failure, with manifestations that include Adie's pupils, orthostatic hypotension with syncope, anhidrosis, and symptoms of gastrointestinal dysmotility [55]. Reduced cardiac ^{123}I-MIBG uptake was noted in two of these patients, and a lack of norepinephrine rise with standing was reported [55].

The potential mechanisms of autonomic nervous system dysfunction in SS are unknown, but there has been some interest in the role of antimuscarinic-3 receptor antibodies [53]. These M3 muscarinic receptors are widely expressed on lacrimal and salivary glands [63], and it has been further hypothesized that antibodies against the M3 muscarinic receptor may lead to autonomic dysfunction through desensitization of receptors, impairment in secondary-messenger pathways, and may cause abnormalities in aquaporin proteins [64].

The 2002 American–European classification criteria are used to establish a diagnosis of SS [52], and require at least four of six items, which include subjective measures of xerophthalmia or xerostomia, objective measures of salivary or lacrimal gland involvement, or elevated antibodies to SS-A or SS-B antibodies [57]. However, establishing a diagnosis of SS can prove challenging given that the sicca symptoms of dry eyes and dry mouth may not exist or may be minimized by patients, and antibodies to SS-A and SS-B may not be detectable in up to 50% of patients with SS [53].

Systemic lupus erythematosus

Systemic lupus erythematosus (SLE) is an autoimmune disorder than can affect multiple organ systems including the nervous system, kidneys, heart, joints, and skin. SLE can affect the central and peripheral nervous system, and may result in autonomic nervous system impairment. The frequency of autonomic nervous system impairment is quite variable, with a reported frequency ranging from 6% to 93% [65–71]. Autonomic nervous system impairment may result from SLE disease activity in the central or peripheral nervous system, could potentially result from medication toxicity, or arise from medical complications resulting from SLE or its treatment (such as corticosteroid-induced diabetes mellitus).

Estimates of the frequency of autonomic symptoms in patients with SLE have been hampered by small sample sizes and inconsistent or incomplete characterization of potential autonomic symptoms. In one series, gastrointestinal symptoms attributed to gastrointestinal dysmotility was reported in 9.8% and abnormal sweating in 5.9% of patients, with no patients reporting symptoms of orthostatic intolerance [72]. In another series, 6 of 17 patients reported orthostatic intolerance, with four patients exhibiting orthostatic hypotension, and all but two patients demonstrating abnormalities on a panel of autonomic tests [69]. Similarly, orthostatic hypotension was noted in nearly 39% of SLE patients in another series, and autonomic testing was graded as being moderately or severely abnormal in nearly 80% of patients tested [73]. Subclinical abnormalities on autonomic testing were noted in 24% of patients in another series, with no patients in this series reporting autonomic symptoms [74]. In a recently reported series, abnormalities on autonomic testing were seen in up to 68% of patients with SLE and these abnormalities did not correlate with disease duration, disease activity, or autoantibody positivity [75]. In their aggregate, these studies would suggest that abnormalities on autonomic testing may occur in the majority of patients, but a minority of patients will report symptoms of autonomic nervous system dysfunction.

It is not clear whether autonomic nervous system dysfunction results from impairment in central or peripheral autonomic pathways. Several authors have reported no correlation between the presence of peripheral neuropathy and autonomic nervous system signs or symptoms [69,72,73]. Furthermore, the presence of autonomic nervous system impairment does not appear to correlate with duration of SLE disease, SLE disease activity, or the presence of autoantibodies [76].

Rheumatoid arthritis

Autonomic nervous system impairment in rheumatoid arthritis (RA) has scarcely been studied. As is true with SLE, autonomic nervous system impairment in RA may result from immune-mediated disruption of autonomic pathways or can potentially result from medications used to treat RA [76]. A sensory polyneuropathy is known to occur in approximately 1/2 of RA patients. Furthermore, vasomotor and sudomotor signs and symptoms are commonly encountered in patients with RA, manifesting as coldness, clamminess, and color change in the extremities [76]. Autonomic nervous system testing was abnormal in 9 of 27 patients with RA, and four of these patients had autonomic symptoms, including three with postural hypotension [77]. In a recently reported study of 36 patients with RA, 75% had abnormalities on autonomic testing [75]. The presence of autonomic nervous system dysfunction does not appear to correlate with duration of RA, rheumatoid factor titer, or presence or severity of articular destruction [73].

Sarcoidosis

Sarcoidosis is an inflammatory disorder that can affect any organ system, including the central and peripheral nervous system. It has been suggested that 5–15% of patients with sarcoidosis have neurological involvement [78], though autopsy studies have suggested that only 50% of those with pathological involvement of the nervous system were diagnosed with neurosarcoidosis prior to death [79]. The frequency of autonomic nervous system involvement by sarcoidosis is not known. As suggested by the aforementioned postmortem study, it is likely that there are a substantial number of patients with subclinical involvement of autonomic pathways. Approximately 15% of patients with neurosarcoidosis develop dysfunction of the peripheral nervous system [80,81], and can manifest as a length-dependent sensorimotor peripheral neuropathy, smallfiber neuropathy, mononeuropathy, and polyradiculopathy.

There is increasing recognition that small fiber neuropathy can occur in patients with sarcoidosis [82–84], and there may be an association between the HLA DQB1 0602 allele positivity and small fiber neuropathy in patients with sarcoidosis [85]. Intraepidermal nerve fiber density was abnormal in 37% of sarcoid patients with symptoms suggestive of small fiber neuropathy. It is conceivable that some patients with neurosarcoidosis may have signs or symptoms of autonomic systemic impairment, and that this may correlate with the presence of small fiber neuropathy; however further studies are needed.

Metabolic disorders

Vitamin B12 deficiency

Peripheral neuropathy, myelopathy, myeloneuropathy, and cognitive dysfunction are widely recognized neurological complications of vitamin B12 deficiency. The most common neurological syndrome associated with vitamin B12 deficiency is subacute combined degeneration of the spinal cord. Orthostatic hypotension has been reported in conjunction with vitamin B12 deficiency [86–91]. Autonomic dysfunction may be a subclinical manifestation in a significant percentage of patients with vitamin B12 deficiency. Autonomic dysfunction may rarely occur without other evidence of neurologic dysfunction [89]. Timely recognition of vitamin B12 deficiency is critical in these patients, as vitamin B12 supplementation may result in resolution of autonomic signs and symptoms [86–88,91].

Orthostatic hypotension may result from damage to central or peripheral autonomic pathways in vitamin B12 deficiency [92]. Autonomic testing on 21 patients with vitamin B12 deficiency demonstrated a significant drop in systolic blood pressure during tilt-table testing with a lack of increase in total peripheral resistance during head-up tilt despite the postural drop in blood pressure [93]. The authors reported similar findings on autonomic testing of a cohort of patients with diabetic autonomic neuropathy.

Uremia

Disturbance in autonomic function is a potential complication of uremia, and may manifest as orthostatic hypotension, diarrhea, constipation, sweating disturbance, and impotence [94]. Gastrointestinal autonomic symptoms have been the most frequent manifestation of autonomic neuropathy in uremia, occurring in up to 42% of patients, with complaints of postural lightheadedness reported in 36% of patients [95]. Autonomic testing in patients with uremia has consistently demonstrated reduced baroreceptor sensitivity [96–99], impairment in cardiovagal function [96,100,101], and abnormalities on tests of sympathetic nervous system function in a number of studies [96,102–104]. Some studies have suggested that autonomic dysfunction in uremia occurs as part of a more generalized uremic polyneuropathy [95,105]. Improvement in autonomic nervous system function is expected following renal transplantation.

Porphyria

The porphyrias result from an enzyme deficiency in the heme biosynthesis pathway, leading to overproduction of toxic heme precursors [106]. During an acute attack, porphyrin precursors are excreted in large amounts by the liver, resulting in neurovisceral signs and symptoms. Porphyrias are primarily autosomal dominant, though autosomal recessive and other patterns of inheritance are possible [106]. The estimated prevalence of porphyria is .5 to 10 per 100,000, and diagnosis may be challenging due to the nonspecific signs and symptoms that may mimic other disorders.

Autonomic nervous system impairment is common in acute intermittent porphyria. Symptoms and signs may include hypertension, tachycardia, bladder dysfunction, disorders of sweating, and constipation [107,108]. Autonomic testing in patients with porphyria has demonstrated abnormalities on both sympathetic and parasympathetic tests [109].

Urinary porphobilinogen is elevated during acute attacks, but may be normal in between attacks, particularly in variegate porphyria and hereditary coproporphyria [106]. DNA testing may be considered in asymptomatic patients with suspected acute intermittent porphyria, variegate porphyria, aminolavulinate dehydratase deficiency, and hereditary coproporphyria. Certain medications, alcohol, infection, fasting, or changes in sex hormone balance may precipitate an acute attack of porphyria. During an acute attack opiates may be helpful to control abdominal and extremity pain, and propranolol has been used to treat hypertension and tachycardia [110].

Paraneoplastic autonomic syndromes

Paraneoplastic neurological syndromes result from an immune-mediated attack on the central or peripheral nervous system, triggered remotely by an underlying neoplasm. Paraneoplastic neurological syndromes occur in less than 1% of patients with cancer [111]. The most common tumors associated with paraneoplastic syndromes include lung (especially small cell lung cancer), breast, ovary, and lymphoma [112].

Neurological manifestations of a paraneoplastic syndrome typically evolve subacutely over weeks to months, and may precede the recognition of cancer or may develop during or after cancer treatment. Potential manifestations of paraneoplastic autonomic nervous system dysfunction include orthostatic hypotension, gastrointestinal dysmotility, bladder dysfunction, secretomotor failure, and sweating impairment. The signs and symptoms of autonomic impairment are quite variable and may range from severe panautonomic failure to relatively selective or predominant involvement of a particular organ system.

Typically, paraneoplastic autonomic dysfunction accompanies other neurological disorders, such as cerebellar degeneration, peripheral neuropathy, Lambert-Eaton syndrome (LEMS), or encephalomyelitis. Three autonomic syndromes typically associated with paraneoplastic autoantibodies are autoimmune autonomic ganglionopathy associated with autoantibodies directed against the alpha3 subunit of the ganglionic acetylcholine receptor; intestinal pseudoobstruction, commonly associated with anti-Hu autoantibodies in patients with small-cell lung carcinoma; and syndromes of sympathetic hyperexcitability, associated with autoantibodies against the voltage-gated potassium channel complex.

Paraneoplastic antibody testing is essential in the diagnostic evaluation of suspected paraneoplastic neurological disorders. However, given the large and ever-expanding array of paraneoplastic antibodies, their role and significance in the evaluation of these disorders requires careful consideration. Most of the paraneoplastic antibodies target intracellular antigens in the nucleus or cytoplasm, yet nervous system impairment appears to result from cell-mediated damage to neurons and axons [113,114]. The paraneoplastic antibodies have been associated with specific neurological syndromes and often specific cancer types, though negative antibody tests do not exclude a paraneoplastic cause [113]. Anti-Hu (ANNA-1) antibodies are most frequently associated with paraneoplastic autonomic neuropathy, and in addition to autonomic dysfunction may be associated with a subacute sensory neuronopathy.

Autoimmune channelopathies affecting autonomic function may or may not be a manifestation of an underlying malignancy. For example, autoantibodies directed against voltage-gated potassium channel complex [115,116] or N-methyl-D-aspartate (NMDA) receptors [117] may elicit syndromes of autonomic hyperactivity in association with other manifestations of encephalopathy. Potassium-channel autoantibodies are associated with Morvan syndrome, which is characterized by sympathetic hyperactivity with hyperhidrosis, neuromyotonia, and insomnia [115], or may produce limbic encephalitis, which may manifest with paroxysmal hypothermia [116]. These autoantibodies may be paraneoplastic in patients with small-cell lung carcinoma or thymoma, but may occur in absence of an underlying neoplasm. It is now recognized that these autoantibodies are not targeting potassium-channel proteins directly, but rather target neuronal autoantigens in the region of voltage-gated potassium channels [118]. Patients with limbic encephalitis associated with voltage-gated potassium channel antibodies have antibodies that predominantly target the leucine-rich, glioma-inactivated protein (Lgi1), whereas seropositive patients with Morvan Syndrome have antibodies that target contactin-associated protein-like 2 (Caspr2) [119,120]. Autonomic instability, together with hypoventilation, is a typical manifestation of anti-NMDA receptor encephalitis, commonly associated with ovarian teratoma.

Gastrointestinal dysmotility is a frequent manifestation of paraneoplastic autonomic neuropathy. This syndrome can occur with other autonomic and neurological signs and symptoms or can be the sole or predominant manifestation of a paraneoplastic syndrome. Anti-Hu (ANNA-1) antibodies are most frequently associated with this syndrome, and small-cell lung carcinoma is the most frequent associated cancer [121]. Pathological studies have demonstrated an inflammatory process affecting the myenteric plexus [122].

The definitive management of paraneoplastic autonomic disorders involves identification and appropriate treatment of the underlying malignancy, which may result in stabilization and even improvement in autonomic signs and symptoms [112]. At times, adjunctive immunotherapeutic agents such as plasma exchange, corticosteroids, intravenous immunoglobulin, and cyclophosphamide have been used with variable success. Symptomatic treatment to treat orthostatic hypotension or gastrointestinal dysmotility may be necessary in some patients.

Infectious diseases

Chagas' disease

Chagas' disease (CD) affects 15 million people in South America and results in at least 20,000 deaths annually in endemic regions [123]. CD results from infection with the hemoflagellate *Trypanosoma cruzi*, an intracellular protozoan, with a propensity to affect cardiac and gastrointestinal function. The disease may be transmitted in endemic areas by the reduviid bug, and in other, nonendemic areas via blood transfusions.

Autopsy studies of patients with intractable congestive heart failure revealed a significant reduction in cardiac parasympathetic neurons [124,125]. A number of studies have confirmed the presence of cardiovagal impairment in patients with CD [126–135]. Cardiopulmonary baroreflex sensitivity may be reduced in patients with CD [136,137]. Gastrointestinal CD may manifest as megaesophagus or megacolon, with symptoms of progressive dysphagia and constipation, and presumably results from impairment of the enteric nervous system [138].

Approximately 30% of patients with CD develop cardiomyopathy, and the clinical manifestations and course of this disease are quite variable. Factors responsible for these variable clinical manifestations are unknown, but some authors hypothesize that autoimmune factors may play some role, particularly in the development of autonomic nervous system dysfunction. Antimuscarinic antibodies have been reported early in the course of CD, and reportedly correlate with abnormal cardiovagal function [131]. Diagnosis of CD is established by detecting antibodies to *T. cruzi* using enzyme-linked immunosorbent assay (ELISA) or utilizing complement fixation immunofluorescence.

HIV

Human immunodeficiency virus (HIV-1) is a retrovirus that infects mononuclear phagocytes and CD4+ T lymphocytes, and if untreated or resistant to treatment, may evolve into acquired immunodeficiency syndrome (AIDS). Neurological dysfunction can affect any component of the nervous system, and may occur at any stage of infection from the time of seroconversion to the development of AIDS [139]. In areas with access to highly active anti-retroviral therapy (HAART), HIV may become a chronic illness, and

249

neurological disorders may result from any number of factors including HIV itself, immunosuppression, other comorbid illnesses and infections, and side effects of HAART and other medications [140].

The prevalence and impact of autonomic neuropathy in HIV is unknown [140]. Retrospective studies from the pre-HAART era suggested that 10% of patients had neurological symptoms at the time of diagnosis, 40% of patients developed neurological signs and symptoms during the course of their illness, and 75% had evidence of neurological disease at autopsy [141–143]. The most common neurological complication of HIV is a distal symmetric polyneuropathy (DSP), which has been estimated to affect at least 50% of patients with advanced HIV [144]. While a DSP may result from HIV, toxic neuropathy secondary to antiretroviral therapy (stavudine, didanosine, zalcitabine), is clinically indistinguishable [140].

Autonomic nervous system impairment may result from central or peripheral complications of HIV-1 infection [145], but given the high prevalence rate of polyneuropathy in HIV patients, peripheral autonomic neuropathy is likely the major source of autonomic dysfunction in these patients. In studies prior to the HAART era, cardiovagal and cardiovascular adrenergic impairment was noted, including an increased resting heart rate in HIV patients relative to controls and orthostatic hypotension in some patients [139,146,147]. Fourteen of 25 patients with HIV had autonomic symptoms in one study, including abnormal sweating in 13 patients, diarrhea or constipation in 6, orthostatic intolerance in 6, and bladder impairment in 1 patient [146]. Autonomic signs and symptoms were reported to be more severe in patients with advanced HIV or AIDS [139,146].

Even less is known about autonomic nervous system impairment in the HAART era. A study of HIV patients from India reported 14 of 30 patients with symptoms of hyperhidrosis and rhinorrhea, and none of the patients in this series had symptoms of orthostatic intolerance, bowel or bladder impairment, or sexual dysfunction [148]. Autonomic testing in this cohort of patients demonstrated impairment in cardiovagal and cardiovascular adrenergic function. A study of 80 HIV-positive patients, including 40 patients with AIDS on HAART, showed significant impairment in cardiac autonomic modulation, with evidence of both sympathetic and parasympathetic dysfunction in these patients compared to normal controls [149]. Generalized autonomic failure with orthostatic hypotension has been reported in a patient with well-controlled HIV on HAART [150].

While HAART is known to cause polyneuropathy, these medications are not known to result in autonomic nervous system dysfunction. Furthermore, given that these medications are effective in controlling HIV, and that autonomic complications correlate with HIV severity, it is likely that HAART therapy is limiting to some extent the severity of autonomic complications in patients with HIV. However, given the paucity of studies on autonomic function in the HAART era, further research is necessary to understand the prevalence, extent, and severity of autonomic nervous system impairment in chronic HIV infection.

Botulism

Botulism is caused by the anaerobic, spore-forming bacterium *Clostridium botulinum*, which consists of at least three genetically distinct organisms that produce a number of neurotoxins with diverse properties [151]. Human botulism results primarily from toxin types A, B, and E. There are four recognized clinical forms of botulism including foodborne botulism, wound botulism, infant botulism, and adult infectious botulism [151]. In the United States, infantile botulism is the most common form, followed by foodborne botulism. Half of the foodborne botulism cases in the United States are caused by type A, which has a more severe phenotype and higher fatality rate than types B and E [151,152]. The botulinum toxin binds to presynaptic nerve terminals at the neuromuscular junction and in the autonomic nervous system, where it inhibits acetylcholine release.

Timely clinical recognition of botulism is crucial in order to administer antitoxin and to provide appropriate cardiorespiratory support. In addition, botulism outbreaks are considered a public health emergency, and in the United States surveillance and control measures have been mandated [151]. Botulism characteristically results in a descending pattern of weakness that first affects the cranial nerves, then the upper limbs and respiratory muscles, followed by lower limb paralysis. Typical onset time is 18–36 h after exposure, and respiratory support is often needed for 2–8 weeks [153,154]. Gastrointestinal symptoms such as abdominal pain, nausea, vomiting, and diarrhea may precede or occur together with neuromuscular disease.

Signs and symptoms of autonomic nervous system dysfunction are commonly present in patients with botulism. A report of a large outbreak of botulism in Thailand following the consumption of home-canned bamboo shoots, indicated that all 18 patients affected had fluctuations in heart rate and blood pressure due to autonomic nervous system dysfunction with urinary dysfunction in most [155]. Autonomic studies performed in five patients who suffered foodborne botulism (with signs of relatively mild neuromuscular impairment) demonstrated markedly decreased baroreceptor sensitivity, cardiovagal dysfunction in all five patients, orthostatic hypotension in three, and absent sympathetic skin responses in one or more extremities in four patients [156]. Another report of nine patients afflicted with botulism B following ingestion of contaminated soft cheese in Switzerland, highlighted prominent autonomic symptoms in these patients with modest neuromuscular disease [157].

Nerve conduction studies (NCS) and needle electromyography (EMG) can be useful in patients with suspected botulism. Typical findings include a low-amplitude compound muscle action potential (CMAP) on routine NCS, and an increment of the CMAP with high-frequency repetitive nerve stimulation. With suspected foodborne botulism, serum and stool specimens should be tested for botulism neurotoxin using the mouse inoculation test [151]. Treatment involves cardiorespiratory support and administration of antitoxin.

Leprosy

Leprosy is caused by the bacterium *Mycobacterium leprae*, and is thought to affect approximately 10 million people worldwide, mostly in developing countries [158]. *M. leprae* has a long incubation period and replicates very slowly, with optimal growth occurring in superficial, cooler areas of the skin, nerves, and testis [158]. Peripheral neuropathy is the most disabling complication of leprosy, and is thought to be the most common treatable neuropathy worldwide [159]. There is some evidence that impairment of autonomic nerves occurs before other clinical signs and symptoms become apparent [160,161]. Autonomic testing in 37 patients with lepromatous leprosy showed cardiovagal impairment as measured by R–R

interval variation and sympathetic dysfunction on sympathetic skin response testing [159]. Laser Doppler flowmetry studies have been reported to be abnormal in patients with leprosy [162,163], indicating that small, unmyelinated nerve fibers responsible for vasomotor function in the extremities are dysfunctional in these patients. Treatment of leprosy involves the use of dapsone and rifampin for 12–24 months.

Drug-induced autonomic neuropathy

Autonomic impairment induced by medications used to treat systemic disease typically accompany peripheral neuropathy or other neurotoxic complications such as ototoxicity or retrobulbar neuritis. Vincristine, which is used in the treatment of hematologic malignancies primarily, can cause peripheral neuropathy and symptoms of autonomic failure. Orthostatic hypotension, constipation, and urinary retention have been reported [164,165]. Autonomic neuropathy with orthostatic hypotension has been reported with cisplatin and paclitaxel [165]. The antiarrhythmic agent amiodarone has been associated with a subacute to chronic sensorimotor peripheral neuropathy, and has rarely been associated with an autonomic neuropathy [166]. Gemcitabine, a chemotherapeutic agent used in the treatment of pancreatic and lung cancer has been associated with peripheral neuropathy, and there has been one reported case of an autonomic neuropathy associated with its use [167].

Alcohol

Chronic alcohol consumption affects nearly all organ systems, including the peripheral sensory, motor, and autonomic nerves. The true prevalence of peripheral neuropathy in long-term alcohol abuse, and the relationship between amount, duration, pattern of drinking, and other nutritional factors has not been definitively established [168]. Prevalence estimates of peripheral neuropathy in patients abusing alcohol range from 25% to 66% [169,170]. Autonomic function was prospectively studied in 107 alcoholic patients, and showed signs of cardiovagal (parasympathetic) nervous system impairment in 24% of patients, with no significant difference in sympathetic nervous system function compared to controls [168].

The authors reported a correlation between autonomic and peripheral neuropathy, an inverse correlation between lifetime dose of alcohol and parasympathetic testing, and no correlation between autonomic neuropathy and age, nutritional status, or other alcohol-related diseases. Pathological changes involving the vagal nerves of chronic alcoholic patients are well described [171,172]. An increased mortality in alcoholics with peripheral neuropathy has been suggested [173].

Alcohol-related peripheral neuropathy was previously attributed to malnutrition or to thiamine deficiency. However, recent work suggests that alcohol-related neuropathy is best characterized as a neuropathy that results from the toxic effects of alcohol, and is potentially modulated by other factors including genetic predisposition, thiamine deficiency, malnutrition, systemic disease, or other impurities such as lead [174].

Secreting neoplasms mimicking autonomic disorders

Pheochromocytoma and paraganglioma

Pheochromocytomas and paragangliomas are rare, catecholamine-secreting tumors that arise from neural-crest cells [174]. Pheochromocytomas arise within the adrenal medulla, and paragangliomas are extra-adrenal tumors that arise from sympathetic and parasympathetic paraganglia. Excessive catecholamine secretion by these tumors result in numerous, typically intermittent symptoms. Pheochromocytomas typically secrete both norepinephrine and epinephrine, but usually secrete norepinephrine predominantly, and may rarely secrete dopa and/or dopamine [175].

Patients with these tumors characteristically suffer from intermittent hyperadrenergic symptoms, which typically last less than 1 h, and may occur multiple times per day or as infrequent as one attack every few months [175]. The most commonly experienced symptoms include headache, sweating, palpitations, and hypertension is present in the majority of patients. Patients may experience a number of other hyperadrenergic symptoms including anxiety, flushing, tremor, chest pain, gastrointestinal symptoms, heat intolerance, and Raynaud's phenomena [176].

Catecholamine hypersecretion is responsible for the majority of symptoms associated with pheochromocytoma and paraganglioma. Rarely syncope and orthostatic hypotension can occur in patients with these tumors [177–179]. Surgical removal of tumor in these patients resulted in resolution of orthostatic hypotension. A number of potential causes of hypotension have been proposed including hypovolemia (reduction in circulating blood volume is common with pheochromocytoma), intermittent catecholamine secretion, abnormal peripheral response to catecholamines, high epinephrine to norepinephrine ratio, and baroreflex impairment [177]. Excessive norepinephrine rise with head-up tilt has been noted in patients with pheochromocytoma [180,181]. In these patients there appeared to be a down-regulation of α-2-adrenergic venous receptors, suggesting that excessive venous pooling may occur with standing in these patients. Heart-rate variability studies in patients with these tumors suggest enhanced parasympathetic (cardiovagal) function and inhibited central, sympathetic outflow [182–184].

These tumors are diagnosed by establishing biochemical evidence of catecholamine excess—either of catecholamines themselves or of their metabolites. Fractionated, 24-h urinary metanephrines are a frequently used screening test, but plasma-free metanephrines have the highest sensitivity (97–99%) with a specificity of 82% [185]. It is important to be certain that patients not be on medications known to interfere with the test assay, or alter catecholamine synthesis, release, or metabolism. Diagnostic localization based on CT or MRI studies have comparable sensitivities in identifying adrenal and extra-adrenal tumors, and ^{123}I-MIBG scintigraphy is highly specific, but less sensitive in identifying these tumors [175]. Positron emission tomography (PET) imaging can be utilized if these imaging modalities fail to reveal a tumor.

Mastocytosis

Systemic mastocytosis is a rare, stem-cell-derived myeloproliferative disorder affecting mast cells [186]. Symptoms result from mast-cell mediator release including flushing, presyncope, diarrhea, and hypotension. Other signs may include urticaria pigmentosa or other skin lesions, bone lesions, bone-marrow involvement with bone marrow mast cells, and splenomegaly [187]. The diagnosis is established by demonstrating elevated serum tryptase and increased 24-h urinary excretion of histamine or prostaglandin D2 metabolites. Management of systemic mastocytosis involves avoidance of triggers of mast-cell degranulation, histamine antagonists, and cromolyn sodium. Refractory case may require treatments with cytoreductive agents such as interferon alpha, 2-chlorordeoxyadenosine, and imatinib mesylate [186].

Conclusion

Autonomic nervous system pathways are diffuse and can be affected by a multitude of systemic diseases through a number of different mechanisms. Recognition of autonomic signs and symptoms can facilitate timely and accurate diagnosis in patients with unexplained symptoms, or can occur as a complication of established, chronic disease. Autonomic nervous system impairment in systemic disease is quite variable, ranging from subclinical dysfunction noted on autonomic nervous system testing to profound autonomic failure. Treatment of the underlying condition often results in improvement in autonomic signs and symptoms, but symptomatic treatment of autonomic dysfunction is frequently necessary.

References

1 World Health Organization. January 2011. Available: www.who.int/diabetes.
2 Low PA, Benrud-Larson LM, Sletten DM, Opfer-Gehrking TL, Weigand SD, O'Brien PC, Suarez GA, Dyck PJ. Autonomic symptoms and diabetic neuropathy. A population-based study. *Diab. Care* 2004;27:2942–2947.
3 Dyck PJ, Kratz KM, Karnes JL, Litchy WJ, Klein R, Pach JM, Wilson DM, O'Brien PC, Melton LJIII, The prevalence by staged severity of various types of diabetic neuropathy, retinopathy, and nephropathy in a population-based cohort: the Rochester Diabetic Neuropathy Study. *Neurology* 1993;43:817–824.
4 Hilsted J, Low PA. In PA Low, editor, *Diabetic Autonomic Neuropathy*, 2nd ed. Philadelphia, PA: Lippincott-Raven Publishers, 1997, pp. 487–508.
5 Rundles RW. Diabetic neuropathy. General review with report of 125 cases. *Medicine* 1945;24:111–160.
6 Schönauer M, Thomas A, Morbach S, Niebauer J, Schönauer U, Thiele H. Cardiac autonomic diabetic neuropathy. *Diab. Vasc. Dis. Res.* 2008;5(4):336–344.
7 Pop-Busui R. Cardiac autonomic neuropathy in diabetes: a clinical perspective. *Diab. Care* 2010;33(2):434–441.
8 Ewing DJ Campbell IW, Clarke FB. The natural history of diabetic autonomic neuropathy. *Q. J. Med.* 1980;49:95–108.
9 Watkins PJ Mackay DJ. Cardiac denervation in diabetic neuropathy. *Ann. Intern. Med.* 1980;92:304–307.
10 Pop-Busui R, Kirkwood I, Schmid H, Marinescu V, Schroeder J, Larkin D, Yamada E, Raffel DM, Stevens MJ. Sympathetic dysfunction in type I diabetes: associ-

Five things to remember about autonomic manifestations of systemic disease

1. Patients with suspected autonomic nervous system impairment should be evaluated for symptoms of orthostatic intolerance such as lightheadedness and syncope, disturbances in sweating, vasomotor signs and symptoms, gastrointestinal impairment, and genitourinary dysfunction.
2. Autonomic nervous system dysfunction is a frequent complication of diabetes mellitus, occurring in up to 73% of patients with type II diabetes and over half of patients with type I diabetes mellitus.
3. Cardiac autonomic neuropathy refers to impairment in parasympathetic (cardiovagal) modulation in patients with diabetes mellitus, and has been associated with a higher mortality than diabetics without this complication.
4. Amyloidosis should be suspected in patients with peripheral neuropathy and autonomic failure, most commonly resulting from primary systemic amyloidosis or familial amyloidosis.
5. Autonomic nervous system impairment is a potential manifestation of paraneoplastic disorders and may precede the clinical recognition of malignancy or may occur in patients with established cancer.

ation with impaired myocardial blood flow reserve and diastolic dysfunction. *J. Am. Coll. Cardiol.* 2004;44:2368–2374.

11 Taskiran M, Rasmussen V, Rasmussen B, Fritz-Hansen T, Larsson HB, Jensen GB, Hilsted J. Left ventricular dysfunction in normotensive type I diabetic patients: the impact of autonomic neuropathy. *Diab. Med.* 2004;21:524–530.

12 Ewing DJ, Campbell IW, Clarke BF. Assessment of cardiovascular effects in diabetic autonomic neuropathy and prognostic implications. *Ann. Intern. Med.* 1980;92:308–311.

13 Navarro X, Kennedy WR, Sutherland DE. Autonomic neuropathy and survival in diabetes mellitus: effects of pancreas transplantation. *Diabetologia* 1991;34(Suppl 1):S108–S112.

14 O'Brien IA, McFadden JP, Corrall RJ. The influence of autonomic neuropathy on mortality in insulin-dependent diabetes. *Q. J. Med.* 1991;79:495–502.

15 Vinik AI, Maser RE, Mitchell BD, Freeman R. Diabetic autonomic neuropathy. *Diab. Care* 2003;26:1553–1579.

16 The effect of intensive diabetes therapy on measures of autonomic nervous system function in the Diabetes Control and Complications Trial (DCCT). *Diabetologia* 1998;41(4):416–423.

17 Albers JW, Herman WH, Pop-Busui R, Feldman EL, Martin CL, Cleary PA, Waberski BH, Lachin JM. Diabetes Control and Complications Trial/Epidemiology of Diabetes Interventions and Complications Research Group. Effect of prior intensive insulin treatment during the Diabetes Control and Complications Trial (DCCT) on peripheral neuropathy in type 1 diabetes during the Epidemiology of Diabetes Interventions and Complications (EDIC) study. *Diab. Care* 2010;33(5):1090–1096.

18 Singer W, Opfer-Gehrking TL, McPhee BR, Hilz MJ, Bharucha AE, Low PA. Acetylcholinesterase inhibition: a novel approach in the treatment of neurogenic orthostatic hypotension. *J. Neurol. Neurosurg. Psychiatry* 2003;74(9):1294–1298.

19 Kyle RA, Greipp PR. Amyloidosis (AL). *Mayo Clin. Proc.* 1983;58:665–683.

20 van der Hilst J. Recent insights into the pathogenesis of type AA amyloidosis. *Sci. World J.* 2011;11:641–650.

21 Simmons Z, Specht CS. The neuromuscular manifestations of amyloidosis. *J. Clin. Neuromusc. Dis.* 2010;11 (3):145–157.

22 Kyle RA, Linos A, Beard CM, et al. Incidence and natural history of primary systemic amyloidosis, in Olmsted County, Minnesota, 1950 through 1989. *Blood* 1992;79:1817–1822.

23 Ando Y, Nakamura M, Araki S. Transthyretin-related familial amyloidotic polyneuropathy. *Arch. Neurol.* 2005;62:1057–1062.

24 Gertz MA, Kyle RA, Thibodeau SN. Familial amyloidosis: A study of 52 North-American born patients examined during a 30-year period. *Mayo Clin. Proc.* 1992;67:428–440.

25 Hwee Kim D, Zeldenrust SR, Low PA. Quantitative sensation and autonomic test abnormalities in transthyretin amyloidosis polyneuropathy. *Muscle Nerve* 2009;40:363–370.

26 Vita G, Mazzeo A, Di leo R, Ferlini A. Recurrent syncope as persistently isolated feature of transthyretin amyloidotic polyneuropathy. *Neuromusc. Disorders* 2005;15:259–261.

27 Makioka K, Ikeda M, Ikeda Y, Nakasone A, Osawa T, Sasaki A, Otani T, Arai M, Okamoto K. Familial amyloid polyneuropathy (Finnish type) presenting multiple cranial nerve deficits with carpal tunnel syndrome and orthostatic hypotension. *Neurol. Res.* 2010;32(5): 472–475.

28 Kiuru S. Familial amyloidosis of the Finnish type (FAF). A clinical study of 30 patients. *Acta Neurol. Scand.* 1992;86:346–353.

29 Kiuru S, Matikainen E, Kupari M, Haltia M, Palo J. Autonomic nervous system and cardiac involvement in familial amyloidosis, Finnish type (FAF). *J. Neurol. Sci.* 1994;126(1):40–48.

30 Wang AK, Fealey RD, Gehrking TL, Low PA. Patterns of neuropathy and autonomic failure in patients with amyloidosis. *Mayo Clin. Proc.* 2008;83(11):1226–1230.

31 Sattianayagam PT, Hawkins PN, Gillmore JD. Systemic amyloidosis and the gastrointestinal tract. *Nat. Rev. Gastroenterol. Hepatol.* 2009;6:608–617.

32 Ohnishi A, Yamamoto T, Murai Y, Ando Y, Ando M, Hoshii Y, Ikeda M. Denervation of eccrine glands in patients with familial amyloidotic polyneuropathy type I. *Neurology* 1998;51(3):714–721.

33 Ishiguchi H, Shimoya K, Ohnishi A, Murai Y, Nakazato M, Hoshii Y. Familial amyloidosis, Finnish type with marked anhidrosis. *Rinsho Shinkeigaku* 1996; 36(3):436–441.

34 Chee CE, Lacy MQ, Dogan LA, Zeldenrust SR, Gertz MA. Pitfalls in the diagnosis of primary amyloidosis. *Clin. Lymphoma, Myeloma Leuk.* 2010;10(3): 177–180.

35 Lachamann HJ, Chir B, Booth Dr, Booth SE, Bybee A, Gilberson JA, Gillmore JD, Pepys MB, Hawkins PN. Misdiagnosis of hereditary amyloidosis as AL (primary) Amyloidosis. *N. Engl. J. Med.* 2002;346(23): 1786–1791.

36 Comezo RL, Zhou P, Fleisher M, et al. Seeking confidence in the diagnosis of systemic AL (Ig light-chain) amyloidosis: patients can have both monoclonal gammopathies and hereditary amyloid proteins. *Blood* 2006;107:3489–3491.

37 Vrana JA, Gamez JD, Madden B.J. et al. Classification of amyloidosis by laser microdissection and mass spectrometry based proteonomic analysis in clinical biopsy specimens. *Blood* 2009;114:4957–4959.

38 Kyle RA, Gertz MA, Greipp PR, et al. A trial of three regimens for primary amyloidosis: colchicine alone, melphalan and prednisone, and melphalan, prednisone, and colchicine. *N. Engl. J. Med.* 1997;336:1202–1207.

39 Kyle RA, Gertz MA, Greipp PR. Response rates and survival in primary systemic amyloidosis. *Blood* 1991;77:257.

40 Dispenzieri A, Kyle RA, Lacy MQ, et al. Superior survival in primary systemic amyloidosis patients undergoing peripheral blood stem cell transplantation: a case-control study. *Blood* 2004;103(10):3960–3963.

41 Gertz MA, Lacy MQ, Dispenzieri A, et al. Stem cell transplantation for the management of primary systemic amyloidosis. *Am. J. Med.* 2002;113:549–555.

42 Sanchorawala V, Wright DG, Seldin DC, et al. An overview of the use of high-dose melphalan with autologous stem cell transplantation for the treatment of AL amyloidosis. *Bone Marrow Transpl.* 2001;28:637–642.

43 Vesole Dh, Perez WS, Reece DE, Akasheh M, Horowitz MM, Bredeson C. High dose therapy with autologous hematopoietic stem cell transplantation (HSCT) for patients with primary systemic amyloidosis (AL): results from the Autologous Blood and Marrow Transplant Registry (ABMTR)(abstract). *Blood* 2003;102:118a.

44 Kumar SK, Gertz MA, Lacy MQ, Dingli D, et al. Recent improvements in survival in primary systemic amyloidosis and the importance of an early mortality risk score. *Mayo Clin. Proc.* 2011;86(1):12–18.

45 Mhaskar R, Kumar A, Behera M, Kharfan-Dabaja MA, Djulbegovic B. Role of high-dose chemotherapy and autologous hematopoietic cell transplantation in primary systemic amyloidosis: a systematic review. *Biol. Blood Marrow Transplant.* 2009;15(8):893–902.

46 Benson MD, Kincaid JC. The molecular biology and clinical features of amyloid neuropathy. *Muscle Nerve* 2007;36:411–423.

47 Holmgren G, Steen L, Ekstedt J, et al. Biochemical effect of liver transplantation in two Swedish patients with familial amyloidotic polyneuropathy (FAP-met30). *Clin Genet.* 1991;40:242–246.

48 Herlenius G, Wilczek HE, Larsson M, et al. Ten years of international experience with liver transplantation for familial amyloidotic polyneuropathy: results from the familial amyloidotic polyneuropathy world transplant registry. *Transplantation* 2004;77(1):64–71.

49 Adams, D, Samuel D, Goulon-Goeau C, Nakazato M, Costa PM, Feray C, Plante V, Ducot B, Ichai P, Lacroix C, Metral S, Bismuth H, Said G. The course and prognostic factors of familial amyloid polyneuropathy after liver transplantation. *Brain* 2000;123:1495–1504.

50 Bergethon PR, Sabin TD, Lewis D, Simms RW, Cohen AS, Skinner M. Improvement in the polyneuropathy associated with familial amyloid polyneuropathy after liver transplantation. *Neurology* 1996;47:944–951.

51 Pomfret EA, Lewis DW, Jenkins RL, Bergethon P, Dubrey SW, Reisinger J, Falk RH, Skinner M. Effect of orthotopic liver transplantation on the progression of familial amyloidotic polyneuropathy. *Transplantation* 1998;65(7):918–925.

52 Vitali C, Bombardieri S, Jonsson R, et al. Classification criteria for Sjögren's syndrome: a revised version of the European criteria proposed by the American–European Consensus Group. *Ann. Rheum. Dis.* 2002;61:554–558.

53 Birnbaum J. Peripheral nervous system manifestations of Sjögren syndrome. *Neurologist* 2010;16(5):287–297.

54 Sakakibara R, Hirano S, Asahina M, et al. Primary Sjögren's syndrome presenting with generalized autonomic failure. *Eur. J. Neurol.* 2004;11:635–638.

55 Mori K, Iijima M, Koike H, et al. The wide spectrum of clinical manifestations in Sjögren's syndrome-associated neuropathy. *Brain* 2005;128:2518–2534.

56 Barendregt PJ, Markusse HM, Man In't Veld AJ. Primary Sjögren's syndrome presenting as autonomic neuropathy. Case report. *Neth. J. Med.* 1998;53:196–200.

57 Chai J, Logigian EL. Neurological manifestations of primary Sjögren's syndrome. *Curr. Opin. Neurol.* 2010;23:509–513.

58 Ramos-Casals M, Solans R, Rosas J. et al. Primary Sjögren syndrome in Spain: clinical and immunologic expression 1010 patients. *Medicine (Balt.)* 2008;87:210–219.

59 Delalande S, de Seze J, Fauchais AL, Hachulla E, et al. Neurologic manifestations in primary Sjögren syndrome: a study of 82 patients. *Medicine* 2004; 83(5):280–291.

60 Font J, Valls J, Cervera R, et al. Pure sensory neuropathy in patients with primary Sjögren's syndrome: clinical, immunological, and electromyographic findings. *Ann. Rheum. Dis.* 1990;49:775–778.

61 Grant IA, Hunder GG, Homburger HA, Dyck PJ, Peripheral neuropathy associated with sicca complex. *Neurology* 1997;48:855–862.

62 Mori K, Koike H, Misu K, et al. Spinal cord magnetic resonance imaging demonstrates sensory neuronal involvement and clinical severity neuronopathy

associated with Sjögren's syndrome. *J. Neurol. Neuro-surg. Psychiatry* 2001;71:488–492.

63 Hocevar A, Tomsic M, Praprotnik S, et al. Para-sympathetic nervous system dysfunction in primary Sjögren's syndrome. *Ann. Rheum. Dis.* 2003;62:702–704.

64 Nguyen KH, Brayer J, Cha S, et al. Evidence for anti-muscarinic acetylcholine receptor antibody-mediated dysfunction in NOD mice. *Arthritis Rheum.* 2001;43:2297–2306.

65 Straub RH, Zeuner M, Lock G, Rath H, Hein U, Scholmerich J, Lang B. Autonomic and sensorimotor neuropathy in patients with systemic lupus erythemato-sus and systemic sclerosis. *J. Rheumatol.* 1996;23:87–92.

66 Magaro M, Mirone L, Altomonle L, Zoli A, Angelosanle S. Lack of correlation between anticardiolipin antibod-ies and peripheral autonomic nerve involvement in sys-temic lupus erythematosus. *Clin. Rheumatol.* 1992;11:231–234.

67 Allomonte L, Mirone L, Zoli A, Magaro M. Autonomic nerve dysfunction in systemic lupus erythematosus: evi-dence for a mild involvement. *Lupus* 1997;6:441–444.

68 Omdal R, Jorde R, Mellgren SI, Hybby G. Autonomic function in systemic lupus erythematosus. *Lupus* 1994;3:413–417.

69 Liote F, Osterland CK. Autonomic neuropathy in sys-temic lupus erythematosus: cardiovascular autonomic function assessment. *Ann. Rheum. Dis.* 1994;53:671–674.

70 Hogarth MB, Judd L, Mathias CJ, Ritchie J, Stephens D, Rees RG. Cardiovascular autonomic function in sys-temic lupus erythematosus. *Lupus* 2002;11:308–312.

71 Gamez-Nava JI, Gonzalez-Lopez L, Ramos-Remus C, Fonseca-Gomez MM, Cardona-Munoz EG, Suarez Almazor ME. Autonomic dysfunction in patients with systemic lupus erythematosus. *J. Rheumatol.* 1998;25:1092–1096.

72 Shalimar, Handa R, Deepak KK, Bhatia M, Aggarwal P, Pandey RM. Autonomic dysfunction in systemic lupus erythematosus. *Rheumatol. Int.* 2006;26:837–840.

73 Stojanovich L, Milovanovich B, de Luka SR, Popovich-Kuzmanovich D, Bisenich V, et al. Cardiovascular auto-nomic dysfunction in systemic lupus, rheumatoid arthri-tis, primary Sjögren syndrome and other autoimmune diseases. *Lupus* 2007;16:181–185.

74 Maule S, Quadri R, Mierante D, Pellerito R.A. et al. Autonomic nervous dysfunction in systemic lupus ery-thematosus (SLE) and rheumatoid arthritis (RA): possible pathogenic role of autoantibodies to autonomic nervous structures. *Clin. Exp. Immunol.* 1997;110:423–427.

75 Aydemir M, Yazisiz I, Basarici I, Avci AB, Erbasan F, Felgi A, Terzioglu E. Cardiac autonomic profile in rheumatoid arthritis and systemic lupus erythematosus. *Lupus* 2010;19:255–261.

76 Stojanovich L. Autonomic dysfunction in autoimmune rheumatic disease. *Autoimmun. Rev.* 2009;8:569–572.

77 Edmonds ME, Jones TC, Saunders WA, Sturrock RD. Autonomic neuropathy in rheumatoid arthritis. *Br. Med. J.* 1979;2:173–175.

78 James DG, Sharma OP. Neurosarcoidosis. *Proc. R. Soc. Med.* 1967;60:1169–1170.

79 Iwai k, Tachibana T, Takemura T, et al. Pathological studies on sarcoidosis autopsy. *Acta Pathol. Jpn.* 1993;43:372–376.

80 Terushkin V, Stern BJ, Judson MA, Hagiwara M, Pra-manik B, Sanchez M, Prystowsky S. Neurosarcoidosis presentations and management. *Neurologist* 2010;16:2–15.

81 Hoitsma E, Faber CG, Drent M, et al. Neurosarcoidosis: a clinical dilemma. *Lancet Neurol.* 2004;3:397–407.

82 Hoitsma E, Marziniak M, Faber CG, Reulen JPH, Sommer C, De Baets M, Drent M. Small fibre neuropa-thy in sarcoidosis. *Lancet* 2002;359:2085–2086.

83 Bakkers M, Faber CG, Drent M, Hermans MCE, van Nes SI, Lauria G, De Baets M, Merkies LSJ. Pain and autonomic dysfunction in patients with sarcoidosis and small fibre neuropathy. *J. Neurol.* 2010;257:2086–2090.

84 Bakkers M, Merkies LSJ, Lauria G, Devigili G, Penza P, Lombardi R, Hermans MCE, van Nes SI, De Baets M, Faber CG. Intraepidermal nerve fiber density and its application in sarcoidosis. *Neurology* 2009;73:1142–1148.

85 Voorter CE, Drent M, Hoitsma E, Faber KG, van den Berg-loonen EM. Association of HLA DQB1 0602 in sarcoidosis patients with small fiber neuropathy. *Sar-coidosis Vasc. Diffuse Lung. Dis.* 2005;22(2):129–132.

86 Puntambekar P, Basha MM, Zak IT, Madhavan R. Rare sensory and autonomic disturbances associated with vitamin B12 deficiency. *J. Neurol. Sci.* 2009;287:285–287.

87 White WB, Reik L, Cutlip DE. Pernicious anemia seen initially as orthostatic hypotension. *Arch. Intern. Med.* 1981;141:1543–1544.

88 Graber JJ, Sherman FT, Kaufmann, Kolodny EH, Sathe S. Vitamin B12-responsive severe leukoencephalopathy with "normal" serum B12 levels. *J. Neurol. Neurosurg. Psych.* 2010;81:1369–1371.

89 Moore A, Watts RJ, et al. Orthostatic intolerance in older patients with vitamin B12 deficiency before and after vitamin B12 replacement. *Clin. Auton. Res.* 2004;14:67–71.

90 Kalbfleisch JM, Woods AH. Orthostatic hypotension associated with pernicious anemia: report of a case with complete recover following vitamin B12 therapy. *J. Am. Med. Assoc.* 1962;182:196–198.

91 Johnson GE, Reversible orthostatic hypotension of pernicious anemia. *J. Am. Med. Assoc.* 1987;257(8):1084–1086.

92 McCombe PA, McLeod JG. The peripheral neuropathy of vitamin B12 deficiency. *J. Neurol. Sci.* 1984;66:117–126.

93 Beitzke M, Pfister P, Fortin J, Skrabal F. Autonomic dysfunction and hemodynamics in vitamin B12 deficiency. *Auton. Neurosci.: Basic Clin.* 2002;97:45–54.

94 Krishnan AV, Kiernan MC. *Muscle Nerve* 2007;35:273–290.

95 Wang SJ, Laio KK, Liou HH, Lee SS, Tsai CP, et al. Sympathetic skin response and R–R interval variation in chronic uremic patients. *Muscle Nerve* 1994;17:411–418.

96 Robinson TG, Carr SJ. Cardiovascular autonomic dysfunction in uremia. *Kidney Int.* 2002;62:1921–1932.

97 Pickering TG, Gribbin B, Oliver Do. Baroreflex sensitivity in patients on long term haemodialysis. *Clin. Sci.* 1972;43:645–657.

98 Lazarus JM, Hampers CL, Lowrie EG, Merril JP. Baroreceptor activity in normotensive and hypertensive uremic patients. *Circulation* 1973;47:1015–1021.

99 Bondia A, Tabernero JM, Macias JF, Martin-Luengo C. Autonomic nervous system in haemodialysis. *Nephrol. Dial. Transplant* 1988;2:174–180.

100 Campese VM, Romoff MS, Levitan D, et al. Mechanisms of autonomic nervous system dysfunction in uremia. *Kidney Int.* 1981;20:246–253.

101 Vita G, Bellinghieri G, Trusso A, et al. Uremic autonomic neuropathy studied by spectral analysis of heart rate. *Kidney Int.* 1999;56:232–237.

102 Heidbreder E, Schafferhans K, Heidland A. Disturbances of peripheral and autonomic nervous system in chronic renal failure: effects of hemodialysis and transplantation. *Clin. Nephrol.* 1985;23:222–228.

103 Ewing DJ, Winney R. Autonomic function in patients with chronic renal failure on intermittent haemodialysis. *Nephron* 1975;15:424–429.

104 Jassal SV, Douglas JF, Stout RW. Prevalence of central autonomic neuropathy in elderly dialysis patients. *Nephrol. Dial. Transplant* 1998;13:1702–1708.

105 Kersh ES, Kronfield SJ, Unger A, Popper RW, et al. Autonomic insufficiency in uremia as a cause of hemodialysis-induced hypotension. *N. Engl. J. Med.* 1974;290:650–653.

106 Kauppinen R. Porphyrias. *Lancet* 2005;365:241–252.

107 Goldberg A. Acute intermittent porphyria. A study of 50 cases. *Q. J. Med.* 1959;28:183–209.

108 Ridley A, et al. Tachycardia and the neuropathy of porphyria. *Lancet* 1968;2:708–710.

109 Laiwah AC, et al. Autonomic neuropathy in acute intermittent porphyria. *J. Neurol. Neurosurg. Psych.* 1995;48:1025–1030.

110 Ropper AH. Management of autonomic storm. In PA Low, editor, *Clinical Autonomic Disorders*, 2nd ed. Philadelphia, PA: Lippincott-Raven Publishers, 1997, pp. 487–508.

111 Andersen NE, et al. Autoimmune pathogenesis of paraneoplastic neurological syndromes. *Crit. Rev. Neurobiol.* 1987;3:245–299.

112 Lorusso L, Hart IK, Ferrari D, Ngonga GK, Gasparetto C, Ricevuti G. Autonomic paraneoplastic neurological syndromes. *Autoimmun. Rev.* 2007;6:162–168.

113 Vernino S. Antibody testing as a diagnostic tool in autonomic disorders. *Clin. Aut. Res.* 2009;19:13–19.

114 Darnell RB. Paraneoplastic neurologic disorders: window into neuronal function and tumor immunity. *Arch. Neurol.* 2004;61:30–32.

115 Josephs KA, Silber MH, Fealey RD, Nippoldt TB, Auger RG, Vernino S. Neurophysiologic studies in Morvan syndrome. *J. Clin. Neurophysiol.* 2004;21:440–445.

116 Misawa T, Mizusawa H. [Anti-VGKC antibody-associated limbic encephalitis/Morvan syndrome]. *Brain Nerve* 2010;62:339–345.

117 Dalmau J, Lancaster E, Martinez-Hernandez E, Rosenfeld MR, Balice-Gordon R. Clinical experience and laboratory investigations in patients with anti-NMDAR encephalitis. *Lancet Neurol.* 2011;10:63–74.

118 Cornelius JR, Pittock SJ, McKeon A, et al. Sleep manifestations of voltage-gated potassium channel complex autoimmunity. *Arch. Neurol.* 2011;68(6):733–738.

119 Irani SR, Alexander S, Waters P, et al. Antibodies to Kv1 potassium channel-complex proteins leucine-rich, glioma inactivated 1 protein and contactin-associated protein-2 in limbic encephalitis, Morvan's syndrome and acquired neuromyotonia. *Brain* 2010;133(9):2734–2748.

120 Lai M, Huijbers MG, Lancaster E, et al. Investigation of LGI1 as the antigen in limbic encephalitis previously attributed to potassium channels: a case series. *Lancet Neurol.* 2010;9(8):776–785.

121 Lee HR, Lennon VA, et al. Paraneoplastic gastrointestinal motor dysfunction: clinical and laboratory characteristics. *Am. J. Gastroenterol.* 2001;96(2):373–379.

122 Chinn JS, Schuffler MD. Paraneoplastic visceral neuropathy as a cause of severe gastrointestinal motor dysfunction. *Gastroenterology* 1988;95:1279–1286.

123 World Health Organization on behalf of the Special Programme for Research and Training in Tropical Diseases. *World Health Organization*, Geneva, 2007, p1–p96.

124 Koberle F. Pathogenesis of Chagas' disease. *Ciba Found. Symp.* 1974;20:137–152.

125 Mott K, Hagstrom JWC. The pathologic lesions of the cardiac autonomic nervous system in chronic chagasic myocarditis. *Circulation* 1965;31:273–276.

126 Iosa D, Dequattro V, Lee DD, Elkayam U, Caeiro T, Palmero H. Pathogenesis of cardiac neuro-myopathy in Chagas' disease and the role of the autonomic nervous system. *J. Auton. Nerv. Syst.* 1990;30(Suppl);S83–S87.

127 Junqueira LF. Jr., Soares JD. Impaired autonomic control of heart interval changes to Valsalva manoeuvre in Chagas' disease without overt manifestation. *Auton. Neurosci.* 2002;97:59–67.

128 Marin-Neto JA, Bromberg-Marin G, Pazin-Filho A, Simoes MV, Maciel BC. Cardiac autonomic impairment and early myocardial damage involving the right ventricle are independent phenomena in Chagas' disease. *Int. J. Cardiol.* 1998;65:261–269.

129 Oliveira E, Ribeiro AL, Assis SF, Torres RM, Rocha MO. The Valsalva maneuver in Chagas disease patients without cardiopathy. *Int. J. Cardiol.* 2002;82:49–54.

130 Ribeiro AL, Ferreira LM, Oliveira E, Cruzeiro PC, Torres RM, Rocha MO. Active orthostatic stress and respiratory sinus arrhythmia in patients with Chagas' disease with preserved left ventricular global systolic function. *Arq. Bras. Cardiol.* 2004;83:40–44.

131 Ribeiro AL, Gimenez LE, Hernandez CC, de Carvalho AC, Teixeira MM, Guedes VC, Barros MV, Lombardi F, Costa Rocha MO. Early occurrence of anti-muscarinic autoantibodies and abnormal vagal modulation in Chagas disease. *Int. J. Cardiol.* 2007;117:59–63.

132 Ribeiro AL, Lombardi F, Sousa MR, Lins Barros MV, Porta A, Costa VBV, Gomes ME, Santana MF, Otavio Costa RM. Power-law behavior of heart rate variability in Chagas' disease. *Am. J. Cardiol.* 2002;89:414–418.

133 Ribeiro AL, Lombardi F, Sousa MR, Rocha MO. Vagal dysfunction in Chagas disease. *Int. J. Cardiol.* 2005;103:225–226.

134 Ribeiro AL, Moraes RS, Ribeiro JP, Ferlin EL, Torres RM, Oliveira E, Rocha MO. Parasympathetic dysautonomia precedes left ventricular systolic dysfunction in Chagas disease. *Am. Heart J.* 2001;141:260–265.

135 Ribeiro AL, Schmidt G, Sousa MR, Lombardi F, Gomes ME, Perez AA, Barros MV, Machado FS, Rocha MO. Heart rate turbulence in Chagas disease. *Pacing Clin. Electrophysiol.* 2003;26:406–410.

136 Villar JC, Leon H, Morillo CA. Cardiovascular autonomic function testing in asymptomatic *T. cruzii* carriers: a sensitive method to identify subclinical Chagas' disease. *Int. J. Cardiol.* 2004;93:189–195.

137 Consolim-Colombo FM, Filho JAB, Lopes HF, et al. Decreased cardiopulmonary baroreflex sensitivity in Chagas' heart disease. *Hypertension* 2000;36:1035–1039.

138 Sousa ACS, Marin-Neto JA, Maciel BC, Gallo L, Amorim DS. Cardiac parasympathetic impairment in gastrointestinal Chagas' disease. *Lancet* 1987;1:985.

139 Freeman R, Roberts MS, Friedman LS, Broadbridge C. Autonomic function and human immunodeficiency virus infection. *Neurology* 1990;40:575–580.

140 Robinson-Papp J, Simpson DM. Neuromuscular diseases associated with HIV-1 infection. *Muscle Nerve* 2009;40:1043–1053.

141 Snider W, Simpson DM, Nielson S, et al. Neurological complications of acquired immunodeficiency syndrome: analysis of 50 patients. *Ann. Neurol.* 1983;14:403–418.

142 Levy RM, Bredesen DE, Rosenblum ML. Neurological manifestations of the acquired immunodeficiency syndrome (AIDS): experience at UCSF and review of the literature. *J. Neurosurg.* 1985;62:475–495.

143 McArthur JC. Neurological manifestations of AIDS. *Medicine* 1986;66:407–437.

144 Morgello S, Estanislao L, Simpson D, et al. HIV-associated distal sensory polyneuropathy in the era of highly active antiretroviral therapy: the Manhattan HIV brain bank. *Arch. Neurol.* 2003;61:546–551.

145 Verma A. Epidemiology and clinical features of HIV-1 associated neuropathies. *J. Peripher. Nervous Syst.* 2001;6:8–13.

146 Ruttimann S, Hilti P, Spinas GA, Dubach UC. High frequency of human immunodeficiency virus-associated autonomic neuropathy and more severe involvement in advanced stages of human immunodeficiency disease. *Arch. Intern. Med.* 1991;151:2441–2443.

147 Cohen JA, Laudenslager M. Autonomic nervous system involvement in patients with human immunodeficiency virus infection. *Neurology.* 1989;39(8):1111–1112.

148 Sakhuja A, Goyal A, Jaryal AK, Wig N, Vajpayee M, et al. Heart rate variability and autonomic function tests in HIV positive individuals in India. *Clin. Auton. Res.* 2007;17:193–196.

149 Correia D, Rodrigues de Resende LAP, Molina RJ, et al. Power spectral analysis of heart rate variability in HIV-infected and AIDS patients. *PACE* 2006;29:53–58.

150 Tank J, Heusser K, Schroeder C, Luft FC, Jordan J. Autonomic failure in a HIV-infected patient. *Clin. Auton. Res.* 2010;20:263–265.

151 Shapiro RL, Hatheway C, Swerdlow DL. Botulism in the United States: a clinical and epidemiologic review. *Ann. Intern. Med.* 1998;129:221–228.

152 Woodruff BA, Griffin PM, McCroskey LM, Smart JF, Wainwright RB, Bryan RG, et al. Clinical and laboratory comparison of botulism toxin types A, B, and E in the United States, 1975–1988. *J. Infect. Dis.* 1992;166:1281–1286.

153 Hughes JM, Blumehtal JR, Merson MH, Lombard GL, Dowell VER, Gangarosa EJ. Clinical features of types A and B food-borne botulism. *Ann. Intern. Med.* 1981;95:442–445.

154 Centers for Disease Control and, Prevention. Botulism in the United States, 1899–1973: *Handbook for Epidemiologists, Clinicians, and Laboratory Workers.* Atlanta: Centers for disease control, 1978, pp. 374–8279/G.

155 Kongsaengdao S, Samintarapanya K, Rusmeechan S, et al. An outbreak of botulism in Thailand: clinical manifestations and management of severe respiratory failure. *Clin. Infect. Dis.* 2006;43:1247–1256.

156 Topakian R, Heibl C, Stieglbauer K, et al. Quantitative autonomic testing in the management of botulism. *J. Neurol.* 2009;256:803–809.

157 Jenzer G, Mumenthaler M, Ludin HP, Robert F. Autonomic dysfunction in botulism B: a clinical report. *Neurology* 1975;25:150–153.

158 Agrawal A, Pandit L, Dalal M, Shetty JP. Neurological manifestations of Hansen's disease and their management. *Clin.l Neurol. Neurosurg.* 2005;107:445–454.

159 Ulvi H, Yoldas T, Yigiter R, Mungen B. R–R interval variation and the sympathetic skin response in the assessment of the autonomic nervous system in leprosy patients. *Acta Neurol. Scand.* 2003;107:42–49.

160 Shetty VP, Mehta NH, Antia NH, Irani PF. Teased fibre study of early nerve lesions in leprosy and contacts, with electrophysiologic correlates. *J. Neurol. Neurosurg. Psych.* 1977;40:708–711.

161 Shetty VP, Mehta NH, Irani PF, Antia NH. Study of evaluation of nerve damage in leprosy. Part 1—Lesions of the index branch of the radial cutaneous nerve in early leprosy. Part 2—Observation on the index branch of the radial cutaneous nerve in contacts of leprosy. *Lepr. India* 1980;52:5–25.

162 Wilder-Smith EPV, Wilder-Smith AJ, Nirkko AC. Skin and muscle vasomotor reflexes in detecting autonomic dysfunction in leprosy. *Muscle Nerve* 2000;23:1105–1112.

163 Abbot NC, Beck JS, Mostofi S, Weiss F. Sympathetic vasomotor dysfunction in leprosy patients: comparison with electrophysiological measurement and qualitative sensation testing. *Neurosci. Lett.* 1996;206:57–60.

164 Legha SS. Vincristine neurotoxicity, pathophysiology, and management. *Medic. Toxic.* 1986;421–427.

165 Low PA, McLeod JG. Autonomic neuropathies. In PA Low, editor, *Clinical Autonomic Disorders,* 2nd ed. Philadelphia, PA: Lippincott-Raven Publishers, 1997, pp. 487–508.

166 Manolis AS, et al. Atypical pulmonary and neurologic complications of amiodarone in the same patient. Report of a case and review of the literature. *Arch. Intern. Med.* 1987;147:1805–1809.

167 Dormann AJ, Grünewald T, Wigginghaus B, Huchzermeyer H. Gemcitabine-associated autonomic neuropathy. *Lancet* 1998;351(9103):644.

168 Monforte R, Estruch R, Valls-Sole J, et al. Autonomic and peripheral neuropathies in patients with chronic alcoholism. *Arch. Neurol.* 1995;52:45–51.

169 Ammendola A, Tat MR, Aurilio C, Ciccone G, et al. Peripheral neuropathy in chronic alcoholism: a retrospective cross sectional study in 76 subjects. *Alcohol* 201; 36:271–275.

170 Mellion M, Gilchrist JM, De La Monte S. Alchol-related peripheral neuropathy: nutritional, toxic, or both? *Muscle Nerve* 2011;43(3):309–316.

171 Novak DJ, Victor M. The vagus and sympathetic nerves in alcoholic polyneuropathy. *Arch. Neurol.* 1974;30:273–284.

172 Guo YP, McLeod JG, Baverstock J. Pathological changes in the vagus nerve in diabetes and chronic alcoholism. *J. Neurol. Neurosurg. Psych.* 1987;50:1449–1453.

173 Johnson RH, Robinson BJ. Mortality in alcoholics with autonomic neuropathy. *J. Neurol. Neurosurg. Psych.* 1988;51:476–480.

174 Waguespack SG, Rich T, Grubbs E, Ying AK, Perrier ND, Ayala-Ramirez M, Jimenez C. A current review of the etiology, diagnosis, and treatment of pediatric pheochromocytoma and paraganglioma. *J. Clin. Endocrinol. Metab.* 2010;95:2023–2037.

175 Reisch N, Peczkowska M, Januszewicz N, Neumann HPH. Pheochromocytoma: presentation, diagnosis, and treatment. *J. Hypertension* 2006;24:2331–2339.

176 Adler JT, Meyer-Rochow GY, Chen H, Benn DE, Robinson BG, Sippel RS, Sidhu SB. Pheochromocytoma: current approaches and future directions. *Oncologist* 2008;13:779–793.

177 Ueda T, Oka N, Matsumoto A, Miyazaki H, Ohmura H, Kikuchi T, Nakayama M, et al. Pheochromocytoma presenting as recurrent hypotension and syncope. *Intern. Med.* 2005;44(3):222–227.

178 Bortnik M, Occhetta E, Marino P. Orthostatic hypotension as an unusual clinical manifestation of pheochromocytoma: a case report. *J. Cardiovasc. Med.* 2008;9:839–841.

179 Parkinson T. Phaeochromocytoma presenting as postural hypotension. *Proc. R. Soc. Med.* 1964;57:673–674.

180 Streeten DH, Anderson Gh. Mechanisms of orthostatic hypotension and tachycardia in patients with pheochromocytoma. *Am. J. Hypertens.* 1996;9:760–769.

181 Harrison TS, Bartlett JD, Seaton JF. Exaggerated urinary norepinephrine response to tilt in

pheochromocytoma. Diagnostic implications. *N. Engl. J. Med.* 1967;277:725–728.

182 Dabrowska B, Dabrowski A, Pruszczyk P, Skrobowski A, Wocial B. Heart rate variability in pheochromocytoma. *Am. J. Cardiol.* 1995;76:1202–1204.

183 Minami J, Todoroki M, Ishimitsu T, Matsuoka H. Changes in heart rate variability before and after surgery in patients with pheochromocytoma. *Auton. Neurosc. Basic Clin.* 2004;111:144–146.

184 Munakata M, Aihara A, Imai Y, Noshiro T, Ito S, Yoshinaga K. Altered sympathetic and vagal modulations of the cardiovascular system in patients with pheochromocytoma their relations to orthostatic hypotension. *Am. J. Hypertens.* 1999;12:572–580.

185 Lenders JW, Pacak K, Walther MM, Linehan WM, et al. Biochemical diagnosis of pheochromocytoma: which test is best? *J. Am. Med. Assoc.* 2002;287:1427–1434.

186 Pardanani A, Tefferi A. Systemic mastocytosis in adults: a review on prognosis and treatment based on 342 Mayo Clinic patients and current literature. *Curr. Opin. Hematol.* 2010;17:125–132.

187 Izikson L, English JC, Zirwas MJ. The flushing patient: differential diagnosis, workup, and treatment. *J. Am. Acad. Dermatol.* 2006;55:193–208.

15 Sleep disorders and systemic disease

Erik K. St. Louis

Mayo Clinic, Rochester, MN, USA

Sleep is a universal yet enigmatic biological imperative for all mammals. Recent evidence suggests that sleep is essential to macromolecule synthesis and that sleep deprivation leads to cellular stress, especially in the brain, for which sleep appears critical for plasticity and optimal cognitive functioning [1–3]. Deprivation of sleep leads to insufficient sleep quantity and quality. Adequate sleep is necessary to ensure optimal daytime functioning since vigilance, cognition, daytime functioning and performance, and overall quality of life are each substantially eroded by disordered sleep [1,3–5]. Unfortunately, insufficient sleep quantity and quality is a widespread public health problem in children and adults worldwide, and primary sleep disorders are a highly prevalent cause of morbidity, an important contributor to mortality, and a public health safety hazard in risk of motor vehicle collisions and catastrophic injuries and accidents in safety-sensitive occupations and situations. This chapter reviews sleep-related symptoms and disorders in patients with systemic diseases, and suggests appropriate diagnostic and treatment strategies for patients with systemic disease who manifest common sleep complaints (Table 15.1).

Endocrine disorders

Endocrine disorders featuring prominent sleep problems include disorders of the thyroid, the hypothalamic–pituitary–adrenal axis, and reproductive/sex-related hormones [6–8]. Thyroid deficiency often presents with fatigue, and hypothyroidism may be associated with obstructive sleep apnea or sleep-related hypoventilation, given resultant physical and anatomic predisposing factors of obesity and macroglossia, and impairment in upper airway function, due to deposition of mucopolysaccharides [7]. Thyroid function test screening by measurement of sensitive thyroid stimulating hormone (sTSH) is a reasonable initial investigation in overweight or obese patients presenting with prominent hypersomnia and cognitive or mood impairments, especially in the context of recent significant weight change. One Italian study found a prevalence of 11.5% for previously undiagnosed hypothyroidism employing TSH screening in a sleep clinic population of obese patients with hypersomnia, all without previously diagnosed thyroid disorders [9]. However, one recent large rigorous case-control study found a relatively weak association between hypothyroidism and obstructive sleep apnea, since OSA patients had an odds-ratio for prior hypothyroidism of just 1.47 (95% CI of 0.8–2.8) [10].

The hypothalamic–pituitary–adrenal (HPA) axis is critical for maintenance of normal alertness and regulation of sleep, since the lateral hypothalamus produces the key alertness modulator hypocretin (orexin), while the principally GABA-ergic ventrolateral preoptic nucleus (VLPO) of the hypothalamus is involved in non-rapid eye movement (NREM) sleep onset and regulation [6,11,12]. Hypothalamic hyperarousal has been suggested as a mechanism for insomnia, while deficient hypocretin (orexin) production causes narcolepsy [6,12]. HPA axis hyperactivity may also contribute to associated complications of OSA

Neurological Disorders due to Systemic Disease, First Edition. Edited by Steven L. Lewis.
© 2013 Blackwell Publishing Ltd. Published 2013 by Blackwell Publishing Ltd.

Table 15.1 Diagnosis and treatment of common sleep problems in systemic disease

Symptom	Diagnostic test	Potential findings	Treatments
Hypersomnia	Polysomnogram	Sleep apnea	Positive airway pressure, positional therapy, oral appliances, surgical approaches
	Multiple sleep latency	Mean sleep latency <8 min, with or without sleep-onset REM periods	Stimulants (modafinil, methylphenidate, amphetamines)
	If encephalopathy too, consider paraneoplastic antibodies	Anti-Ma positivity	Malignancy workup, stimulants
Parasomnia	Video-polysomnography	REM sleep without atonia (REM sleep behavior disorder)	Melatonin, clonazepam
	Video–EEG–PSG	NREM parasomnias, nocturnal epilepsies	Clonazepam, anticonvulsants
Restless leg syndrome	Ferritin	>50 μg/L	Pramipexole, ropinirole, carbidopa–levodopa, gabapentin, tramadol
		<50 μg/L	Iron-replacement therapy alone if mild symptoms; symptomatic management with dopaminergic agents
	Creatinine		Treat underlying cause of renal insufficiency
Insomnia	Generally none; with encephalopathy consider paraneoplastic antibodies	VGKC+, malignancy workup	Hypnotics

Note: VGKC, anti-voltage-gated potassium channel antibody.

including insulin resistance, hypertension, depression, and insomnia. Acromegaly also commonly leads to development of sleep-disordered breathing, most commonly OSA, due to anatomical factors such as thickened soft tissues in the oropharyngeal airway, and central sleep apnea may also occur.

Gonadal hormones may have significant effects on sleep and sleep-disordered breathing. Testosterone-replacement therapy at supraphysiologic doses has been reported to cause or aggravate OSA, although the frequency and consistency of this complication are debated [13]. Medroxyprogesterone is a respiratory stimulant, acting via the hypothalamic estrogen-dependent progesterone receptor, and has been applied therapeutically for this purpose [14,15]. Sleep quality may be affected by menses, with increased spindle frequency and reduced REM sleep during the luteal phase, but the timing and composition of

sleep are otherwise largely unaffected by the menstrual cycle [16]. Hot flashes associated with menopause cause insomnia in up to 80% of women having severe vasomotor instability, and sleep-disordered breathing and restless leg symptoms are also frequent in post-menopausal women [17,18].

Pregnant women have a two- to threefold higher risk for developing restless legs syndrome (RLS), which has a 11–27% prevalence during pregnancy [19]. Symptoms typically worsen as pregnancy progresses, and may be worst during the last trimester and resolve in the postpartum state. Increased prolactin and gonadal hormone fluctuations, as well as iron and folate deficiency, have been proposed as causes [19].

Women are more vulnerable than men to the development of insomnia [20]. Menstrual associated sleep disorders include premenstrual insomnia, or hypersomnia related to the late luteal phase of menses, or to menopause, and the causes are unknown [20,21]. Insomnia during late pregnancy and the postpartum state is also common [22]. Premenstrual hypersomnia is characterized by recurrent episodic hypersomnia preceding menses by about 1 week, and may be treated with hormonal contraceptives. Menopausal insomnia is associated with nocturnal hyperhidrosis and "hot flashes" ascribed to estrogen deficiency, with recurrent spontaneous arousals. Symptoms are usually treated effectively by hormone-replacement therapy, but a recently published trial has shown that eszopiclone is also effective in relieving nighttime hot flashes and sleep disturbance [22,23].

Disturbed or reduced sleep is also associated with increased risk for evolution of diabetes, the most common endocrine disorder. Short (<5–6 h nightly) or long (>8–9 h nightly) sleep duration, as well as insomnia with difficulty initiating or maintaining sleep, are each associated with increased incident type 2 diabetes [24,25]. Selective disruption of slow wave sleep also reduces glucose clearance and increases insulin resistance, suggesting a possible mechanism for increased diabetes risk in older age and in obese individuals with OSA [26,27]. Sleep-disordered breathing, especially obstructive sleep apnea (OSA), may also lead to insulin resistance and the metabolic syndrome [28].

Electrolyte and other metabolic disorders

While electrolyte disturbances such as severe hyponatremia, hypoglycemia, and hypercalcemia may cause altered mental status with encephalopathy and drowsiness, dyselectrolytemias are relatively uncommon causes of chronic sleep problems. This section briefly reviews those electrolyte disturbances that have been linked with chronic sleep disturbances, including altered glucose levels with hyperglycemia or hypoglycemia, the impact of ammonia on sleep, primary hyperparathyroidism with hypercalcemia as a cause of restless legs, nocturnal leg cramps as associated with dyselectrolytemias, and the relationship of sleep disturbances to metabolism.

Alterations in glucose levels can affect vigilance levels through the modulation of hypothalamic function. Hyperglycemia inhibits hypocretin cell firing,

decreasing alertness, and reducing locomotor activity and feeding behavior, while hypoglycemia increases the electrical firing of hypothalamic hypocretin cells, mediating opposite effects of increased alertness, locomotor activity, and feeding behavior [29].

One distinctive and unusual cause of restless legs syndrome is hypercalcemia associated with primary hyperparathyroidism. Treatment with parathyroidectomy resulted in normalization of parathyroid hormone and calcium levels, and an effective cure of RLS symptoms in one reported case [30].

Sleep-related leg cramps are a common and enigmatic problem affecting 7–10% of children, and up to 70% of elderly adults, and are frequently blamed on electrolyte deficiencies although they are most often idiopathic [31]. Testing for electrolyte abnormalities such as hypokalemia, hypocalcemia, hypomagnesemia, and hyponatremia can be considered; standard laboratory testing is usually of extremely low yield, but correction of any identified electrolyte dyscrasias should still be attempted. Unfortunately, despite their extremely common occurrence and impact on the quality of life of cramp sufferers, little is known about the pathophysiology or treatment of this condition. Cramps are painful, involuntary, sustained muscle contractions lasting 2–10 min, affecting unilateral or bilateral calves, thighs, or feet, with residual tenderness of the affected muscle, lasting up to an hour or longer. The clinical approach to sleep-related leg cramps is to first determine whether they are also present during daytime. If daytime cramping is prominent, exclusion of a precipitating neuromuscular disorder is paramount, including amyotrophic lateral sclerosis, peripheral neuropathy, myositis, or cramp-fasciculation syndrome. In elderly males, peripheral vascular disease and other systemic medical comorbidities are also common. A neurological examination should be conducted on all cramp sufferers, and those having sensorimotor findings, fasciculations, or pathological reflex findings should be referred for electromyography and undergo serum creatinine kinase or additional blood and urine testing for exclusion of symptomatic causes of neuropathy as appropriate. When examination findings are normal, and cramps are isolated to the sleep state, further diagnostic workup can usually be avoided. Symptomatic treatment measures for sleep-related leg cramps include tonic water with lemon, and advising adequate hydration and nightly stretching of the calves and thighs. For refractory cramp sufferers, a sodium-channel blocking anticonvulsant such as carbamazepine or oxcarbazepine may also be considered; the United State Food and Drug Administration (FDA) has issued a warning against the use of the antimalarial agent quinine for leg cramps, due to the risk of potential life-threatening hematologic side effects [32].

Metabolism is governed by both sleep and circadian factors [33,34]. Molecular clock genes control the timing of transcription in both central hypothalamic suprachiasmatic nuclear and peripheral tissues including liver, muscle, adipose, heart, and the vasculature, playing key roles in lipid and cholesterol biosynthesis, carbohydrate metabolism and transport, oxidative phosphorylation, and detoxification pathways [34]. Insufficient sleep amount and poor sleep quality may have adverse effects on metabolism [33]. The metabolic syndrome is a constellation of related metabolic derangements including central obesity, hypertension, insulin resistance, and hyperlipidemia, promoting the development of atherosclerosis. Sleep-disordered breathing, especially OSA, has been associated with several components of the metabolic syndrome, especially insulin resistance with hyperglycemia and dyslipidemia [28,35].

Systemic autoimmune disorders

Autoimmune disorders often have prominent fatigue and sleep complaints, especially systemic lupus erythematosis (SLE) and rheumatoid arthritis. While not autoimmune disorders per se, the closely related, enigmatic and traditionally rheumatological disorders of fibromyalgia and chronic fatigue syndromes are also considered in this section. The autoimmune encephalopathy Morvan syndrome is also discussed since it has prominent sleep dysfunction and accompanying systemic features including autonomic instability and neuropathy.

Most patients with SLE report fatigue and poor sleep quality, especially those with active disease, functional disability, and those receiving prednisone therapy [36,37]. Comorbid depression appears to be a significant mediator of sleep problems in SLE patients [37]. In one case-control study, SLE patients had more frequent daytime hypersomnia, as well as more frequent respiratory and movement disorders during polysomnography [38]. Sleepiness in SLE has been related to sleep fragmentation due to increased arousal index and stage transitions, decreased sleep efficiency, and decreased delta sleep [37].

Sleep complaints are seen in up to half of rheumatoid arthritis (RA) patients, and fatigue and risk for sleep-disordered breathing are more frequent in RA than control subjects [39,40]. Interestingly, improvements in sleep and alertness in RA following treatment with the monoclonal antibody infliximab appear independent of direct joint discomfort amelioration, and instead may be related to inhibition of proinflammatory cytokines such as tumor necrosis factor (TNF)-alpha, which have also been implicated in mediating hypersomnia in sleep-disordered breathing [41,42]. Patients with RA have more frequent periodic leg movements of sleep and alpha-intrusion in NREM sleep (a nonspecific finding but one that has been correlated with nonrestorative sleep) than controls, and symptoms of pain and morning stiffness are related to increases in wake time and possibly to alpha-intrusion into NREM sleep in RA and ankylosing spondylitis, suggesting a homeostatic bodily reaction to joint inflammation [39,43–46]. Disturbed sleep and sleep-disordered breathing have also been correlated with cognitive impairments in reaction time and sustained visual attention in children with juvenile idiopathic arthritis, who have been shown to have disturbed sleep microarchitecture with increases in the NREM cyclic alternating pattern (CAP) sleep rate in comparison to controls [47,48].

Chronic fatigue syndrome involves intense physical and mental fatigue lasting longer than 6 months and unassociated with a known underlying medical or physical cause. The diagnosis is one of exclusion, and presumes an appropriate preceding appropriate evaluation to exclude medical diseases, or possible sleep disorders that may cause fatigue. A combined multidisciplinary treatment approach is usually necessary and frequently unsuccessful [49].

Fibromyalgia is a chronic musculoskeletal pain disorder with prominent features of fatigue and complaints of nonrestorative sleep [43]. Abnormalities have been identified at multiple levels in the peripheral, central, and sympathetic nervous systems, involving polymorphisms of genes in the serotoninergic, dopaminergic, and catecholaminergic systems, resulting in amplified pain transmission and interpretation [50]. Exercise and cognitive behavioral therapy, and pain medications including pregabalin, duloxetine, and milnacipran are the usual therapies for this enigmatic disorder [51].

Morvan syndrome (Morvan's fibrillary chorea) is an autoimmune encephalopathy involving continuous muscle fiber activity of neuromyotonia, prominent complete insomnia (agrypnia excitata), variable hypersomnia, hallucinosis with altered behavior, and hyperhidrosis with autonomic instability [52–54]. A severe course progressing to death is classic, yet more recent literature suggests a more benign course. Morvan syndrome has been classically associated with anti-voltage-gated potassium channel antibodies, and more recently found to be associated with antibodies to proteins closely associated to the voltage-gated potassium channel, specifically contactin-associated protein- 2 (CASPR-2) [54]. Other common clinical features include muscle pain, cramping, slow relaxation, and stiffness. There may be inherited and acquired forms associated with malignancies (including thymoma) or myasthenia gravis [53].

Organ dysfunction and failure

Pulmonary disease

A continuum of sleep-disordered breathing disorders result from upper airway obstruction; this can range from mild snoring, to limited airflow resulting in reduced tidal volume (hypopnea), to airflow cessation (apnea). Some patients demonstrate a predisposing narrowed nasal or oropharyngeal anatomy, including problems such as nasal septal deviation, a low-lying palate or redundant soft palate tissue, thickened tongue base, or narrowed hypopharynx.

OSA can be considered a systemic disorder since it has many potential systemic consequences including endocrinologic abnormalities and metabolic syndrome, as well as systemic inflammation and coagulation–fibrinolysis imbalances that may confer cardiovascular risk [55]. OSA is an extremely common health problem present in 2–4% of the general population, and has been linked to development of hypertension and an increased prevalence of coronary artery disease, heart failure, and stroke [56]. OSA typically presents with a history of loud disruptive snoring, with or without snort arousals, witnessed apneic periods during sleep, and daytime sleepiness. OSA has been associated with the development of hypertension, and

is a risk factor for incident development of stroke, coronary artery disease, congestive heart failure, and atrial fibrillation. OSA has been shown to be associated with a wide variety of endothelial and metabolic abnormalities that favor vascular disease, and when patients with moderate to severe OSA are compared to normal or treated OSA patients, they appear to have a higher mortality and cardiovascular event frequency [57]. The main reasons to diagnose and treat OSA are for symptom improvement and to limit associated cardiovascular consequences.

The initial diagnostic approach for a patient with suspected OSA is polysomnography; this is the preferred diagnostic investigation for patients with a complaint of hypersomnia unexplained by insufficient sleep quantity, as well as for patients with a history of snoring or abnormal body movements in sleep [58]. OSA severity is rated by the polysomnographic apnea–hypopnea index (AHI), the rate of apneas and hypopneas occurring hourly averaged over the total sleep time. AHI of 4 per hour or less is normal, while mild OSA severity is indicated by an AHI of 5–14 per hour, moderate OSA by an AHI of 15–29 per hour, and severe OSA with an AHI of 30 per hour or greater. The AHI is also determined during NREM and REM sleep stages and during supine and nonsupine body positions.

The upper airway resistance syndrome (UARS) is the mildest form of OSA, and is characterized by a clinical complaint of hypersomnia, usually accompanied by snoring, but lacking a significant frequency of overt apneas or hypopneas [59]. Polysomnography demonstrates repetitive respiratory effort-related arousals (RERAs) that fragment sleep and reduce sleep quality. Treatment is similar to more severe forms of OSA.

Treatments for snoring and OSA include reducing nasal congestion or obstruction, positional therapies, nasal continuous positive airway pressure (nCPAP), oral appliances, or surgical management. Positional therapy involves use of a strategy to encourage sleep in a nonsupine body position, usually on the side. A "tennis-ball t-shirt" or body pillows are usual methods, although long-term adherence or compliance remains relatively poor [60]. Weight loss reduces oropharyngeal compression by decreasing soft tissue in the neck. Positive airway pressure (PAP) is the mainstay of treatment for OSA for the majority of patients [61]. Continuous PAP (CPAP) delivers a continuous set pressure between 5 and 20 cmH$_2$O. If an optimal pressure cannot be determined by laboratory titration or data is not available to guide prescription of a specific pressure for a patient, an auto-titrating PAP (APAP) device may be considered. CPAP is delivered through a nasal mask, nasal pillows, or a full face mask interface. Bilevel positive airway pressure (BPAP) may also be employed at higher treatment pressures if CPAP is not well tolerated. Setting a pressure delta of 3–6 cm between the inspiratory and expiratory pressure is useful as positive pressure ventilation for patients with sleep-related hypoventilation from intrinsic pulmonary disease or neuromuscular respiratory muscle weakness. Oral appliances advance the mandible, opening the oropharyngeal airway and obviating apneas and hypopneas, and are most effective for mild to moderate severity OSA, and generally less effective for severe OSA. Surgical options can also be considered when PAP is poorly tolerated.

Central sleep apnea (CSA) is associated with an unstable ventilatory drive during sleep, resulting in periods of insufficient ventilation and compromised gas exchange despite patency of the oropharyngeal airway. CSA causes similar symptoms to OSA but more frequently involves insomnia than hypersomnia. CSA may be idiopathic, or related to high-altitude induced periodic breathing, neurological diseases, Cheyne–Strokes breathing, or narcotic drugs. When caused by congestive heart failure (CHF), the presence of central sleep apnea syndrome or Cheyne–Stokes breathing implies a poor prognosis, and CHF further disrupts sleep quality due to insomnia, paroxysmal nocturnal dyspnea, and nocturia. CPAP improves cardiac functioning but does not reduce mortality in CHF patients [62]. Unfortunately, CSA is often at least partially resistant to treatment with conventional nasal CPAP therapy; although CPAP improves oxygenation and cardiac functioning, frequent arousals that fragment sleep often continue.

Complex sleep apnea syndrome (CompSAS) occurs in as many as 4–15% of those with OSA, and is characterized by OSA together with unstable ventilation typical of CSA when CPAP is administered [63]. CompSAS patients have frequent physiological sleep onset/postarousal central apneic events that may or may not later resolve with continued longitudinal exposure to CPAP. When central apneic events continue to occur at a frequency of more than five times per hour, a suboptimal treatment outcome of persisting hypersomnia and medical risk results. Alternative

PAP modes such as adaptive servoventilation (ASV) may be more effective for the treatment of both CompSAS and CSA, but definitive trials comparing these modalities remain in progress [64].

Sleep-related hypoventilation results when ventilation fails to achieve adequate oxygenation or CO_2 clearance, resulting in hypoxia and hypercapnea [65]. Causes of sleep-related hypoventilation include primary pulmonary parenchymal disorders such as chronic obstructive pulmonary disease (COPD), neuromuscular conditions affecting bellows musculature (such as amyotrophic lateral sclerosis or severe myopathies), or restrictive physiology of the chest wall accompanying obesity or kyphoscoliotic disorders [65–67]. Each of these disorders can ultimately also cause daytime hypoventilation, but recumbency during supine sleep and REM sleep stage (which involves relative chest-wall paralysis and dependency on diaphragmatic respiratory effort) usually lead to exclusive or initial sleep-related hypoventilation with subsequent medical risk consequent to suboptimal nocturnal oxygenation [65]. Failure to identify and treat significant sleep-related hypoventilation could result in sequelae of hypoxemia such as polycythemia, cor pulmonale with pulmonary hypertension and right heart failure, or hypercapnic respiratory failure. Treatment involves non-invasive positive pressure ventilation (NIPPV), such as bilevel positive airway pressure therapy [65]. Unopposed oxygen therapy in severe COPD or neuromuscular causes of sleep-related hypoventilation is a particular danger, since the hypoxic drive to breathe may become the principle factor supporting continued ventilatory effort as ventilation fails and hypercapnea mounts (which blunts the CO_2 sensitive chemoreceptor driven breathing drive); in some cases, masking the hypoxic breathing drive by oxygen administration may precipitate acute respiratory failure. A morning arterial blood gas on room air following initiation of NIPPV is indicated to assess for potential hypercapnea and assess the impact of ventilatory support. In the context of severe hypercapnea (i.e., PCO_2 of 55 mmHg or greater), serial arterial blood gases to monitor the effects of ventilatory support, oxygenation, and accumulating hypercapnea may be helpful to determine whether nocturnal mechanical ventilatory support is indicated.

Pulmonary conditions such as asthma may become exacerbated during sleep and additionally complicate obstructive sleep-disordered breathing and lead to further sleep-related hypoxia. Pulmonary function varies in a circadian rhythm, with peak lung function occurring in the late afternoon and a nadir in lung function occurring in the early morning hours. Nocturnal asthma is due to an apparent exaggeration of these circadian changes in pulmonary function, and is associated with greater morbidity and inadequate asthma control, gastroesophageal reflux disease, and obesity [68]. Effective treatment of asthma with long-acting beta-agonist or steroid inhalers can reduce nighttime symptoms, improve psychometric outcomes, and improve QOL.

Cardiac disease

The relationship between cardiac disease and sleep-disordered breathing is bidirectional [69]. Obstructive sleep apnea, particularly when moderately severe or severe, is associated with incident atrial fibrillation and a higher risk of recurrence of paroxysmal atrial fibrillation, although there is conflicting evidence on the value of nasal CPAP therapy in reducing recurrent atrial fibrillation [70,71]. More than half of patients with CHF have sleep-disordered breathing, placing additional strain on cardiac functioning since normal reductions in sympathetic tone and increases in vagal parasympathetic tone are blunted [72]. OSA may contribute to reduced cardiac function through apnea-induced hypoxemia and hypercapnea, negative intrathoracic pressures, and repetitive arousals leading to hypertension, endothelial shearing, and accelerated atherosclerosis, while effective treatment of OSA may favorably impact these influences and improve cardiac systolic contractility [72]. CSA with Cheyne–Stokes respirations result from CHF given delayed circulation time from failing cardiac output. Improvement of cardiac functioning is the best means of treating CSA associated with CHF, although CPAP is of additional benefit in improving oxygenation, and no good evidence has as yet shown that CPAP impacts mortality associated with CHF.

Cardiac dysrhythmias from the SCN5A channelopathies (which include long QT syndrome type 3 (LQT3), idiopathic familial ventricular fibrillation, and cardiac conduction defects) occur most often during sleep, but the relationship of this effect remains poorly understood [73].

Renal disease

Sleep-associated symptoms and excessive daytime sleepiness are common in patients with chronic renal insufficiency, especially those receiving hemodialysis or peritoneal dialysis, which have a prevalence of sleep disturbances of approximately 80% [74–76]. OSA may occur 10-fold more frequently in uremic patients compared to the general population, affecting as many as 30–80% of those dialyzed [74,76,77]. Hypersomnia is seen in about 50% of dialysis patients, and has been associated with the severity of uremic encephalopathy and somnogenic cytokines, in addition to impaired sleep efficiency [76,77]. Insomnia affects 70% of dialysis patients, while restless legs syndrome and periodic limb movement disorder affect approximately 30% and may improve following dialysis or renal transplantation [76]. Sleep apnea associated with renal failure may be improved by nocturnal hemodialysis [77].

Gastrointestinal disease

Gastroesophageal reflux (GERD) may be promoted by several sleep-related factors, including a recumbent and supine sleep position, decreased arousal threshold, mechanical effects of the abdomen, and comorbid OSA which may generate negative intrathoracic pressures that aggravates GERD, and may lead to refractory GERD with prominent nocturnal or early morning symptoms [78,79]. Peptic ulcer disease may also be worsened by sleep loss [80]. Nonalcoholic fatty liver disease has also been recently associated with metabolic syndrome and hypoxia related to OSA [81].

Systemic cancer and paraneoplastic disorders

Fatigue and disturbed sleep are prominent issues accompanying most forms of cancer and its therapies, affecting between 25% and 99% of patients during the course of their illness, and fatigue often persists for years following completion of treatment [82–84]. Insomnia is common and a predictor of fatigue in cancer patients, and polysomnography demonstrates reduced sleep efficiency, prolonged initial sleep latency, and increased wake time during the night [85–87]. Disturbed sleep with frequent nocturnal awakenings and flattened circadian cortisol rhythms have been shown to predict increased mortality in metastatic colorectal cancer [88].

Causes of sleep disturbance in cancer are multifactorial, and include altered circadian rhythms due to daytime fatigue and daytime inactivity with resultant disturbed nighttime sleep, psychological stress, altered mood, and pain. However, there is also evidence that reactive inflammatory processes and neuroendocrine responses to cancer and its treatments play a key role, suggested by altered levels of C-reactive protein (CRP), cytokines (especially interleukin 6 which prolongs sleep latency and decreases slow wave sleep), and cortisol secretion [89,90].

Paraneoplastic disorders have recently gained attention as a rare but distinctive cause of insomnia, hypersomnia, and parasomnias. The clinical manifestations of typical Morvan syndrome were previously discussed under idiopathic autoimmune disorders, but there is also a spectrum of paraneoplastic sleep disorders classically associated with antivoltage-gated potassium channel (VGKC) antibodies and now known to be due to the CASPR-2 epitope, which may include insomnia, hypersomnia, and parasomnia behavior (especially REM sleep behavior disorder) [54,91]. Accompanying neurological and systemic manifestations occurring in patients with VGKC antibodies may also include cognitive impairment, extrapyramidal dysfunction, seizures, brain stem/cranial nerve dysfunction, dysautonomia, myoclonus, and peripheral neuropathy and/or hyperexcitability (neuromyotonia or continuous muscle fiber activity) [92]. Underlying malignancies reported in association with VGKC antibodies include carcinomas, thymoma, and hematologic malignancy, so it is crucial to screen all patients found to have VGKC antibody positivity for occult malignancy, such as with positron emission tomography (PET) and computed tomography (CT) of the body [53,54,92]. Hyponatremia is seen in over one-third of patients, and other organ-specific autoantibodies in nearly half, with a coexisting autoimmune disorder in one-third (especially thyroiditis and type 1 diabetes), and 89% of patients in one large series benefited from immunotherapy [92].

REM sleep behavior disorder (RBD) may also be associated with paraneoplastic disorders, most often VGKC antibodies with or without associated limbic encephalitis [91,93]. RBD typically presents with variable recall of frightening dream content (characteristically involving fighting off attackers or defending oneself against assailants), together with the objective correlate of witnessed dream enactment manifested most often by violent thrashing movements and screaming or shouting vocalization in sleep [94,95]. While RBD patients rarely leave the bed and sleep walk, falls or other injurious behavior to self or the bed partner are frequent. Importantly, elderly patients newly diagnosed with RBD harbor a 40–50% risk of developing parkinsonism within 10–12 years of symptom onset, so all patients with otherwise idiopathic RBD require serial neurological examinations and follow-up [96]. Diagnosis of RBD is by clinical history as well as confirmatory evidence for heightened muscle tone evident on polysomnographic electromyogram (EMG) leads in the chin and limbs (so called REM sleep without atonia) [97]. Treatment options include melatonin, initially at doses of 3 mg and gradually titrating toward 12 mg nightly as needed to suppress visible behavior, or clonazepam 0.5–1.0 mg as initial doses that can be increased to 2–3 mg nightly. Great care should be taken to first exclude comorbid OSA in such patients prior to use of clonazepam, a potential respiratory and upper airway suppressant.

A similar clinical sleep syndrome with a prominent narcoleptic phenotype is seen with anti-Ma 2 paraneoplastic antibodies, including symptoms of RBD and encephalopathy with cognitive impairment, parkinsonism, and gaze palsy [98]. Brain magnetic resonance imaging (MRI) shows damaged dorsolateral midbrain, amygdala, and paramedian thalami [98]. Supportive evidence for symptomatic narcolepsy has been reported in a patient with hypersomnia and anti-Ma 2 antibody positivity, with multiple sleep latency testing demonstrating four sleep onset REM periods and severe reduction of CSF hypocretin [98].

Central hypoventilation has also been reported in brain stem encephalitides associated with the paraneoplastic anti-Hu antibody [99]. Severe inflammatory infiltrates and neuronal loss in the medulla were seen in an autopsied patient.

Systemic infectious diseases

General systemic infection

Not surprisingly, poor sleep habits with reduced sleep duration and efficiency in otherwise healthy individuals in the weeks directly prior to exposure are associated with a higher risk of evolving the common cold [100]. Sleep problems occur commonly in a variety of systemic infections; insomnia is a prominent initial symptom in influenza and following influenza vaccination, sleep disturbances occur in 60–65% of those with hepatitis C infection, and cystic fibrosis patients with pulmonary infectious exacerbations have increased wake after sleep onset time, lower REM percentage, and poorer neuro-behavioral task performance than control cystic fibrosis patients with stable disease [101,102]. Sleep architecture is influenced by microbial products such as endo-toxin as well as endogenous immune signaling cytokines, although effects across species and even at varying concentrations are inconsistent [103]. Cyto-kines, including interleukin 1b and TNF-alpha, and brain neurotransmitters including the serotonergic sys-tem, are amplified during infection and may play a role in fever generation [103–106].

Trypanosomiasis (sleeping sickness)

Trypanosomiasis is caused by *Trypanosoma brucei*, a parasite transmitted by the painful bite of the tsetse fly. Two different strains exist, East African *T.b. rhode-siense* and West African *T.b. gambiense* [107]. The East African variety has been diagnosed in the United States in individuals with a history of travel to Eastern Africa, especially Uganda, Tanzania, Malayi, and Zambia [107]. There are between 15 and 20,000 new cases of trypanosomiasis reported every year to the World Health Organization, but the true prevalence is proba-bly between 50 and 70,000 cases a year, and unfortunately no preventive strategies or vaccinations exist. Major early symptoms of the disorder are chancre formation at the bite site, with ensuing fever, rash, swelling, headaches, fatigue, myalgias, arthralgias, pru-ritis, lymphadenopathy, and weight loss as the disease unfolds, followed ultimately by late-stage encephalo-pathic alterations including irritability, extreme fatigue and hypersomnia, and personality changes with pro-gressive confusion. Without treatment, usually with either suramin, pentamidine, melarsoprol, and eflorni-thine, progression to death is relentless [107].

Human immunodeficiency virus

Insomnia in reported in approximately 70% of human immunodeficiency virus (HIV) patients, and is reported during all stages of infection [108,109]. Psy-chological comorbidity, cognitive impairment, and treatment with efavirenz appear to be the most

significant risk factors [109]. Poor nighttime sleep quality has been significantly correlated with fatigue intensity and daytime sleepiness [110]. Physiologic coupling between TNF-alpha and delta sleep EEG amplitude has been found to be reduced in HIV-infected patients, possibly relating to fatigue-related symptoms [111].

Fatal familial insomnia

Fatal familial insomnia (FFI) is an extremely rare auto-somal dominant condition involving progressive insom-nia with prominent autonomic nervous system dysfunction, including symptoms of hyperhidrosis, hyperthermia, tachycardia, and hypertension, followed by ataxia with myoclonus and pyramidal dysfunction. FFI is caused by the conversion of the constitutively expressed prion protein, PrP(C), into an abnormally aggregated isoform, called PrP(Sc). Most prion diseases are sporadic, although about 10–15% of patients are affected by a genetic form and carry either a point mutation or an insertion of octapeptide repeats in the prion protein gene [112]. Disease onset is in the middle age between 30 and 60 years in most individuals, with a typical course between 6 and 25 months. Pathologically, all cases have shown severe atrophy of the anterior ventral and mediodorsal thalamic nuclei, and most cases also have cortical gliosis with or without spongy degen-eration, moderate cerebellar atrophy with "torpedoes," and severe inferior olivary nuclear atrophy [113].

Whipple disease

Whipple disease is caused by *Tropheryma whippelii*. Neurological involvement is seen in approximately 40% of patients, and hypersomnia or insomnia with agrypnia mimicking fatal familial insomnia may be an initial presenting symptom of the disorder in rarely reported cases, presumably due to disruption of normal hypothalamic functioning, and impaired hypocretin pro-duction has been documented in one case [114,115].

Complications due to transplantation

There remains a relative dearth of data concerning transplantation and sleep complaints or disorders. Sleep problems associated with renal disease reviewed in a previous section of this chapter also impact kidney transplant recipients. Insomnia and restless legs prevalence is reduced in kidney-transplanted patients compared to dialysis patients, although sleep apnea remains frequent and is seen in about 30% of these patients [116]. The late adverse effects of hematopoietic stem cell transplantation (HSCT) include sleep disorders in approximately 26% of patients, especially those of female gender and those who received previous busulfan-cyclophosphamide conditioning [117].

Complications of critical medical illness

Disturbances of sleep are nearly universal and multifactorial in cause in critically ill patients, including environmental factors (such as noise within intensive care units (ICUs), frequent caregiver assessments, and light exposure); endogenous patient issues related to the type and severity of underlying and comorbid illnesses (i.e., pain, sepsis, and metabolic, immune, inflammatory, neurological, and respiratory illnesses); and other treatment-related factors (including intravenous drug therapies, mechanical ventilator treatments, and diagnostic procedures) [118–122]. Detrimental impacts of sleep deprivation in the ICU setting may include cardiovascular stimulation, increased gastric secretion, pituitary and adrenal stimulation, suppression of the immune system and wound healing, and possible contribution to delirium [118].

Studies concerning sleep timing, quality, and disruption in the ICU setting remain relatively limited, given the difficulty of applying polysomnographic techniques and interpretation of sleep scoring in critically ill patients [123]. Sleep schedules become irregular with approximately half of total sleep time occurring during daytime, and circadian entrainment is lost in many patients [123]. Polysomnographic studies of critically ill patients suggest prolonged sleep latencies, reductions in sleep efficiency, altered sleep architecture with increased light NREM stages N1 and N2 and reduced restorative slow wave NREM and REM sleep stages, and increased arousal index with a degree of sleep fragmentation comparable to that of obstructive sleep apnea [120–124]. Patients receiving neuromuscular blockade have shown longer sleep durations and increased slow wave sleep, possibly related to age, drugs, or metabolic factors [125].

Approximately 20% of arousals appear to be due to environmental noise, and 10% of arousals have been related to patient care activities, but the cause for the majority of remaining arousals in critically ill patients remains unclear, suggesting the need for further active investigation into other causes of sleep disruption in the environment, care, or underlying illnesses [123,126].

Given the difficulty of applying traditional sleep scoring techniques in critically ill patients receiving sedative medications and manifesting encephalopathic generalized or regional slowing of the electroencephalogram, alternative techniques for assessing sleep have been assessed [127–129]. Subjective nurse/caregiver and patient sleep assessment methods consistently overestimate sleep duration and cannot assess sleep quality and the degree of sleep fragmentation accurately [123,129]. EEG spectral analysis, bispectral index score (BIS), and actigraphy have been attempted as surrogate measures for sleep quality, but currently remain investigational [127–129].

Sleep disruption induces sympathetic activation and leads to blood pressure elevation, which could lead to further cardiovascular and cerebrovascular complications. However, it is currently unknown if disturbed sleep in ICU patients independently predicts poor outcomes such as difficulty with weaning, prolonged recovery times, or morbidity/mortality, or is simply a manifestation of cerebral and bodily dysfunction [124]. Sleep disruption may be related to development of delirium and the effects of sedative/hypnotic medications [130–132]. Delirium is a predictor of increased morbidity and mortality, so reduction of sleep disruption that reduces the frequency of delirium could significantly improve ICU outcomes [132].

Considerable further research is needed to evaluate strategies for sleep enrichment and its bearing on clinical outcomes, since evidence-basis for sleep promotion interventions is currently lacking [133]. Other general strategies to improve the quantity and quality of sleep in critically ill patients include consideration of the mode of mechanical ventilation utilized, decreasing environmental noise, limiting nursing and caregiver assessments to enrich sleep, and judicious use of sedative agents [123]. Frequent evaluation of neurological status is necessary to avoid excessive or prolonged sedation.

Hypnotic agents such as benzodiazepines can increase total sleep time, but they alter sleep architecture by eroding restorative sleep stages of slow wave and REM sleep. Decreased melatonin production is seen in critically ill patients, and melatonin levels may decrease following procedures. There have been reports of successful treatment of sleep problems and delirium with melatonin in hospitalized patients, and there is additional rationale for use of melatonin in critically ill patients given its antioxidant activity, offering potential to reduce reperfusion injury, prevent multiorgan failure, and treat sepsis [134,135]. However, limited data exists for routine melatonin supplementation currently, although a recently published pilot controlled trial of high-dose melatonin in critically ill patients improved measures of sleep duration and efficiency [136].

Optimizing ventilatory support is an important consideration in minimizing sleep disruption in critically ill patients. Early recognition and treatment of sleep-disordered breathing in nonventilated patients, utilizing screening tools like the STOP–BANG (Snoring, Tiredness, Observed apnea, and high blood Pressure–Body mass index, Age, Neck circumference, and Gender) questionnaire or screening portable overnight oximetry may be helpful in selecting patients who would benefit from inpatient polysomnography, or empiric noninvasive positive airway pressure therapy trials, for treatment of obstructive or central sleep apnea and sleep-related hypoventilation associated with chronic obstructive pulmonary disease, neuromuscular disorders, or obesity [137,138]. In patients receiving mechanical ventilation, the mode of ventilation and appropriate ventilator settings need to be carefully considered to minimize a deleterious impact on sleep. Spontaneous pressure support ventilatory modes have been thought to contribute to sleep fragmentation, and it has been shown that avoiding overventilation when utilizing spontaneous ventilatory modes is helpful to avoid induction of hypocapnia and resultant central apneas that may mediate further arousal and promote ineffective effort [139–141]. However, one recent study found no difference in arousal index when comparing assist control with clinically or automatically adjusted pressure support modes of mechanical ventilation [142]. Noninvasive ventilation in elderly patients with acute hypercapnic respiratory failure has also been associated with disturbed sleep, including abnormal EEG patterns and reduced REM sleep [143].

One recent study showed that earplugs and eye mask use in a simulated ICU environment benefited sleep by increasing REM time, reducing arousal index, and increasing melatonin levels [144]. Another study examining the impact of a masking white noise in simulated ICUs found that the intervention increased arousal thresholds and reduced the arousal index apparently by reducing differences between background noise and peak noise [145].

Insomnia is characterized by repeated complaints of difficulties falling or staying asleep, poor sleep quality, or waking undesirably early despite an adequate time and opportunity sleep, and resultant daytime impairment. Insomnia affects between 30% and 80% of hospitalized patients for multiple reasons, including the impact of underlying illness, environmental factors of noise and care activities, medications, and comorbid anxiety and mood disorders [146,147]. Chronic insomnia may be preceded in predisposed individuals by precipitating factors such as illness or stress, and may be propagated by behavioral or maladapted cognitive factors. Patients should be asked what amount of their insomnia is ascribable to an active mind or worries, restless legs, or body pain. In most cases of insomnia, precipitating and/or propagating influences may be found through careful interview, and help to establish a secure diagnosis. Treatment of insomnia is directed at optimizing treatment for the underlying medical disorders including effective pain relief, reduction of environmental sleep disruption, and behavioral and hyponotic medication therapies directed at psychophysiologic insomnia factors. The main behavioral therapies for insomnia are addressing aspects of inadequate sleep hygiene and cognitive-behavioral therapies [148,149]. Patients often respond best to combined modalities. Patients should be encouraged to maintain a regular sleep schedule, avoid lying sleepless in bed, avoid clock-watching behavior, and to schedule planning, thinking, or worry time at least 2 hours prior to sleep.

There are now several highly effective, safe, and tolerable hypnotic medications available for short-term, intermittent, as well as chronic use. The class of nonbenzodiazepine receptor agonists (the so-called "Z" drugs: zolpidem, zaleplon, and ezopiclone) are preferred by most sleep specialists, but remain costlier than the older generation choices including the benzodiazepines, which have adverse effects on sleep architecture, and trazadone which has less specific sleep-promoting effects and more adverse effects and drug–drug interactions, especially in elderly patients. An excellent recent evidence-based review has been published on the subject of pharmacotherapy in insomnia, to which the interested reader is referred [150].

There is limited evidence concerning long-term outcomes of poor sleep following recovery from acute illness in the context of ICU care. Poor sleep quality may continue following discharge and become a chronic disorder. In one small study of seven survivors of acute respiratory distress syndrome (ARDS) reporting difficulty sleeping 6 months following discharge from the hospital, five patients had chronic insomnia, one patient had parasomnia, and one had OSA [151].

Sleep disturbances are a common sequelae of traumatic brain injury, occurring in 25–72% of patients [152–155]. Incident sleep problems following trauma are especially common, with about 28% of patients having hypersomnia within 6 months following a head injury, 22% having an increased need for longer sleep [152]. The substrate of many such cases may be symptomatic narcolepsy, as mean sleep latencies are pathologically brief with sleep onset REM periods in 25–32% of patients, and CSF hypocretin was found reduced in up to 93% of patients acutely following head injury, with hypocretin levels persistently reduced in 19% of patients after 6 months [152,155,156]. Insomnia is seen in another 25%, and parasomnias may also be seen in up to 25% following head injury, with REM sleep behavior disorder seen in up to 8% of these patients [155]. Sleep problems are also frequently chronically enduring, with approximately 25% of patients having persistent hypersomnia 3 years following head injury, and 10% having insomnia linked to mood disturbances [153,157]. Modafinil may be effective in treating posttraumatic hypersomnia [158].

Drugs, toxins (including alcohol), and vitamin and mineral deficiencies

Dreaming, nightmares, and dream enactment, and their relationship to drugs and medications

Nightmares represent undesirable, disturbing dream content that leads to sudden arousal from sleep with heightened autonomic sequelae of sweating, hypervigilance, tachycardia, and tachypnea. Nightmares and vivid dreaming are present in 10–50% of normal young children and in about 50% of adults, but become abnormally disturbing in content or frequency in a substantially less frequent subset of individuals, and the true prevalence of nightmare disorder remains unknown. Patients who present with a chief complaint of frequent nightmares should be reassured as to their biological nature and receive a detailed physical and neurological history and examination to exclude potential provoking comorbid causes such as a recent medication change in type or dosage, mood or anxiety disorder, or primary sleep disorder such as sleep-disordered breathing [159]. If no certain readily reversible triggering cause may be identified, referral for consideration of hypnosis, cognitive restructuring technique, imagery rehearsal therapy, or pharmacotherapy with clonazepam may be helpful in some cases.

Patients and their bedpartners should be questioned carefully regarding the potential of dream enactment when they present with prominent dreaming or nightmares, particularly those involving fighting off animals or persons, since REM sleep behavioral disorder (RBD) in young adults may be associated with antidepressant medications, especially the tricyclic antidepressants and selective serotonin reuptake inhibitors (SSRIs), and these drugs should be avoided whenever possible in patients with RBD [160,161]. Removal of the offending drug may lead to resolution of dream enactment in selected patients, but clonazepam or melatonin therapy can also reduce the behaviors.

Alcohol

Alcohol is a double-edged sword in relation to sleep. Despite being initially sedating in moderate doses for a short timeframe, alcohol eventually disrupts sleep persistently in as few as 3 days of continued use [162]. Initially, alcohol decreases sleep latency, and acutely it may increase N1 and slow wave NREM sleep during the first half of the night (in some cases, the latter effect may increase the risk of sleepwalking behaviors); as the night progresses and the sedating impact wears off, alcohol typically further fragments sleep by reducing restorative slow wave and REM sleep percentages and sleep efficiency, promoting alpha frequency intrusion, leading to increased wakefulness and decreasing total sleep duration, as well as causing disruptive symptoms of tachycardia and sweating [163–168]. Even when ingested several hours prior to sleep during the late afternoon hours, the disturbing effects of alcohol on nocturnal sleep remain [169]. The mechanism of disruptive effects of sleep by alcohol is probably multifactorial and multilevel, mediated by gamma-aminobutyric acid (GABA), serotonin (5-hydroxytryptamine; 5-HT), adenosine, or other neurotransmitter systems, and decreases in melatonin secretion have also been documented with moderate alcohol exposure [165,170]. The direct sedating effects and deleterious impact on cognitive performance mediated by alcohol is well known, and perhaps not surprisingly it has been found that alcohol interacts with sleep deprivation to exacerbate daytime sleepiness and alcohol-induced performance impairments [167,171]. Alcohol abuse is associated with problems falling asleep and decreased total sleep time during drinking periods and withdrawal, and abstinent alcoholics often still experience persistent prominent sleep abnormalities [165,172]. Prominent beta band power is seen in alcohol-dependent patients during sleep [173]. Alcohol can also exacerbate primary sleep disturbances such as obstructive sleep apnea, by reducing upper airway tone and causing sedation, thereby contributing to excessive daytime sleepiness [174,175]. As there is evidence that comorbid sleep disorders may impact relapse risk, identification and treatment of sleep disorders in alcohol-dependent and abstinent patients is important, including treatment of insomnia, and it is generally recommended to concentrate on behavioral approaches while avoiding benzodiazepines in these patients [176,177].

Illicit drugs

Illicit recreational drugs of abuse such as cocaine, ecstasy, and marijuana have prominent impact on sleep [178]. Cocaine increases wakefulness and suppresses REM, and its withdrawal disturbs sleep and may produce unpleasant dream content. 3,4-Methylenedioxymethamphetamine (MDMA; "ecstasy") also has arousing properties similar to those of cocaine, and long-term MDMA abuse may lead to persistent sleep disturbances, including a possible elevated risk for evolving obstructive sleep apnea, possibly due to serotonin neural toxicity induced by MDMA [179,180]. Cannabis increases drowsiness, reduces REM, and increases Stage 4 (slow wave) sleep. Withdrawal of marijuana may cause insomnia and unusual dreams,

with prolonged initial sleep latency, reduced N3, and REM sleep rebound.

Caffeine

Caffeine is ubiquitous and has significant benefit toward maintaining alertness, wakefulness, and performance, as well as a deleterious effect on sleep [181]. Caffeine has been well studied and found to enhance vigilance and performance following sleep deprivation and circadian sleep disturbances such as shift work. Dependence may develop at low doses following brief durations of regular use. Sleep disturbance and daytime sleepiness are associated with chronic caffeine use, possibly by reducing sleep propensity and efficiency, as well as by disrupting homeostatic adenosinergic regulation of nonREM slow-wave sleep duration and intensity, especially disrupting the restorative effects of enriched recovery sleep following sleep deprivation [182–187].

Nicotine

Nicotine use, withdrawal, and replacement therapy may also lead to sleep disturbance, with insomnia associated with prolonged initial sleep latency, sleep fragmentation, and decreased slow-wave and REM sleep with reduced sleep efficiency [188,189]. Sleep disturbance is also commonly reported by recently abstinent smokers, and nicotine-replacement therapy (NRT) or bupropion can further worsen sleep quality in these patients [188].

Prescription medications

Prescription medications including beta blockers, antidepressants, anticonvulsants, anti-inflammatory drugs (especially prednisone and interferons), antiarrythmics, and pain medications (especially opiate analgesics) may have prominent sleep-related symptoms including insomnia, hypersomnia, or excessive or bizarre dreams. Several of these medications, particularly psychotropic drugs and anticonvulsants, disturb sleep architecture prominently, while a few newer antiepileptic and psychotropic drugs may have favorable impacts on sleep quality. A review of these effects is beyond the scope of this chapter and the reader is referred to other recent resources [190,191].

273

Iron deficiency and restless legs syndrome

The hematologic dyscrasia of iron deficiency, even when only relative, and with serum ferritin measures that remain in the normal range, has been associated with the restless leg syndrome and periodic leg movements of sleep [192–194]. Diagnosis of restless leg syndrome (RLS) is based completely on the clinical history, and typically requires four central elements to the described symptoms: (1) urge to move the legs, with or without uncomfortable leg sensations; (2) temporary relief by movement; (3) symptoms occur solely or predominantly at rest; and (4) nocturnal worsening of symptoms [195,196]. The nature of the symptoms as described by the patient may be quite variable with regard to the symptom quality, location or distribution, temporal occurrence, frequency, and severity. RLS symptoms are usually described as uncomfortable, although not really painful, with a sense of a creepy-crawly or prickling discomfort, often below the knees and centered about the shins or calves, but sometimes more proximally in the thighs, or even isolated to the feet and ankles. Symptoms may occur in the arms as well, especially proximally near the shoulders. The much feared but little-understood phenomena of augmentation involves a worsening of the symptoms in temporal expression, severity, and distribution, with symptoms changing from intermittent to constant, with growing intensity and frequency, occurring earlier in the day, and spreading up the legs to the trunk and arms.

About 50% of patients with RLS will carry a positive family history of the disorder, but positive family history is not necessary for the diagnosis. Pedigrees suggest an autosomal-dominant transmission with high penetrance. Genetic loci associated with RLS include those on chromosomes 12q, 14q, 9p, 2q, 20p, and 16p [196]. Restless leg syndrome has been linked to deficient iron stores and dopaminergic neurotransmission in the brain, and symptomatic forms of the condition occur commonly in patients with pregnancy or chronic renal insufficiency. The condition is also common in those with neurological conditions such as parkinsonism, multiple sclerosis, and epilepsy.

While periodic leg movements of sleep (PLMS) are seen in 80–90% of RLS patients, PLMs are not necessary for the diagnosis of RLS. Furthermore, PLMS are also extremely frequent in the general population, seen in 5–15% of younger adults and as many as 45% of elderly individuals. Recently, the common variant intron BTBD9 on chromosome 6p21 has been associated with susceptibility to periodic limb movements in sleep, with an inverse correlation of the variant with serum iron stores, consistent with iron depletion as a mechanism for PLMD [193,194]. Periodic limb movement disorder (PLMD) is diagnosed when PLMs are thought causative of daytime hypersomnia.

Nonpharmacologic treatments including warm or cool baths, massage, or stretching, and application of spontaneous compression devices has even been reported to be effective anecdotally and in small case series; however, evidence basis for these measures remains poor, and most patients seeking medical care for the symptom have severe enough symptoms to merit pharmacologic treatment.

Iron deficiency, or even low normal body iron stores, may worsen or precipitate RLS symptoms [192,197,198]. The hypothesis of brain iron insufficiency as a mechanism for RLS symptom generation has been advanced due to several lines of converging evidence including neuroimaging data, cerebrospinal fluid studies, autopsy, and evidence of effective prompt relief with intravenous iron treatment [192]. It is thought that some RLS patients have brain iron stores that become inadequate, either dependent upon, or independent of, peripheral iron access or amount [192].

Measuring a serum ferritin should be considered early in all RLS patients, with iron-replacement therapy begun if serum ferritin values are less than 50 µg/L. Iron therapy can be constipating or cause GI distress, and the formulation of ferrous gluconate with added vitamin C is often well tolerated by those who cannot stomach ferrous sulfate.

Carbidopa–levodopa may be used for patients with only intermittently disturbing symptoms, but chronic nightly use of carbidopa–levodopa, especially above a dosage of 200 mg daily, may raise the risk of augmentation. For nightly use, the dopaminergic agonist medications pramipexole or ropinirole are the mainstay of treatment. Pramipexole may be initiated at 0.125–0.25 mg nightly and titrated every few days to the 0.35–0.50 mg range or beyond if needed for symptom control. Doses beyond 1.0 mg are typically not additionally effective. Ropinirole may be initiated at 0.5–1.0 mg with gradual upward titration to the 4–6 mg range as

Five things to remember about sleep disorders due to systemic disease

1. Patients with hypersomnia that is not adequately explained by insufficient sleep quantity, especially when associated with snoring or abnormal movements in sleep, should be investigated with diagnostic polysomnography to exclude sleep-disordered breathing and periodic limb movement disorder.
2. The main treatments for OSA include continuous positive airway pressure (nCPAP), positional therapy, and mandibular advancement devices; of these options, CPAP is usually superior in those who can tolerate and comply with the treatment.
3. Symptomatic causes for restless leg syndrome include iron deficiency, chronic renal insufficiency, and pregnancy; when serum ferritin is lower than 50 µg/L, iron supplementation should be provided and treatment with a dopamine agonist or gabapentin may provide further relief of symptoms.
4. Paraneoplastic sleep disorders are a relatively rare but critically important cause of sleep disturbances, causing symptoms of prominent insomnia, hypersomnia, and REM sleep behavior disorder parasomnias. Consider evaluation with paraneoplastic antibody panels, especially including anti-voltage-gated potassium channel and anti-Ma antibodies, in patients with a history of malignancy, concurrent encephalopathy, or neuropathy of unknown cause, or an atypical subacute onset.
5. Sleep disruption is nearly universal in critically ill patients, especially those in intensive care unit settings; considerations to minimize sleep disruption in these patients include decreasing environmental noise, limiting nursing and caregiver assessments, altering the mode of mechanical ventilation utilized, and judicious use of sedative agents.

needed and tolerated. Generally, dosing 1 h prior to bedtime is sufficient, but if earlier evening or late-afternoon symptoms emerge, cautious application of divided doses may be utilized with precautions to the patient regarding the possibility of augmentation. Another newer dopamine agonist, rotigotine, was recently approved for treatment of restless legs syndrome, offering a convenient transdermal delivery system associated with relatively low levels of clinically significant augmentation. [199, 200] With dopamine agonists, there is also a risk of impulse control disorders (e.g., pathological gambling or shopping behaviors), requiring cessation of treatment. [201,202]. For patients intolerant or resistant to the dopaminergic drugs, gabapentin has become the preferred second-line medication, dosed 300–1200 mg qhs as needed and tolerated. For patients unresponsive to these measures, opiate treatment with oxycodone 5–15 mg qhs, hydromorphone, or in severe refractory cases, methadone [203] is frequently effective, and other alternatives for refractory RLS cases may include tramadol, clonazepam, zolpidem, carbamazepine, oxcarbazepine, and lamotrigine, but despite widespread use of some

of these agents, a Movement Disorders Society Task Force of leading authorities on RLS considered these treatments investigational [204]. The impact of comorbid OSA should also be considered, as optimization of treatment for sleep-disordered breathing may improve both subjective RLS symptoms as well as PLMD frequency in many patients.

References

1 Frank MG. The mystery of sleep function: current perspectives and future directions. *Rev. Neurosci.* 2006;17:375–392.
2 Mackiewicz M, Naidoo N, Zimmerman JE, et al. Molecular mechanisms of sleep and wakefulness. *Ann. N. Y. Acad. Sci.* 2008;1129:335–349.
3 Walker MP, Stickgold R. Sleep, memory, and plasticity. *Annu. Rev. Psychol.* 2006;57:139–166.
4 Pilcher JJ, Huffcutt, AI. Effects of sleep deprivation on performance: a meta analysis. *Sleep* 1996;19:318–326.
5 Van Dongen HP, Maislin G, Mullington JM, et al. The cumulative cost of additional wakefulness: dose–response effects on neurobehavioral functions and sleep

physiology from chronic sleep restriction and total sleep deprivation. *Sleep* 2003;26:117–126.

6 Buckley TM, Schatzberg AF. On the interactions of the hypothalamic–pituitary–adrenal (HPA) axis and sleep: normal HPA axis activity and circadian rhythm, exemplary sleep disorders. *J. Clin. Endocrinol. Metab.* 2005;90:3106–3114.

7 Linn CC, Tsan KW, Chen PJ. The relationship between sleep apnea syndrome and hypothyroidism. *Chest* 1992;102:1663–1667.

8 Saaresranta T, Polo O. Hormones and breathing. *Chest* 2002;122:2165–2182.

9 Resta O, Pannacciulli N, Di Gioia G, et al. High prevalence of previously unknown subclinical hypothyroidism in obese patients referred to a sleep clinic for sleep disordered breathing. *Nutr. Metab. Cardiovasc. Dis.* 2004;14:248–253.

10 Kapur VK, Koepsell TD, deMaine J, et al. Association of hypothyroidism and obstructive sleep apnea. *Am. J. Respir. Crit. Care Med.* 1998;158:1379–1383.

11 Sakurai T, Mieda M, Tsujino N. The orexin system: roles in sleep/wake regulation. *Ann. N. Y. Acad. Sci.* 2010;1200:149–161.

12 Szymusiak R, McGinty D. Hypothalamic regulation of sleep and arousal. *Ann. N. Y. Acad. Sci.* 2008;1129:275–286.

13 Hanafy HM. Testosterone therapy and obstructive sleep apnea: is there a real connection? *J Sex. Med.* 2007;4:1241–1246.

14 Bayliss, DA, Millhorn, DE. Central neural mechanisms of progesterone action: application to the respiratory system. *J. Appl. Physiol.* 1992;73:393–404.

15 Kim, SH, Eisele, DW, Smith, PL, et al. Evaluation of patients with sleep apnea after tracheotomy. *Arch. Otolaryngol. Head Neck Surg.* 1998;124:996–1000.

16 Baker FC, Driver HS. Circadian rhythms, sleep, and the menstrual cycle. *Sleep Med.* 2007;8:613–622.

17 Ohayon MM. Severe hot flashes are associated with chronic insomnia. *Arch. Intern. Med.* 2006;166:1262–1268.

18 Parish JM. Sleep-related problems in common medical conditions. *Chest* 2009;135:563–572.

19 Manconi M, Govoni V, De Vito A, et al. Pregnancy as a risk factor for restless legs syndrome. *Sleep Med.* 2004;5:305–308.

20 Krystal AD. Insomnia in women. *Clin. Cornerstone* 2003;5:41–50.

21 Miller EH. Women and insomnia. *Clin. Cornerstone* 2004;6(Suppl 1B):S8–S18.

22 Moline ML, Broch L, Zak R, et al. Sleep in women across the life cycle from adulthood through menopause. *Sleep Med. Rev.* 2003;7:155–177.

23 Joffe H, Petrillo L, Viguera A, et al. Eszopiclone improves insomnia and depressive and anxious symptoms in perimenopausal and postmenopausal women with hot flashes: a randomized, double-blinded, placebo-controlled crossover trial. *Am. J. Obstet. Gynecol.* 2010;202:171.e1–171.e11.

24 Cappuccio FP, D'Elia L, Strazzullo P, et al. Quantity and quality of sleep and incidence of type 2 diabetes: a systematic review and meta-analysis. *Diab. Care* 2010;33:414–420.

25 Zizi F, Jean-Louis G, Brown CD, et al. Sleep duration and the risk of diabetes mellitus: epidemiologic evidence and pathophysiologic insights. *Curr. Diab. Rep.* 2010;10:43–47.

26 Dijk DJ. Slow-wave sleep, diabetes, and the sympathetic nervous system. *Proc. Natl. Acad. Sci. USA* 2008;105:1107–1108.

27 Tasali E, Leproult R, Ehrmann DA, et al. Slow-wave sleep and the risk of type 2 diabetes in humans. *Proc. Natl. Acad. Sci. USA* 2008;105:1044–1049.

28 Bopparaju S, Surani S. Sleep and diabetes. *Int. J. Endocrinol.* 2010;2010:759509.

29 Burdakov D, Luckman SM, Verkhratsky A. Glucose-sensing neurons of the hypothalamus. *Philos. Trans. R. Soc. Lond. B Biol. Sci.* 2005;360:2227–2235.

30 Lim LL, Dinner D, Tham KW, et al. Restless legs syndrome associated with primary hyperparathyroidism. *Sleep Med.* 2005;6:283–285.

31 Monderer RS, Wu WP, Thorpy MJ. Nocturnal leg cramps. *Curr. Neurol. Neurosci. Rep.* 2010;10:53–59.

32 FFDA Drug Safety Communication: new risk management plan and patient Medication Guide for Qualaquin (quinine sulfate); Available on line at http://www.fda.gov/Drugs/DrugSafety/PostmarketDrugSafetyInformationforPatientsandProviders/ucm218202.htm#sa; accessed 9/19/2011 at 0850.

33 Balkin TJ, Rupp T, Picchioni D, et al. Sleep loss and sleepiness: current issues. *Chest* 2008;134:653–660.

34 Marcheva B, Ramsey KM, Affinati A, et al. Clock genes and metabolic disease. *J. Appl. Physiol.* 2009;107:1638–1646.

35 Kono M, Tatsumi K, Saibara T, et al. Obstructive sleep apnea syndrome is associated with some components of metabolic syndrome. *Chest* 2007;131:1387–1392.

36 Tench CM, McCurdie I, White PD, et al. The prevalence and associations of fatigue in systemic lupus erythematosus. *Rheumatol. (Oxf.)* 2000;39:1249–1254.

37 Valencia-Flores M, Resendiz M, Castano VA, et al. Determinants of sleep quality in women with systemic lupus erythematosus. *Arthritis Rheum.* 2005;53:272–278.

38 Valencia X, Alcocer J, Ramos GG, et al. Objective and subjective sleep disturbances in patients with systemic

lupus erythematosus. *Arthritis Rheum.* 1999;42:2189–2193.

39 Drewes AM, Jennum P, Andreasen A, et al. Self-reported sleep disturbances and daytime complaints in women with fibromyalgia and rheumatoid arthritis. *J. Musculoskel. Pain* 1994;2:15–31.

40 Reading SR, Crowson CS, Rodeheffer RJ, et al. Do rheumatoid arthritis patients have a higher risk for sleep apnea? *J. Rheumatol.* 2009;36:1869–1872.

41 Vgontzas AN, Zoumakis E, Lin HM, et al. Marked decrease in sleepiness in patients with sleep apnea by etanercept, a tumor necrosis factor-alpha antagonist. *J. Clin. Endocrinol. Metab.* 2004;89:4409–4413.

42 Zamarron C, Maceiras F, Mera A, et al. Effect of the first infliximab infusion on sleep and alertness in patients with active rheumatoid arthritis. *Ann. Rheum. Dis.* 2004;63:88–90.

43 Drewes AM. Pain and sleep disturbances with special reference to fibromyalgia and rheumatoid arthritis. *Rheumatol. (Oxf.)* 1999;38(11):1035–1038.

44 Drewes AM, Svendsen L, Taagholt SJ, et al. Sleep in rheumatoid arthritis: a comparison with healthy subjects and studies of sleep/wake interactions. *Br. J. Rheumatol.* 1998;37:71–81.

45 Drewes AM, Nielsen KD, Hansen B, et al. A longitudinal study of clinical symptoms and sleep parameters in rheumatoid arthritis. *Rheumatol. (Oxf.)* 2000;39:1287–1289.

46 Jamieson AH, Alford CA, Bird HA, et al. The effect of sleep and nocturnal movements on stiffness, pain, and psychomotor performance in ankylosing spondylitis. *Clin. Exp. Rheumatol.* 1995;13:73–78.

47 Lopes MC, Guilleminault C, Rosa A, et al. Delta sleep instability in children with chronic arthritis. *Braz. J. Med. Biol. Res.* 2008;41:938–943.

48 Ward TM, Archbold K, Lentz M, et al. Sleep disturbance, daytime sleepiness, and neurocognitive performance in children with juvenile idiopathic arthritis. *Sleep* 2010;33:252–259.

49 Avellaneda Fernandez A, Perez Martin A, Izquierdo Martinez M, et al. Chronic fatigue syndrome: aetiology, diagnosis and treatment. *BMC Psychiatry* 2009;9(Suppl 1):S1.

50 Buskila D. Developments in the scientific and clinical understanding of fibromyalgia. *Arthritis Res. Ther.* 2009;11:242.

51 Chong YY, Ng BY. Clinical aspects and management of fibromyalgia syndrome. *Ann. Acad. Med. Singapore* 2009;38(11) 967–973.

52 Josephs KA, Silber MH, Fealey RD, et al. Neurophysiologic studies in Morvan syndrome. *J. Clin. Neurophysiol.* 2004;21:440–445.

53 Vernino S, Geschwind M, Boeve B. Autoimmune encephalopathies. *Neurologist* 2007;13:140–147.

54 Irani SR, Alexander S, Waters P, Kleopa KA, Pettingill P, Zuliani L, Peles E, Buckley C, Lang B, Vincent A. Antibodies to Kv1 potassium channel-complex proteins leucine-rich, glioma inactivated 1 protein and contactin-associated protein-2 in limbic encephalitis, Morvan's syndrome and acquired neuromyotonia. *Brain* 2010;133(9):2734–2748.

55 Zamarron C, Garcia Paz V, Riveiro A. Obstructive sleep apnea syndrome is a systemic disease. Current evidence. *Eur. J. Intern. Med.* 2008;19:390–398.

56 Young T, Peppard PE, Gottlieb DJ. Epidemiology of obstructive sleep apnea: a population health perspective. *Am. J. Resp. Crit. Care Med.* 2002;165:1217–1239.

57 Khayat R, Patt B, Hayes DJr. Obstructive sleep apnea: the new cardiovascular disease. Part I: obstructive sleep apnea and the pathogenesis of vascular disease. *Heart Fail. Rev.* 2009;14:143–153.

58 Kushida CA, Littner MR, Morgenthaler T, et al. Practice parameters for the indications for polysomnography and related procedures: an update for 2005. *Sleep* 2005;28:499–521.

59 Bao G, Guilleminault C. Upper airway resistance syndrome—one decade later. *Curr. Opin. Pulm. Med.* 2004;10:461–467.

60 Chan AS, Lee RW, Cistulli PA. Non-positive airway pressure modalities: mandibular advancement devices/positional therapy. *Proc. Am. Thorac. Soc.* 2008;5:179–184.

61 Loube DI, Gay PC, Strohl KP, et al. Indications for positive airway pressure treatment of adult obstructive sleep apnea patients: a consensus statement. *Chest* 1999;115:863–866.

62 Arzt M, Bradley TD. Treatment of sleep apnea in heart failure. *Am. J. Respir. Crit. Care Med.* 2006;173:1300–1308.

63 Pusalavidyasagar SS, Olson EJ, Gay PC, et al. Treatment of complex sleep apnea syndrome: a retrospective comparative review. *Sleep Med.* 2006;7:474–479.

64 Allam JS, Olson EJ, Gay PC, et al. Efficacy of adaptive servoventilation in treatment of complex and central sleep apnea syndromes. *Chest* 2007;132:1839–1846.

65 Casey KR, Cantillo KO, Brown LK. Sleep-related hypoventilation/hypoxemic syndromes. *Chest* 2007;131:1936–1948.

66 Fanfulla F, Cascone L, Taurino AE. Sleep disordered breathing in patients with chronic obstructive pulmonary disease. *Minerva Med.* 2004;95:307–321.

67 Powers MA. The obesity hypoventilation syndrome. *Respir. Care* 2008;53:1723–1730.

68 Calhoun WJ. Nocturnal asthma. *Chest* 2003;123:399S–405S.

69 Schoonderwoerd BA, Smit MD, Pen L, et al. New risk factors for atrial fibrillation: causes of "not-so-lone atrial fibrillation". *Europace* 2008;10:668–673.

70 Gami AS, Hodge DO, Herges RM, et al. Obstructive sleep apnea, obesity, and the risk of incident atrial fibrillation. *J. Am. Coll. Cardiol.* 2007;49:565–571.

71 Kanagala R, Murali NS, Friedman PA, et al. Obstructive sleep apnea and the recurrence of atrial fibrillation. *Circulation* 2003;107:2589–2594.

72 Naughton MT, Lorenzi-Filho G. Sleep in heart failure. *Prog. Cardiovasc. Dis.* 2009;51:339–349.

73 Head C, Gardiner M. Paroxysms of excitement: sodium channel dysfunction in heart and brain. *Bioessays* 2003;25:981–993.

74 De Santo RM, Perna A, Di Iorio BR, et al. Sleep disorders in kidney disease. *Minerva Urol. Nefrol.* 2010;62:111–128.

75 Gul A, Aoun N, Trayner EMJr. Why do patients sleep on dialysis? *Semin. Dial.* 2006;19:152–157.

76 Merlino G, Gigli GL, Valente M. Sleep disturbances in dialysis patients. *J. Nephrol.* 2008;21(Suppl 13):S66–S70.

77 Hanly P. Sleep apnea and daytime sleepiness in end-stage renal disease. *Semin. Dial.* 2004;17:109–114.

78 Collop N. The effect of obstructive sleep apnea on chronic medical disorders. *Cleve. Clin. J. Med.* 2007;74:72–78.

79 Foresman BH. Sleep-related gastroesophageal reflux. *J. Am. Osteopath. Assoc.* 2000;100:S7–S10.

80 Levenstein S. Peptic ulcer at the end of the 20th century: biological and psychological risk factors. *Can. J. Gastroenterol.* 1999;13:753–759.

81 Ahmed MH, Byrne CD. Obstructive sleep apnea syndrome and fatty liver: association or causal link? *World J. Gastroenterol.* 2010;16:4243–4252.

82 Cella D, Davis K, Breitbart W, et al. Cancer-related fatigue: prevalence of proposed diagnostic criteria in a United States sample of cancer survivors. *J. Clin. Oncol.* 2001;19:3385–3391.

83 Poulson MJ. Not just tired. *J. Clin. Oncol.* 2001;19:4180–4181.

84 Servaes P, Verhagen C, Bleijenberg G. Fatigue in cancer patients during and after treatment: prevalence, correlates and interventions. *Eur. J. Cancer* 2002;38:27–43.

85 Lee K, Cho M, Miaskowski C, et al. Impaired sleep and rhythms in persons with cancer. *Sleep Med. Rev.* 2004;8:199–212.

86 Savard J, Simard S, Blanchet J, et al. Prevalence, clinical characteristics, and risk factors for insomnia in the context of breast cancer. *Sleep* 2001;24:583–590.

87 Savard J, Morin CM. Insomnia in the context of cancer: a review of a neglected problem. *J. Clin. Oncol.* 2001;19:895–908.

88 Mormont MC, Waterhouse J, Bleuzen P, et al. Marked 24-h rest/activity rhythms are associated with better quality of life, better response, and longer survival in patients with metastatic colorectal cancer and good performance status. *Clin. Cancer Res.* 2000;6:3038–3045.

89 Miller AH, Ancoli-Israel S, Bower JE, et al. Neuroendocrine-immune mechanisms of behavioral comorbidities in patients with cancer. *J. Clin. Oncol.* 2008;26:971–982.

90 Schubert C, Hong S, Natarajan L, et al. The association between fatigue and inflammatory marker levels in cancer patients: a quantitative review. *Brain Behav. Immun.* 2007;21:413–427.

91 Cornelius JC, Pittock SJ, Lennon VA, Aston P, McKeon A, Josephs K, Silber MH. Sleep manifestations of voltage-gated potassium channel autoimmunity. *Sleep* 2010;33:A283.

92 Tan KM, Lennon VA, Klein CJ, et al. Clinical spectrum of voltage-gated potassium channel autoimmunity. *Neurology* 2008;70:1883–1890.

93 Iranzo A, Graus F, Clover L, et al. Rapid eye movement sleep behavior disorder and potassium channel antibody-associated limbic encephalitis. *Ann. Neurol.* 2006;59:178–181.

94 Olson EJ, Boeve BF, Silber MH. REM sleep behaviour disorder: demographic, clinical, and lab findings in 93 cases. *Brain* 2000;123:331–339.

95 Mahowald MW, Schenck CH. REM sleep behavior disorder—past, present, and future. *Schweiz. Arch. Neurol. Psychiatr.* 2003;154:363–368.

96 Postuma RB, Gagnon JF, Vendette M, et al. Quantifying the risk of neurodegenerative disease in idiopathic REM sleep behavior disorder. *Neurology* 2009;72:1296–1300.

97 Montplaisir J, Gagnon JF, Fantini ML, et al. Polysomnographic diagnosis of idiopathic REM sleep behavior disorder. *Mov. Disord.* 2010;25:2044–2051.

98 Compta Y, Iranzo A, Santamaria J, et al. REM sleep behavior disorder and narcoleptic features in anti-Ma2-associated encephalitis. *Sleep* 2007;30:767–769.

99 Gomez-Choco MJ, Zarranz JJ, Saiz A, et al. Central hypoventilation as the presenting symptom in Hu associated paraneoplastic encephalomyelitis. *J. Neurol. Neurosurg. Psychiatry* 2007;78:1143–1145.

100 Cohen S, Doyle WJ, Alper CM, et al. Sleep habits and susceptibility to the common cold. *Arch. Intern. Med.* 2009;169:62–67.

101 Dobbin CJ, Bartlett D, Melehan K, et al. The effect of infective exacerbations on sleep and neurobehavioral function in cystic fibrosis. *Am. J. Respir. Crit Care Med* 2005;172:99–104.

102 Sockalingam S, Abbey SE, Alosaimi F, et al. A review of sleep disturbance in hepatitis C. *J. Clin. Gastroenterol.* 2010;44:38–45.

103 Marshall L, Born J. Brain–immune interactions in sleep. *Int. Rev. Neurobiol.* 2002;52:93–131.

104 Imeri L, Opp MR. How (and why) the immune system makes us sleep. *Nat. Rev. Neurosci.* 2009;10:199–210.

105 Lorton D, Lubahn CL, Estus C, et al. Bidirectional communication between the brain and the immune system: implications for physiological sleep and disorders with disrupted sleep. *Neuroimmunomodulation* 2006;13:357–374.

106 Opp MR. Cytokines and sleep. *Sleep Med. Rev.* 2005;9:355–364.

107 Kennedy PG. Human African trypanosomiasis of the CNS: current issues and challenges. *J. Clin. Invest.* 2004;113:496–504.

108 Omonuwa TS, Goforth HW, Preud'homme X, et al. The pharmacologic management of insomnia in patients with HIV. *J. Clin. Sleep Med.* 2009;5:251–262.

109 Reid S, Dwyer J. Insomnia in HIV infection: a systematic review of prevalence, correlates, and management. *Psychosom. Med.* 2005;67:260–269.

110 Salahuddin N, Barroso J, Leserman J, et al. Daytime sleepiness, nighttime sleep quality, stressful life events, and HIV-related fatigue. *J. Assoc. Nurses AIDS Care* 2009;20:6–13.

111 Darko DF, Miller JC, Gallen C, et al. Sleep electroencephalogram delta-frequency amplitude, night plasma levels of tumor necrosis factor alpha, and human immunodeficiency virus infection. *Proc. Natl. Acad. Sci. USA.* 1995;92:12080–12084.

112 Capellari S, Strammiello R, Saverioni D, et al. Genetic Creutzfeldt–Jakob disease and fatal familial insomnia: insights into phenotypic variability and disease pathogenesis. *Acta Neuropathol.* 2011;121(1):21–37.

113 Manetto V, Medori R, Cortelli P, et al. Fatal familial insomnia: clinical and pathologic study of five new cases. *Neurology* 1992;42:312–319.

114 Maia LF, Marta M, Lopes V, et al. Hypersomnia in Whipple disease: case report. *Arq. Neuropsiquiatr.* 2006;64:865–868.

115 Voderholzer U, Riemann D, Gann H, et al. Transient total sleep loss in cerebral Whipple's disease: a longitudinal study. *J Sleep Res.* 2002;11:321–329.

116 Molnar MZ, Novak M, Mucsi I. Sleep disorders and quality of life in renal transplant recipients. *Int. Urol. Nephrol.* 2009;41:373–382.

117 Faulhaber GA, Furlanetto TW, Astigarraga CC, et al. Association of busulfan and cyclophosphamide conditioning with sleep disorders after hematopoietic stem cell transplantation. *Acta Haematol.* 2010;124:125–128.

118 BaHammam A. Sleep in acute care units. *Sleep Breath* 2006;10:6–15.

119 Drouot X, Cabello B, d'Ortho MP, et al. Sleep in the intensive care unit. *Sleep Med. Rev.* 2008;12:391–403.

120 Friese RS. Sleep and recovery from critical illness and injury: a review of theory, current practice, and future directions. *Crit. Care Med.* 2008;36:697–705.

121 Gabor JY, Cooper AB, Hanly PJ. Sleep disruption in the intensive care unit. *Curr. Opin. Crit. Care* 2001;7:21–27.

122 Weinhouse GL, Schwab RJ. Sleep in the critically ill patient. *Sleep* 2006;29:707–716.

123 Parthasarathy S, Tobin MJ. Sleep in the intensive care unit. *Intensive Care Med.* 2004;30:197–206.

124 Hardin KA. Sleep in the ICU: potential mechanisms and clinical implications. *Chest* 2009;136:284–294.

125 Hardin KA, Seyal M, Stewart T, et al. Sleep in critically ill chemically paralyzed patients requiring mechanical ventilation. *Chest* 2006;129:1468–1477.

126 Gabor JY, Cooper AB, Crombach SA, et al. Contribution of the intensive care unit environment to sleep disruption in mechanically ventilated patients and healthy subjects. *Am. J. Respir. Crit. Care Med.* 2003;167:708–715.

127 Ambrogio C, Koebnick J, Quan SF, et al. Assessment of sleep in ventilator-supported critically III patients. *Sleep* 2008;31:1559–1568.

128 Bourne RS, Minelli C, Mills GH, et al. Clinical review: sleep measurement in critical care patients: research and clinical implications. *Crit. Care* 2007;11:226.

129 Watson PL. Measuring sleep in critically ill patients: beware the pitfalls. *Crit. Care* 2007;11:159.

130 Figueroa-Ramos MI, Arroyo-Novoa CM, Lee KA, et al. Sleep and delirium in ICU patients: a review of mechanisms and manifestations. *Intensive Care Med.* 2009;35:781–795.

131 Mistraletti G, Carloni E, Cigada M, et al. Sleep and delirium in the intensive care unit. *Minerva Anestesiol.* 2008;74:329–333.

132 Weinhouse GL, Schwab RJ, Watson PL, et al. Bench-to-bedside review: delirium in ICU patients—importance of sleep deprivation. *Crit. Care* 2009;13:234.

133 Redeker NS. Challenges and opportunities associated with studying sleep in critically ill adults. *AACN Adv. Crit. Care* 2008;19:178–185.

134 Bourne RS, Mills GH. Melatonin: possible implications for the postoperative and critically ill patient. *Intensive Care Med.* 2006;32:371–379.

135 Hanania M, Kitain E. Melatonin for treatment and prevention of postoperative delirium. *Anesth. Analg.* 2002;94:338–339.

136 Bourne RS, Mills GH, Minelli C. Melatonin therapy to improve nocturnal sleep in critically ill patients: encouraging results from a small randomised controlled trial. *Crit. Care* 2008;12:R52.

137 Gay PC. Sleep and sleep-disordered breathing in the hospitalized patient. *Respir. Care* 2010;55:1240–1254.

138 Olson EJ, Simon PM. Sleep–wake cycles and the management of respiratory failure. *Curr. Opin. Pulm. Med.* 1996;2:500–506.

279

139 Cabello B, Parthasarathy S, Mancebo J. Mechanical ventilation: let us minimize sleep disturbances. *Curr. Opin. Crit. Care* 2007;13:20–26.

140 Ozsancak A, D'Ambrosio C, Garpestad E, et al. Sleep and mechanical ventilation. *Crit. Care Clin.* 2008;24:517–531, vi–vii.

141 Parthasarathy S, Tobin MJ. Effect of ventilator mode on sleep quality in critically ill patients. *Am. J. Respir. Crit. Care Med.* 2002;166:1423–1429.

142 Cabello B, Thille AW, Drouot X, et al. Sleep quality in mechanically ventilated patients: comparison of three ventilatory modes. *Crit. Care Med.* 2008;36:1749–1755.

143 Roche Campo F, Drouot X, Thille AW, et al. Poor sleep quality is associated with late noninvasive ventilation failure in patients with acute hypercapnic respiratory failure. *Crit. Care Med.* 2010;38:477–485.

144 Hu RF, Jiang XY, Zeng YM, et al. Effects of earplugs and eye masks on nocturnal sleep, melatonin and cortisol in a simulated intensive care unit environment. *Crit. Care* 2010;14:R66.

145 Stanchina ML, Abu-Hijleh M, Chaudhry BK, et al. The influence of white noise on sleep in subjects exposed to ICU noise. *Sleep Med.* 2005;6:423–428.

146 Berlin RM. Management of insomnia in hospitalized patients. *Ann. Intern. Med.* 1984;100:398–404.

147 Flaherty JH. Insomnia among hospitalized older persons. *Clin. Geriatr. Med.* 2008;24:51–67, vi.

148 Chesson AL, Anderson WM, Littner M, et al. Practice parameters for the nonpharmacologic treatment of chronic insomnia. *Sleep* 1999;22:1128–1133.

149 Smith MT, Huang MI, Manber R. Cognitive behavior therapy for chronic insomnia occurring within the context of medical and psychiatric disorders. *Clin. Psychol. Rev.* 2005;25:559–592.

150 Carson S, Yen PY, McDonagh MS. Drug Class Review on Newer Drugs for Insomnia: Final Report [Internet]. Portland, OR: Oregon Health & Science University Drug Class Reviews, 2006.

151 Lee CM, Herridge MS, Gabor JY, et al. Chronic sleep disorders in survivors of the acute respiratory distress syndrome. *Intensive Care Med.* 2009;35:314–320.

152 Baumann CR, Werth E, Stocker R, et al. Sleep–wake disturbances 6 months after traumatic brain injury: a prospective study. *Brain* 2007;130:1873–1883.

153 Kempf J, Werth E, Kaiser PR, et al. Sleep–wake disturbances 3 years after traumatic brain injury. *J. Neurol. Neurosurg. Psychiatry* 2010;81:1402–1405.

154 Mellman TA, Hipolito MM. Sleep disturbances in the aftermath of trauma and posttraumatic stress disorder. *CNS Spectr.* 2006;11:611–615.

155 Verma A, Anand V, Verma NP. Sleep disorders in chronic traumatic brain injury. *J. Clin. Sleep Med.* 2007;3:357–362.

156 Castriotta RJ, Wilde MC, Lai JM, et al. Prevalence and consequences of sleep disorders in traumatic brain injury. *J. Clin. Sleep Med.* 2007;3:349–356.

157 Watson NF, Dikmen S, Machamer J, et al. Hypersomnia following traumatic brain injury. *J. Clin. Sleep Med.* 2007;3:363–368.

158 Castriotta RJ, Atanasov S, Wilde MC, et al. Treatment of sleep disorders after traumatic brain injury. *J. Clin. Sleep Med.* 2009;5:137–144.

159 Spoormaker VI, Schredl M, van den Bout J. Nightmares: from anxiety symptom to sleep disorder. *Sleep Med. Rev.* 2006;10:19–31.

160 Gagnon JF, Postuma RB, Montplaisir J. Update on the pharmacology of REM sleep behavior disorder. *Neurology* 2006;67:742–747.

161 Teman PT, Tippmann-Peikert M, Silber MH, et al. Idiopathic rapid-eye-movement sleep disorder: associations with antidepressants, psychiatric diagnoses, and other factors, in relation to age of onset. *Sleep Med.* 2009;10:60–65.

162 Stein MD, Friedmann PD. Disturbed sleep and its relationship to alcohol use. *Subst. Abus.* 2005;26:1–13.

163 Ehlers CL, Slawecki CJ. Effects of chronic ethanol exposure on sleep in rats. *Alcohol* 2000;20:173–179.

164 Feige B, Gann H, Brueck R, et al. Effects of alcohol on polysomnographically recorded sleep in healthy subjects. *Alcohol Clin. Exp. Res.* 2006;30:1527–1537.

165 Landolt HP, Gillin JC. Sleep abnormalities during abstinence in alcohol-dependent patients. Aetiology and management. *CNS Drugs* 2001;15:413–425.

166 Pressman MR, Mahowald MW, Schenck CH, et al. Alcohol-induced sleepwalking or confusional arousal as a defense to criminal behavior: a review of scientific evidence, methods and forensic considerations. *J. Sleep Res.* 2007;16:198–212.

167 Roehrs T, Roth T. Sleep, sleepiness, and alcohol use. *Alcohol Res. Health* 2001;25:101–109.

168 Van Reen E, Jenni OG, Carskadon MA. Effects of alcohol on sleep and the sleep electroencephalogram in healthy young women. *Alcohol Clin. Exp. Res.* 2006;30:974–981.

169 Landolt HP, Roth C, Dijk DJ, et al. Late-afternoon ethanol intake affects nocturnal sleep and the sleep EEG in middle-aged men. *J. Clin. Psychopharmacol.* 1996;16:428–436.

170 Rupp TL, Acebo C, Seifer R, et al. Effects of a moderate evening alcohol dose. II: performance. *Alcohol Clin. Exp. Res.* 2007;31:1365–1371.

171 Rupp TL, Acebo C, Carskadon MA. Evening alcohol suppresses salivary melatonin in young adults. *Chronobiol. Int.* 2007;24:463–470.

172 Brower KJ. Alcohol's effects on sleep in alcoholics. *Alcohol Res. Health* 2001;25:110–125.

173 Feige B, Scaal S, Hornyak M, et al. Sleep electroencephalographic spectral power after withdrawal from

alcohol in alcohol-dependent patients. *Alcohol Clin. Exp. Res.* 2007;31:19–27.

174 Aldrich MS, Shipley JE, Tandon R, et al. Sleep-disordered breathing in alcoholics: association with age. *Alcohol Clin. Exp. Res.* 1993;17:1179–1183.

175 Aldrich MS, Brower KJ, Hall JM. Sleep-disordered breathing in alcoholics. *Alcohol Clin. Exp. Res.* 1999;23:134–140.

176 Arnedt JT, Conroy DA, Brower KJ. Treatment options for sleep disturbances during alcohol recovery. *J. Addict. Dis.* 2007;26:41–54.

177 Roth T. Workshop Participants. Does effective management of sleep disorders reduce substance dependence? *Drugs* 2009;69(Suppl 2):65–75.

178 Schierenbeck T, Riemann D, Berger M, et al. Effect of illicit recreational drugs upon sleep: cocaine, ecstasy and marijuana. *Sleep Med. Rev.* 2008;12:381–389.

179 Allen RP, McCann UD, Ricaurte GA. Persistent effects of (+/−)3,4-methylenedioxymethamphetamine (MDMA, "ecstasy") on human sleep. *Sleep* 1993;16:560–564.

180 McCann UD, Sgambati FP, Schwartz AR, et al. Sleep apnea in young abstinent recreational MDMA ("ecstasy") consumers. *Neurology* 2009;73:2011–2017.

181 Roehrs T, Roth T. Caffeine: sleep and daytime sleepiness. *Sleep Med. Rev.* 2008;12:153–162.

182 Carrier J, Paquet J, Fernandez-Bolanos M, et al. Effects of caffeine on daytime recovery sleep: a double challenge to the sleep–wake cycle in aging. *Sleep Med.* 2009;10:1016–1024.

183 LaJambe CM, Kamimori GH, Belenky G, et al. Caffeine effects on recovery sleep following 27 h total sleep deprivation. *Aviat. Space Environ. Med.* 2005;76:108–113.

184 Landolt HP, Werth E, Borbely AA, et al. Caffeine intake (200 mg) in the morning affects human sleep and EEG power spectra at night. *Brain Res.* 1995;675:67–74.

185 Landolt HP, Retey JV, Tonz K, et al. Caffeine attenuates waking and sleep electroencephalographic markers of sleep homeostasis in humans. *Neuropsychopharmacology* 2004;29:1933–1939.

186 Landolt HP. Sleep homeostasis: a role for adenosine in humans? *Biochem. Pharmacol.* 2008;75:2070–2079.

187 Retey JV, Adam M, Gottselig JM, et al. Adenosinergic mechanisms contribute to individual differences in sleep deprivation-induced changes in neurobehavioral function and brain rhythmic activity. *J. Neurosci.* 2006;26:10472–10479.

188 Colrain IM, Trinder J, Swan GE. The impact of smoking cessation on objective and subjective markers of sleep: review, synthesis, and recommendations. *Nicotine Tob. Res.* 2004;6:913–925.

189 Jaehne A, Loessl B, Barkai Z, et al. Effects of nicotine on sleep during consumption, withdrawal and replacement therapy. *Sleep Med. Rev.* 2009;13:363–377.

190 Brown WD. The effect of medication on sleep. *Respir. Care Clin. N. Am.* 2006;12:81–99, ix.

191 Qureshi A, Lee-Chiong TJr. Medications and their effects on sleep. *Med. Clin. N. Am.* 2004;88:751–766, x.

192 Allen RP, Earley CJ. The role of iron in restless legs syndrome. *Mov. Disord.* 2007;22(Suppl 18):S440–S448.

193 Stefansson H, Rye DB, Hicks A, et al. A genetic risk factor for periodic limb movements in sleep. *N. Engl. J. Med.* 2007;357:639–647.

194 Trotti LM, Bhadriraju S, Rye DB. An update on the pathophysiology and genetics of restless legs syndrome. *Curr. Neurol. Neurosci. Rep.* 2008;8:281–287.

195 Gamaldo CE, Earley CJ. Restless legs syndrome: a clinical update. *Chest* 2006;130:1596–1604.

196 Ekbom K, Ulfberg J. Restless legs syndrome. *J. Intern. Med.* 2009;266:419–431.

197 Allen R. Dopamine and iron in the pathophysiology of restless legs syndrome (RLS). *Sleep Med.* 2004;5:385–391.

198 Connor JR, Wang XS, Allen RP, et al. Altered dopaminergic profile in the putamen and substantia nigra in restless leg syndrome. *Brain* 2009;132:2403–2412.

199 Beneš H, García-Borreguero D, Ferini-Strambi L, Schollmayer E, Fichtner A, Kohnen R. Augmentation in the treatment of restless legs syndrome with transdermal rotigotine. *Sleep Med.* 2012;13:697.

200 Oertel W, Trenkwalder C, Beneš H, Ferini-Strambi L, Högl B, Poewe W, Stiasny-Kolster K, Fichtner A, Schollmayer E, Kohnen R, García-Borreguero D; SP710 study group. Long-term safety and efficacy of rotigotine transdermal patch for moderate-to-severe idiopathic restless legs syndrome: a 5-year open-label extension study. *Lancet Neurol.* 2011;10(8):710–20. Epub 2011 Jun 24.

201 Cornelius JR, Tippmann-Peikert M, Slocumb NL, Frerichs CF, Silber MH. Impulse control disorders with the use of dopaminergic agents in restless legs syndrome: a case-control study. *Sleep* 2010;33(1):81–7.

202 Voon V, Schoerling A, Wenzel S, Ekanayake V, Reiff J, Trenkwalder C, Sixel-Döring F. Frequency of impulse control behaviours associated with dopaminergic therapy in restless legs syndrome. *BMC Neurol* 2011;11:117.

203 Silver N, Allen RP, Senerth J, Earley CJ. A 10-year, longitudinal assessment of dopamine agonists and methadone in the treatment of restless legs syndrome. *Sleep Med.* 2011;12(5):440–444.

204 Trenkwalder C, Hening WA, Montagna P, Oertel WH, Allen RP, Walters AS, Costa J, Stiasny-Kolster K, Sampaio C. Treatment of restless legs syndrome: an evidence-based review and implications for clinicalpractice. *Mov. Disord.* 2008;23(16):2267–2302.

Index

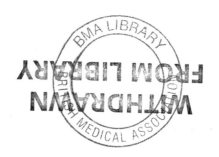